Grundmann · Geller

Histopathology

Color Atlas of Organs and Systems

EDITED BY

Ekkehard Grundmann and Stephen A. Geller

CONTRIBUTORS

Hans-Werner Altmann, Chlodwig Beck, Leonardo Bianchi, Georg Dhom,
Ekkehard Grundmann, Filippo Gullotta, Christoph Hedinger,
J. Heinrich Holzner, Oskar Klinge, Günther Klöppel, Hans-Jürgen Knieriem,
Günter Könn, Antonio Llombart-Bosch, Egon Macher, Klaus-Michael Müller,
Hugo Noetzel, Wolfgang Oehlert, Wolfgang Remagen, Wolfgang Rotter,
Wolfgang Saeger, Hans-Eckart Schaefer, Wilfried Schilli, Fritz Städtler,
Fereydoun Vakilzadeh, Martin Vogel, Klaus Wolff

TRANSLATED BY

Stephen A. Geller

830 Color Illustrations

Urban & Schwarzenberg · Munich–Baltimore

Urban & Schwarzenberg GmbH
Pettenkoferstraße 18
D-8000 München 2
Federal Republic of Germany

Urban & Schwarzenberg, Inc.
7 East Redwood Street
Baltimore, Maryland 21202
U.S.A.

Editors' addresses:
Prof. Dr. med. *Ekkehard Grundmann*
Gerhard-Domagk-Institut für Pathologie
der Universität, Domagkstraße 17
D-4400 Münster
F.R.G.

Stephen A. Geller, M.D.
Director, Department of Pathology and
Laboratory Medicine
Cedars-Sinai Medical Center
Adjunct Professor of Pathology, UCLA
Los Angeles, California 90048
U.S.A.

Contributors' addresses:
Prof. Dr. med. h.c. *Hans-Werner Altmann,* Pfalzstr. 22,
   D-8700 Würzburg
Prof. Dr. med. *Chlodwig Beck,* Universitäts-Hals-Nasen- und
   Ohren-Klinik, Killianstr., D-7800 Freiburg
Prof. Dr. med. *Leonardo Bianchi,* Institut für Pathologie der
   Universität, Schönbeinstr. 40, CH-4003 Basel
Prof. Dr. med. *Georg Dhom,* Pathologisches Institut der
   Universität des Saarlandes, D-6650 Homburg
Prof. Dr. *Filippo Gullotta,* Lehrstuhl für Neuropathologie der
   Universität, Domagkstr. 17, D-4400 Münster
Prof. Dr. med. h.c. *Christoph Hedinger,* Institut für Pathologie der
   Universität, Schmelzbergstr. 12, CH-8091 Zürich
Prof. Dr. med. *J. Heinrich Holzner,* Institut für Pathologische
   Anatomie der Universität, Spitalgasse 4, A-1090 Wien
Prof. Dr. med. *Oskar Klinge,* Institut für Pathologie,
   Städt. Kliniken, Mönchebergstr. 41–43, D-3500 Kassel
Prof. Dr. med. *Günther Klöppel,* Fak. Geneeskunde en Farmacie,
   Lab. Pathol. Outleedkunde, Laarbeeklaan 101,
   B-1090 Brussels/Belgium
Prof. Dr. med. *Hans-Jürgen Knieriem,* Institut für Pathologie,
   Ev. Krankenhaus Bethesda, Heerstr. 219, D-4100 Duisburg
Prof. Dr. med. *Günter Könn,* Am Reichenberg 40,
   D-5340 Bad Honnef
Prof. Dr. med. *Antonio Llombart-Bosch,* Dept. of Patologia,
   Facultat de Medicina, Av. Blasco Ibanez, E-17 Valencia 10,
   Spain
Prof. Dr. med. *Egon Macher,* Universitäts-Hautklinik,
   von-Esmarch-Str. 56, D-4400 Münster

Prof. Dr. med. *Klaus-Michael Müller,* Institut für Pathologie,
   Krankenanstalten „Bergmannsheil", Hunscheidtstr. 1,
   D-4630 Bochum 1
Prof. Dr. med. *Hugo Noetzel,* Jos-Fritz-Str. 34,
   D-7800 Freiburg-Lehen
Prof. Dr. med. *Wolfgang Oehlert,* Institut für Pathologie,
   Rosastr. 9, D-7800 Freiburg
Prof. Dr. med. *Wolfgang Remagen,* Institut für Pathologie der
   Universität, Schönbeinstr. 40, CH-4003 Basel
Prof. Dr. med. *Wolfgang Rotter,* Bierbrauerweg 4,
   D-6050 Offenbach
Prof. Dr. med. *Wolfgang Saeger,* Abt. f. Pathologie des
   Marienkrankenhauses, Alfredstr. 9, D-2000 Hamburg 76
Prof. Dr. med. *Hans-Eckart Schaefer,* Pathologisches Institut der
   Universität, Albertstr. 19, D-7800 Freiburg
Prof. Dr. med. *Wilfried Schilli,* Zentrum für Zahn-, Mund- und
   Kieferheilkunde der Universität, Hugstetter Str. 55,
   D-7800 Freiburg
Prof. Dr. med. *Fritz Städtler,* Pathologisches Institut,
   Am Schwarzen Meer 134/136, D-2800 Bremen 1
Prof. Dr. med. *Fereydoun Vakilzadeh,* Dermatologische Klinik des
   Städt. Krankenhauses, Weinberg 1, D-3200 Hildesheim
Prof. Dr. med. *Martin Vogel,* Augenklinik der Universität,
   Robert-Koch-Str. 40, D-3400 Göttingen
Prof. Dr. med. *Klaus Wolff,* I. Univ.-Hautklinik,
   Allgemeines Krankenhaus der Stadt Wien, Alserstr. 4,
   A-1090 Wien

CIP-Kurztitelaufnahme der Deutschen Bibliothek

Histopathology / Grundmann ; Geller. Ed. by Ekkehard Grundmann and Stephen A. Geller. Contributors Hans-Werner Altmann ... Transl. by Stephen A. Geller. – Munich ; Baltimore : Urban and Schwarzenberg.
   Dt. Ausg. u.d.T.: Spezielle Pathologie

NE: Grundmann, Ekkehard [Hrsg.]; Altmann, Hans-Werner [Mitverf.]

Color atlas of organs and systems / Grundmann ; Geller. Ed. by Ekkehard Grundmann and Stephen A. Geller. Contributors Hans-Werner Altmann ... Transl. by Stephen A. Geller. – Munich ; Baltimore : Urban and Schwarzenberg, 1988
   (Histopathology)
   Dt. Ausg. u.d.T.: Farbatlas der makroskopischen und mikroskopischen Pathologie
   ISBN 3-541-70721-6

NE: Grundmann, Ekkehard [Hrsg.]; Altmann, Hans-Werner [Mitverf.]

Printed in Germany

92	91	90	89
5	4	3	2	1	0

ISBN 3-541-70721-6 (Munich)

ISBN 0-8067-0721-6 (Baltimore)

Foreword

This Atlas presents the pathomorphologic characteristics of the most important diseases in splendid, full-color photographs. It is intended to complement textbooks of Systemic Pathology, and to be used in conjunction with them. Since each textbook stresses different aspects, every chapter of this Atlas features a short introduction explaining the major features of the figures that follow.

The figures have been selected for their didactic value. Inclusion of all facets of Systemic Pathology would have exceeded didactic requirements, and have made the book too expensive for most students. With this in mind, electron microscopy and immunohistochemistry are reviewed only briefly.

Despite the considerable progress in printing techniques in the past few years, reproductions of photographs can never be superior to the originals. Every effort has been made to select the bestquality illustrations available, not excluding the respective authors' personal preferences.

Editorial intervention was occasionally necessary to achieve a homogeneous impression of the entire volume. The authors were always very cooperative, although they were sometimes requested to omit figures or alter the legends.

The English version of this Atlas required some revision of the introductory texts and the legends. Nevertheless, this did not mean sacrificing the original concept, for the most important feature of an Atlas is its figures.

Having now completed the task, I should like to thank all contributors and the staff members of the publishing and printing companies. Above all my gratitude is due to Stephen A. Geller, who not only translated the German text, but also carefully inserted the English scientific terminology relevant for the English-speaking readers.

Ekkehard Grundmann
Münster, December 1988

Preface

This atlas is the English language version of a book that was originally published in German. Professor Ekkehard Grundmann developed the atlas to demonstrate what he and his colleagues felt to be the most important lesions. Clearly they could not illustrate all diseases and conditions of importance to man.

This English language edition attempts to relay the scientific judgements of the original German authors in terms that will be useful for the English-speaking student. The strength of this publication lies principally in the excellent illustrations which have been superbly reproduced. This atlas cannot stand by itself as a means of learning pathology but is certainly of great value as a means of review for those already familiar with the pathology of human diseases. For those who are just learning pathology, this atlas can be useful if studied in conjunction with one of the standard textbooks. The photographs are of the highest quality and can certainly provide a strong foundation for the beginning student who wants to understand the morphologic basis of the many conditions that affect man.

The original atlas was the product of many experts whose contributions were molded into a coherent, relatively uniform, instructional product by Professor Grundmann. We have attempted to maintain the special viewpoints of the original authors, while adjusting the emphasis and terminology. To a great degree the judgement of the original authors, and the quality of the original illustrations, can stand alone as a foundation for a fine book. We hope that our efforts have not significantly reduced the value of this atlas, and that they have been equal to the fine work of the original authors and the publisher. Ms. Elaine Mudrick provided expert secretarial support. Special appreciation is due to Mr. Braxton D. Mitchell, President of Urban & Schwarzenberg in Baltimore, who has been both encouraging and patient beyond anyone's expectations.

Stephen A. Geller, M.D.
Los Angeles, 1988

Contents

A. Heart

E. Grundmann, H.-J. Knieriem, K.-M. Müller

Heart disease remains the leading cause of morbidity and mortality in industrial nations. Disorders of the heart can affect all other organ systems. When the heart is damaged, decompensation can lead to physiological and even structural changes in the lungs, liver, kidneys, and other organs. Congestive heart failure is the term used for the clinical syndrome resulting from reduced cardiac stroke volume, resulting in lower cardiac output than venous return. The fundamental derangement might be impaired contractility, as in intrinsic myocardial disease, or increased workload, as in valvular incompetence. Often multiple factors are operative.

The exact incidence of congenital heart disease is unknown, but it may be as high as nine cases per 100,000 births. Inherited heart defects can be present with virtually every conceivable embryologic variation; the most practical way of classifying them is in terms of the type of shunt. Congenital defects with a predominant left-to-right shunt include atrial-septal or ventricular-septal defects, and patent ductus arteriosus. A right-to-left shunt is associated with tetralogy of Fallot and transposition of the great vessels, among others. One common congenital defect is aortic coarctation, which is not associated with shunting.

More prevalent than congenital heart defects are acquired disorders of the heart. For instance, a variety of changes can affect the endocardium, particularly the valves. Most of these affect the left heart. In addition to age-related degeneration of the valves, there are various forms of endocarditis, both infective and noninfective. Infective endocarditis might occur as a complication of rheumatic heart disease, but can also develop in association with congenital anomalies or degenerative changes of aging, and even in normal valves. Historically, rheumatic heart disease was a major cause of chronic valvular heart disease. This disorder has become less common in industrialized countries as the use of antibiotics has become widespread. Both acquired and congenital valvular disorders may be treated successfully with the use of artificial valves.

Atherosclerotic changes of the coronary arteries contribute to coronary deficiency and, subsequently, to myocardial infarction. The characteristically thickened intima, lipid deposits, and fibrosis narrow the lumen. Rarely, coronary artery disease can follow arteritides. The clinical, and associated histologic, changes of myocardial infarction following coronary insufficiency are well known.

A varied group of nonischemic myocardial disorders can be classified as cardiomyopathies. These can be primary, or can follow a systemic condition such as hypertension. The cardiomyopathies have in common enlargement of the heart and ultimately, heart failure. Among the causes of cardiomyopathy are viral agents, such as Coxsackie, alcoholism, and congenital metabolic disorders.

The most important disease of the pericardium is fibrinous pericarditis. This condition also might be related to primary cardiac disease, or might be the result of extracardiac disease. For example, fibrinous pericarditis is common in uremic patients. It can also follow viral infections or be a reaction to metastatic tumor. In many cases pericarditis leads to the production of a pericardial effusion, which compromises diastolic filling and ultimately, results in heart failure. Cardiac tamponade also occurs as a sequela of myocardial infarction when there is perforation of the heart and leakage of blood into the pericardial sac.

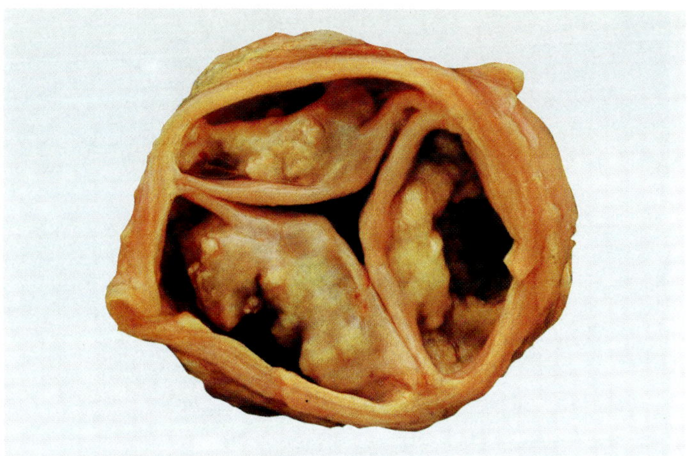

Endocarditis (A8–A17)
E. Grundmann

Fig. A8. Senile calcification of the aortic valve (seen from above). All three cusps show nodular calcifications. Aortic stenosis is a sequela of this kind of vascular sclerosis since, as in this example, the nodular masses restrict the motion of the cusp during systole. This condition is morphologically distinct from rheumatic aortic valvulitis. In the latter disorder, the commissures are fused whereas, in this case, they are distinctly separate.

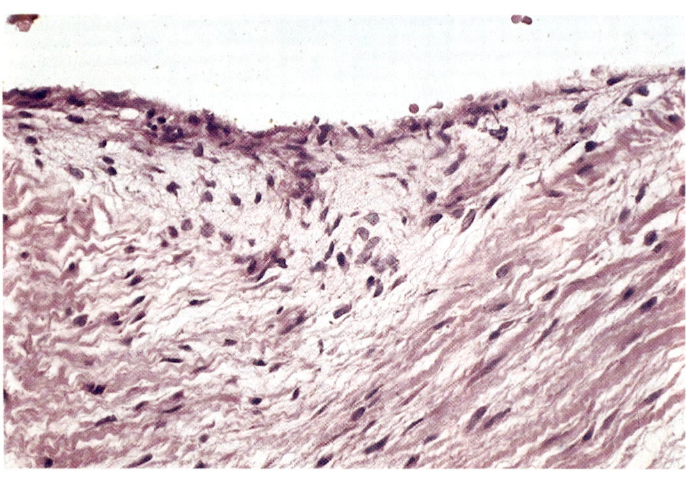

Fig. A9. Myxomatous degeneration of the mitral valve. The plump connective tissue cells beneath the degenerating endothelium have foamy cytoplasm. This morphologic finding is often seen, and might not have any clinical manifestation. In some patients, however, it is associated with the mitral valve prolapse syndrome ("floppy valve syndrome").   (hematoxylin-eosin)

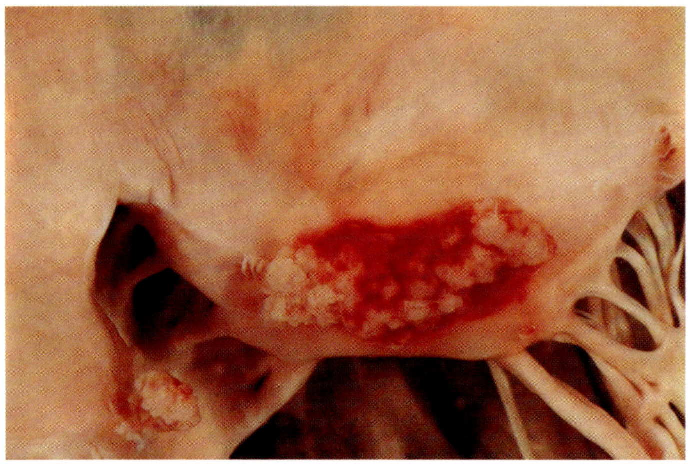

Fig. A10.   Recurrent rheumatic endocarditis of the mitral valve. Multiple grey, warty (verrucous) excrescences at the line of closure of the valve are surrounded by recently deposited fibrin (red). Evidence of prior rheumatic endocarditis is seen not only as opacity of the normally transparent cusp and distortion and thickening of the line of closure, but also in chordae tendinae which show the characteristic thickening, shortening, and fusion. These latter changes reflect fibrosis with contraction of collagen fibrils (thickening and shortening) and surface fibrin deposition, which leads to fusion.

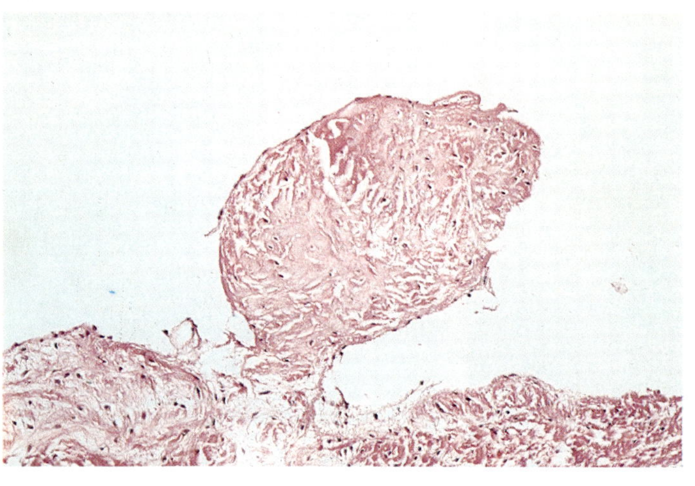

Fig. A11. Histologic appearance of verrucous rheumatic endocarditis. A warty excresence, consisting primarily of fibrin and platelets, protrudes from the endocardial surface. In places, it is partially covered by newly formed endothelium.   (hematoxylin-eosin)

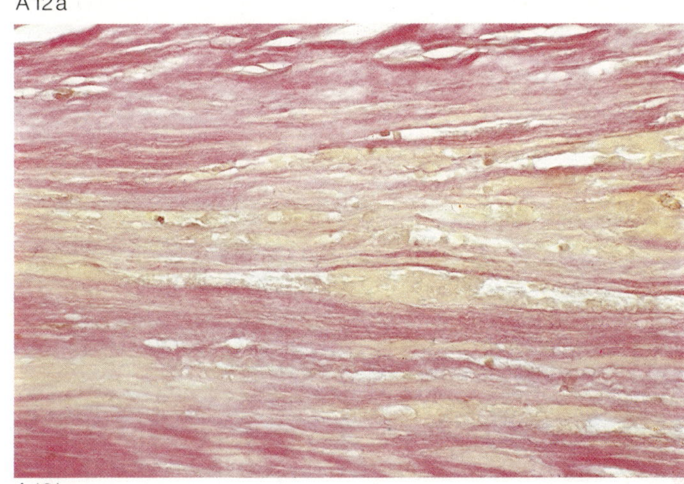

A 12 a

Fig. A 12 a. Recent rheumatic endocarditis. The rheumatic verruca consists of fibrin on the surface and subendothelial deposition of fibrin interspersed with connective tissue. Fibrinoid material is seen in

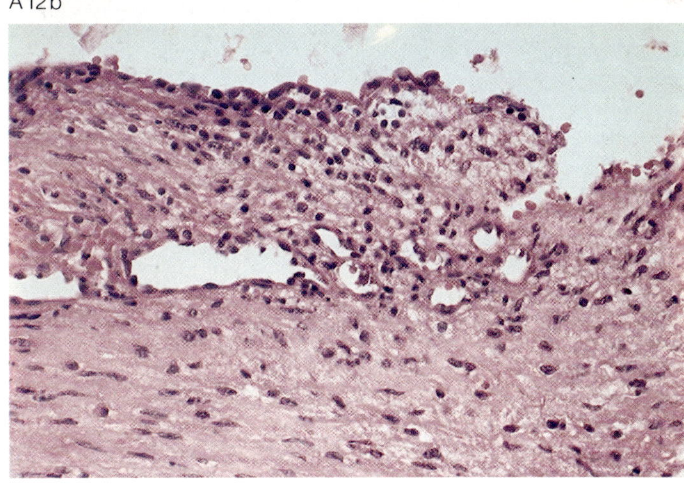

A 12 b

Fig. A 12 b. as yellow brown staining between the red stained collagen. (van Gieson)

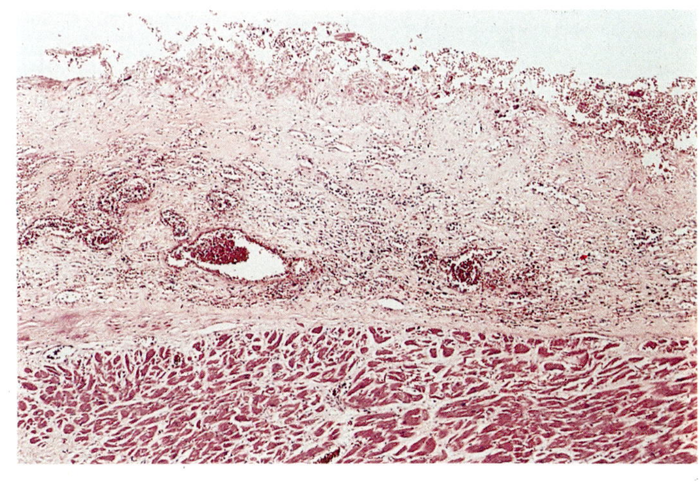

Fig. A 13. Verrucous rheumatic endocarditis in the stage of organization. The persisting warty excresence, which was previously composed of fibrin and platelets *(see Fig. A 11)* now consists of granulation tissue with lymphocytes and histiocytes, and is partially covered by newly formed endothelium. (hematoxylin-eosin)

Fig. A 14. Fibroblastic endocarditis. This follows endomyocarditis involving the mural endocardium, in this case of the left ventricle, with involvement of the myocardium. Within the capillary-rich granulation tissue there are sheets of eosinophils. (hematoxylin-eosin)

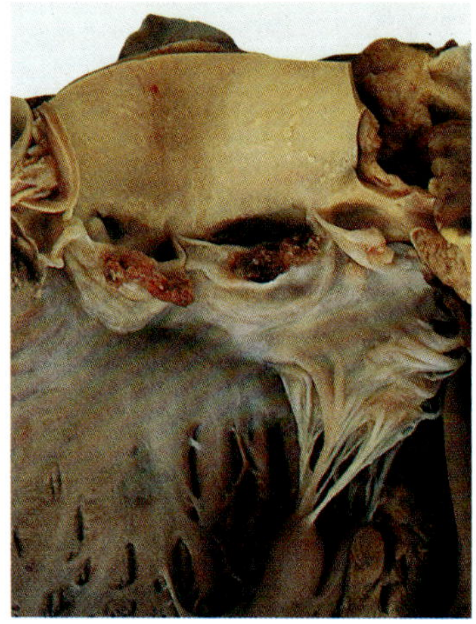

Fig. A 15. Infective endocarditis. A fresh, polypoid thrombotic mass ("vegetation") is at the line of closure of the aortic valve. Infective endocarditis is fatal if untreated. Manifestations can be similar regardless of whether the infecting organism is a bacterium, fungus, rickettsia, or protozoa; they depend on the site and complications of the infection.

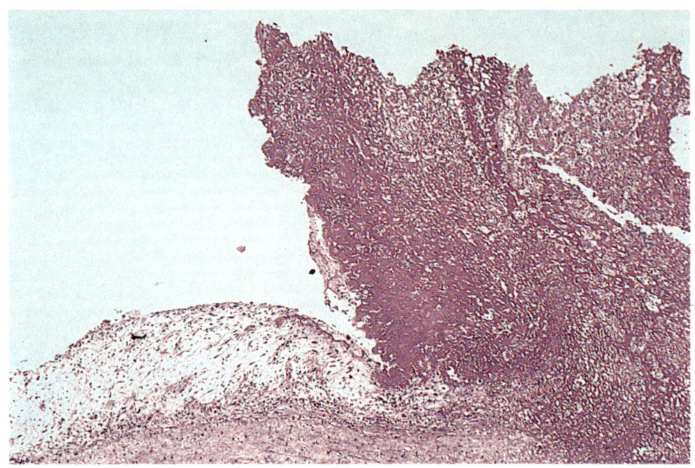

Fig. A 16. Histologic appearance of infective endocarditis. The endocardium in the left portion of the photomicrograph is markedly edematous and the intermixture of fibrin and platelets, forming a thrombus, is infiltrated by numerous polymorphonuclear leukocytes. This vegetation is extremely friable, as seen at the right of the photomicrograph, where it is partially disrupted. Vegetations can break off and embolize to various parts of the body. (hematoxylin-eosin)

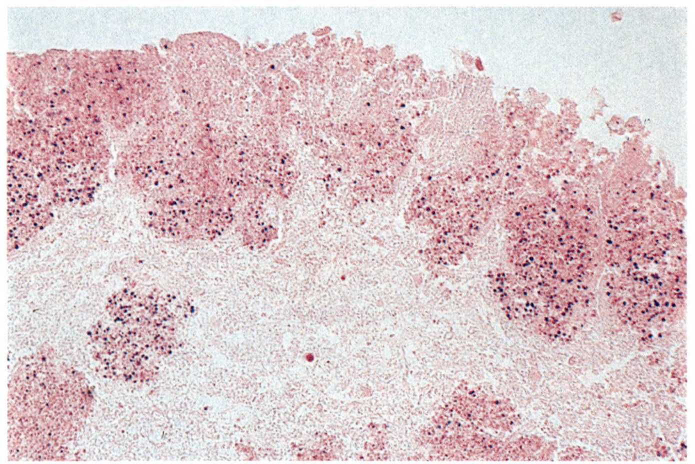

Fig. A 17. Infective endocarditis. Many gram positive cocci are seen within this vegetation on the surface of the aortic valve. (Gram)

Acquired Heart Disease   (A 18–A 23)
E. Grundmann

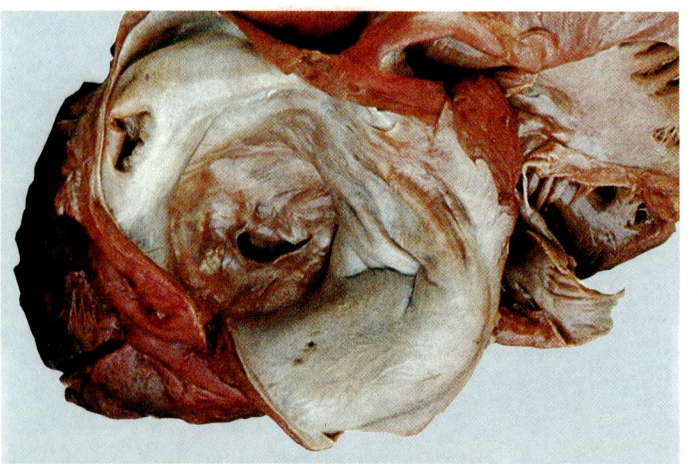

Fig. A 18. Mitral stenosis, with a characteristic "fish mouth" deformity, seen from the atrial aspect. This is a late sequela of rheumatic endocarditis. The opened left atrium is markedly dilated and fibrotic. Rheumatic fever is an immunologically mediated inflammatory disease that occurs as a delayed sequela to pharyngitis caused by Group A, β-hemolytic streptococci. The acute phase, shown in Figs. *A 10–A 13,* is a diffuse, nonspecific inflammatory process affecting all layers of the heart. Chronic rheumatic heart disease becomes manifest 10–20 years after the acute episode and typically consists of deformed, fibrotic valves which show collagenization, increased vascularity, and, in late stages, calcification.

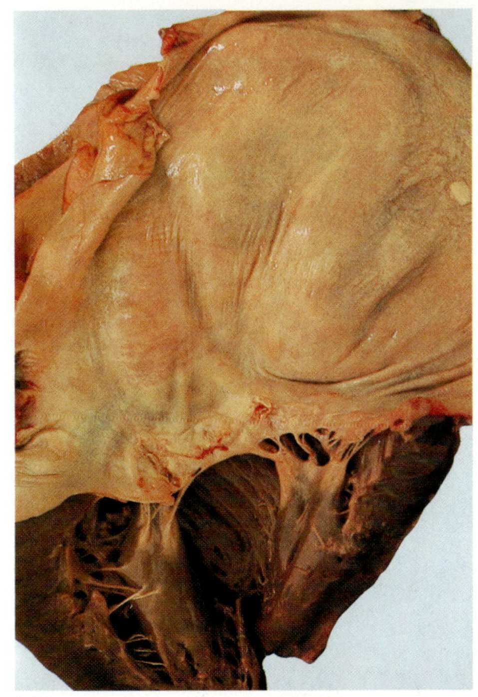

A 19

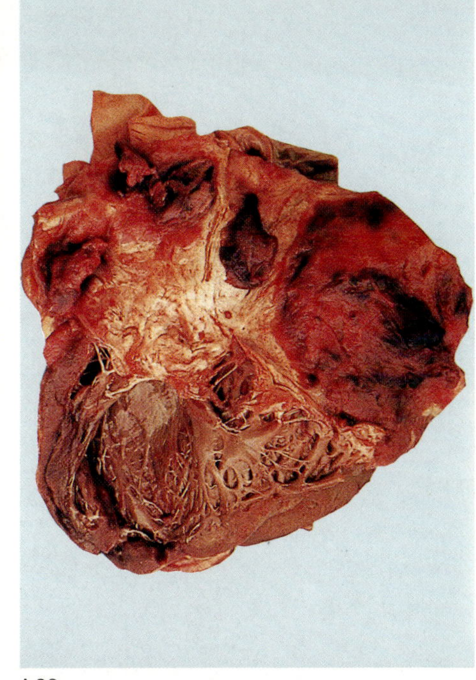

A 20

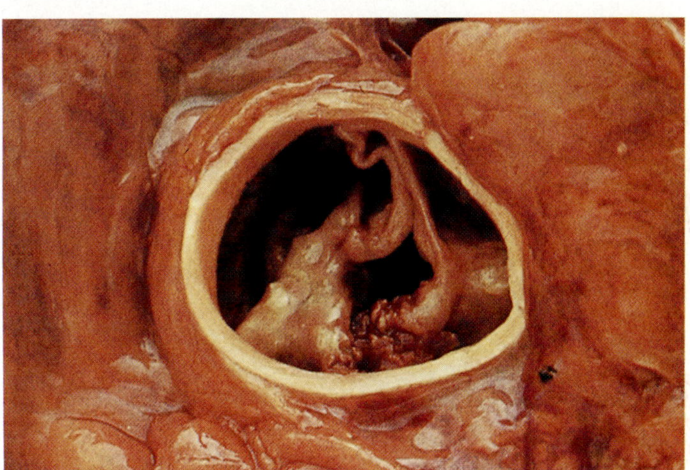

Fig. A 19. Mitral stenosis seen with the left lateral aspect of the heart incised. The left atrium is massively dilated with fibrosis and atheromatous plaques above the tapering left ventricle. The mitral valve is fibrotic and opaque, the commissures are obliterated, and the chordae tendinae are shortened and fused. In rheumatic heart disease the mitral valve is involved most often (48%); combined mitral and aortic involvement is second most common (42%).

Fig. A 20. Combined mitral stenosis and mitral insufficiency following severe, destructive (ulcerating) infective endocarditis. The left ventricle (below) is dilated. The left atrium (above) is also greatly dilated and fibrotic, with marked deposition of lipids and calcium salts, which appear yellow. Multiple large mural thrombi cover the left atrial endocardium.

Fig. A 21. Aortic stenosis following endocarditis. The coronary ostia are obstructed and there is marked thickening and deformity of the semilunar valves. In one area there is a recently formed infective vegetation as evidence of the recurrent nature of the septic endocarditis. (Compare this picture with *Fig. A 8,* which shows aortic stenosis which did not follow infectious endocarditis.) This valvular deformity can be difficult to distinguish from bicuspid aortic valve, a relatively common anomaly that is hemodynamically abnormal and more likely than aortic stenosis to demonstrate degenerative changes leading to fibrosis. The bicuspid semilunar valve is more susceptible to infective endocarditis.

Fig. A 22. Aortic stenosis following endocarditis, with subsequent massive left ventricular hypertrophy. The heart has been sectioned frontally so that the right ventricle (which is to the left of this photograph) can be compared to the left. The right ventricular wall is not altered. The left ventricular hypertrophy is concentric, as evidenced by the equal thickening of the septum and the lateral wall.

Fig. A 23. Aortic insufficiency following endocarditis. The aortic valve has been partially destroyed by an extensive ulcerating and vegetative endocarditis *(arrow).* The left ventricle is massively dilated and hypertrophied, the morphologic expression of the greatly increased workload.

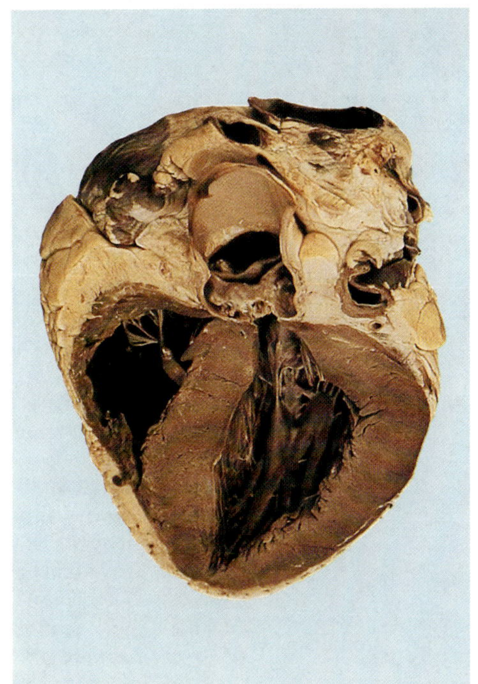

A 22

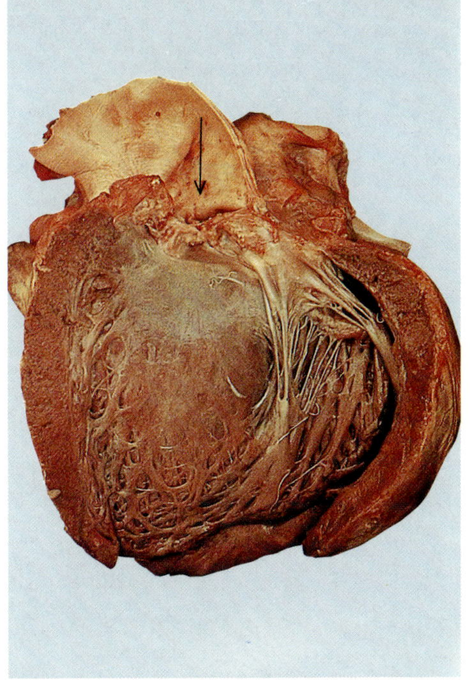

A 23

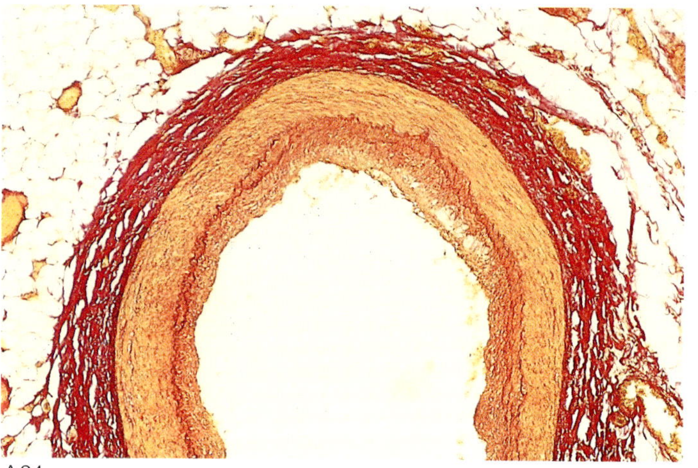

A24

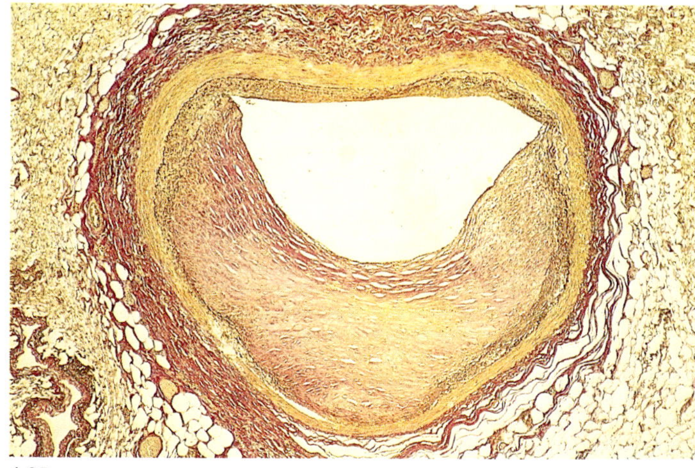

A25

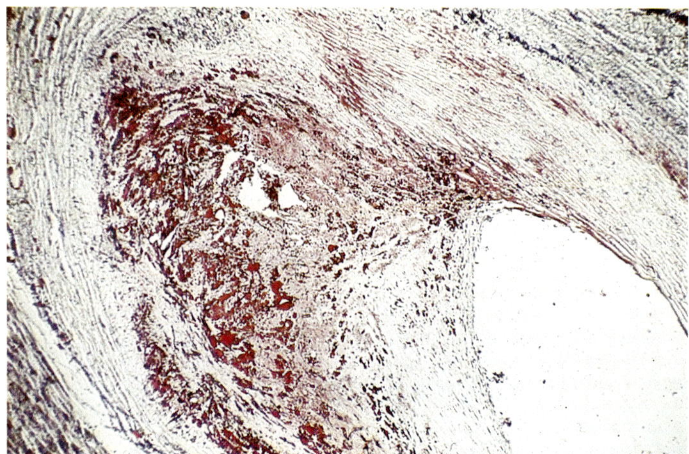

A26

Coronary Artery Disease   (A24–A31)
K.-M. Müller

Fig. A24.   Early changes associated with coronary atherosclerosis in a 15-year-old girl. Focal intimal changes are due to the insudation of plasma and lipids. The media and adventitia are unchanged. (elastica-van Gieson)

Fig. A25.   Advanced coronary artery atherosclerosis. Note the markedly thickened, fibrotic wall, with approximately 70% lumen obliteration. The thickening of the wall is due to a proliferation of fibroblasts and smooth muscle cells, as well as to the formation of new collagen fibers. The muscular wall is narrowed in areas and the adventitia fibers are disrupted.   (elastica-van Gieson)

Fig. A26.   High grade stenosis of a coronary artery with only a small area of relatively normal arterial wall (upper right). Red-stained fat and cholesterol deposits are in the sclerotic portion (left). (hematoxylin-Sudan III)

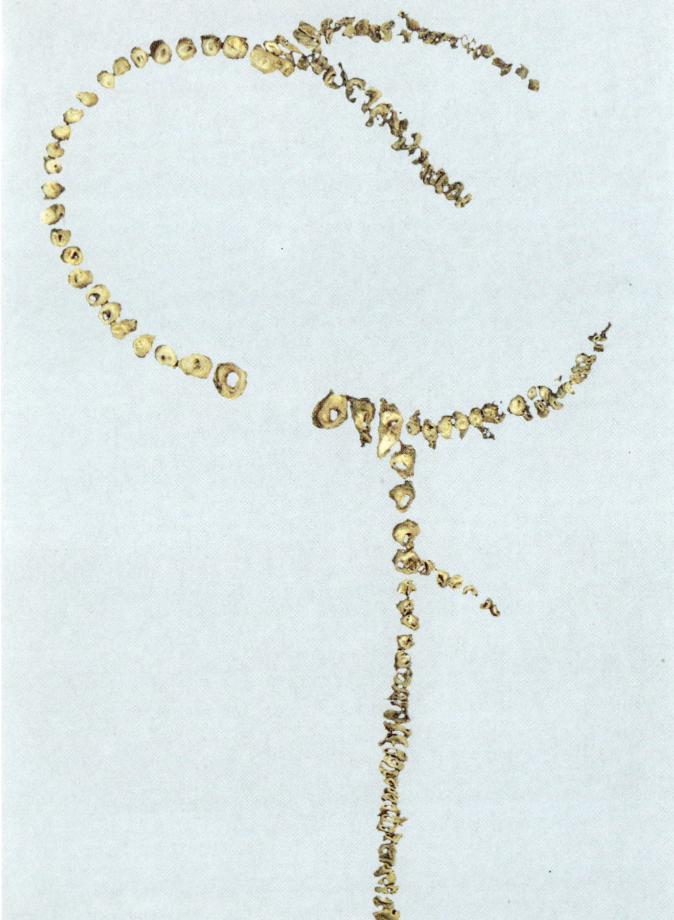

Fig. A27.   High grade, generalized, three-vessel coronary atherosclerosis from a 75-year-old hypertensive patient. The coronary arteries have been laid out in the usual configuration and have been cross-sectioned. There is considerable variation in the degree of changes seen, with some segments showing complete obliteration of the lumen, and others less severely changed. The right coronary artery (to the left and above) is, in this case, the dominant artery and is particularly affected. The site of myocardial infarction varies with the coronary vessels involved. When the left anterior descending coronary artery is severely involved, infarction occurs in the anterior left ventricle or anteroseptum; the bundle of His and right bundle branch can also be affected. When the circumflex is involved, the posterior or lateral left ventricle can show ischemic changes, and the atrioventricular node might be damaged. With right coronary disease, as is particularly prominent in this case, the posterior left ventricle or posteroseptum is usually involved, in addition to the posterior right ventricle. The conduction system might show multiple areas of involvement, including the sino-atrial node, the atrioventricular node, and the bundle of His.

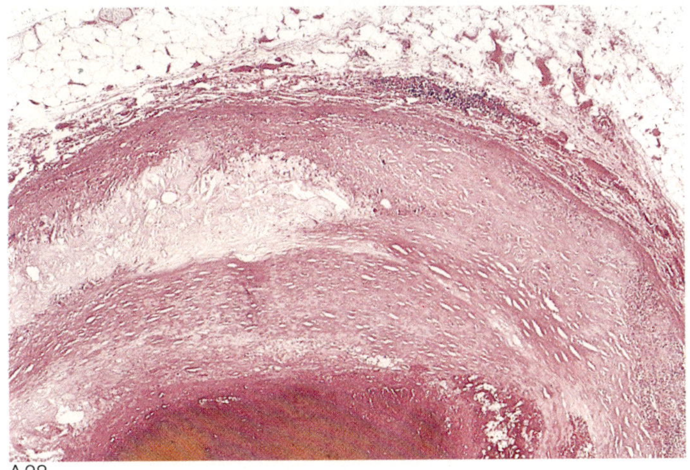

A28

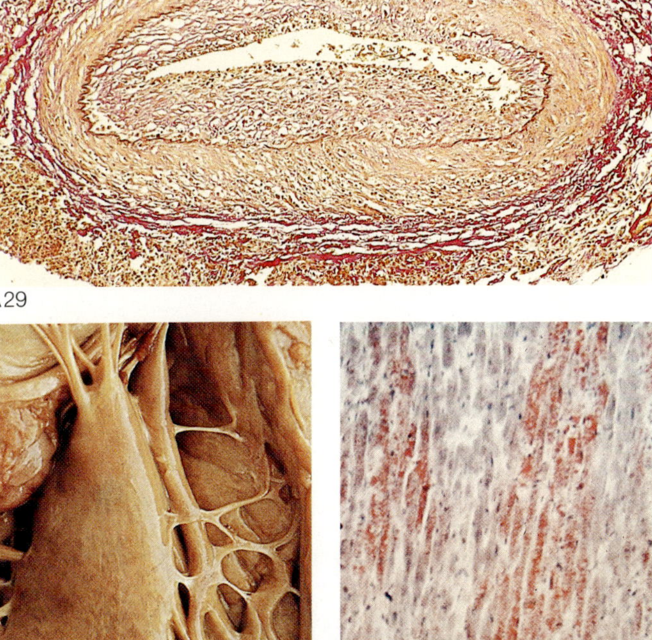

A29

Fig. A28. Section of a coronary artery showing a laminated pattern of atherosclerotic change, with completely fibrotic areas, a pale lipid-laden area, and, at the lower edge of the photograph, a fresh mural thrombus completely covering the intima and obliterating the lumen. (hematoxylin-eosin)

Fig. A29. Polyarteritis ("periarteritis") nodosa of a coronary artery branch showing extensive and severe inflammation of the intima, with partial destruction of the elastica in the media, seen in the lower portion of the photomicrograph. Marked inflammatory cell infiltration is seen throughout the media in the adventitia. This is a relatively rare cause of coronary artery disease. (elastica-van Gieson).

Fig. A30a. Fatty degeneration ("tigering") of the myocardium. This is seen as yellow flecks in the right ventricular muscle. Fatty degeneration can follow chronic coronary insufficiency or protracted anemia.

Fig. A30b. Histologic section of fatty degeneration of the myocardium showing sudanophilia (red) of the lipid material within myocardial fibers. (hematoxylin-Sudan III)

A30a

A30b

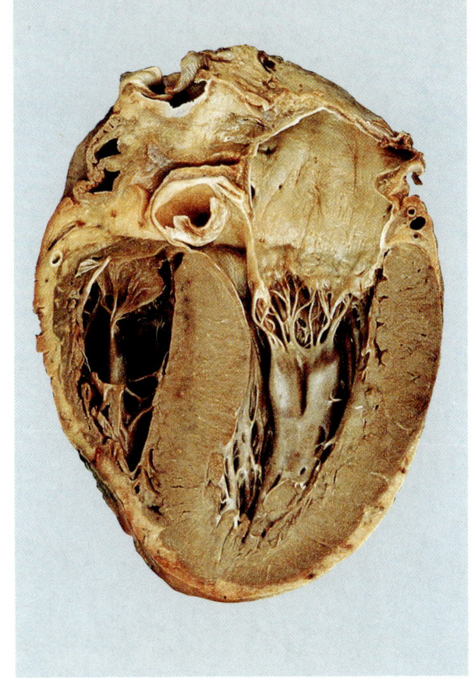

Fig. A31. Marked, concentric left ventricular hypertrophy associated with essential hypertension. This is the typical appearance of longstanding hypertension. The right ventricle (to the left, in this photograph) is unchanged. The septal and lateral left ventrical myocardia are greatly thickened and the papillary muscles are particularly prominent, as a compensation for the increased left-sided peripheral resistance. Note that the mitral valve itself is unremarkable; compare these chordae tendinae to those of rheumatic heart disease *(Figs. A 10, A 19).*

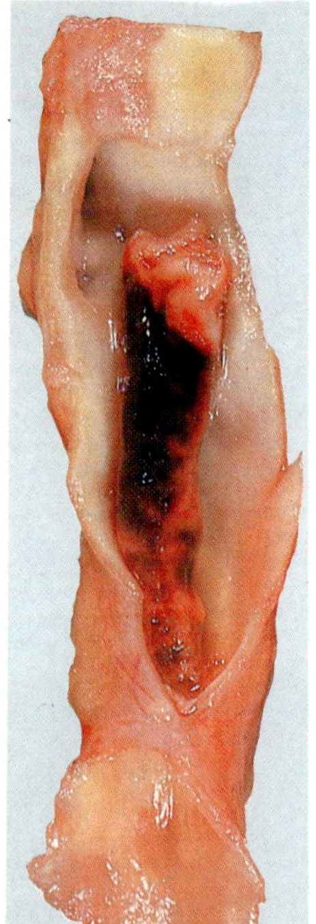

A32

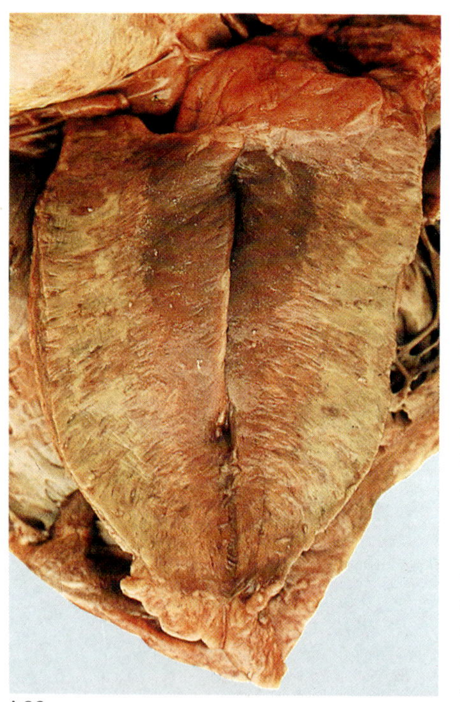

A33a

Myocardial Infarction *(A32–A37)*
K.-M. Müller

Fig. A32. This partially opened coronary artery is almost completely filled by a recently formed thrombus which is adherent to an atherosclerotic plaque. This patient had a fresh myocardial infarction. The upper aspect of the thrombus consists mostly of lipids, whereas the lower portion of the thrombus demonstrates the characteristic ("Zahn's") lines of organization.

Fig. A33a. Myocardial infarction approximately 18 hours after coronary thrombosis. The clay-colored portion is the area of necrosis and is delineated relatively sharply from the intact red-brown myocardium. The most central portion of the infarct shows complete obliteration of fiber detail and is seen as a relatively homogeneous area of discoloration.

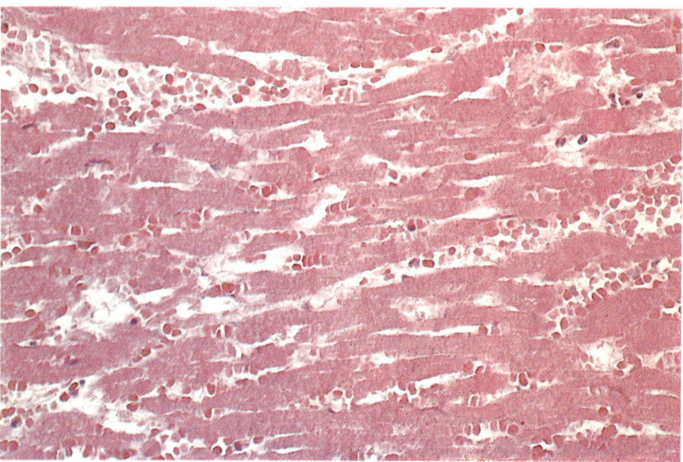

A33b

Fig. A33b. Histologic section of acute myocardial infarction. The usual cardiac fiber striations are obliterated and the cytoplasm is homogeneous. The interstitium is widened because of edema. (hematoxylin-eosin)

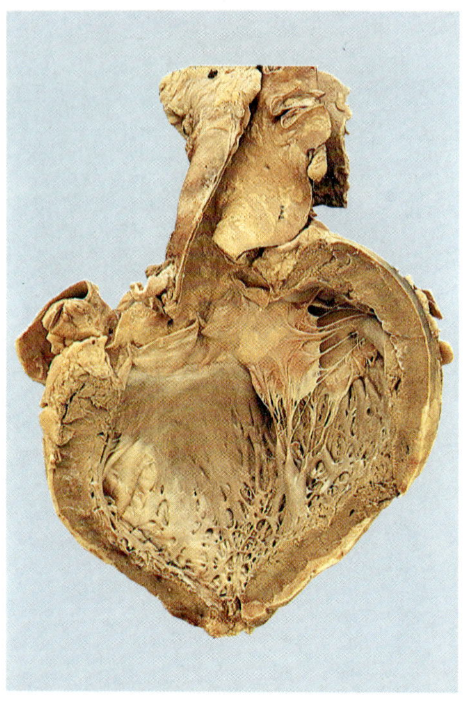

Fig. A34. Old anteroseptal myocardial infarction. The myocardium is replaced by grey-white scar tissue in this dilated left ventricle. This followed a prior surgical resection of a postinfarction ventricular aneurysm.

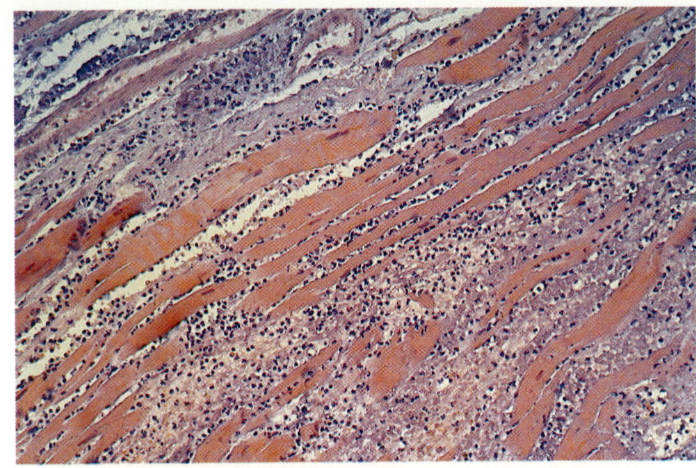

Fig. A35. Myocardial infarction approximately 24 hours after the onset of chest pain. The myocardial fibers show coagulative necrosis and there is infiltration by many polymorphonuclear leukocytes.

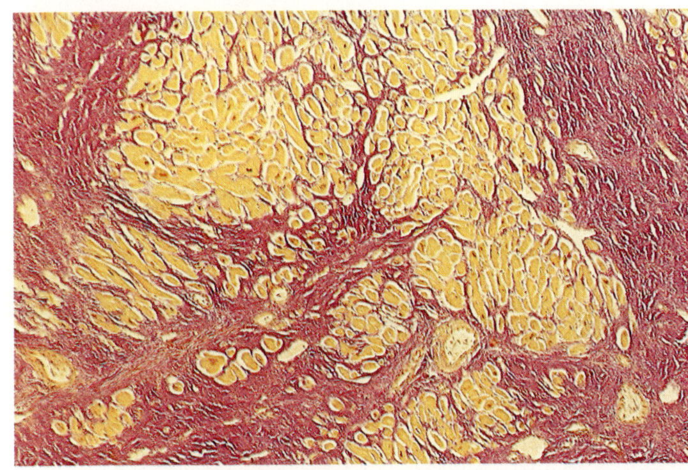

Fig. A36. Partial myocardial replacement after an acute myocardial infarction. In this photomicrograph the residual muscle fibers are yellow, and are incompletely surrounded by red stained collagen. (van Gieson)

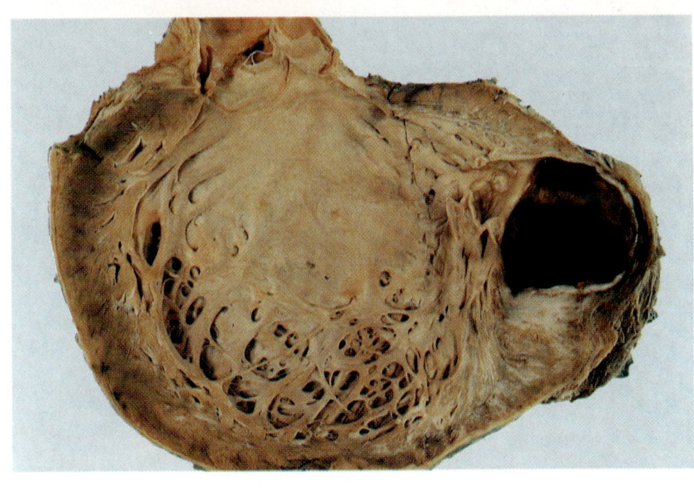

Fig. A37. Large saccular aneurysm of the left ventricle after a clinically silent myocardial infarction. The aneurysm is seen as a dark cavity. The myocardium below this is replaced by grey-white fibrosis.

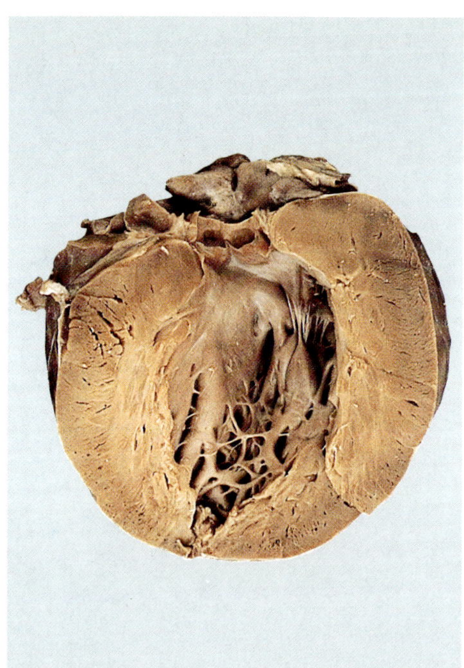

Idiopathic Cardiomyopathies *(A 38–A 43)*
H.-J. Knieriem

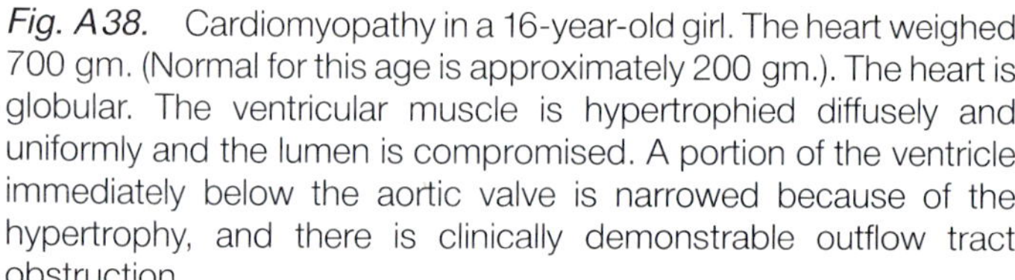

Fig. A38. Cardiomyopathy in a 16-year-old girl. The heart weighed 700 gm. (Normal for this age is approximately 200 gm.). The heart is globular. The ventricular muscle is hypertrophied diffusely and uniformly and the lumen is compromised. A portion of the ventricle immediately below the aortic valve is narrowed because of the hypertrophy, and there is clinically demonstrable outflow tract obstruction.

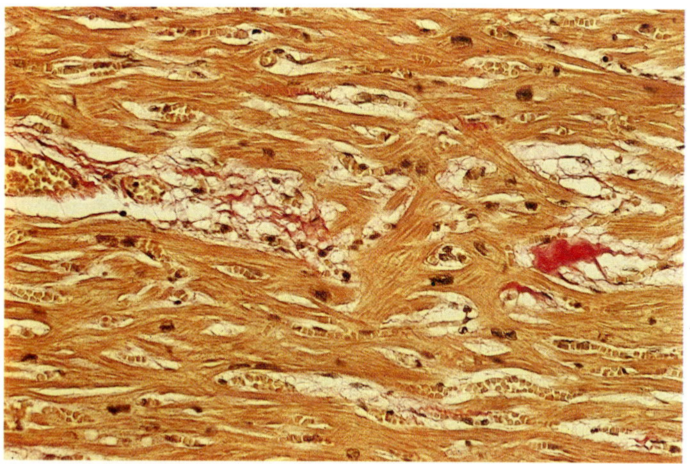

Fig. A39. Histologic section from a case of hypertrophic cardiomyopathy with a distinctive alteration of the myocardial architecture, which is seen in this two-dimensional representation as branching fibers. The nuclei are enlarged and hyperchromatic. In addition, interstitial fibrosis is present, contributing to diminished contractibility.   (elastica-van Gieson)

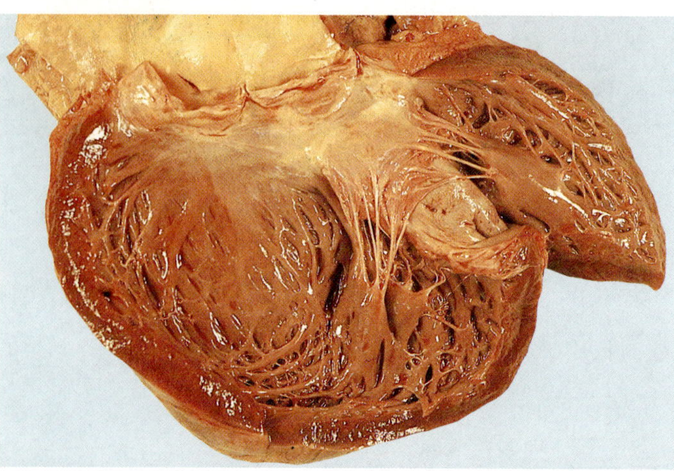

A40

Fig. A40. Dilated cardiomyopathy. The left ventricle of this 34-year-old patient is massively dilated two years after she had viral myocarditis. Small mural thrombi are between the trabeculae carnae. Note the massive enlargement of the papillary muscles, particularly the one to the right of the picture. This is strong evidence that the entire heart was hypertrophied prior to the onset of cardiac failure. With failure, the chamber became dilated and the wall thinned. Had the patient survived longer, the papillary muscles would have become completely flattened. Note also the dilation of the aortic valve ring leading to secondary aortic insufficiency, further complicating the ventricular dilation and contributing to heart failure.

Fig. A41. Transmission electron microscopy of a myocardial biopsy from a patient with congestive cardiomyopathy. Branching of the myocardial fiber is obvious. The nucleus is central and is surrounded by many mitochondria and lipofuschin granules. Interstitial fibrosis is represented, in this picture, by fibrocytes to the left and above the myocardial fibrils.   (magnification 5,760×)

Fig. A42. Transmission electron microscopy of heart muscle resected from a patient with congestive cardiomyopathy. The myofibrils are divided at the inner portion of the sarcoplasm. There is also Z-band distortion and loss of organelles. Small mitochondria, some of which show degenerative changes, are adjacent to the myofibrils. Other mitochondria are enlarged and abnormally formed. (magnification 18,700×)

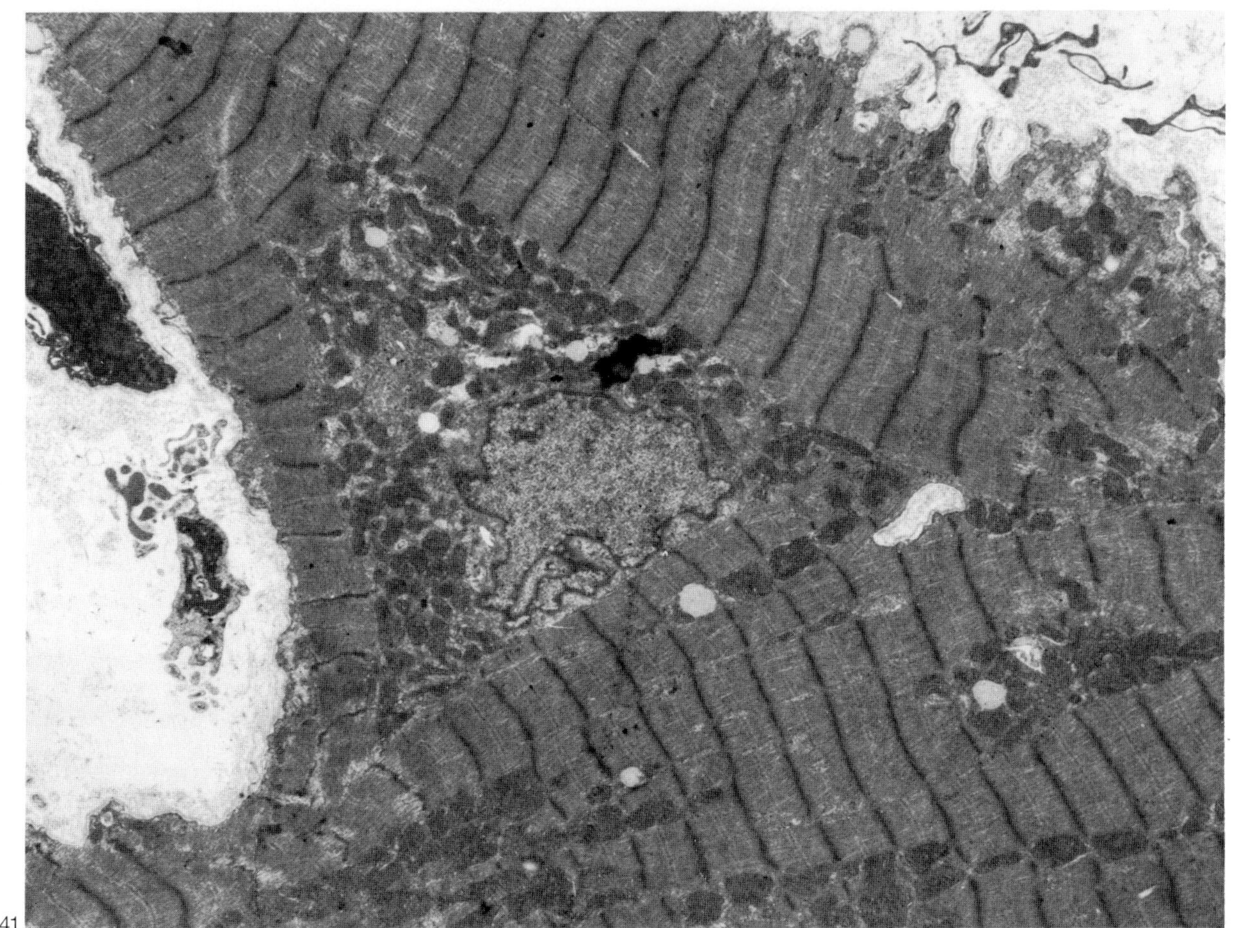

A41

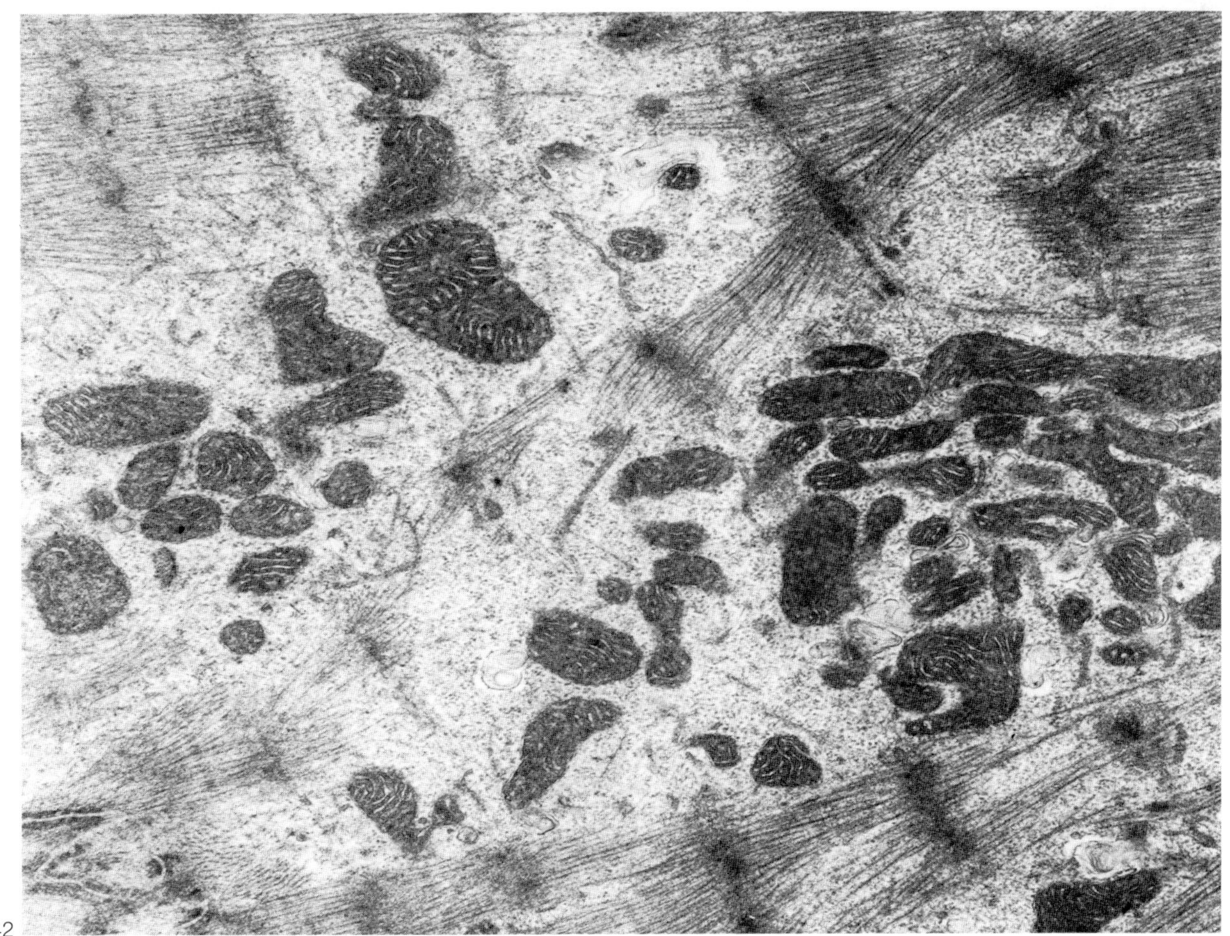

A42

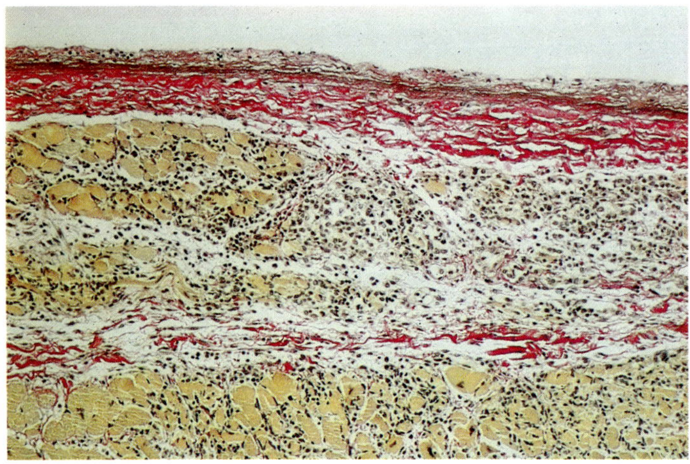

Fig. A 49. Viral myocarditis in a 23-year-old woman with complete AV block. The extensive granulocytic and lymphocytic inflammatory infiltrate particularly involved the left-sided conduction system and caused reduced cardiac output. Many necrotic myocardial fibers are seen. The left conduction bundle is marked by the collagen fibers which appear as a distinct layer under the thin endocardium. (elastica-van Gieson)

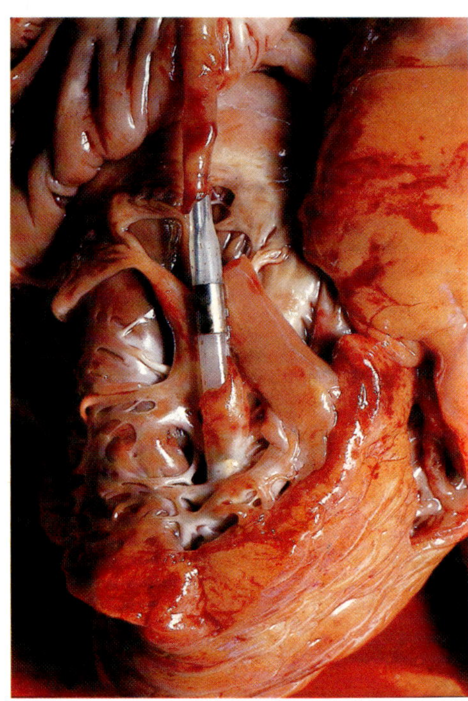

Fig. A 50. Electrodes from a transvenous pacemaker in the trabecular muscles of the right ventricle, with adherent organized thrombotic material covering parts of the electrode wire. The thrombotic material at the upper portion of the wire extended into the right atrium.

Pericardium *(A 51–A 52)*
H.-J. Knieriem

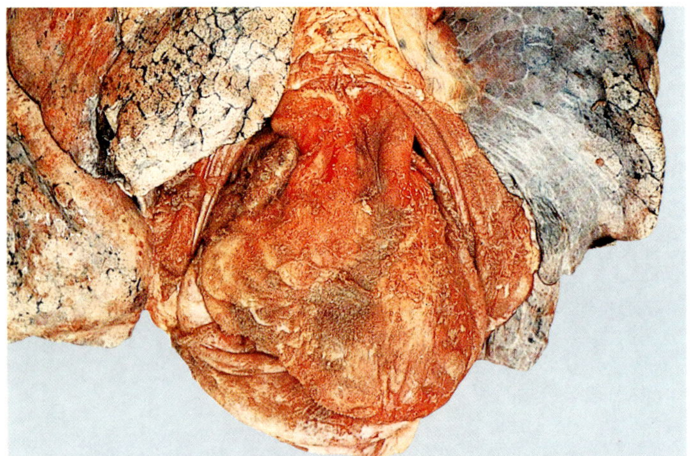

Fig. A 51. Fibrinous pericarditis from a 61-year-old man who died of uremia. The hemorrhagic fibrin deposits cover the epicardium and the parietal pericardium which is peeled away from the anterior heart. The epicardium and parietal pericardium were loosely adherent. The heart is relatively unchanged, and only the pericardial sac has been incised. The fibrin is relatively sticky and, because of the rubbing together of the epicardium and pericardium, a "friction rub" can be heart on auscultation of the heart.

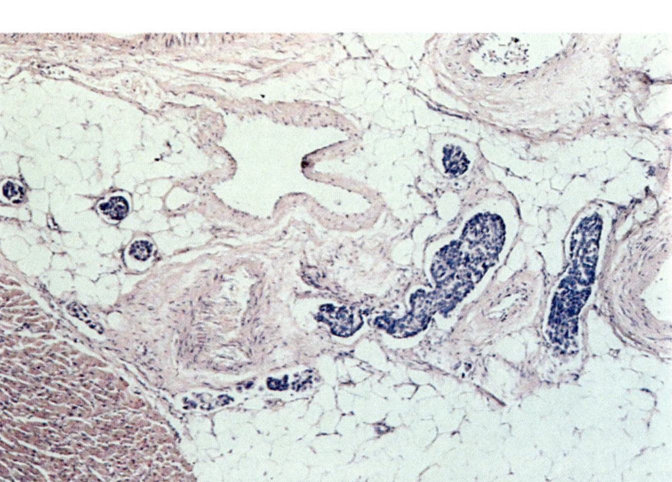

Fig. A 52. Photomicrograph of a metastatic breast carcinoma in pericardial lymphatics, from a 39-year-old woman. The tumor cells have hyperchromatic nuclei and are seen easily. Adjacent small arteries and a dilated vein are not infiltrated, and there is no inflammatory response. Metastatic carcinoma can mimic the clinical and morphologic picture of fibrinous pericarditis. (hematoxylin-eosin)

B. Vascular System

A. Llombart-Bosch

In addition to the heart, the cardiovascular system includes the great vessels, their tributaries, and the venous system, all of which can be affected by degenerative, inflammatory, traumatic, and, to a lesser extent, neoplastic conditions.

The most frequent, and therefore the most important, disease affecting the vascular system is arteriosclerosis. The term arteriosclerosis actually designates a group of degenerative diseases of the large arteries, the most important of which is atherosclerosis. Atherosclerosis is characterized by the deposition of lipids, complex carbohydrates, and blood and its products in vessel walls, with subsequent complicating fibrosis, calcification, and other sequelae. Arteries tend to degenerate because of constant tension, relative lack of intramural capillaries (with resultant limitation of repair), and an inability to "rest." Atherosclerosis begins during youth and becomes clinically manifest during the later years of life, when the lesions are complicated by ulceration, mural thrombosis, and aneurysm formation, as well as fibrosis and calcification.

Inflammatory disorders can also affect the blood vessels. Such conditions can be nonspecific or related to a specific etiologic agent. Immunologic mechanisms in particular have been incriminated in this group of disorders. At one time syphilis was a major cause of vascular inflammation and many associated complications. Fortunately, however, the advanced stages of syphilis, which affect blood vessels, have become rare. Indeed, except for atherosclerosis, all of the conditions affecting the blood vessels are relatively uncommon.

Tumors of vasoformative tissue are not common. In general, they do not derive from large vessels.

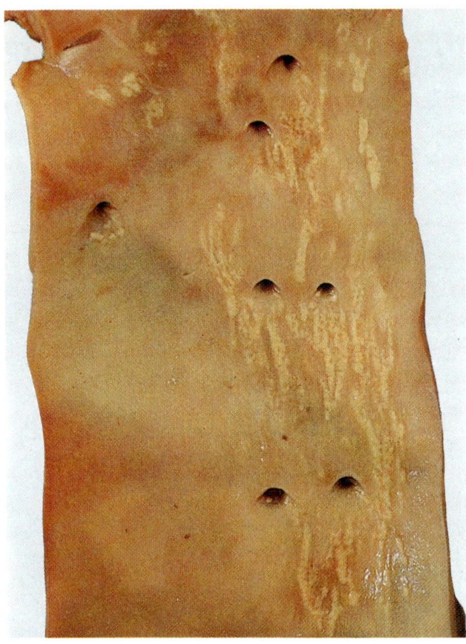

Fig. B1. This aorta, from a 19-year-old, shows typical fatty streaks of early atherosclerosis. In some areas the fatty streaks show beginning coalescence.

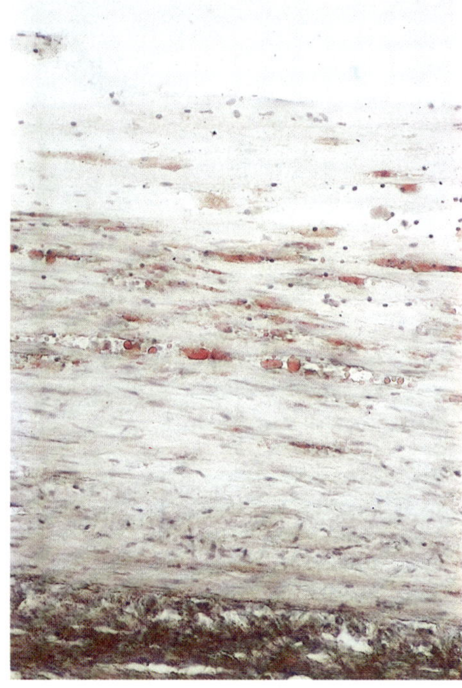

Fig. B2. Photomicrograph of early deposition of lipid in the arterial intima. Fatty streaks are macroscopic representations of this accumulation of lipid in cells of the aortic intima. The interstition in this photomicrograph is edematous. (hematoxylin-Sudan red)

Fig. B3. Complicated lesion of atherosclerosis with fibrous tissue (F) beneath the thickened intima. There is intense lipid deposition (L) and partial interruption of the inner muscle fibers of the media (M). (hematoxylin-Sudan red)

Fig. B4a. Scanning electron micrograph of an atherosclerotic ▷ coronary artery. The endothelial surface is marked by an adherent microthrombus (M). There is obvious intimal thickening (S). (magnification 40×)

Fig. B4b. Scanning electron micrograph of the endothelium of an ▷ atherosclerotic coronary artery. The surface irregularity is due to the ongoing endothelial damage, and organized microthrombi (M) are completely adherent to the surface, with attachment at the junction between adjacent endothelial cells. (magnification 2,500×)

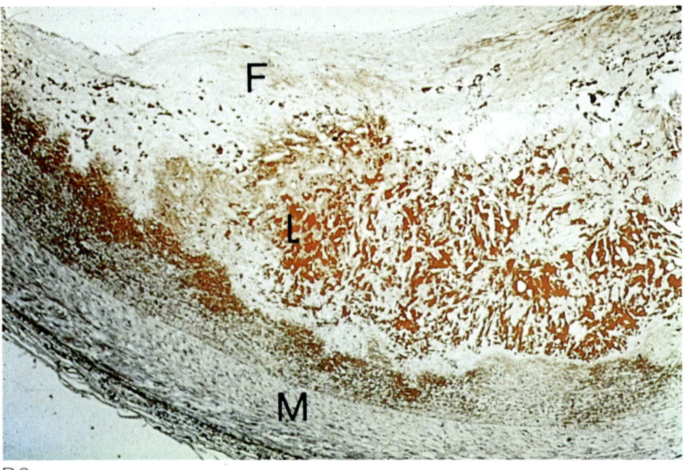

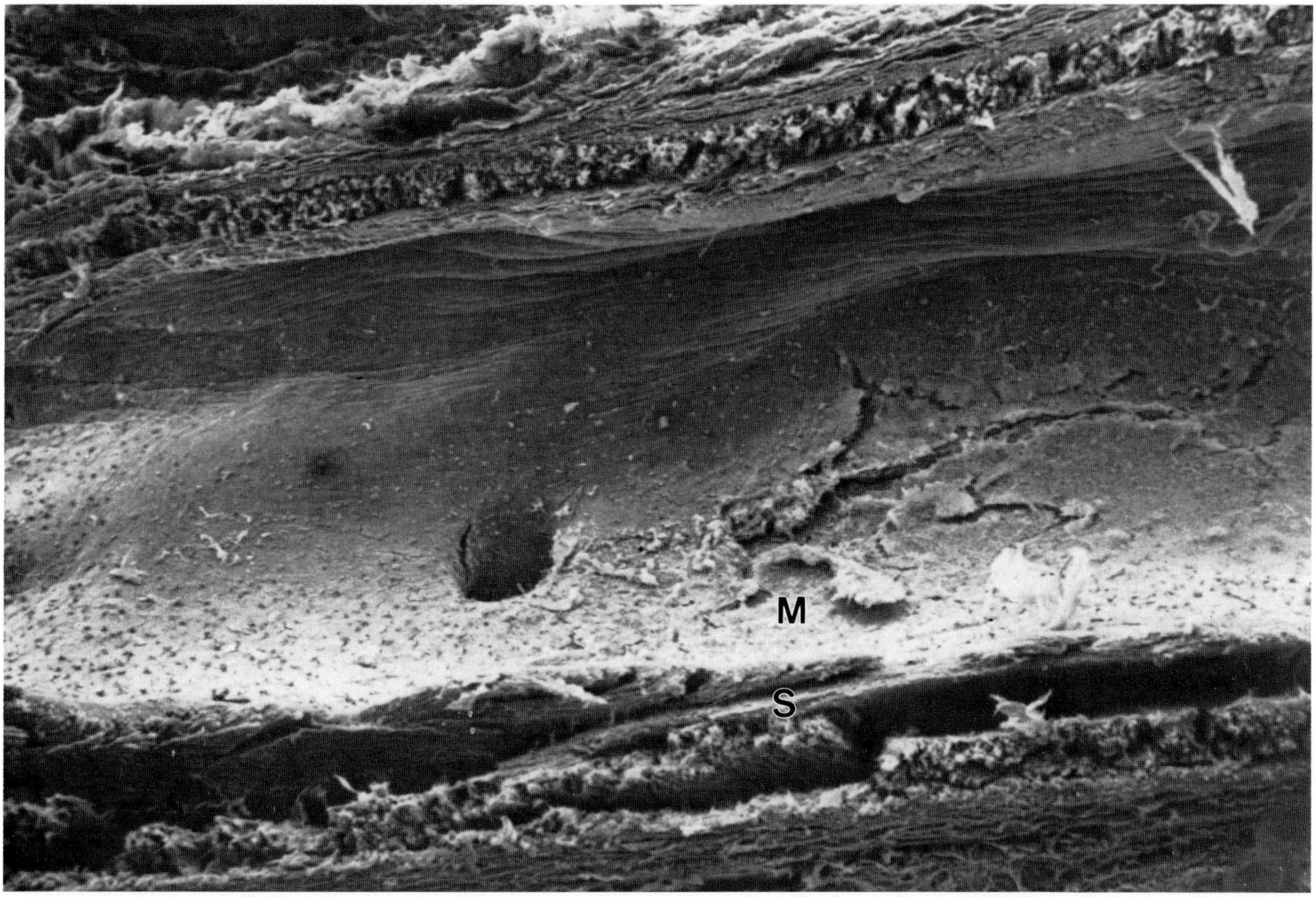

B4a
M
S

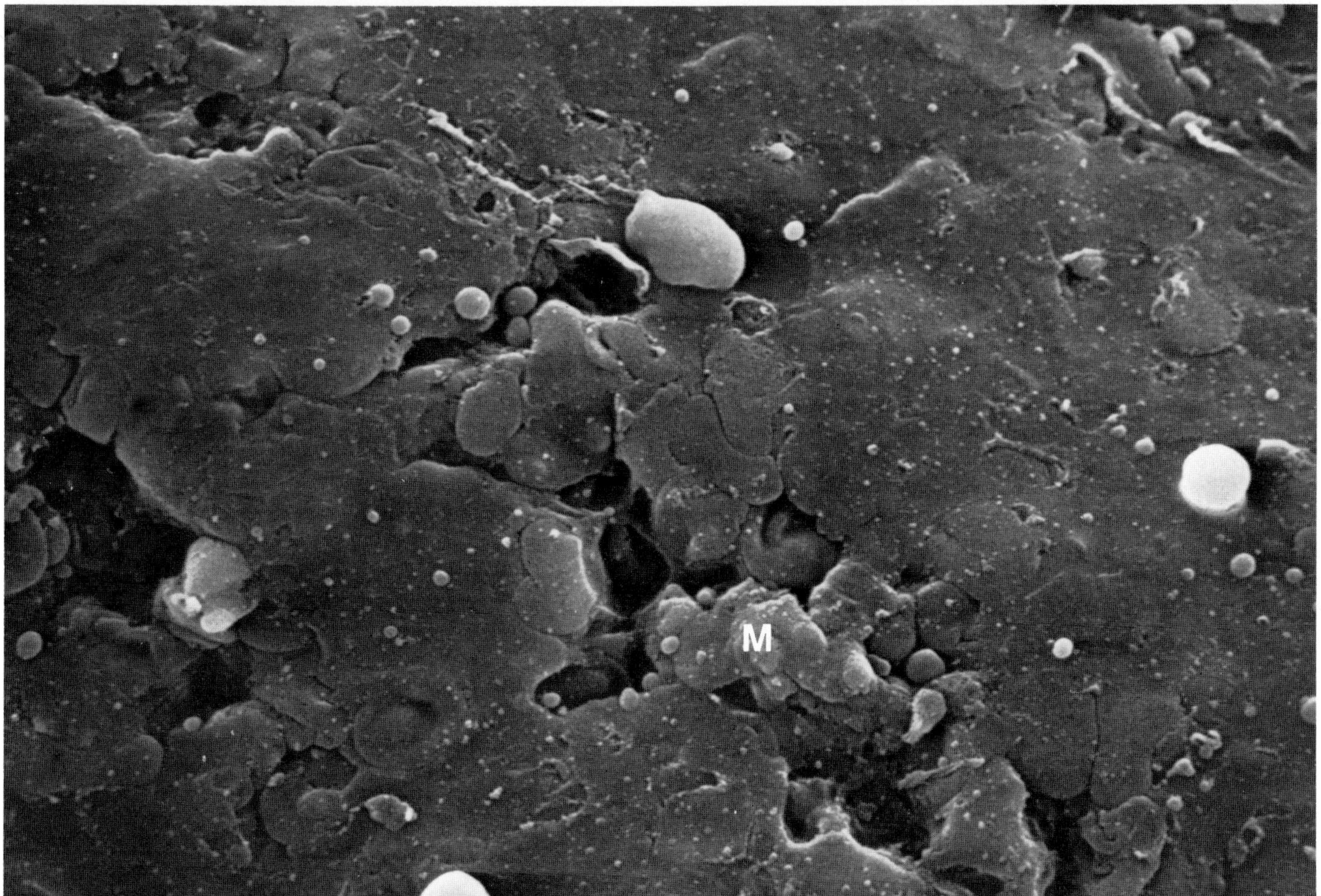

B4b
M

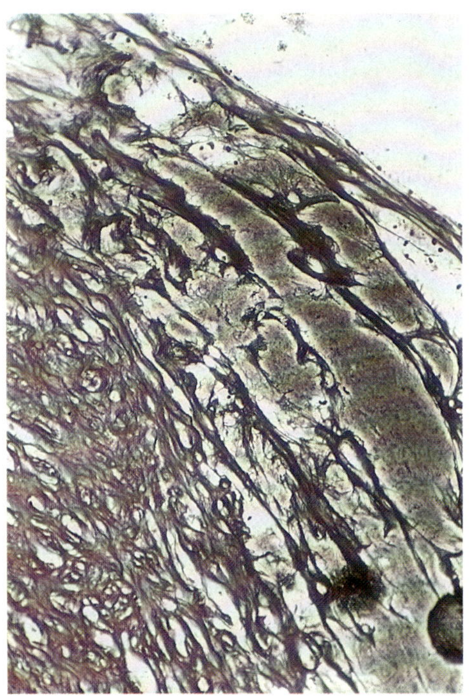

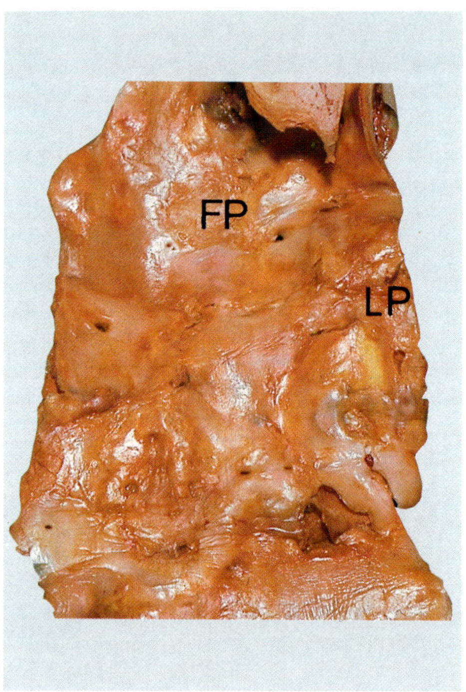

Fig. B5.   Subendothelial edema with splitting of fibers of the intima and inner media, with early subintimal fibrosis. This lesion would resemble a blister macroscopically.
(silver impregnation, Rio-Hortega)

Fig. B6.   Fibrous plaques (FP) and lipid-rich deposits (LP) of the aorta. These complicated lesions surround intercostal arterial ostia and, in some areas, are coalescent. Lipid deposits were stained by immersing the specimen in Sudan red solution for 72 hours.

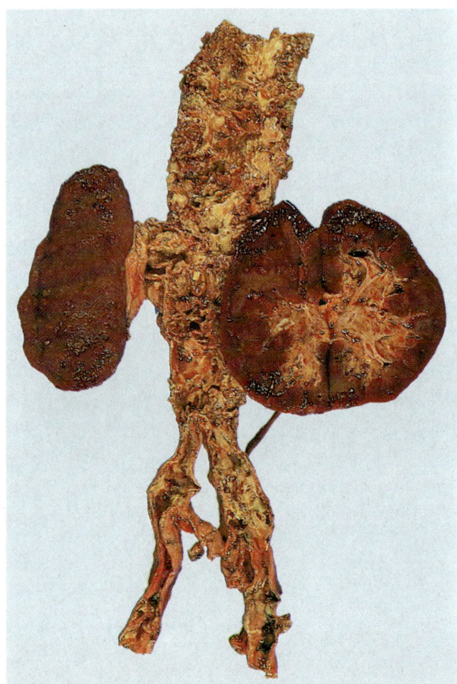

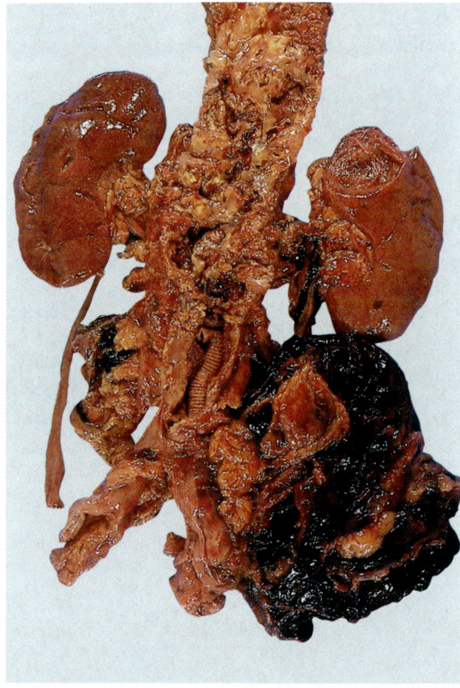

Fig. B7.   Severe atherosclerosis of the abdominal aorta and iliac arteries. Ulcers and thrombi are present in the iliac artery. The kidneys are nephrosclerotic, as evidenced by the irregular, coarsely granular surfaces.

Fig. B8.   Massive, fatal hemorrhage from an atherosclerotic aneurysm at the aortic bifurcation.

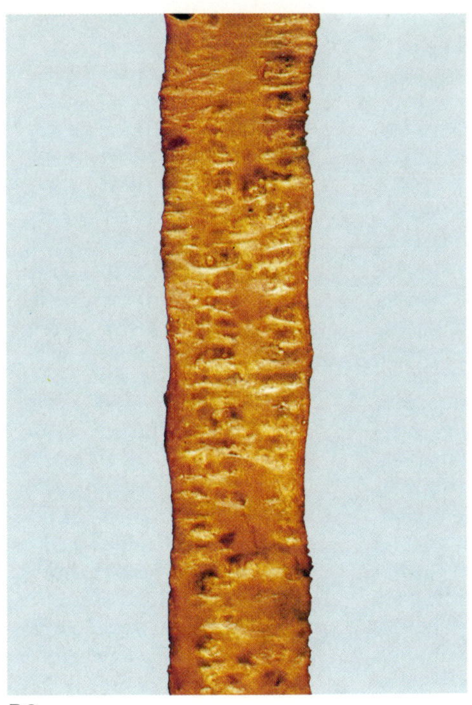

B 9

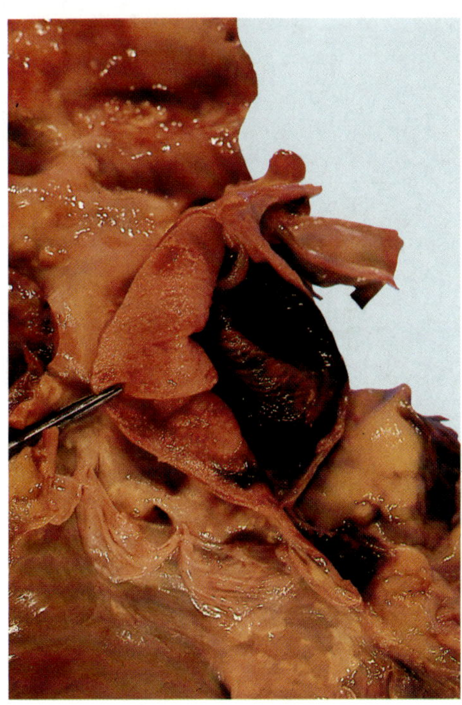

Fig. B 10. Nephrosclerosis. There is severe occlusion by lipid-rich hyaline material of the afferent arteriole leading to a glomerulus. (hematoxylin-Sudan red)

Fig. B 9. Monckeberg's medial calcific sclerosis in a medium sized lower extremity artery. The transverse ridges are reflections of the predominantly circular accumulations of calcifications.

Aneurysms   *(B 11 – B 15)*

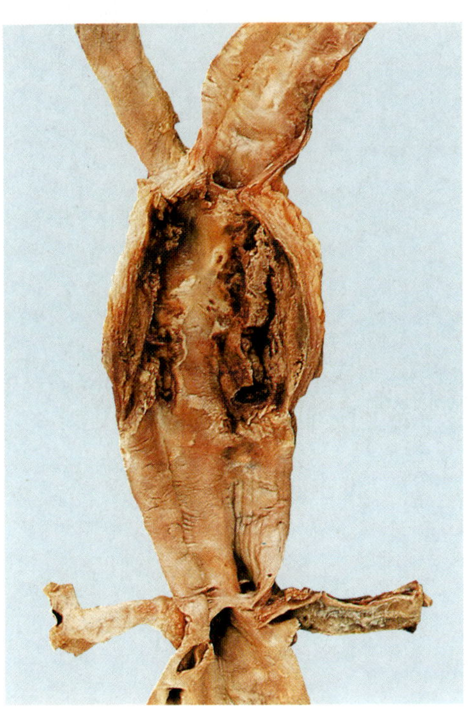

above

Fig. B 11. Large, fusiform aneurysm at the bifurcation of the aorta, with secondary thrombus formation. The iliac arteries are at the upper part of the photograph.

Fig. B 12. Dissecting aneurysm. Clotted blood is seen between the intima and the media. Most cases of dissecting aneurysm occur in the 6–7th decade of life, generally in men. Hypertension is commonly associated.

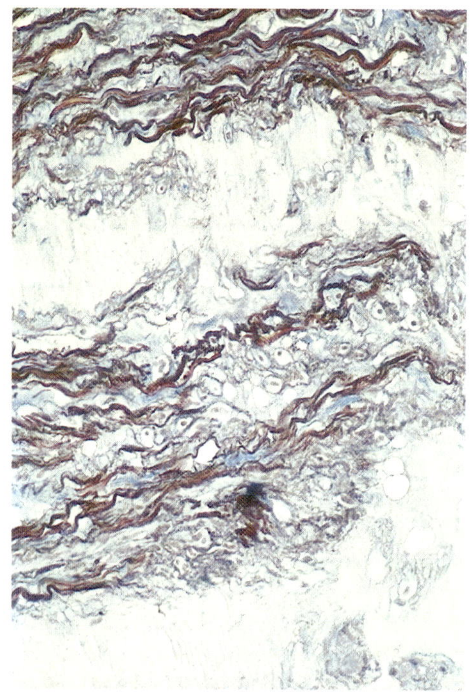

Fig. B 13. So-called "cystic medial necrosis" of Erdheim, with partial destruction of the elastic lamella. The name is misleading since the condition is not cystic, is not always limited to the media, and does not show true necrosis. Instead there is an irregular accumulation of mucopolysaccharides. This condition can be associated with the development of dissecting aneurysm. (elastica, Gallego)

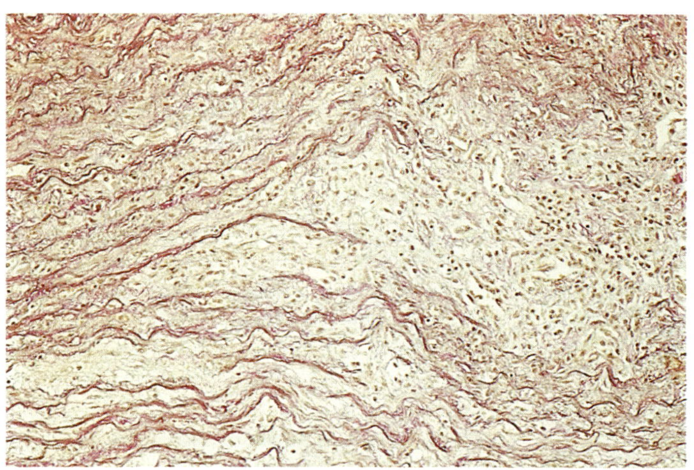

Fig. B 14. Syphilitic aortitis with disruption of the elastic and muscle fibers of the aorta. To the right is perivascular accumulation of lymphocytes and plasma cells.

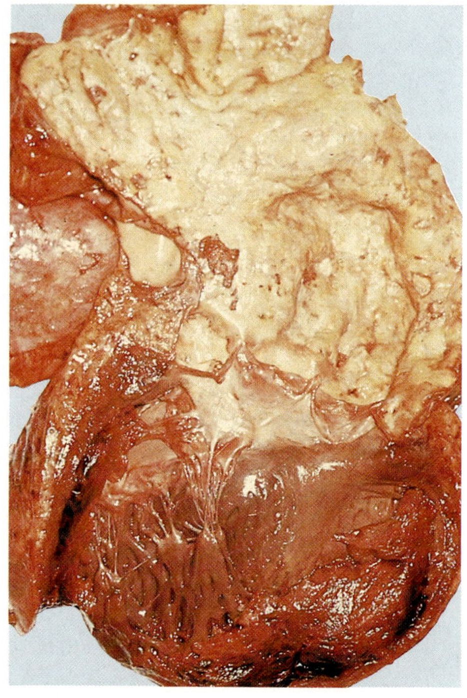

Fig. B 15. Syphilitic aneurysm of the ascending aorta, with superimposed aortic atherosclerosis. Coronary ostia are almost completely obliterated. Note the wrinkled ("tree bark") appearance of the intima. At one time syphilis was the most common cause of aneurysm of the ascending aorta. Now this condition is rare; atherosclerotic aneurysms are most often seen.

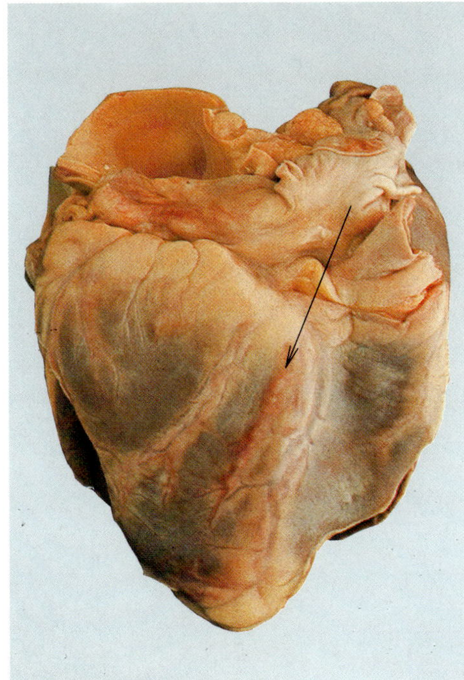

Fig. B 16.   Periarteritis nodosa. Nodular, erythematous nodules are seen along the right coronary artery on the posterior heart *(arrow)*, reflecting the inflammatory changes of the blood vessels in this condition.

Fig. B 17.   Periarteritis nodosa with fibrinoid necrosis (involving the media and intima) and infiltration by lymphocytes, plasma cells, and histiocytes in all layers of the arterial wall.

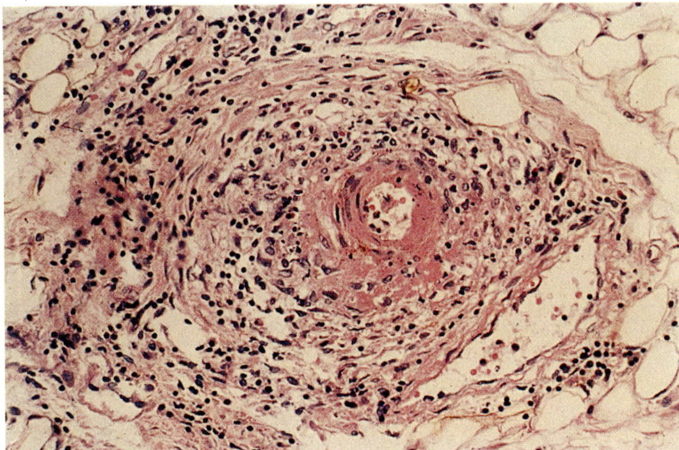

Fig. B 18.   Granulomatous ("temporal") arteritis. The lumen is almost completely obliterated because of the granulomatous inflammatory reaction. Multinucleated giant cells with peripheral nuclei, resembling Langhans cells, are seen, and there is partial destruction of the elastica and marked adventitial fibrosis.

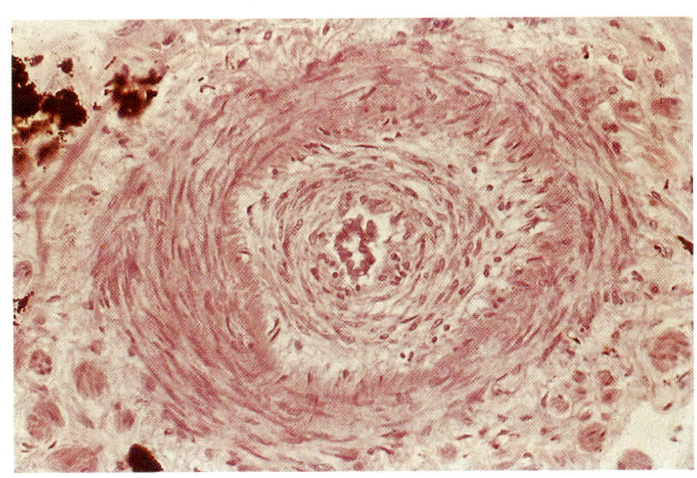

Fig. B 19.   Chronic angiitis obliterans, with fibrous thickening of the intima and media and almost complete occlusion.

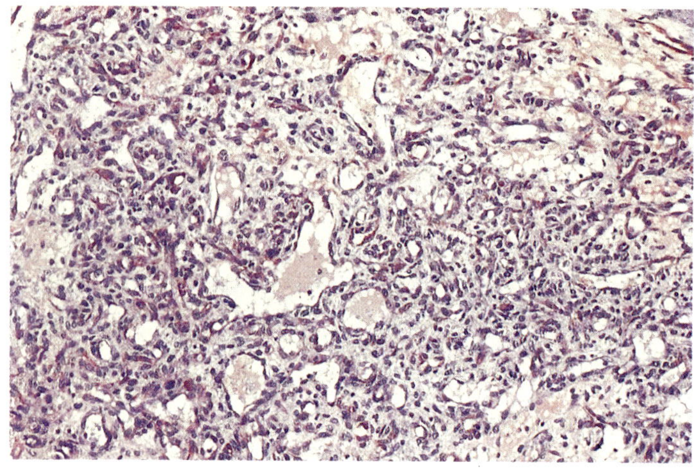

Fig. B20a.   Capillary hemangioma of the skin showing thin-walled, irregular vascular spaces lined by plump endothelial cells. These skin tumors are often present at birth and appear as bright red, granular, "raspberry" lesions.

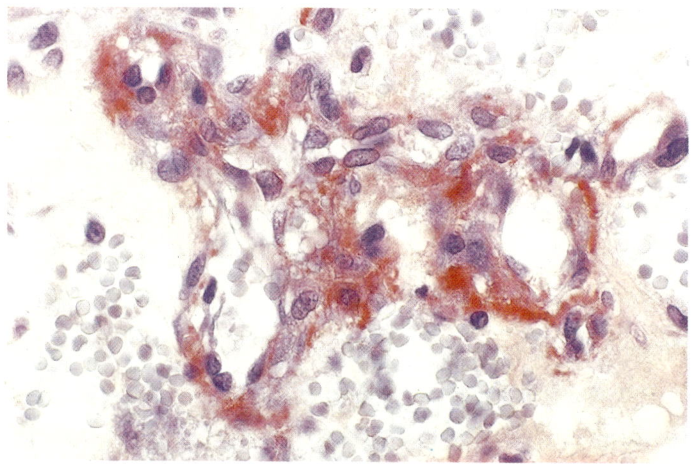

Fig. B20b.   Capillary hemangioma of the skin, stained for the presence of Factor VIII antigen, which is seen as the cytoplasmic red fine granularity.   (peroxidase-antiperoxidase)

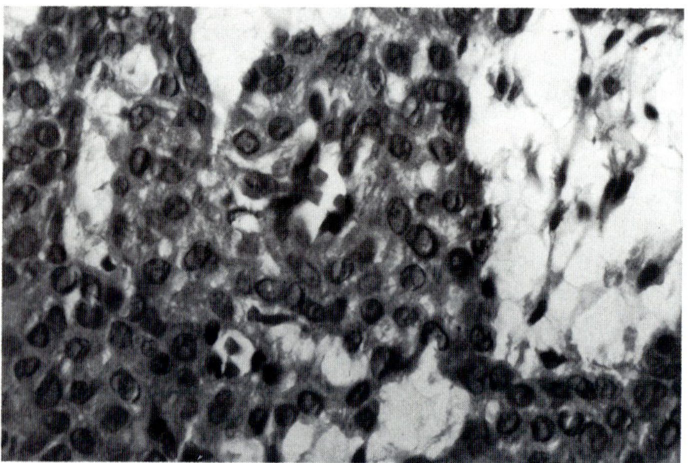

Fig. B21.   Glomus tumor (paraganglioma). The tumor consists of epithelioid glomus cells arranged around capillaries. These tumors can be exquisitely sensitive to touch.

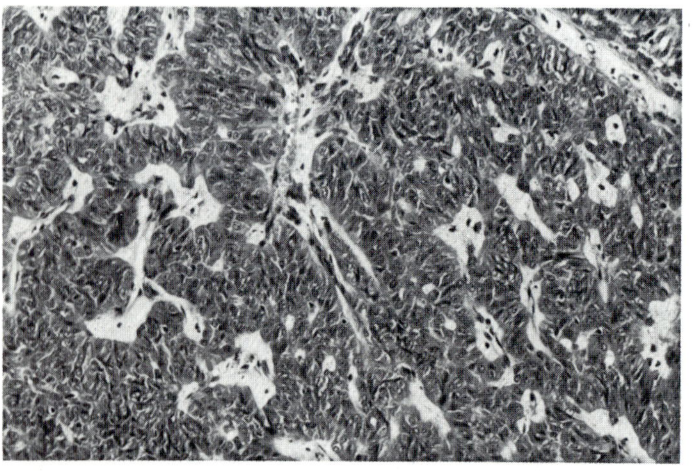

Fig. B22a.   Hemangiopericytoma in subcutaneous tissues. Nests of pericytic cells surround capillaries. These nests tend to be cuboid, cylindrical, or polygonal, with a palisaded arrangement.

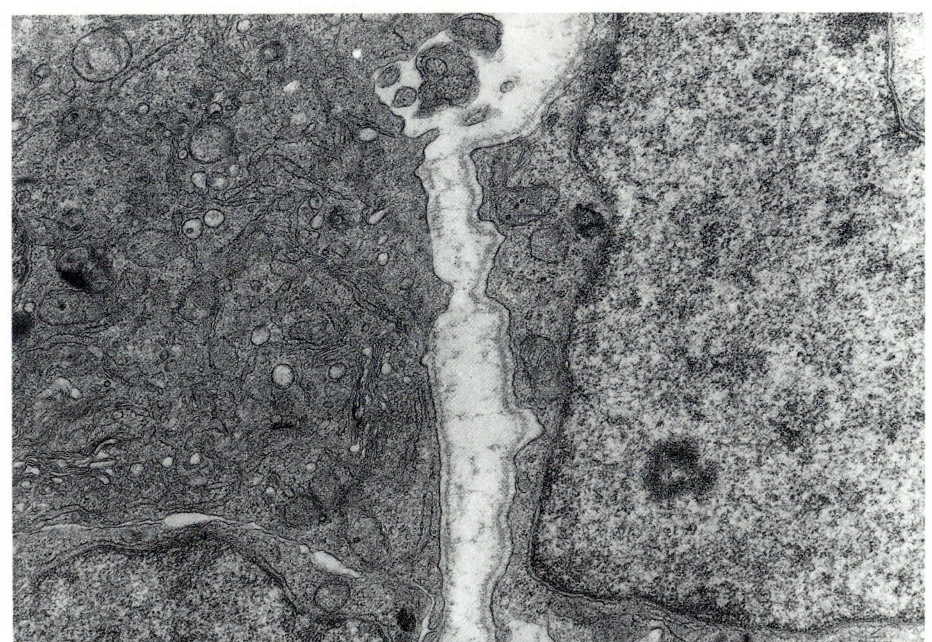

Fig. B22b. Transmission electron micrograph of the hemangiopericytoma showing two adjacent pericytic cells. Basal lamina, seen as a uniform, thin gray line, surrounds each cell. (magnification 7,500×)

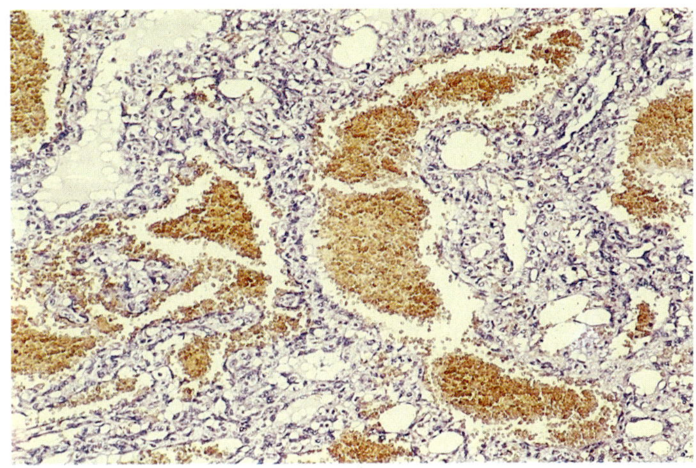

Fig. B23. Angiosarcoma showing disordered growth, with atypical endothelial cells and proliferation of new vessels. Red blood cells fill many of the vascular channels.

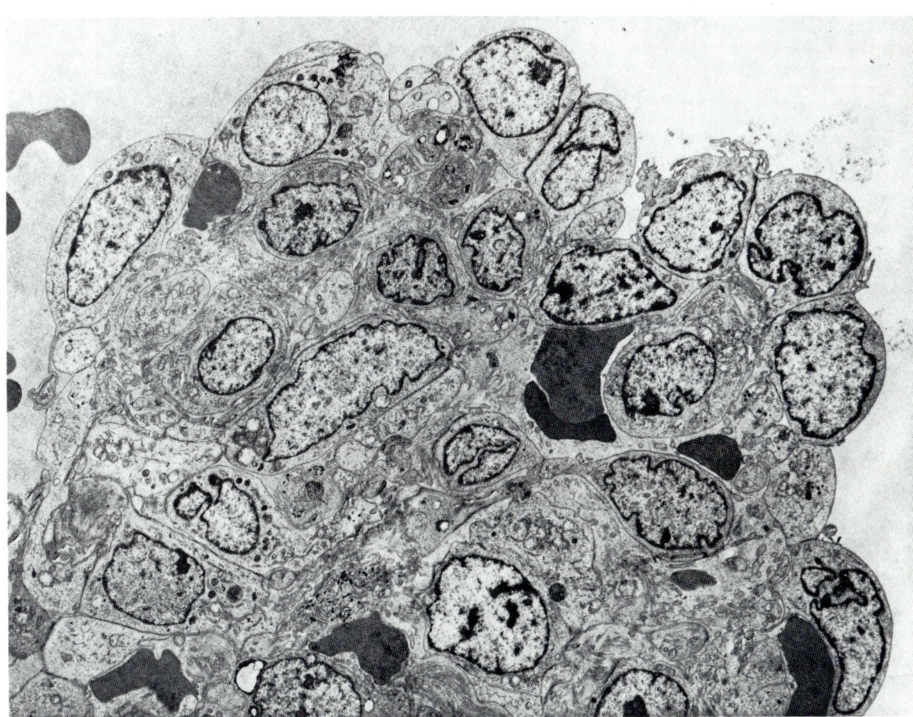

Fig. B24. Transmission electron micrograph of angiosarcoma. Proliferating endothelial cells impart an epithelial appearance, resembling a papillary formation. Red blood cells are seen within poorly formed vascular spaces. (magnification 3,500×)

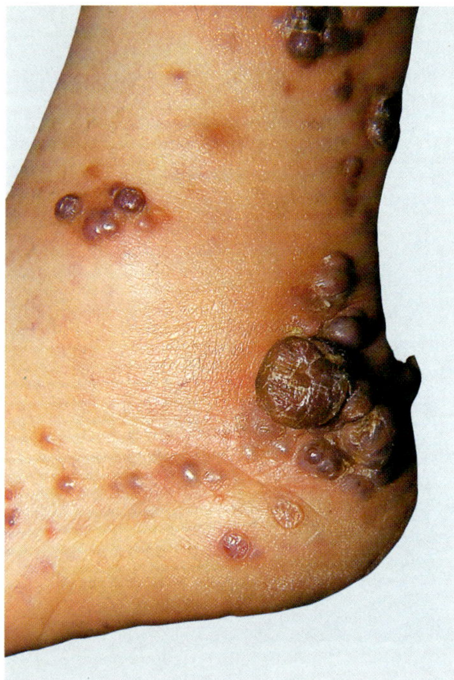 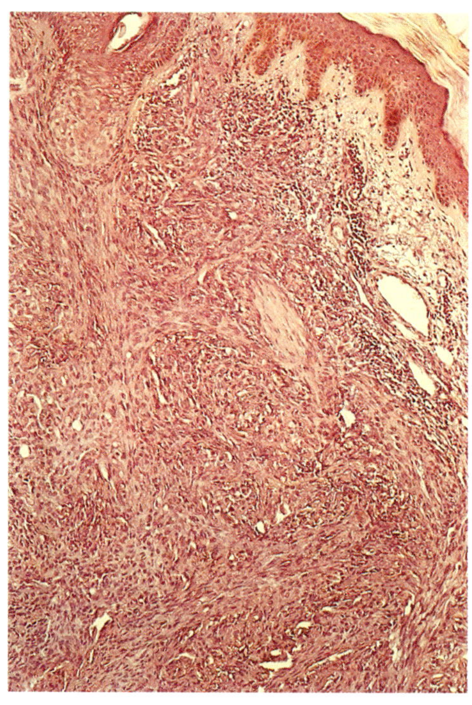

Fig. 25a. Kaposi's sarcoma of the skin, with multiple isolated and confluent tumors, on the foot of a 61-year-old man. This form of Kaposi's sarcoma is not associated with the acquired immune deficiency syndrome (AIDS) and tends to be a relatively indolent malignancy, occurring particularly in elderly men of Mediterranean origin.

Fig. B25b. Kaposi's sarcoma. This is the typical appearance: vascular spaces, a general lack of obvious endothelial cells, and sheets of interlacing spindle cells. Plasma cells and lymphocytes are scattered throughout, and erythrocytes are extravasated among the spindle cells.

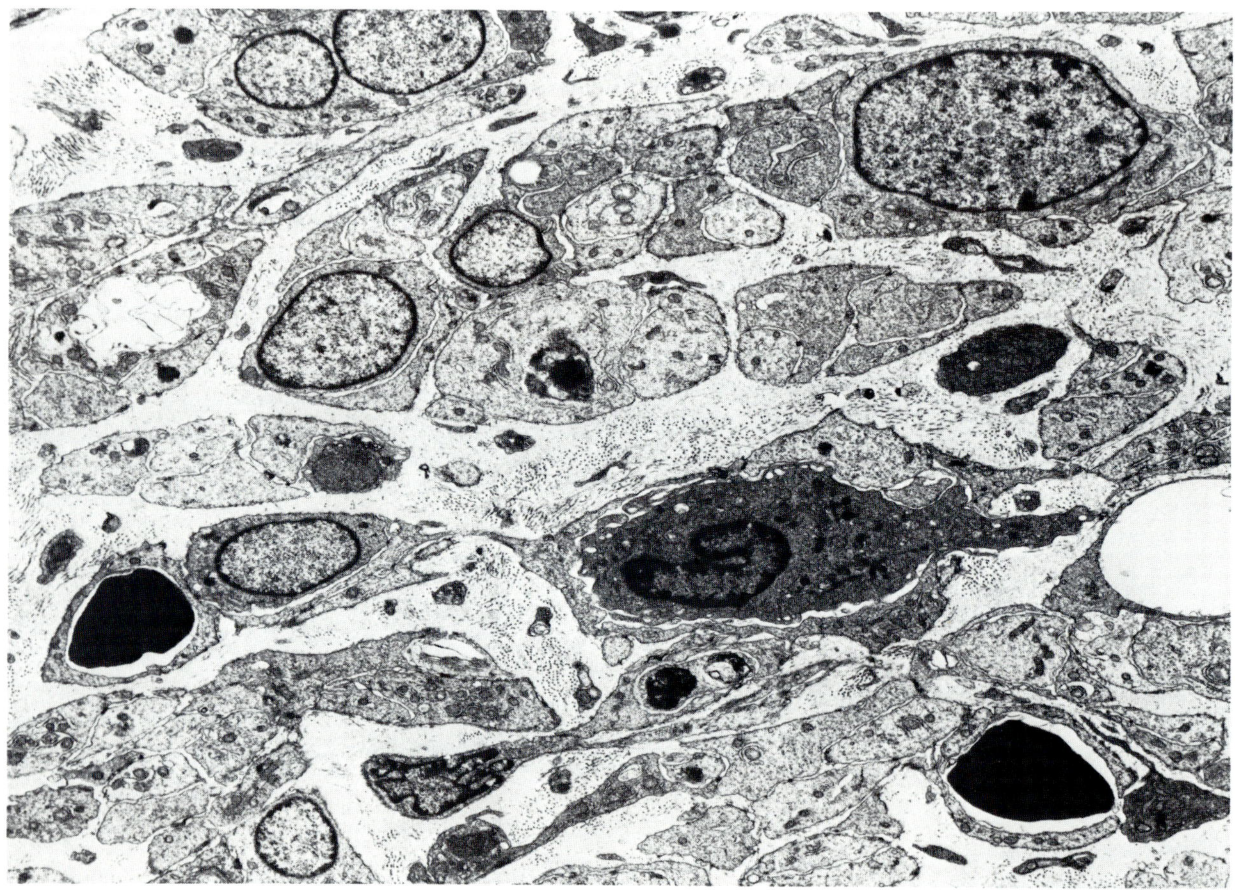

Fig. B25c. Transmission electron micrograph of Kaposi's sarcoma. There is a proliferation of malignant endothelial cells with some epithelial features. The dark cell is a reactive macrophage and there are intracytoplasmic erythrocyte fragments.

C. Blood, Bone Marrow, and Lymphoid Tissues

E. Grundmann

These organs are grouped together. Conditions affecting them fall under the relatively new designation of "hematopathology". This classification allows ready recognition of the fact that disorders of one of these systems might be due to, or might affect, another. The bone marrow is certainly critical to understanding these conditions. It is, of course, the site of most blood cell formation, and can become hyperplastic as a result of the proliferation of one or all of its elements.

A variety of erythropoietic disorders, including almost all of the anemias, can affect the bone marrow. Megaloblastic and iron deficiency anemias can produce characteristic bone marrow changes associated with the consequences of impaired absorption of iron. The various hemolytic anemias are accompanied by increased erythropoiesis and are associated with characteristic changes in the spleen. Marrow hypoplasia is always associated with the diminished formation of blood cells; in many cases, all of the blood forming lines can be involved. Certain cytotoxic drugs can affect white blood cell forming tissues selectively, as can immunologic disorders.

The myeloproliferative disorders are neoplastic proliferations of blood forming cells. One or more cell lines can predominate, and can resemble the usual forms of malignant tumors. This group of disorders includes polycythemia vera, myelofibrosis, and the granulocytic (myelogenous) leukemias.

Illnesses characterized by the increased appearance in the blood of specific immunoglobulins are grouped together as monoclonal gammopathies. These include myeloma, with its various manifestations, and Waldenstrom's macroglobulinemia.

Malignant lymphomas are characterized by autonomous proliferation of the cells of the lymphocyte series. The most common lymphoma is Hodgkin's disease, which has four histologic variants. Classification of the non-Hodgkin's lymphomas remains confusing because of the plethora of established categories. This chapter tends to use the terms most appropriate to each particular illustration, and has not scrupulously followed any single classification system. For practical purposes, the non-Hodgkin's lymphomas can be thought of as proliferations of lymphocytic cells which may have low- or high-grade malignant behavior.

Immunologic disorders are, of course, based in the cells of the lymphoid tissues. Consequently, morphologic changes indicative of these reactions are seen. Correct interpretation of the disorders requires an understanding of the functional organization of the lymph nodes. Lymphadenitis can be specific or nonspecific; pathogenesis is often determined solely on the basis of histological examination.

The spleen is involved in all of the myeloproliferative disorders, as well as in isolated diseases of the red cell series or of the platelets. Tumors originating in the spleen are rare, as are metastases to the spleen.

As a primary organ of the immunologic system, the thymus participates in a large number of illnesses, particularly the autoimmune disorders. Thymomas are usually epithelial in nature, although they can have a significant lymphocytic component. Other tumors of the thymus are rare.

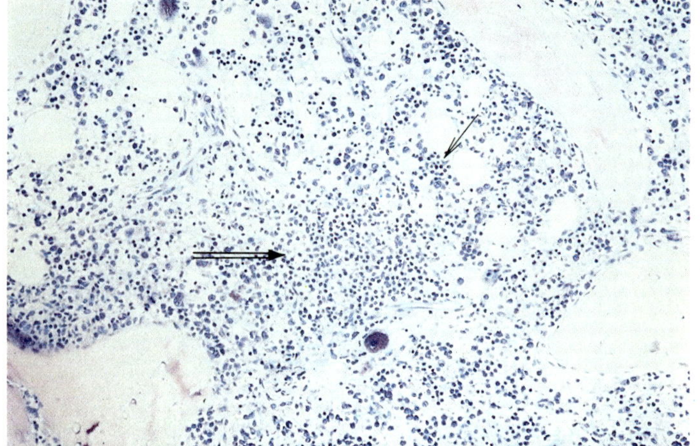

Fig. C1a.   Normal human bone marrow. Islands of hematopoietic cells are between the pale-staining bony trabeculae. Red blood cell precursors (single arrow) are seen as collections of uniform, hyperchromatic cells with indistinct cytoplasm. They are surrounded primarily by granulocyte precursors. The larger cells, with prominent nuclei, are megakaryocytes. Near the center of the photomicrograph (double arrow) is a lymphoid aggregate. The round empty spaces are fat cells.

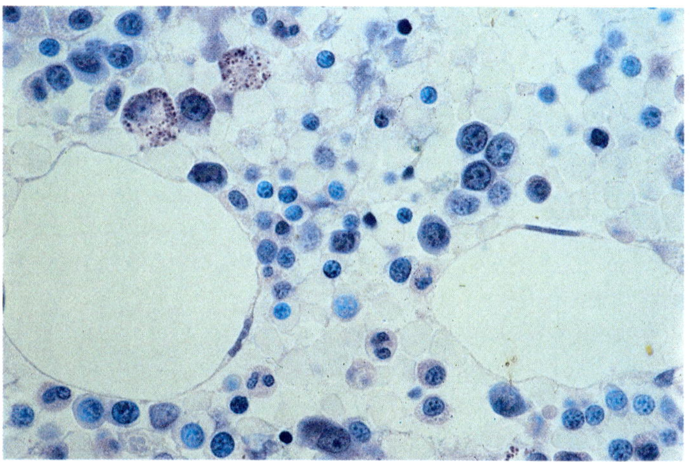

Fig. C1b.   Normal bone marrow at higher magnification. A hematopoietic area is between two fat cells (seen here as optically clear spaces). The four prominent cells with large open nuclei and small nucleoli, to the right of center, are proerythroblasts. The small round cells to the left of center are erythroblasts. The two granular cells at the upper left are granulocyte precursors. Two mature granulocytic cells, with bilobed nuclei, are in the lower portion of the middle of the photographic field. Various other hematopoietic cells are also seen.   (Giemsa)

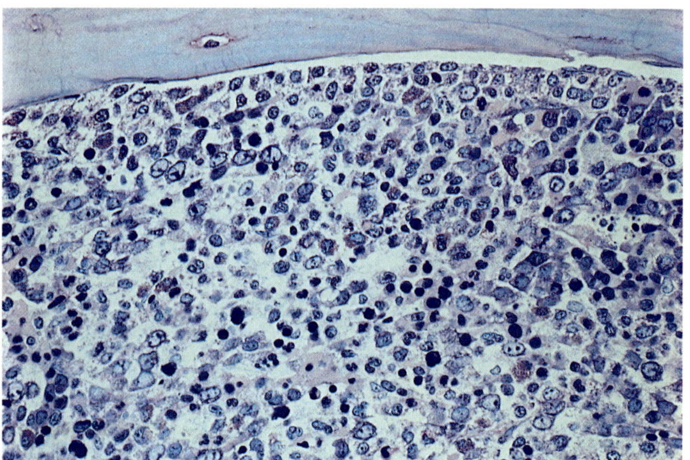

Fig. C2a.   Bone marrow of a patient with megaloblastic anemia. The hyperplastic marrow is almost completely cellular, with no obvious fat; many enlarged ("megaloblastic") and irregular immature cells are obvious. Between the megaloblasts are small, dark, round erythroblasts. Megaloblastic anemia is due to vitamin B_{12} and/or folic acid deficiency, either because of dietary inadequacy or interference with absorption. Many patients display a characteristic triad of manifestations: weakness, sore tongue, and numbness and tingling in the extremities.

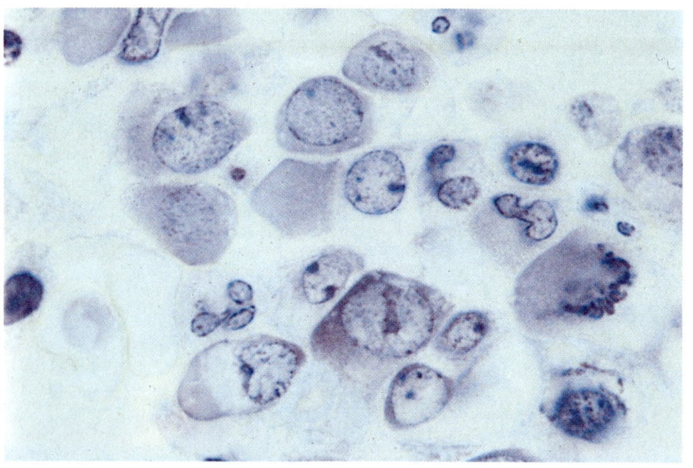

Fig. C2b.   Megaloblastic anemia at higher magnification. The megaloblasts have pale-stained nuclei with finely granular chromatin and moderately enlarged nucleoli. The cytoplasm is pale basophilic. In some of the cells red-violet areas of hemoglobin can be seen. A cell in mitosis is seen to the right. Two segmented granulocytes are to the right of center and a trilobed granulocyte is slightly to the left of center. Hypersegmentation of granulocytes is characteristic of megaloblastic anemia.

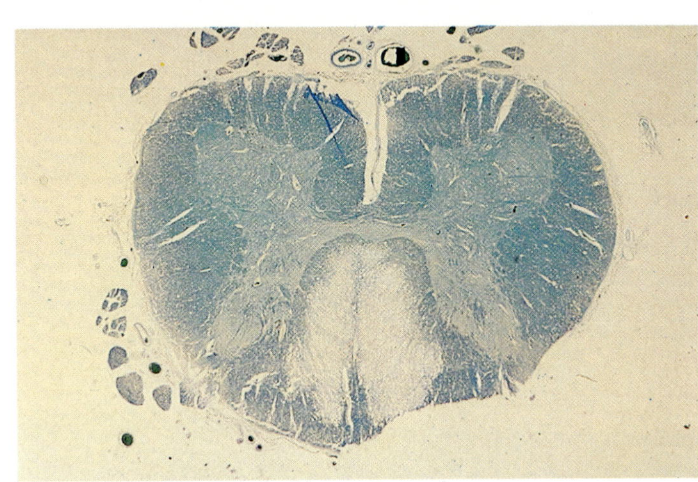

Fig. C3. Degeneration of the posterior column (poorly stained areas) of the spinal cord in a patient with megaloblastic anemia. Lateral columns can also be affected. Histologically, loss of myelin is seen first, followed by loss of oligodendroglia, and eventually of axons. These changes are the morphologic basis of the lower extremity sensory phenomena characteristic of megaloblastic anemias.

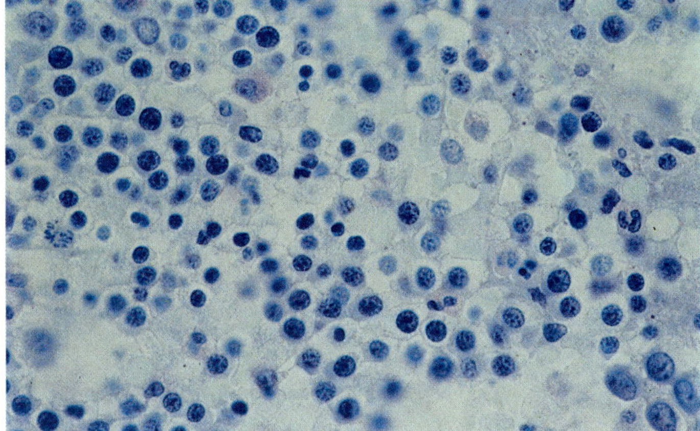

C4

Fig. C4. Marked increase of erythropoietic cells in the bone marrow following anemia due to chronic blood loss. There are clusters of proerythroblasts (lower right) and, particularly prominent, dark, uniform erythroblasts (middle and upper left). (Giemsa)

Fig. C5. Bone marrow in sideroblastic anemia. Sideroblasts are red blood cell precursors containing granules of nonheme iron pigment, seen here with the Prussian blue reaction. A ring sideroblast is near the center. Proerythroblasts are seen, along with somewhat elongated macrophages. Sideroblastic anemias are a heterogeneous group of disorders in which hypochromic, microcytic erythrocytes circulate in the blood.

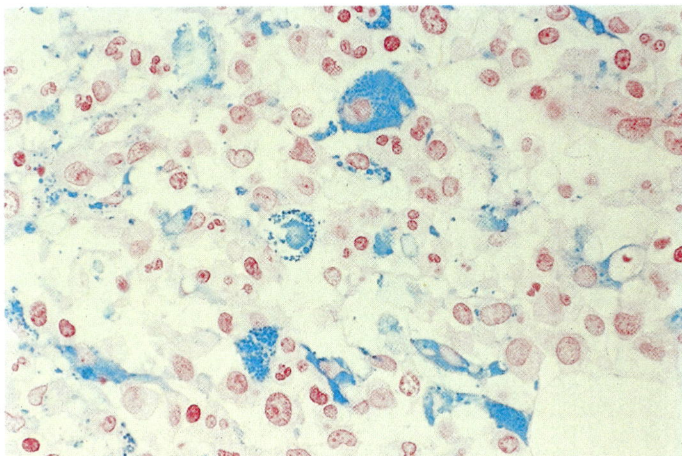

C5

Fig. C6a. Spleen from a patient with spherocytic hemolytic anemia. The cords of Billroth are congested with spheroid erythrocytes (PM). The sinusoids (S), in contrast, are generally empty and characterized, as seen in this photomicrograph, by hyperplasia of endothelial cells.

Fig. C6b. Spleen from a hereditary non-spherocytic hemolytic anemia. In comparison to spherocytosis *(Fig. C6a)* the sinuses contain many erythrocytes, and the cords of Billroth are relatively pale and bloodless.

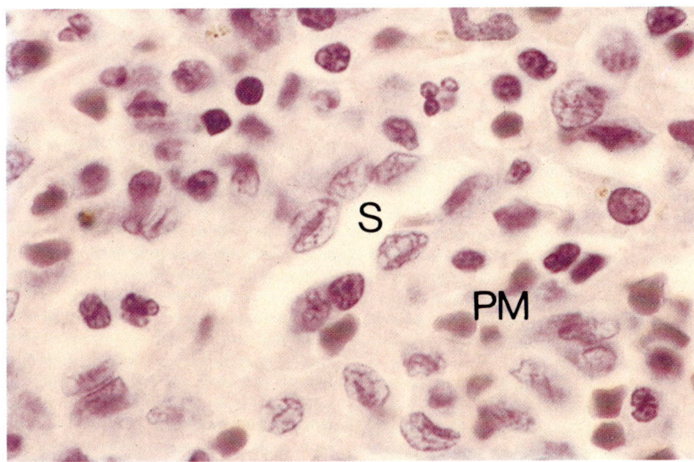

C6a

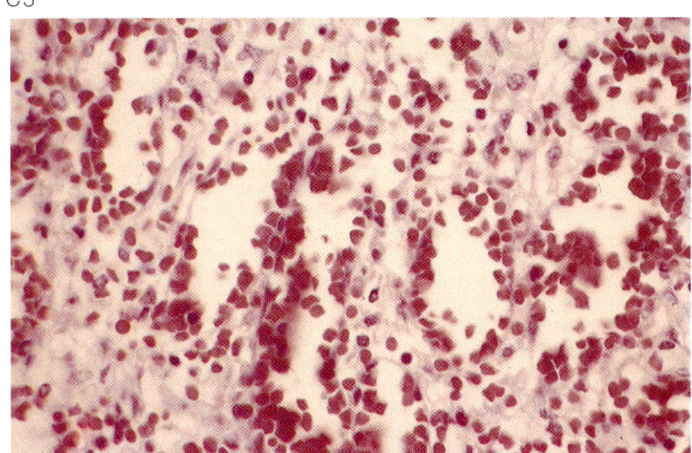

C6b

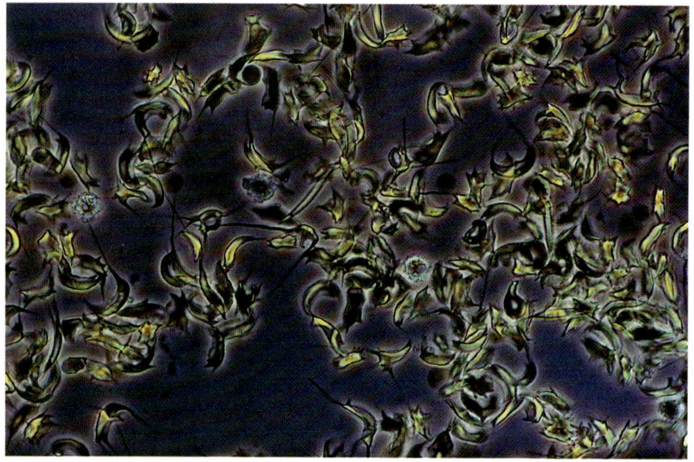

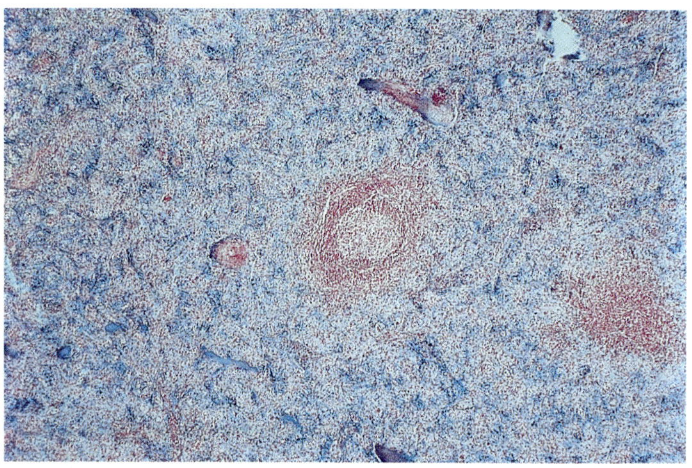

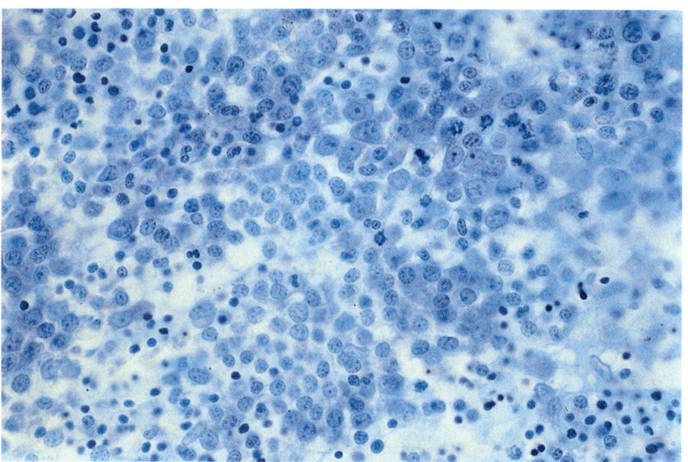

Fig. C 9. Severe bone marrow hyperplasia, consisting almost entirely of red cell precursors, in immune-mediated hemolytic anemia. The marrow consists mostly of proerythroblasts with large nuclei and many mitoses. Clusters of small round erythroblasts are scattered between the sheets of proerythroblasts.   (Giemsa)

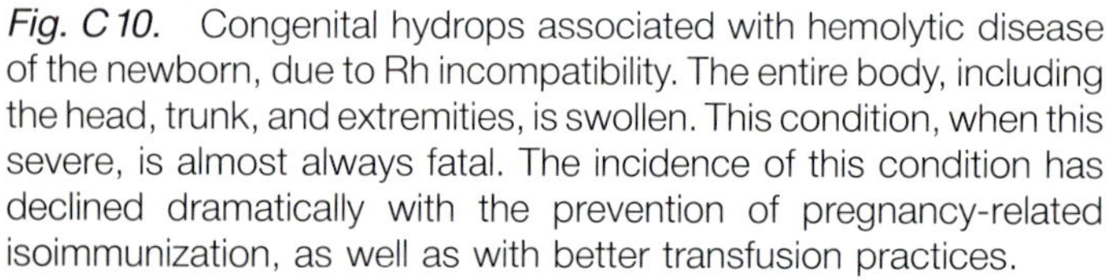

Fig. C 10. Congenital hydrops associated with hemolytic disease of the newborn, due to Rh incompatibility. The entire body, including the head, trunk, and extremities, is swollen. This condition, when this severe, is almost always fatal. The incidence of this condition has declined dramatically with the prevention of pregnancy-related isoimmunization, as well as with better transfusion practices.

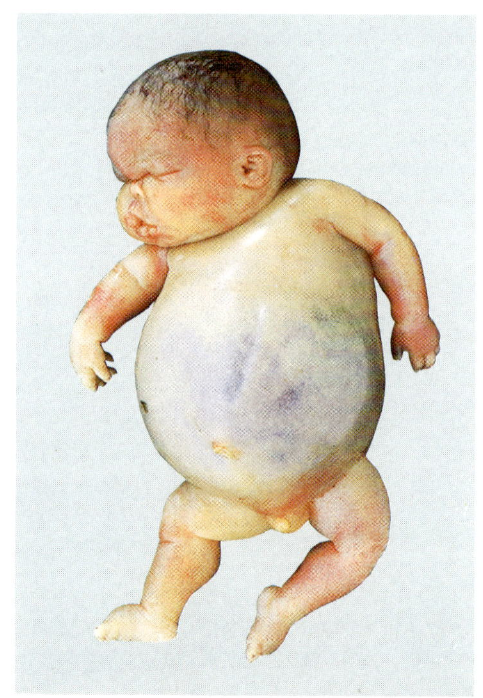

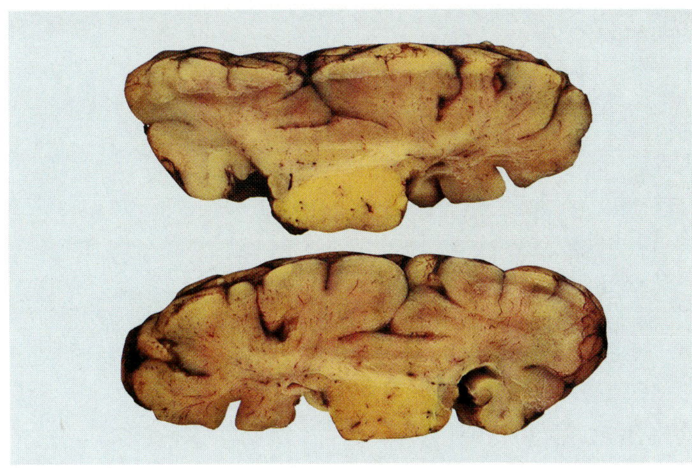

Fig. C 11.   Liver in hemolytic disease of the newborn. The hepatic sinusoids are filled with erythroblasts and proerythroblasts. The hepatocytes contain gold-brown hemosiderin and greenish bilirubin. Both pigments accumulate with the breakdown of hemoglobin. A few hepatocytes contain small fat vacuoles because of hypoxia. (hematoxylin-eosin)

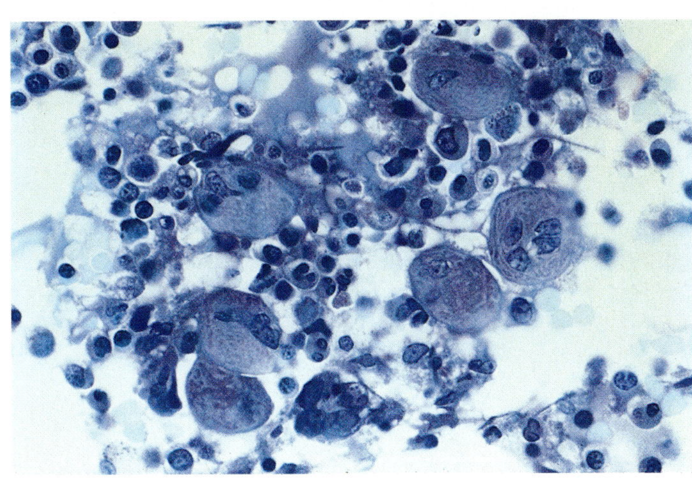

Fig. C 12.   Kernicterus, from an infant with hemolytic disease of the newborn. Abnormally high concentrations of lipid-soluble, unconjugated bile pigments have collected in the globus pallidus, subthalamic nucleus, hippocampus, and dentate and inferior olivary nuclei. In severe cases the cerebral and cerebellar cortices can be affected.

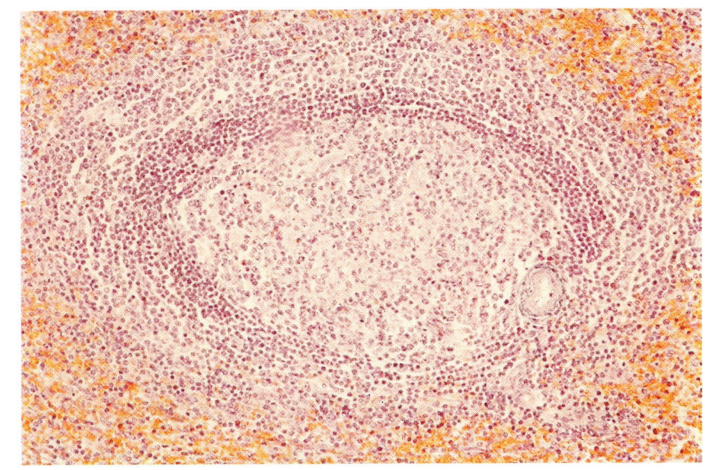

Fig. C 13.   Bone marrow in idiopathic thrombocytopenia purpura (ITP). There are increased numbers of megakaryocytes, easily seen among the other marrow cells. Normally there is only one megakaryocyte per high magnification field *(see Fig. C 1 a).*   (Giemsa)

Fig. C 14.   Spleen in ITP. The lymphoid follicle of the white pulp is greatly enlarged, with a markedly hyperplastic germinal center and a relatively narrow rim of mature lymphocytes. The lumen of the follicle artery is to the right of the germinal center.   (hematoxylin-eosin)

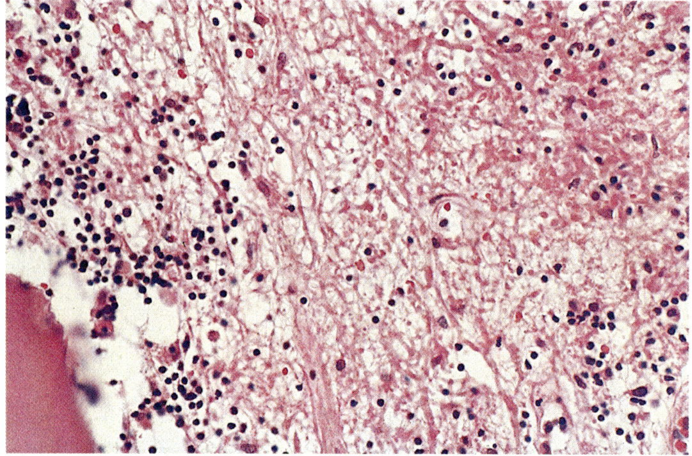

Fig. C 15. Acute marrow depression ("myelophthisis") following therapy with a folic acid antagonist, aminopterin. A bone trabeculum is at the lower left and there are a few remaining hematopoietic cells at the left and right sides of the photomicrograph. Most of the marrow has been replaced by fibrin which appears as eosinophilic fibrillary material.   (hematoxylin-eosin)

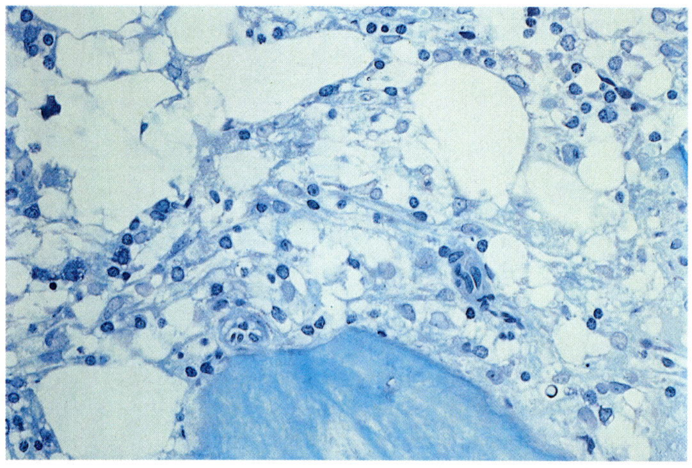

Fig. C 16. Acute marrow depression following radiation. There is marked reduction of the usual hematopoietic elements and beginning replacement by fibrosis.   (Giemsa)

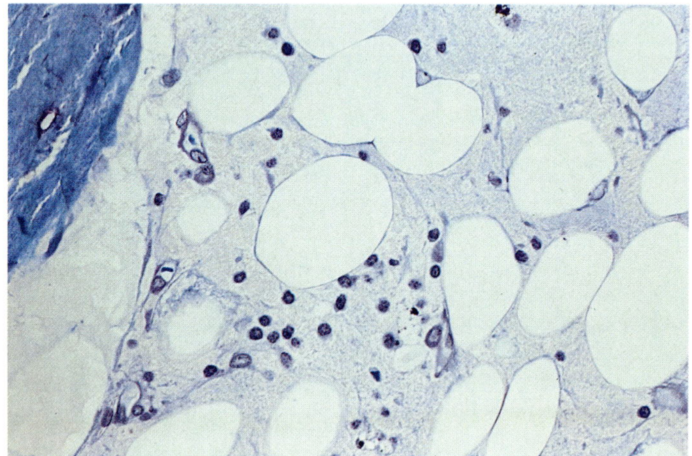

Fig. C 17. Marrow atrophy following chemotherapy with an antineoplastic agent. The hematopoietic cells are almost completely absent and there are a few, mostly scattered, lymphocytes. The fat is separated by pale basophilic mucinous ("gelatinous") material. (Giemsa)

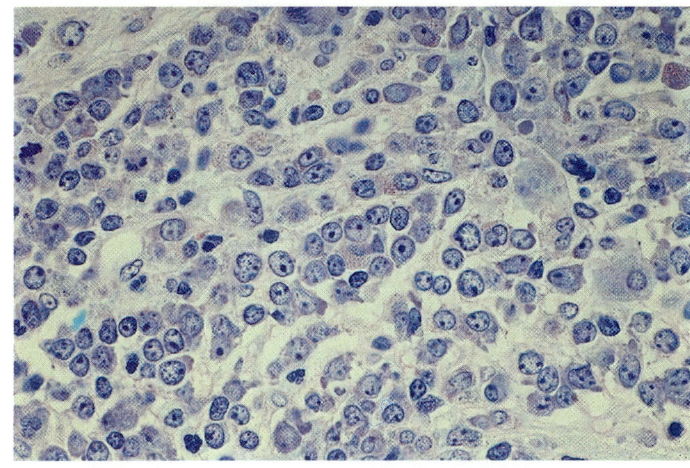

Fig. C 18.   Increased numbers of granulocytic precursors as a reaction to a preceding agranulocytosis. The marrow is filled with promyelocytes, the granules of which stain intensely red with the chloroacetate-esterase reaction.

Fig. C 19.   The acute ("blastic") phase of chronic myelogenous (granulocytic) leukemia. The marrow is filled with atypical myeloblasts. Between the blasts are a few red blood cell precursors, with vesicular round nuclei; these are most obvious at the lower left. (Giemsa)

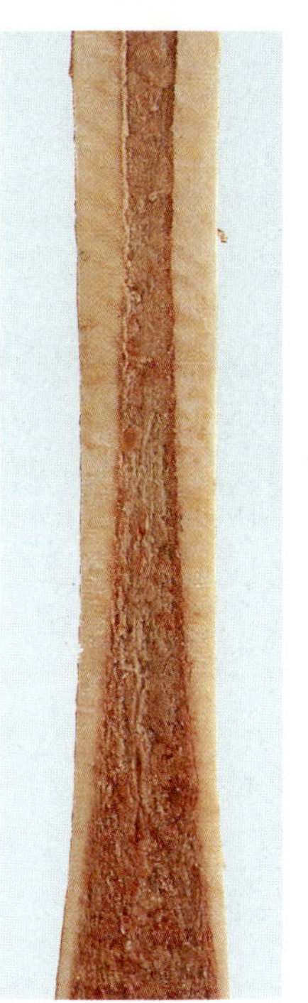

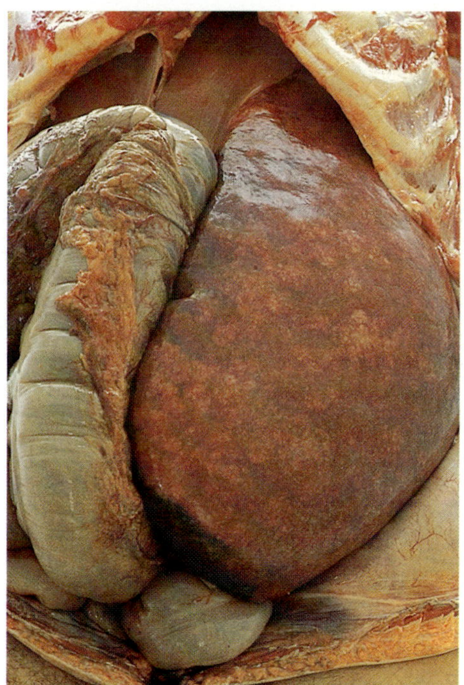

Fig. C20.   Bone marrow in chronic myelogenous leukemia. In normal adults the marrow of the long bones is yellow, consisting mostly of fat, with relatively few hematopoietic cells. In this form of leukemia, however, the marrow is usually packed with cells and appears homogeneous red-brown.

Fig. C21.   Massive splenomegaly in chronic myelogenous leukemia. The ribs are seen above. The spleen fills the entire left side of the abdomen, pushing the descending colon to the right side of the abdomen. The spleen in this case weighed 4,200 gm (normal = 150 gm).

C20   C21

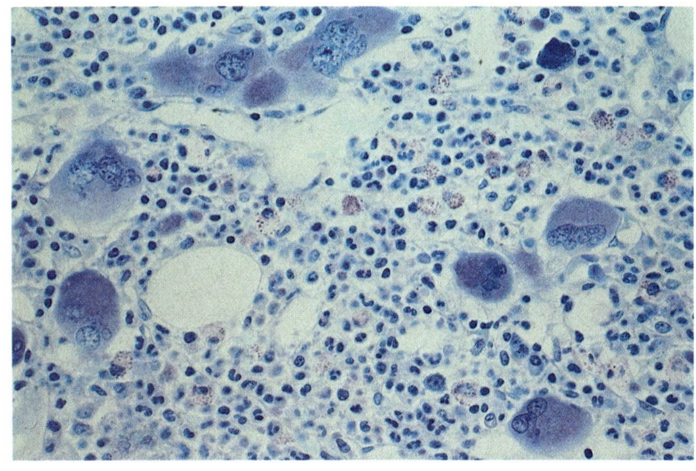

Fig. C22. Myeloproliferative disorder. The marrow is markedly hypercellular, with increased numbers of megakaryocytes, some atypical, which cluster together. In addition, the erythroid and granulocytic elements are also increased ("panmyelosis"). (Giemsa)

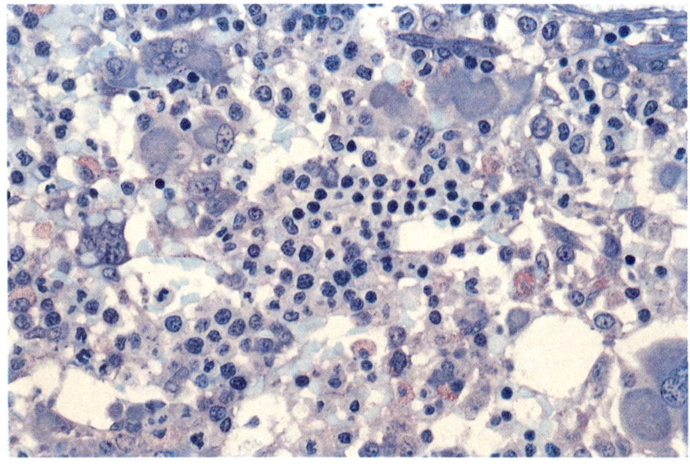

Fig. C23. Polycythemia vera. The marrow is almost completely cellular. The number of erythroid precursors is increased; they are most easily seen as a large erythropoietic aggregate in the center of the photomicrograph. There is also a general panmyelosis, with increased numbers of megakaryocytes and granulocyte precursors. (Giemsa)

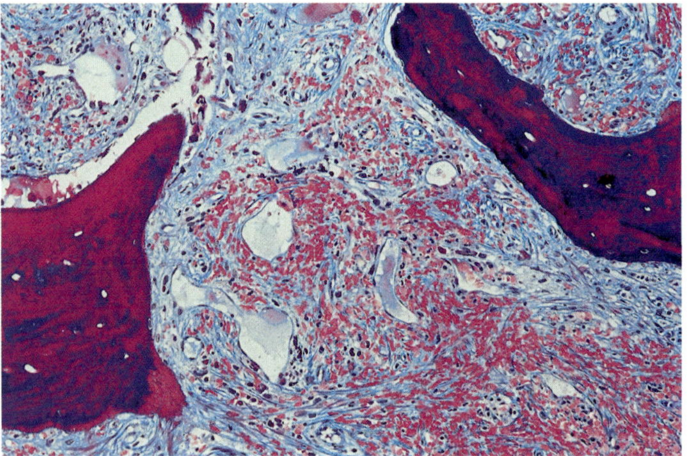

Fig. C24a. Myelofibrosis. Most of the marrow space is replaced by collagen fibers, which appear blue in this connective tissue stain, and there is a proliferation of capillaries and fibroblasts. Only a few remnants of hematopoietic activity remain. Nonmineralized bone trabeculae can be seen, as red-stained osteoid matrix, at both sides of the photographic field. This is evidence of the reactive bone growth and progression to osteosclerosis. (Ladewig)

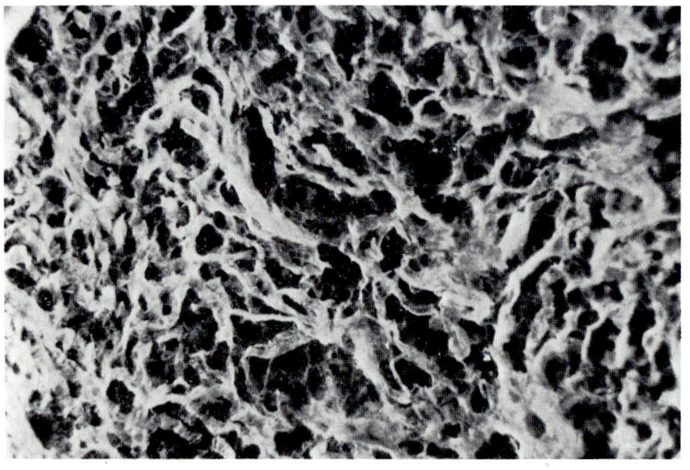

Fig. C24b. Osteosclerosis. This photomicrograph shows immunohistochemical demonstration of type I collagen. The honeycomb pattern is typical.

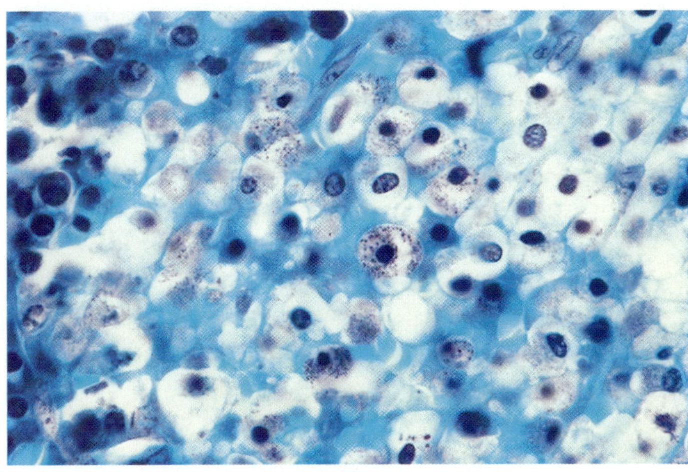

Fig. C25a. Systemic mastocytosis. The marrow is infiltrated by atypical mast cells. The cells are characterized by small, uniform, hyperchromatic nuclei, with ample, almost optically clear cytoplasm containing typical mast cell granules. The clinical course of patients with this condition might resemble leukemia.
(toluidine blue, pH 5.8)

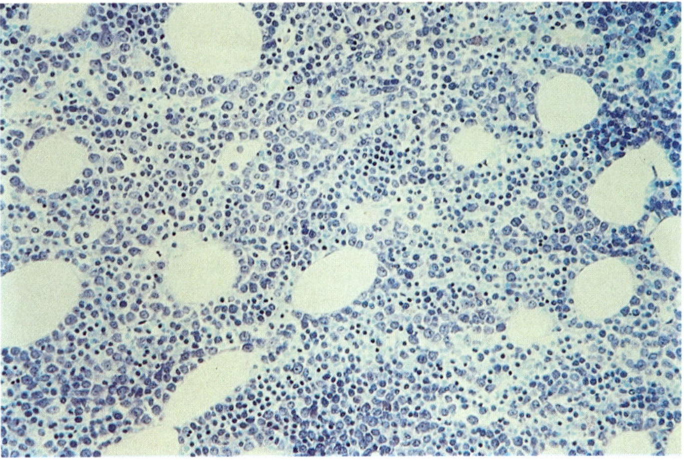

Fig. C25b. Systemic mastocytosis. The mast cells, seen here infiltrating a lymph node, stain brilliant red with the chloroacetate-esterase reaction. Systemic mastocytosis can be associated with flushing, urticaria, edema, pruritus, headache, tachycardia, and hypotension, presumably related to the release of histamine by the proliferating mast cells.

Fig. C26. Acute erythroleukemia. Most of the bone marrow is replaced by erythroid precursors at varying degrees of maturity. Mature erythroblasts are seen as nests of uniform, small, dark stained cells. The larger immature erythropoietic cells have large, pale nuclei with small distinct nucleoli and are seen as irregular sheets. The amount of marrow fat is reduced slightly.   (Giemsa)

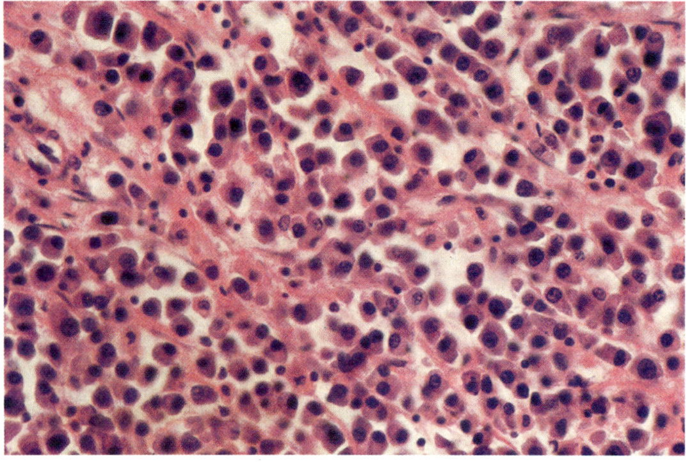

Fig. C27.   Myeloma. The marrow is largely replaced by abnormal plasma cells. These are characterized by relatively large, eccentrically placed nuclei, with a paranuclear clear ("Hof") zone. The clear zone represents the Golgi substance.   (hematoxylin-eosin)

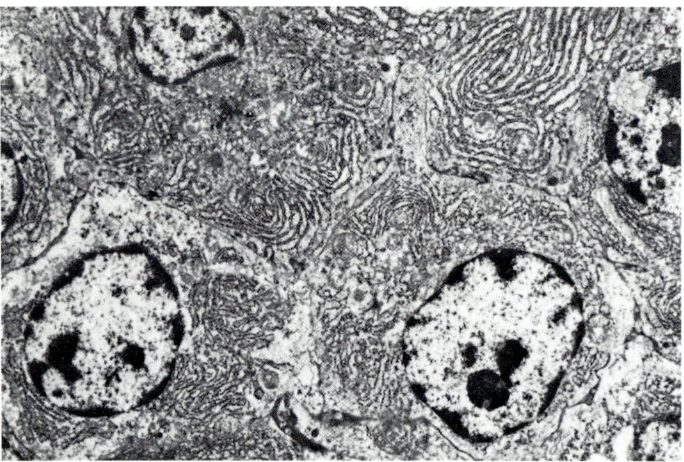

Fig. C28.   Ultrastructure of a myeloma cell. The cytoplasm is filled with parallel stacks of endoplasmic reticulum. The nucleus has peripherally distributed chromatin and distinct nucleoli.

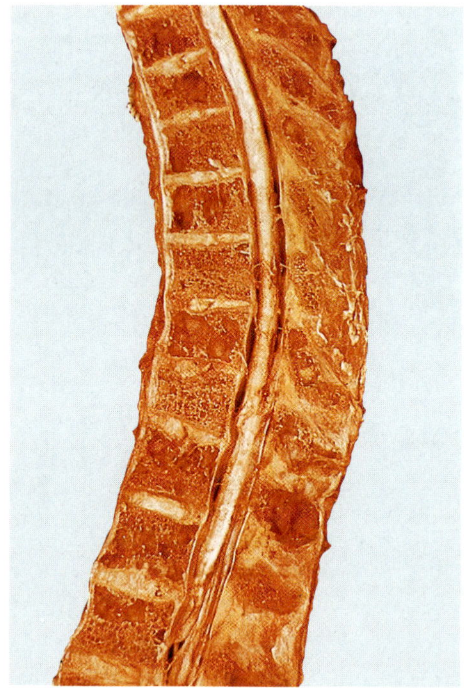

Fig. C29.   Hemisection of the vertebral column from a patient with myelomatosis. The vertebral bodies are to the left of the spinal cord, and the spinous processes to the right. The normal appearance of the bone is best seen in the 4th vertebral body from the bottom and, to a lesser extent, the 6th. The other bodies show varying degrees of bone replacement by a soft infiltrate. This condition is typically multifocal and is associated with dysproteinemias.

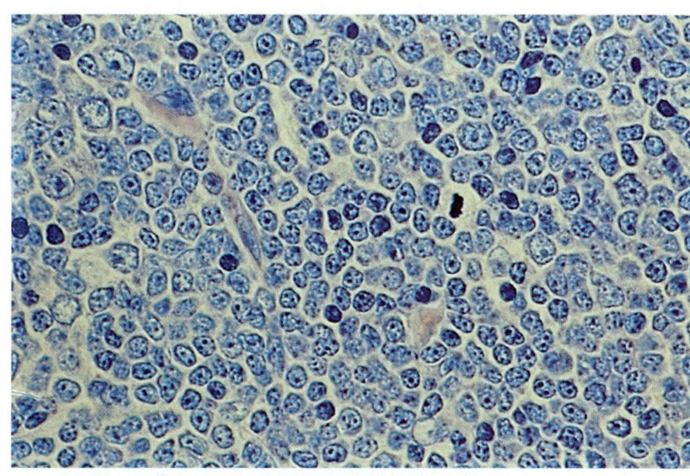

Fig. C30.   Chronic lymphocytic leukemia completely replacing the bone marrow. There is marked proliferation of small atypical lymphocytes and lymphoblasts, many with mitoses. This form of leukemia usually affects elderly people and can have a relatively benign course for many years.   (Giemsa)

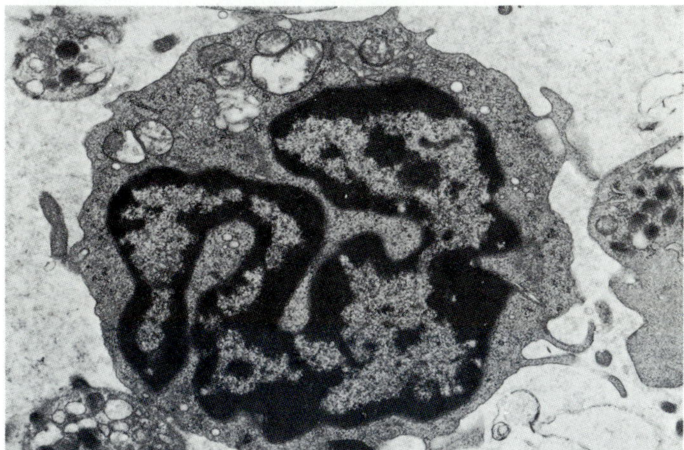

Fig. C31.   Typical Sezary cell. This cell, characterized by a convoluted nucleus with peripherally distributed chromatin, is an abnormal T-lymphocyte, and is seen in Sezary's syndrome and mycosis fungoides.

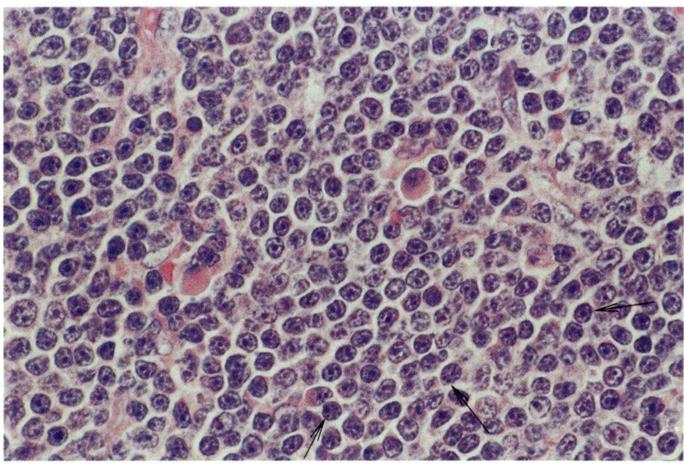

Fig. C32.   Well-differentiated lymphocytic lymphoma, diffuse type, with many plasma cells (lymphoplasmacytoid immunocytoma) in a lymph node with mature plasma cells (arrows) as well as some lymphoblastic cells with large nuclei. Two large cells with ample pink cytoplasm are present; these most likely contain immunoglobulin. Patients with this form of lymphoma might have a monoclonal macroglobulinemia.   (hematoxylin-eosin)

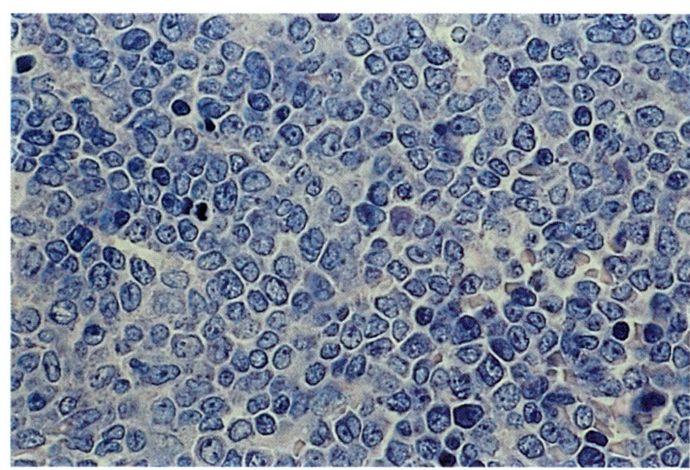

Fig. C33.   Malignant lymphoma, poorly differentiated, lymphocytic (small cleaved cell lymphoma). The entire lymph node is infiltrated uniformly by small-to medium-sized lymphoid cells with indented ("cleaved") nuclei and peripherally located nucleoli. This is one of the most common of the types of non-Hodgkin's lymphoma.   (Giemsa)

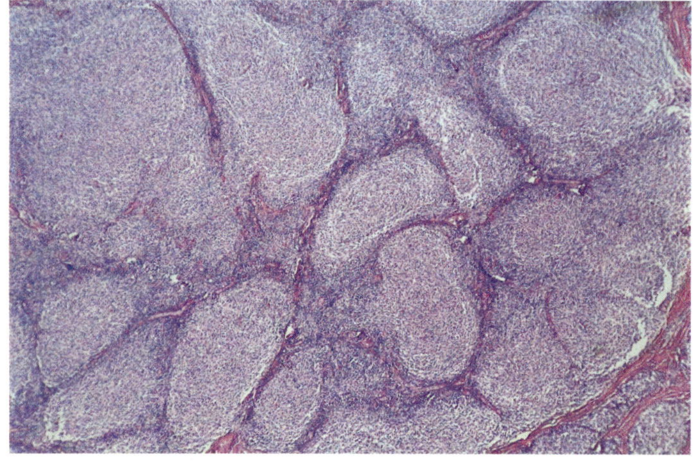

Fig. C34. Malignant lymphoma, nodular, mixed small (cleaved) cell and large lymphoid cell (mixed lymphocytic-"histiocytic" lymphoma, nodular). The usual lymph node architecture is replaced by follicle-like collections of lymphoma cells. Patients whose lymphomas display a nodular pattern tend to have a better prognosis than those presenting with a diffuse pattern.

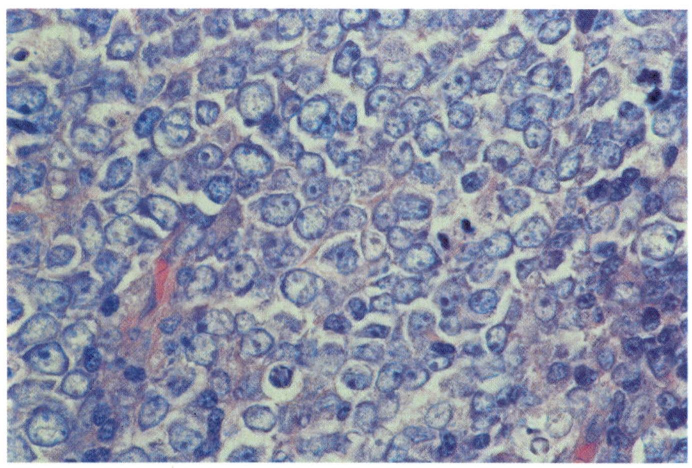

Fig. C35. Lymphoblastic lymphoma. This is an unsatisfactory name, since the cells do not display all the features characteristic of blasts. These relatively large cells have vesicular nuclei with fine chromatin as well as generally peripheral nucleoli. Mitoses can be abundant. This tumor affects adolescents primarily. In a high percentage of cases, it arises in the thymus and has a leukemia component. This is a T-cell lymphoma.   (Giemsa)

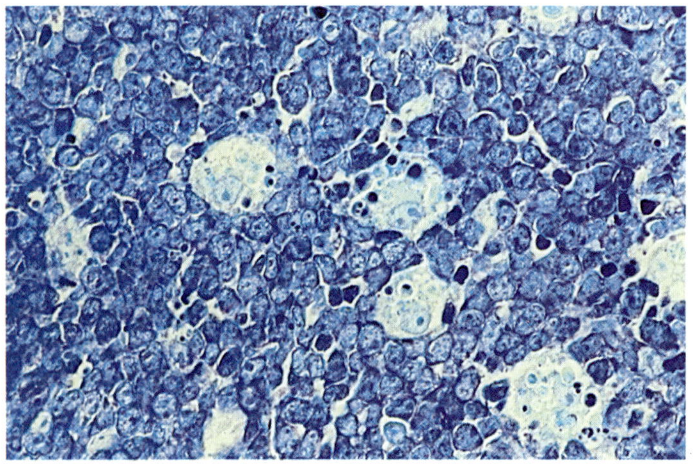

Fig. C36. Burkitt's lymphoma. In this lymphoma there are cohesive, tightly packed lymphoblastic cells with deeply basophilic cytoplasm and multiple nucleoli. Large, benign macrophages containing digested debris are scattered throughout, imparting a "starry sky" appearance. This type of lymphoma occurs most often in African children and affects the facial structures, such as the bones of the jaw and the orbit.   (Giemsa)

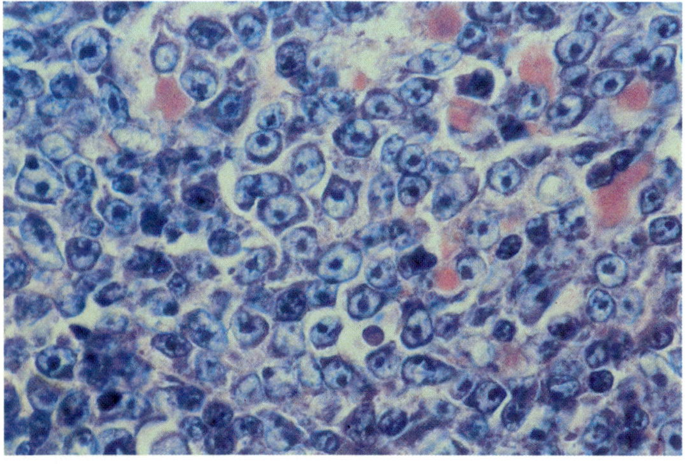

Fig. C37. Immunoblastic sarcoma (malignant lymphoma, "histiocytic", diffuse). The tumor cells have a deeply basophilic cytoplasm, and relatively clear nuclei with large, distinct, central nucleoli. These tumors may be either B- or T-cell derived, whereas most other adult lymphomas are B-cell derived.   (Giemsa)

Fig. C38. Angioimmunoblastic lymphadenopathy. The normal lymph node structure is effaced by a heterogeneous population of lymphocytes, immunoblasts, plasma cells, and epithelioid histiocytes, irregularly separated, as seen in this photomicrograph, by branching twig-like venules. This entity can present with fever, night sweats, weight loss, and skin rash, in addition to lymphadenopathy and splenomegaly, and can be associated with a polyclonal hypergammaglobulinemia and a hemolytic anemia.   (Giemsa)

Fig. C39. Ultrastructure of cells of hairy cell leukemia. The nucleus of the typical cell has a distinct nucleolus. A characteristic cytoplasmic inclusion, the ribosomal-lamellar complex, is seen in cross section at the upper left of the electron micrograph. The cellular origin of this disorder has not been elucidated completely. The onset is insidious, with massive splenomegaly often seen.

Fig. C40. Extensive increase of reticulin fibers in the bone marrow infiltrated by hairy cell leukemia. Pancytopenia is frequently associated and a "dry tap" or hypocellular specimen is obtained on bone marrow aspiration.   (Gomori's)

Fig. C41. Spleen infiltrated by hairy cell leukemia. Typically the cords of Billroth are infiltrated, rather than the sinuses. Despite the presence of splenic involvement, the prognosis is relatively good and some patients do quite well after splenectomy only. The course is often poor after chemotherapy.

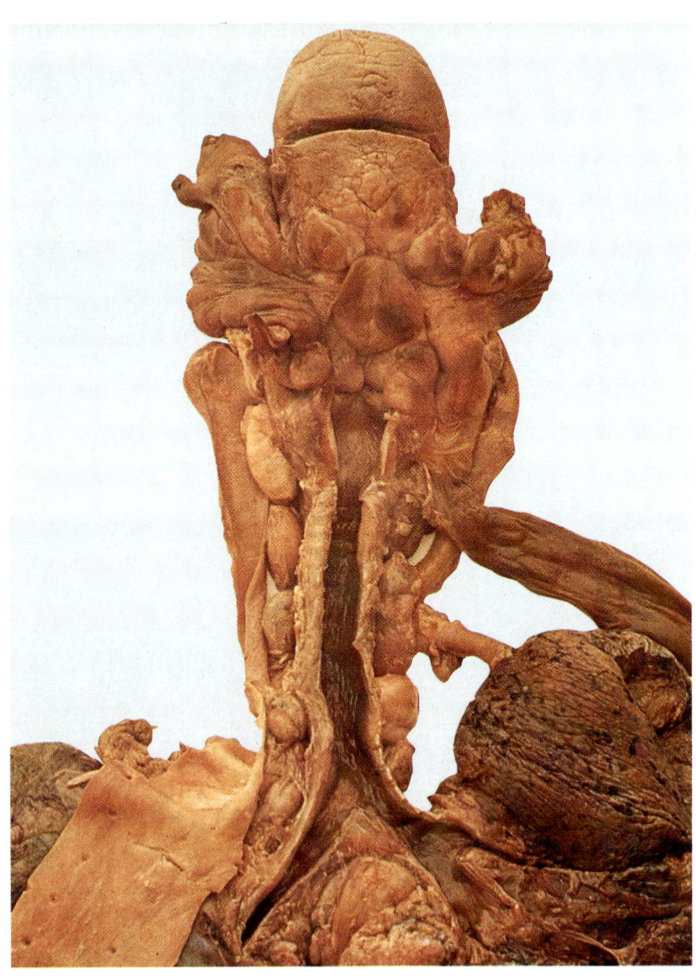

Fig. C42. Hodgkin's disease, with massive involvement of the lymphoid structures of the neck. Large lymph nodes are obvious at both sides and at the bifurcation of the trachea. Typically, in Hodgkin's disease, in contrast to the non-Hodgkin's lymphomas, the nodes tend to remain discrete.

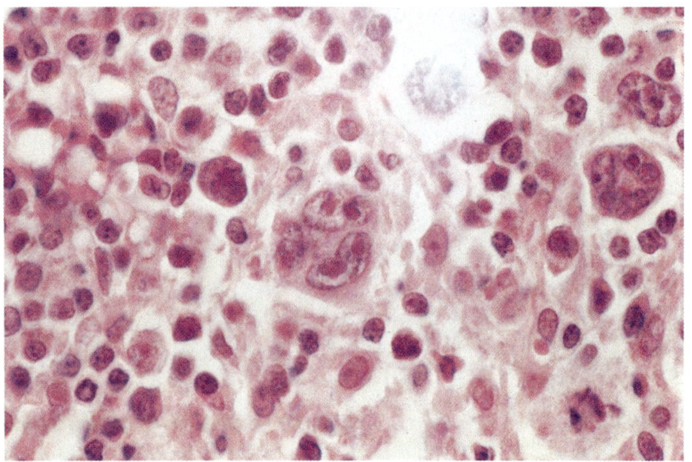

Fig. C43. Hodgkin's disease, mixed cellular type. A characteristic Reed-Sternberg cell is seen in the midfield. This large cell typically has a bilobed nucleus with a distinct chromatin border and prominent, amphophilic nucleoli. To the right are other, less typical Reed-Sternberg cells. Between these cells is the usual heterogeneous population of lymphocytes, plasma cells, histiocytic cells, and eosinophils.   (hematoxylin-eosin)

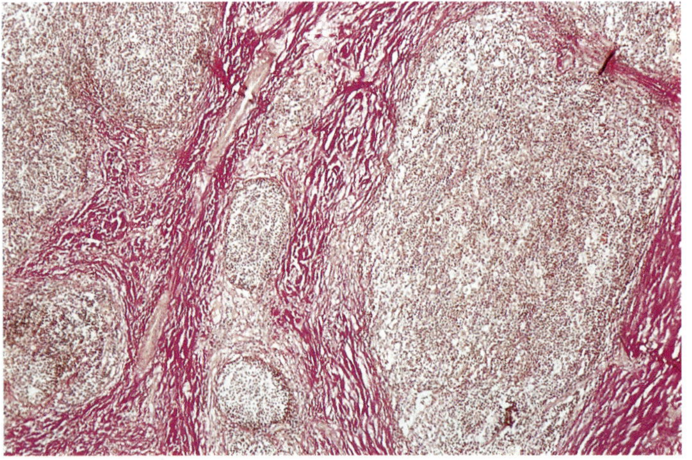

Fig. C44. Hodgkin's disease, nodular sclerosis type. Broad bands of collagen, stained red in this connective tissue preparation, distort the structure of the lymph node, forming distinct nodules. Within these nodules there are lymphoid cells with scattered, atypical, usually monolobed, Reed-Sternberg-like cells in clear spaces ("lacunar cells").   (van Gieson)

Reticulohistiocytoses   (C45–C46)

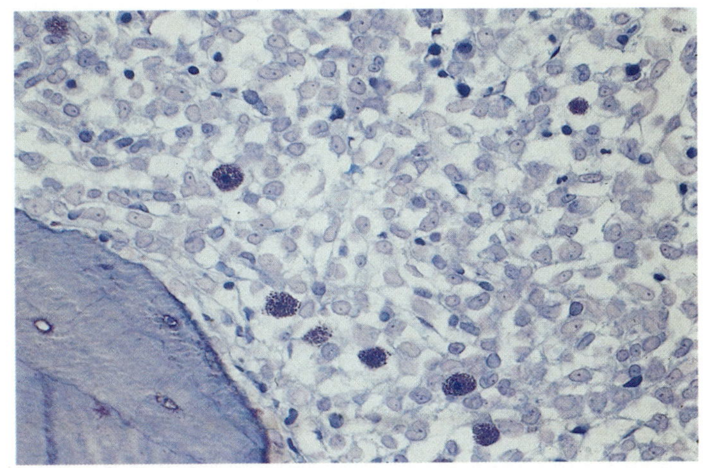

Fig. C45.   Malignant histiocytosis. The bone marrow is almost completely replaced by atypical histiocytes with generally oval, delicate nuclei and clear cytoplasm which, in this case, contains lipid. Near the bone (lower left) are five mast cells with basophilic granules. This fatal disorder often presents with fever, weight loss, lymphadenopathy, hepatosplenomegaly, jaundice, and pancytopenia. (Giemsa)

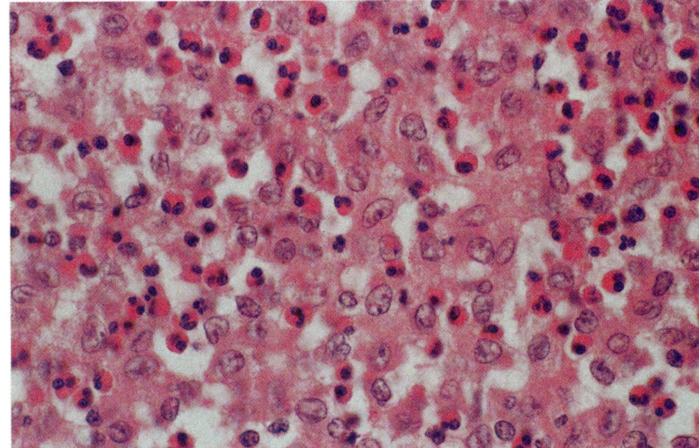

Fig. C46.   Eosinophilic granuloma involving bone. Between the larger atypical histiocytes, which have relatively clear cytoplasm, are many bilobed and polymorphonuclear leukocytes in which there are prominent eosinophilic granules. This solitary, bone-destroying lesion usually occurs in children.   (hematoxylin-eosin)

Benign Reactive Changes of Lymph Nodes   (C47–C55)

Fig. C47.   Lymph node changes following cell-mediated ("delayed hypersensitivity") immune reaction caused by immunization with BCG (bacille Calmette-Guerin). There is marked hyperplasia of the paracortex because of the increased numbers of T-lymphocytes stained brown with the α-naphthylacetate-esterase reaction. The cortex is narrow and virtually free of T-lymphocytes, and there are no germinal centers.

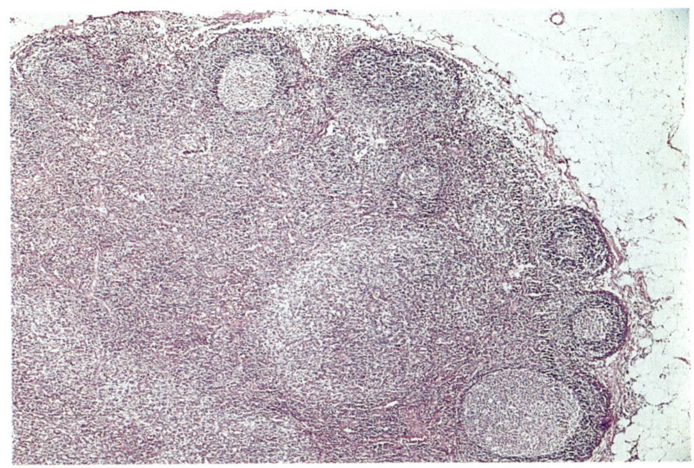

Fig. C48.   Lymph node after a complex immune reaction. The follicles are enlarged markedly, with prominent germinal centers and intervening broad sheets of lymphocytes, all characteristic of an antibody-mediated response with B-cell activation. In the midfield, beneath a T-cell tertiary follicle, there is also a poorly defined paracortical collection of lymphocytes. This lymph node was from the mesentery of a patient undergoing colonic resection for adenocarcinoma. There was no evidence of metastasis. (hematoxylin-eosin)

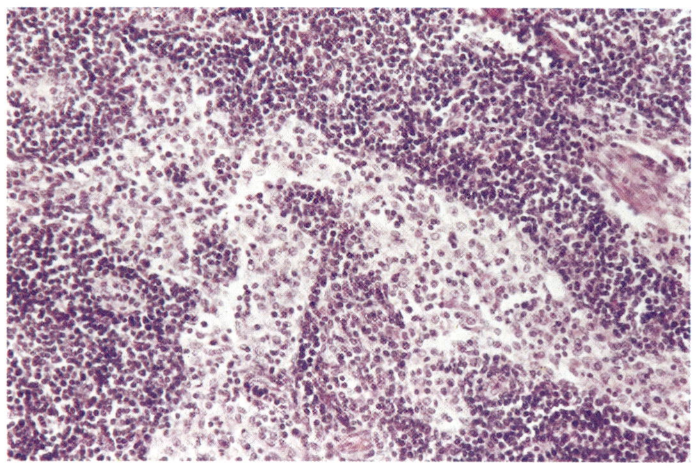

Fig. C49. Sinus histiocytosis. The lymph node sinuses are filled with histiocytes and the endothelial cells are hyperplastic. These nonspecific changes, when found in the draining axillary lymph nodes, have been associated with a better prognosis for breast cancer patients.   (hematoxylin-eosin)

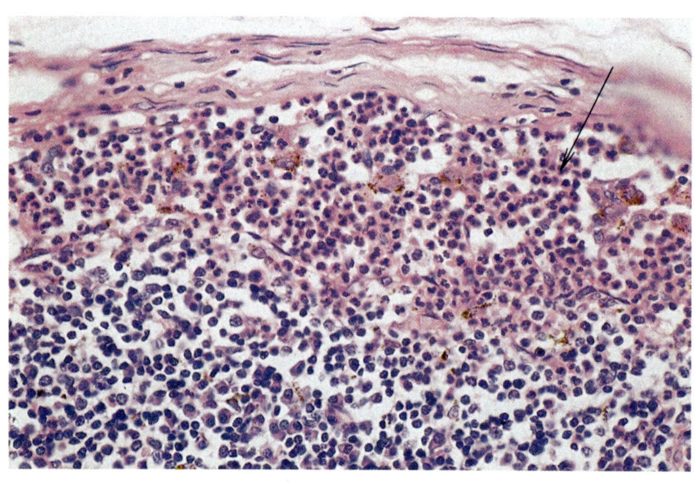

Fig. C50. Acute lymphadenitis. The peripheral sinus of the lymph node is distended with polymorphonuclear neutrophilic leukocytes *(arrow).* (hematoxylin-eosin)

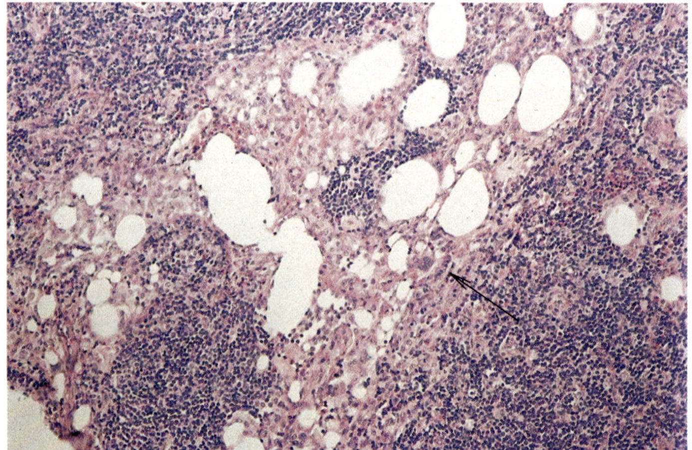

Fig. C51. Lymph node reaction after lymphangiography. In addition to the large lipid vacuoles within the lymph node sinus, the endothelial cells are hyperplastic and there are foreign body giant cells *(arrow).* (hematoxylin-eosin)

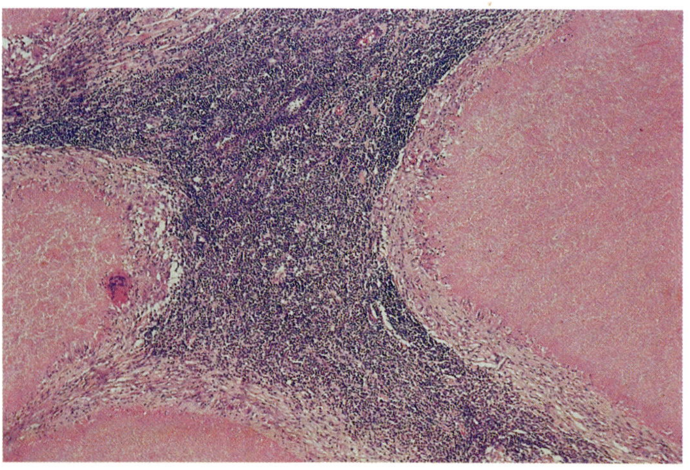

Fig. C52. Caseating granulomas of tuberculosis. There are three distinct zones of caseous necrosis seen as relatively homogeneous eosinophilic material around which there is a rim of epithelioid histiocytes, lymphocytes, Langhans giant cells (left), and fibroblasts. (hematoxylin-eosin)

Fig. C53. Lymph node from a patient with sarcoidosis. There are many noncaseating epithelioid and giant cell granulomata. A Langhans giant cell is present *(arrow).* This disease occurs worldwide, most often affecting adults and usually involving thoracic organs, including lymph nodes.   (hematoxylin-eosin)

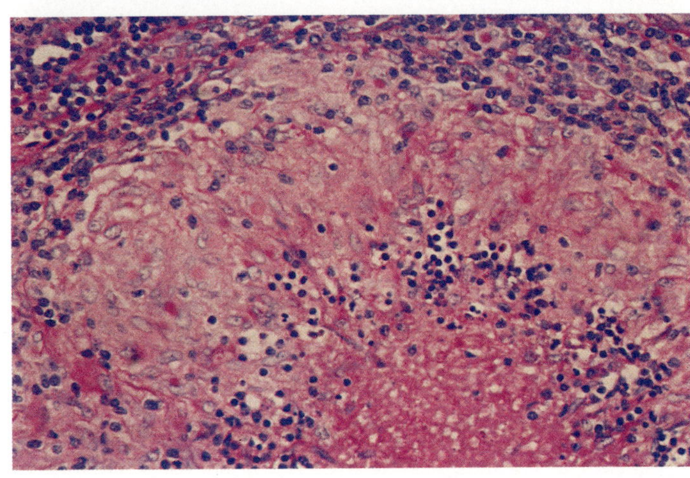

Fig. C54. Cat-scratch disease. This regional lymphadenopathy is characterized by a central necrotic area (lower right) infiltrated by polymorphonuclear neutrophilic leukocytes surrounded by palisaded epithelioid histiocytes with occasional giant cells. Recently, pleomorphic Gram-negative bacilli have been found in some of these cases. This histologic picture can also be seen in mesenteric lymphadenitis associated with *Yersinia enterocolitica,* with lymphogranuloma venereum, tularemia, and other infections. (hematoxylin-eosin)

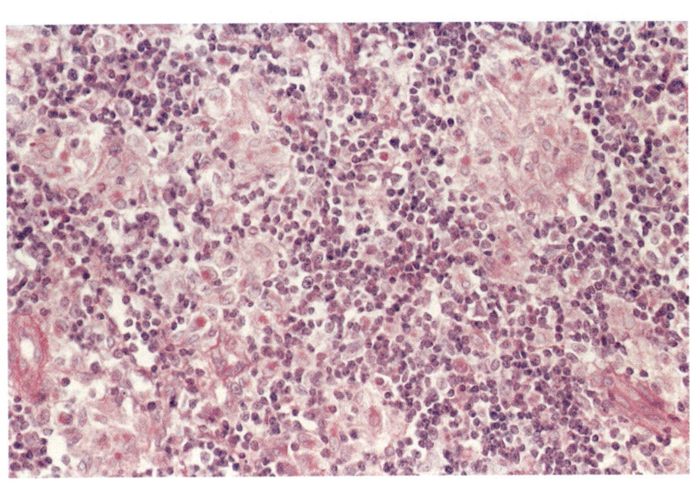

Fig. C55. Toxoplasmosis. In this case the lymph node architecture is almost completely effaced by clusters of epithelioid histiocytes, usually without necrosis or giant cells. Toxoplasma lymphadenitis generally involves cervical lymph nodes and toxoplasmic cysts are found only rarely.   (hematoxylin-eosin)

Spleen   *(C56)*

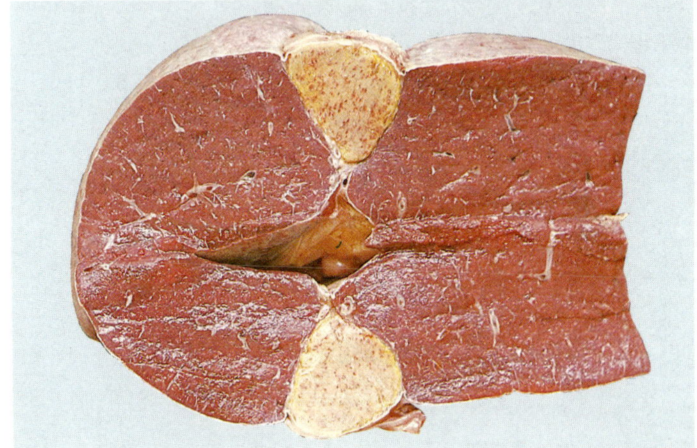

Fig. C56. Splenic infarct. The spleen has been bisected to demonstrate a well delineated, wedge shaped, pale yellow, old infarct which occurred because of embolization in a patient with endocarditis.

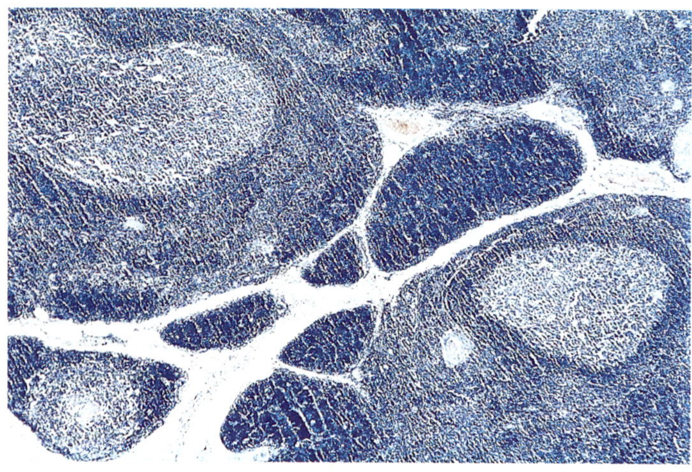

Fig. C57.   Thymus from a patient with myasthenia gravis, showing prominent germinal centers in the thymic lymphoid tissue. In many patients with these changes, thymectomy leads to marked clinical improvement.   (Giemsa)

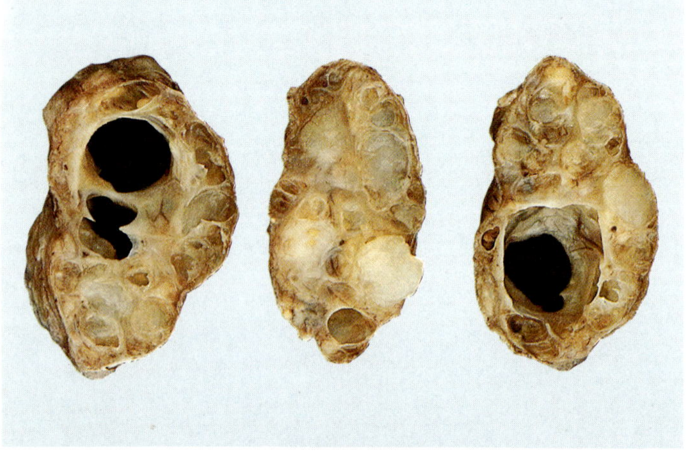

Fig. C58.   Cystic thymoma. Homogeneous white material is seen within the cysts in these cross sections. The thymoma cells are present in this material.

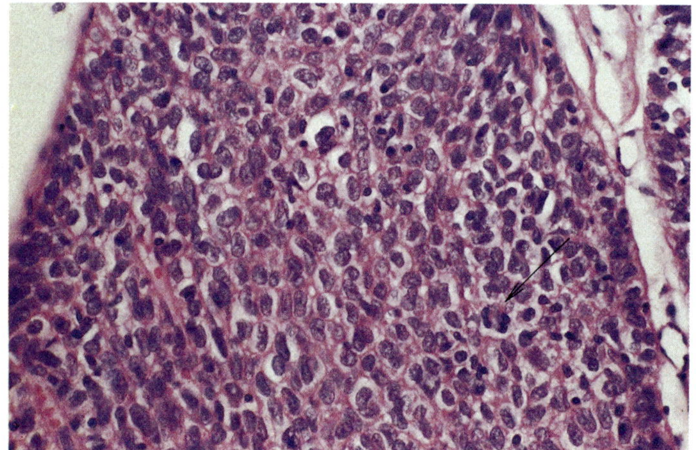

Fig. C59.   Spindle-cell thymoma. Predominant in the epithelial cell component are elongated, spindle-cell forms. There are occasional mitoses *(arrow)* and scattered lymphocytes.   (hematoxylin-eosin)

D. Ear, Nose, Throat, and Larynx

Ch. Beck

The most important conditions affecting the middle ear are inflammatory. They produce characteristic functional and morphologic changes that are most often studied in the clinical setting, rather than through resected specimens. The inner ear can undergo degenerative changes; the most prominent and clinically important of which is otosclerosis. The organ of Corti can undergo changes which impair sound conduction.

The nose can be the site of various malformations and defects that can contribute to impaired breathing. The mucous membranes of the nasal passages are the site of the most common of human inflammations, the cold. The nose can also be the site of a distinct form of dermatitis.

The most characteristic inflammation of the pharynx is tonsillitis, which can be of either specific or nonspecific etiology. Cysts of the neck can result from the congenital persistence of embryologic structures.

Tumors are the most important lesions affecting the larynx. Benign tumors or tumor-like growths can interfere with phonation and breathing. Smokers are particularly prone to the development of laryngeal carcinoma, which is almost always squamous cell in nature.

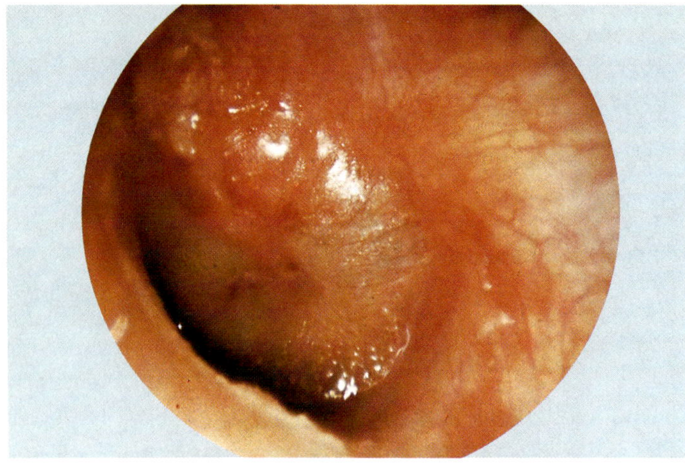

Fig. D1.   Markedly inflamed tympanic membrane in acute purulent otitis media. The membrane is reddened, edematous, and thickened, and the otic canal is narrowed.

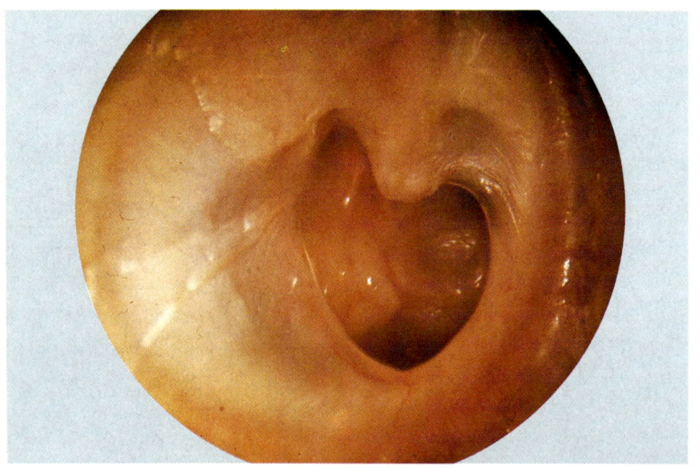

Fig. D2.   Central perforation of the tympanic membrane in chronic otitis media.

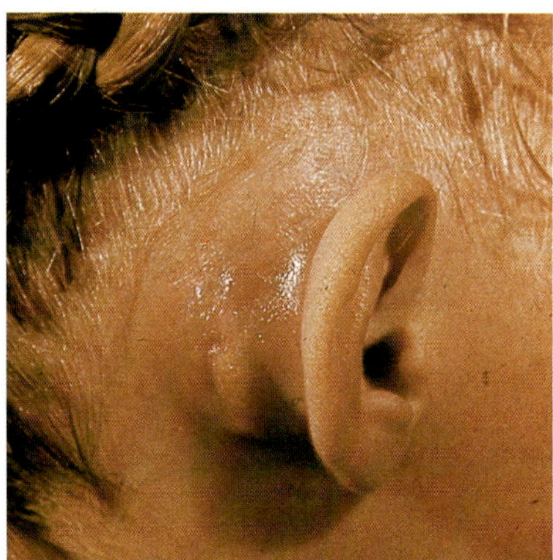

Fig. D3.   Retroauricular cutaneous penetration of a mastoiditis associated with purulent otitis media.

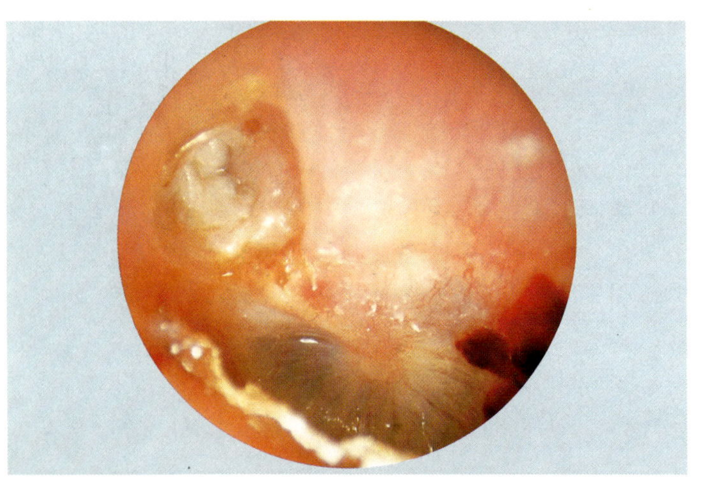

Fig. D4.   Cholesteatoma (keratoma) is generally a complication of acute or chronic otitis media. Accumulations of cream-colored exudate containing keratin are seen, and there is a peripheral perforation of the tympanic membrane.

Fig. D5. Histologic section of a cholesteatoma. The cholesteatoma consists of both keratin and histiocytes surrounding cholesterol crystals (hence, "cholesteatoma"). It can destroy adjacent bone
and ear canal structures as it proliferates. A covering stratified
squamous epithelium is seen at the top.

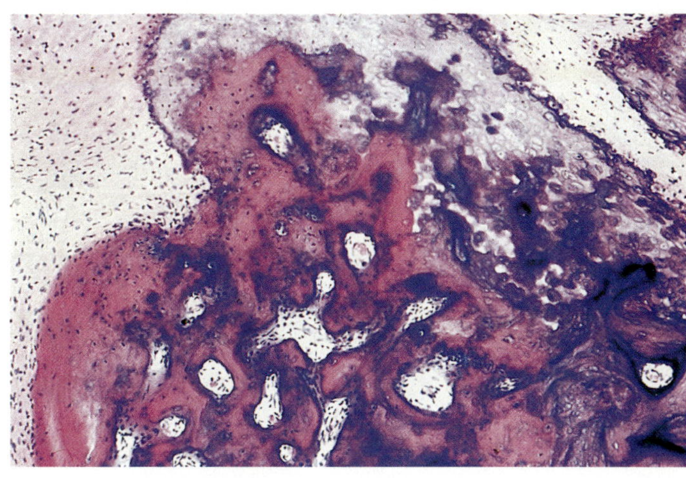

Fig. D6. Otosclerosis (inactive stage), in which there has been
considerable overgrowth of temporal bone anterior to the oval
window. Mosaic lines of new bone formation are seen. Note at the
upper left and right white cartilage and lamellar bone formation
between the cartilage and dense bone.   (hematoxylin-eosin)

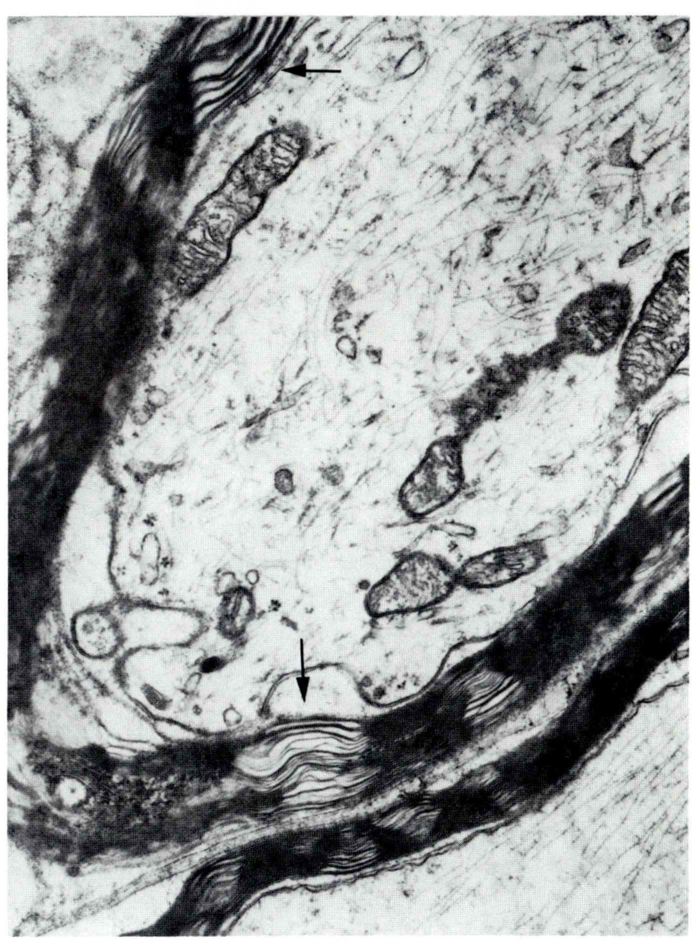

Fig. D7. Electron micrograph of secondary, retrograde degeneration of a nerve as a result of destruction of the organ of Corti. The
central portion of the myelin bundle is split segmentally *(arrow).*

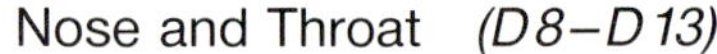

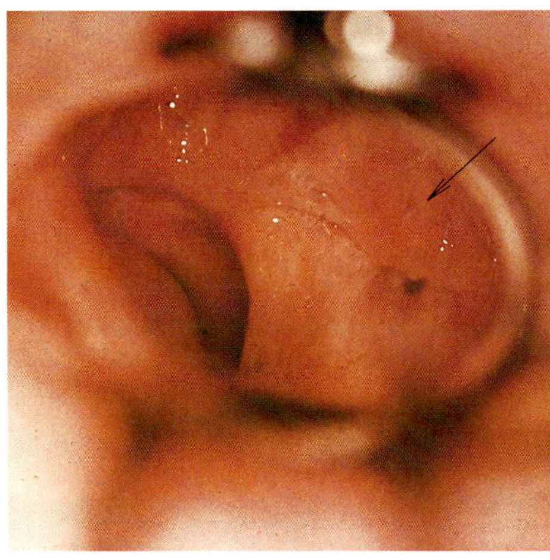

Fig. D8.   Unilateral choanal atresia. The left nasal passage is obstructed by a membrane *(arrow),* probably due to a persistence of the bucconasal membrane that normally disappears during fetal development. Choanal atresia occurs in about one of 7,000 births and is a familial disorder.

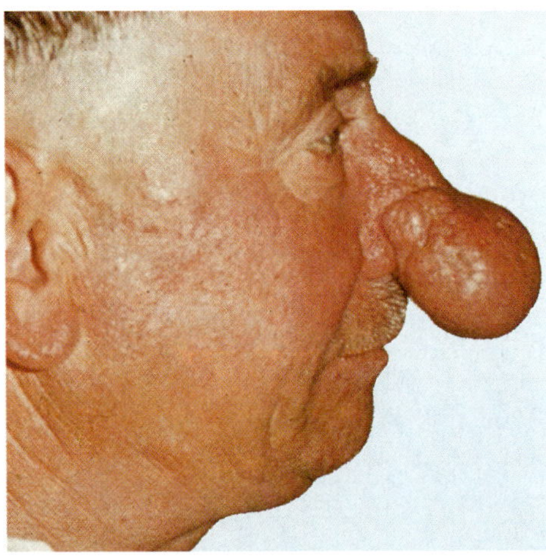

Fig. D9.   Rhinophyma. This term is used for the hyperplastic glandular form of acne rosacea affecting the nose. There is bulbous enlargement of the tip of the nose with marked telangiectasia imparting the red appearance.

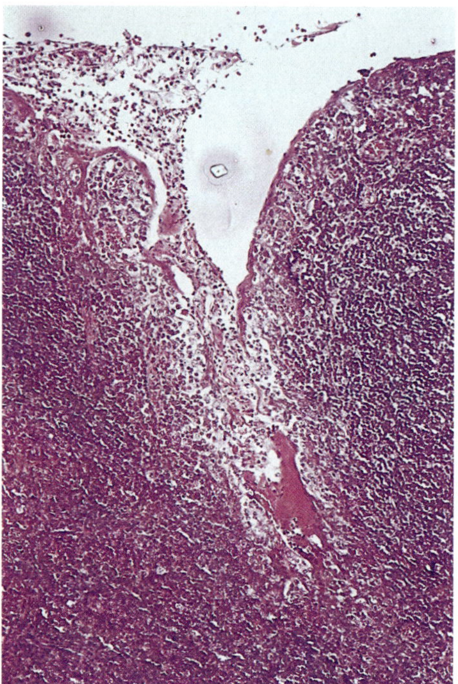

Fig. D10.   Catarrhal pharyngitis. There is loss of epithelium, infiltration by acute inflammatory cells, and accumulation of fibrin in tonsillar crypts.

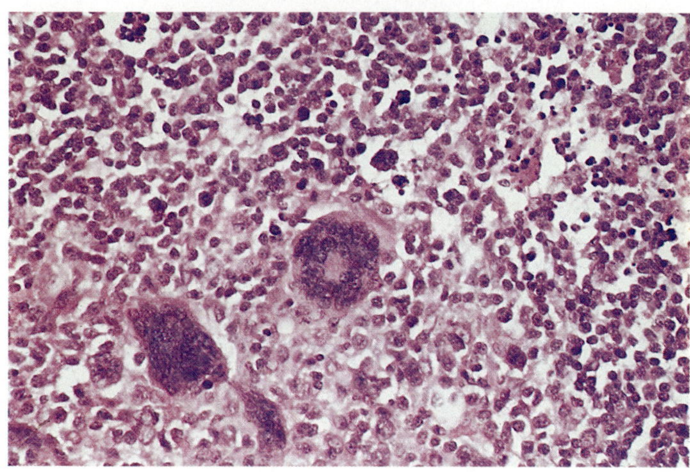

Fig. D 11. Chronic tonsillitis with enlargement of lymphoid germinal centers. The pharyngeal stratified squamous mucosa is to the left and above. The lymphoid tissue in this area is partially lost and there is granulation tissue and early scar formation.

Fig. D 12. Warthin-Finkeldey giant cells in the palatine tonsil. This form of giant cell is characteristic of measles (rubeola).

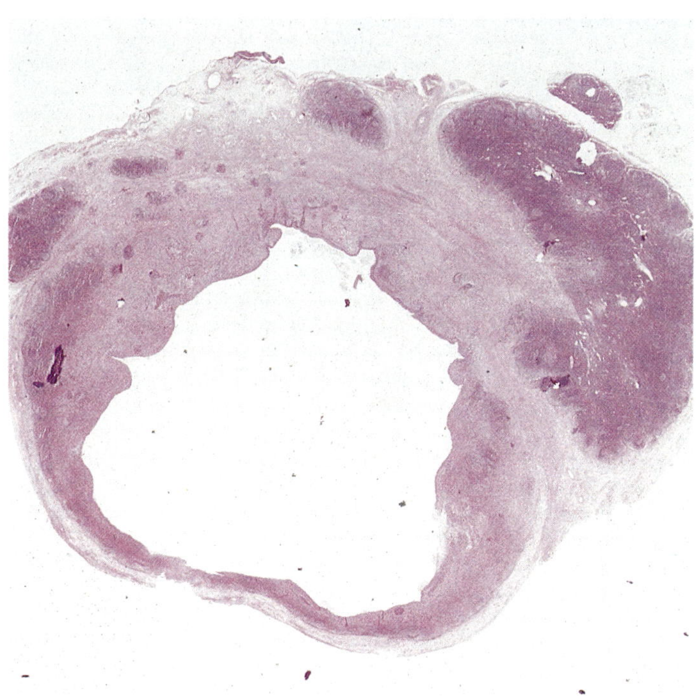

Fig. D 13. Branchial cleft cyst. The cyst can be lined by respiratory-type or stratified squamous epithelium (upper portion of cyst) and surrounded by abundant lymphoid tissue. The fibrosis immediately surrounding the cysts is due to prior infection.

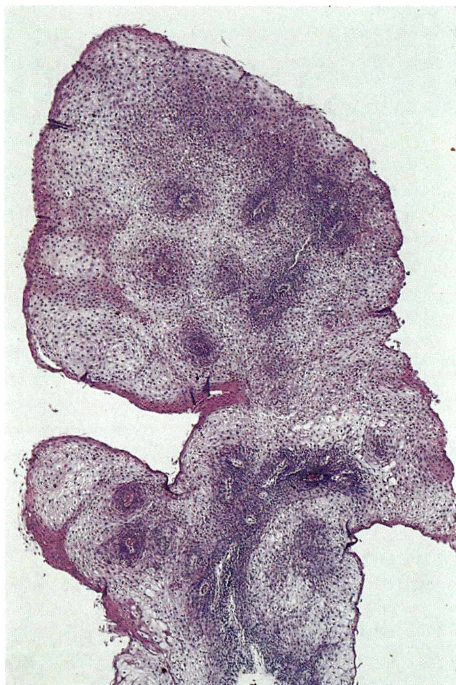

Fig. D14.   Laryngeal squamous papilloma. There is a papillary growth of squamous epithelium with compressed, revascularized stroma.

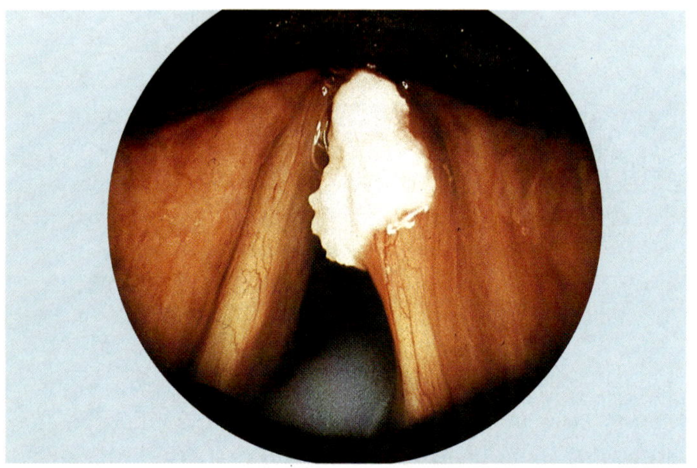

Fig. D15a.   Laryngoscopic view of a carcinoma of the right vocal cord. The white appearance is typical of keratinizing squamous cell carcinoma.

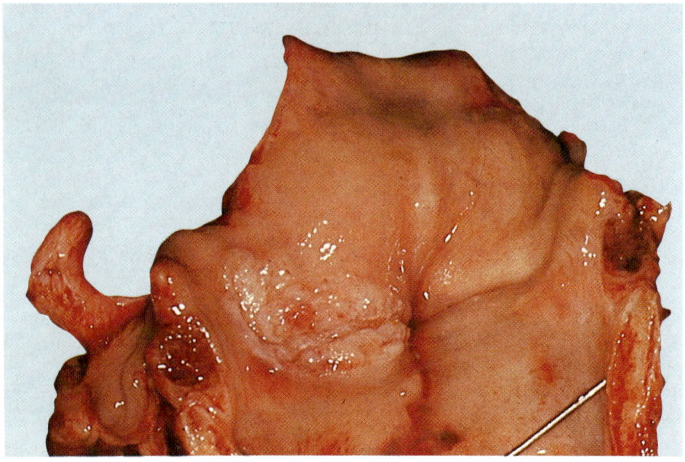

Fig. D15b.   Resected larynx showing a carcinoma of the left false vocal cord with extension to the vestibular fold of the true vocal cord and the subglottic region.

E. Lungs

G. Könn

The lungs are very susceptible to environmental damage, both because they have the largest inner surface area and, more particularly, because of their direct contact with the environment. Bacterial or viral inflammations of the trachea, bronchi, and bronchioles are particularly common. In the acute phase they are associated with a polymorphonuclear leukocyte inflammatory process which can result in production of considerable purulent material. They can also become chronic and, with secondary pulmonary changes, can cause severe respiratory impairment as well as secondary heart damage due to increased resistance in the pulmonary circulation. In addition, the lungs are the sole organs of pulmonary circulation, and most of the disorders of the left heart are reflected in characteristic pulmonary change from both acute and chronic passive congestion.

Other circulatory disorders can also affect the lungs. Pulmonary emboli can be deadly or, when the emboli are small and recurrent, can cause chronic cor pulmonale. Cor pulmonale, or severe right ventricular hypertrophy, can also result from a variety of acquired respiratory disorders, as well as from congenital lesions. The lungs can, of course, become acutely airless (atelectasis) or, through various mechanisms, the air spaces can become dilated (emphysema).

Bacterial pneumonias can occur with varying degrees of severity, and can occur as broncho- or lobar pneumonia. The pattern of pneumonia is, to a large degree, a reflection of the characteristics of the particular causative organism. In bronchopneumonia, the lung shows inflammatory lesions in various stages and is not necessarily affected uniformly. In lobar pneumonia, in contrast, an entire lobe, or multiple lobes, can be involved, and the involvement tends to be fairly uniform in terms of its stage of development. Both forms of pneumonia can, of course, lead ro respiratory insufficiency. Specific morphologic features are found in some of the viral pneumonias as well as in tuberculosis. The pneumoconioses have been recognized increasingly in recent years and many pathogenic factors, including inspiration of various fiber materials, have been identified.

Carcinoma of the lung remains a particularly important health problem. The most common central carcinoma, arising in large bronchi, is squamous cell carcinoma. The most common peripheral carcinoma, arising from terminal bronchiolar or alveolar epithelium, is adenocarcinoma. Squamous cell carcinoma, because of its central location and associated bronchial obstruction, is often associated with bronchopneumonia.

The pleura can be affected by a variety of inflammatory conditions. One of the most common is fibrinous pleuritis, which can lead to pleural fibrosis and obliteration. Pleural empyema is due to the presence of a pyogenic organism on the pleural surface. The major tumor originating on the pleura (rather than metastasizing to) is mesothelioma. Mesothelioma's association with occupational exposure to asbestos has been well documented.

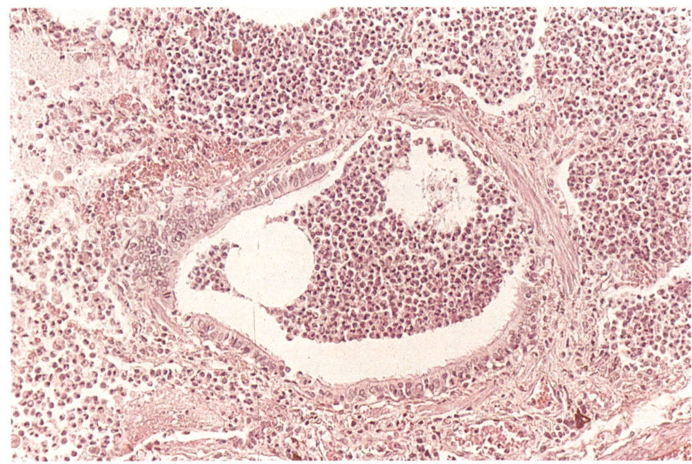

Fig. E1.   Acute pyogenic bronchiolitis. The lumen of the bronchiole is filled with acute imflammatory cells, with extension into the surrounding alveoli.   (hematoxylin-eosin)

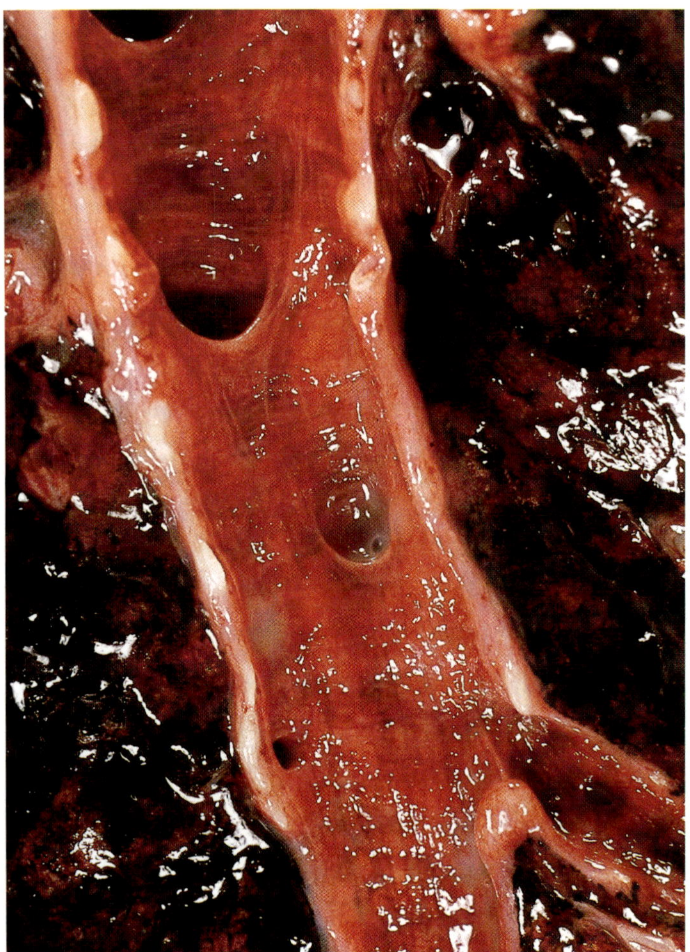

Fig. E2.   Chronic hypertrophic bronchitis. The mucosa is reddened and slightly thickened and there are scattered collections of mucous secretions.

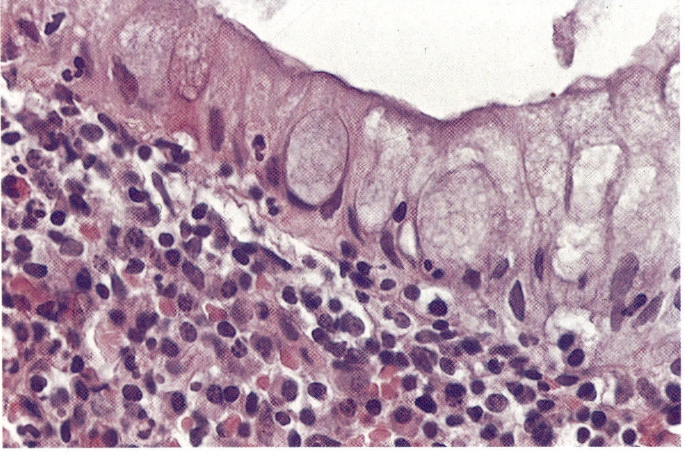

Fig. E3.   Bronchial epithelium from a patient with bronchial asthma. There is marked increase of goblet cells. The basement membrane is thickened, and there is a heavy accumulation of chronic inflammatory cells, including lymphocytes, plasma cells, and eosinophils, in the submucosa.   (hematoxylin-eosin)

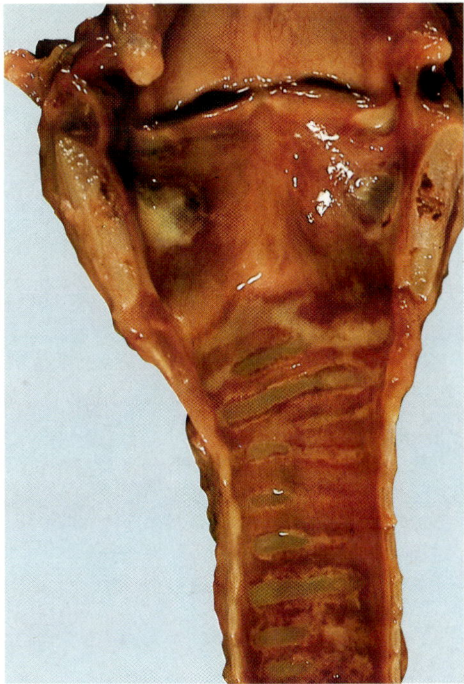

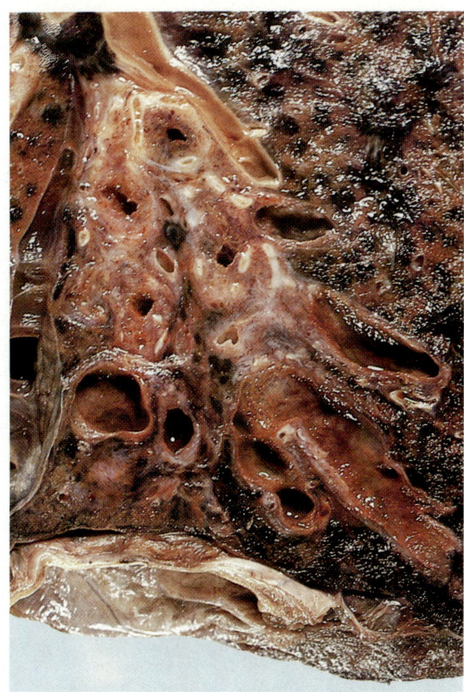

Fig. E4. Chronic ulcerated laryngotracheitis following intubation with an indwelling airway. The tracheal cartilagenous rings are evident where the mucosa is ulcerated.

Fig. E5. Cylindrical bronchiectasis in the lower lobe of the lung. The bronchi are greatly enlarged and can be opened easily to their termination immediately beneath the pleura. Normally bronchi are invisible beyond the inner two-thirds of the lung. The pleura is seen in the figure; it is thickened and adherent, evidence of preceding pleuritis.

Circulatory Disturbances *(E6–E11)*

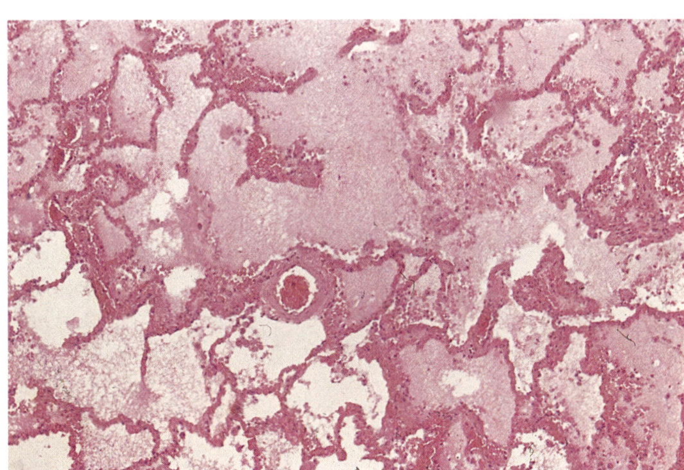

Fig. E6. Pulmonary edema, following acute left-sided heart failure. The alveoli are filled with a homogeneous, generally acellular, eosinophilic fluid. In some alveoli the material appears as delicate fibrillary strands. Red blood cells are in some alveoli and the alveolar capillaries and small blood vessels are distended with blood. (hematoxylin-eosin)

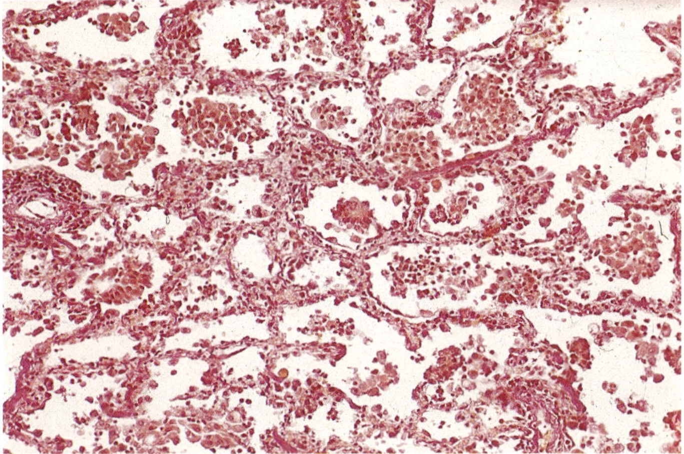

Fig. E7. Chronic congestion of the lungs. The alveolar septa are fibrotic and the alveoli contain many iron-laden macrophages ("heart-failure cells"). Macroscopically these lungs are brown and indurated. This type of lung was seen more commonly in years past, when rheumatic mitral stenosis was more prevalent, and was often described as "mitral lungs".   (hematoxylin-eosin)

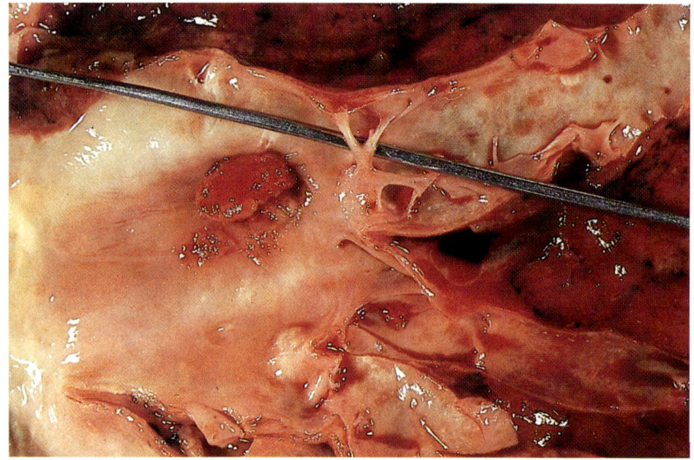

Fig. E8. Pulmonary arterial webs, evidence of prior pulmonary thromboembolism. A probe elevates fibrous strands indicating the position of the old thromboembolus. Slightly to the left of this, and below the probe, a recently formed red thromboembolus fills an arterial branch.

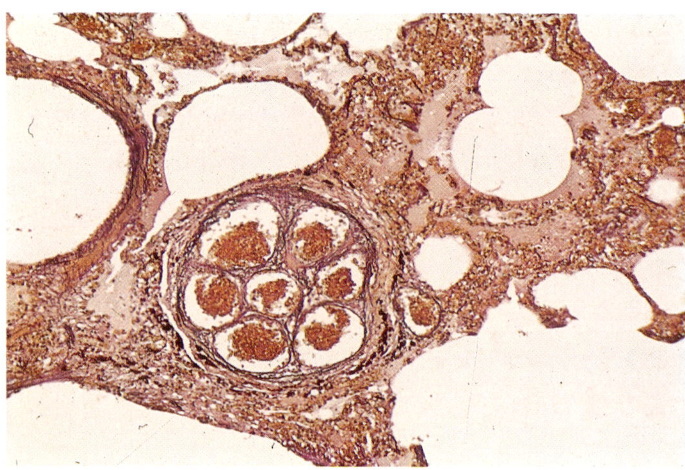

Fig. E9. Old, recanalized thromboembolus in pulmonary artery branch. (elastica-van Gieson)

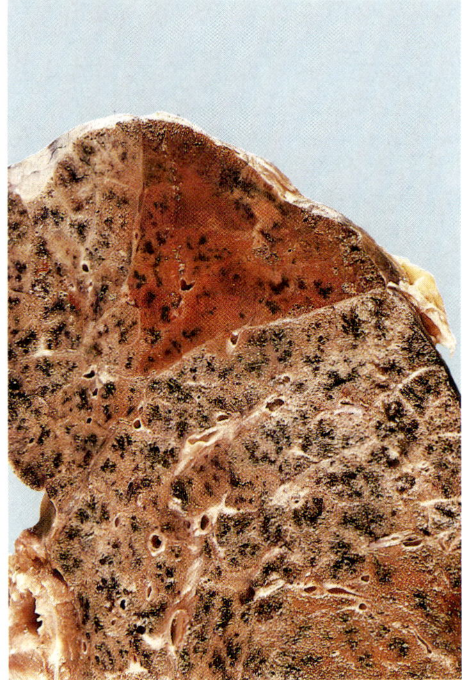

Fig. E10. Hemorrhagic pulmonary infarct. A red, wedge-shaped zone, firmer than the surrounding lung, is obvious. The overlying parietal pleura is adherent and there is a fibrinous pleuritis. Pulmonary infarcts generally do not occur, even when the thromboembolism is large, unless there is concomitant heart failure. Since the lung has a dual circulation, with both pulmonary and bronchial arteries, both circulations must be compromised to produce an infarct.

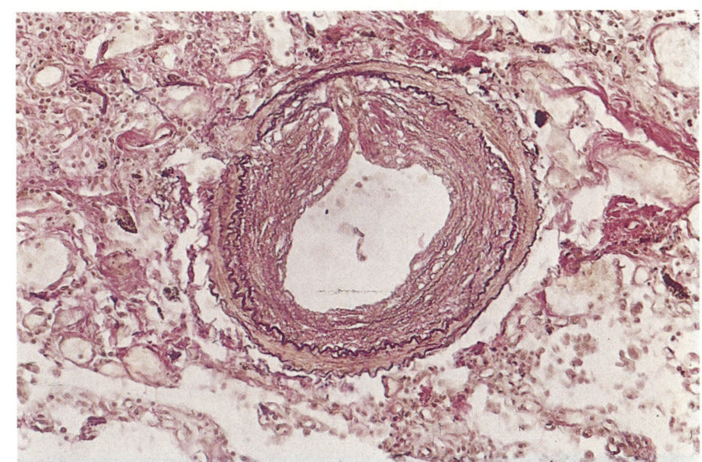

Fig. E11.   Small pulmonary artery branch showing medial thickening and stenosing intimal fibrosis as sequelae to chronic pulmonary hypertension.   (elastica-van Gieson)

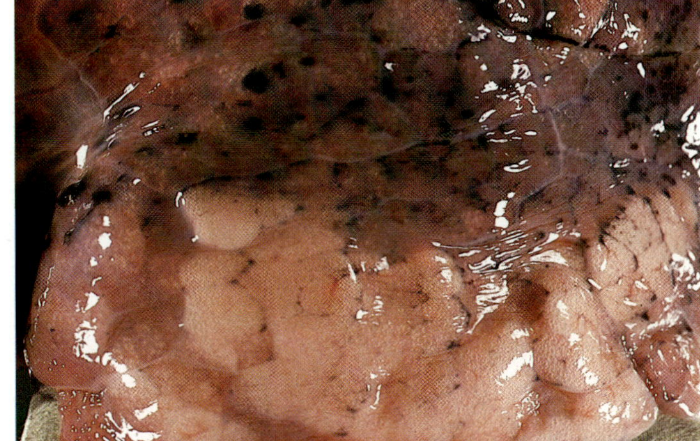

Atelectasis and Emphysema   *(E 12 – E 13)*

Fig. E12.   Atelectasis. At the upper portion of the specimen the lung is depressed and dark, and the pleura is focally wrinkled, without evidence of pleuritis. The depressed area has a well-defined irregular border and is sharply delineated from the adjacent lung which is well expanded and pink.

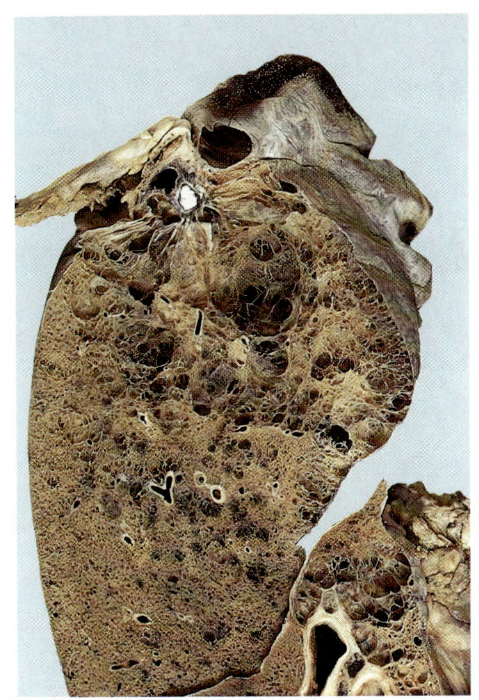

Fig. E13.   Small enlarged emphysematous spaces are seen as a sequela to bronchial obstruction due to old, caseating tuberculosis (seen as a chalky, white nodule at the upper portion of the photograph). The tuberculosis has caused localized scarring, including fibrosis and adherence of the pleura.

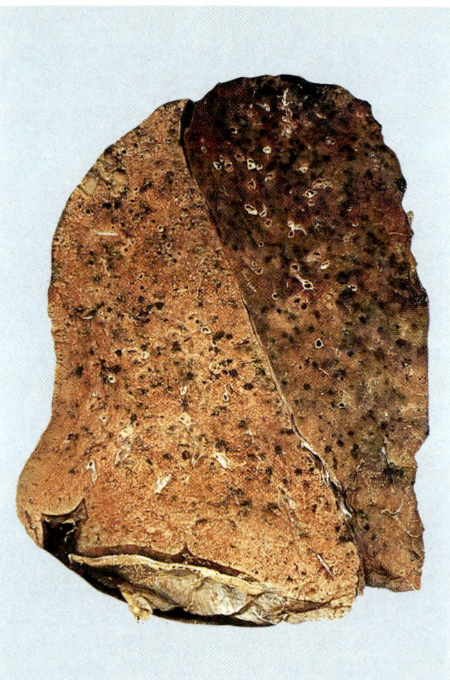

Fig. E 14 a. Lobar pneumonia of the left lower lobe. The lower lobe is consolidated and is light brown, in contrast to the upper lobe which appears normal. The black flecks are inhaled environmental pigments deposited in macrophages. The pleura at the base is adherent.

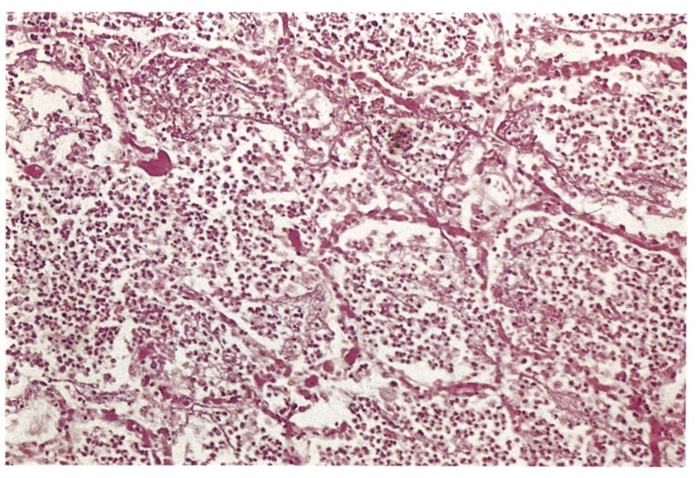

Fig. E 14 b. Histopathology of the lobar pneumonia demonstrated in *Fig. E 14 a.* The alveoli are filled with polymorphonuclear neutrophilic leukocytes. Between these acute inflammatory cells there are delicate fibrin strands.   (hematoxylin-eosin)

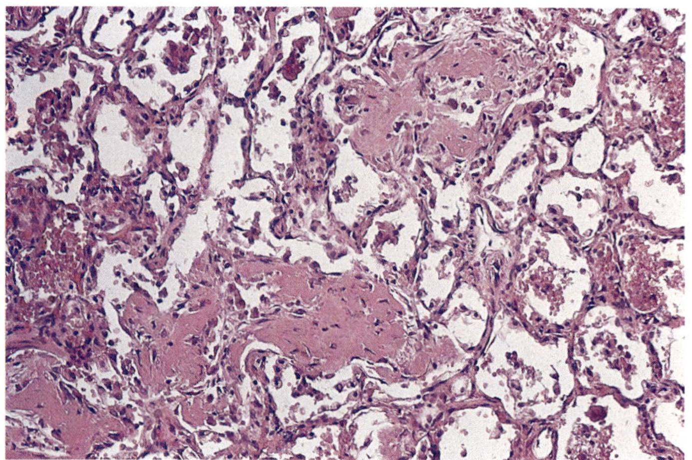

Fig. E 15. Organizing pneumonia. Some of the alveoli are filled with fibrin in which fibroblasts can be seen. This process will, if continued, result in fibrous tissue replacing the fibrin.   (hematoxylin-eosin)

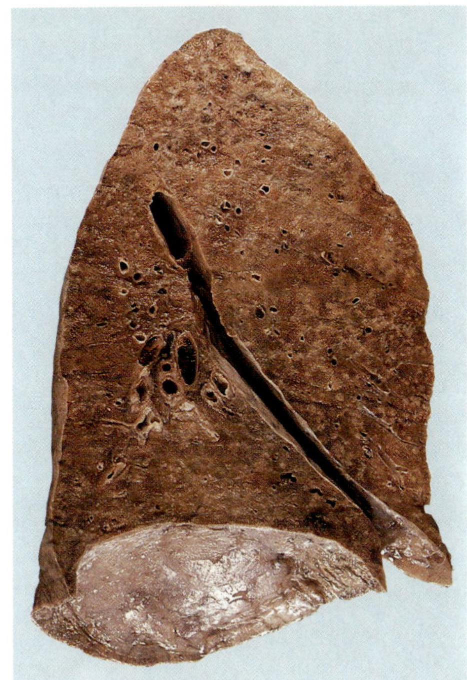

Fig. E 16. Bronchopneumonia. Scattered tan and grey, poorly defined nodular areas mottle the lung parenchyma in both lobes.

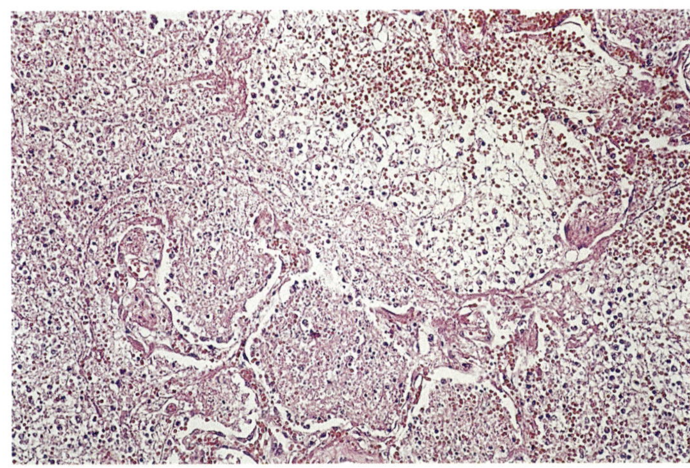

Fig. E 17. Aspiration bronchopneumonia. The alveoli are filled with a poorly formed fibrin network within which there are white and red blood cells. In the upper portion of the photomicrograph the architecture is distorted because of the destruction of alveolar septa by aspirated gastric juices.   (hematoxylin-eosin)

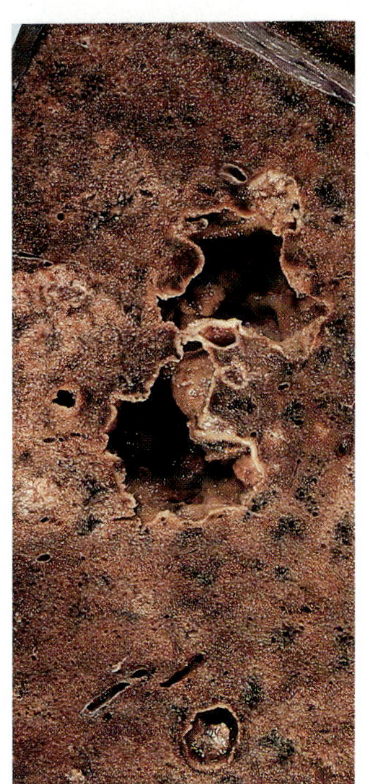
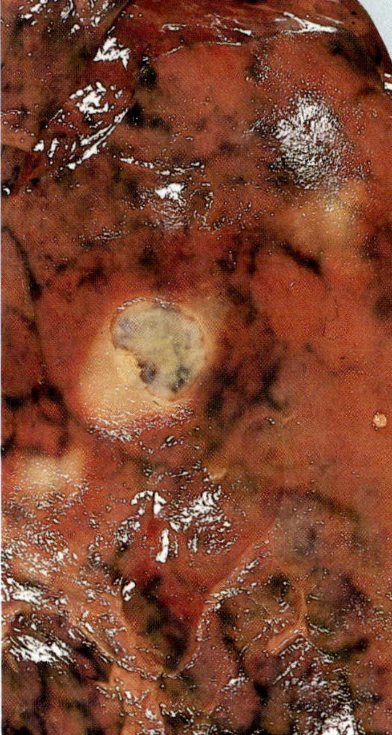

Fig. E 18a. Cut surface of the lung with an abscess cavity. Tan and grey areas of bronchopneumonia are in the surrounding parenchyma, best viewed to the left of the abscess.

Fig. E 18b. Abscess formation and bronchopneumonia from systemic staphylococcal infection. The yellow abscess, with its red inflammatory border, is at the visceral pleural surface of the lung. Surrounding this abscess, the pleura is granular because of the deposition of fibrin as the beginning stage of a purulent pleuritis.

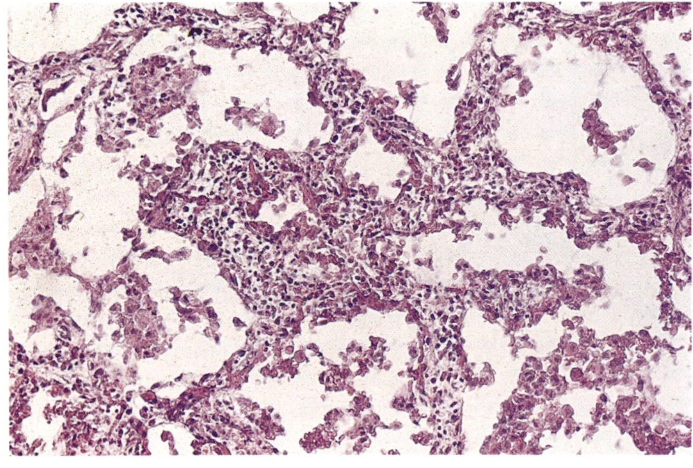

Fig. E19. Interstitial pneumonitis. The alveolar septa are widened because of the accumulation of lymphocytes. The alveolar lining cells are hyperplastic and the alveolar spaces contain many macrophages.   (hematoxylin-eosin)

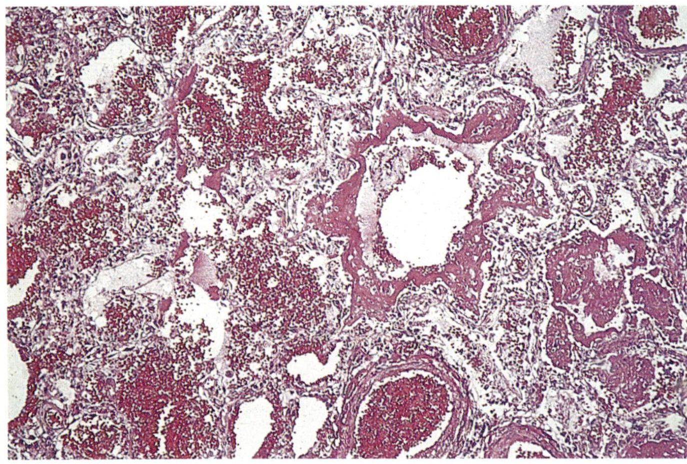

Fig. E20. Viral pneumonia. There is a hemorrhagic pneumonia with accumulation of fibrin and inflammatory cell infiltration. Hyaline membrane formation is seen lining the relatively empty alveolar space slightly to the right of the middle of the photomicrograph. (hematoxylin-eosin)

Pulmonary Fibrosis and Pulmonary Mycosis   *(E21–E22)*

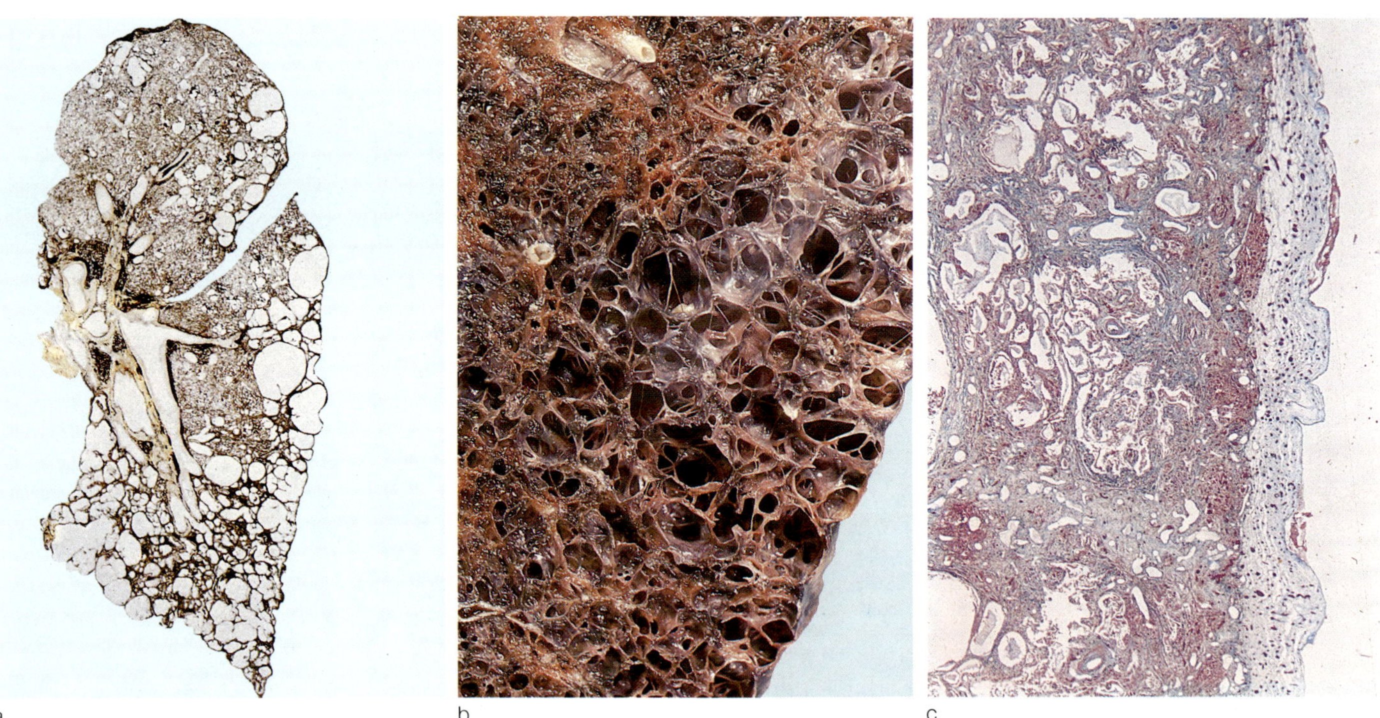

Fig. E21. Interstitial fibrosis of the lung. In the lung section to the left *(a)* and the close-up photograph *(b)*, markedly enlarged air spaces separated by thickened alveolar septal walls are easily seen. This is the picture of "honeycomb" lung. Histologically *(c)* the normal lung structure is not seen. Instead there are large, irregular air spaces with intervening fibrotic walls in which there is abundant collagen (blue). The pleura is also thickened (right).   (Goldner trichrome)

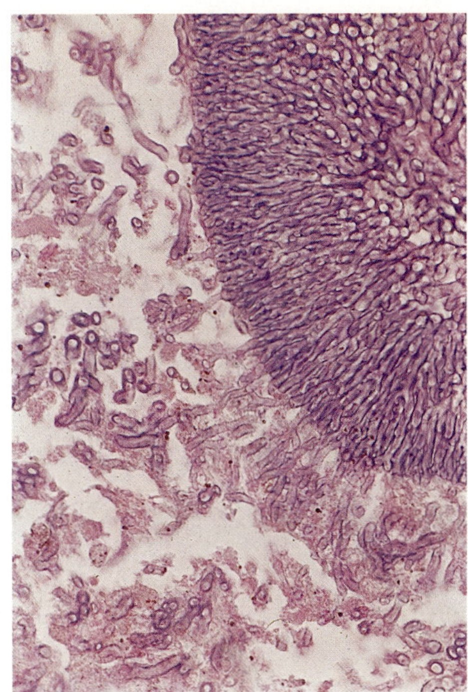

Fig. E22.   Pulmonary aspergillosis. This biopsy is from a patient who was clinically and radiologically diagnosed as having pulmonary carcinoma. To the right of the photomicrograph there is a nodular mass of uniform, narrow, regularly septated hyphal forms which are seen more discretely in the surrounding lung tissue.   (PAS)

Pulmonary Tuberculosis   *(E23–E25)*

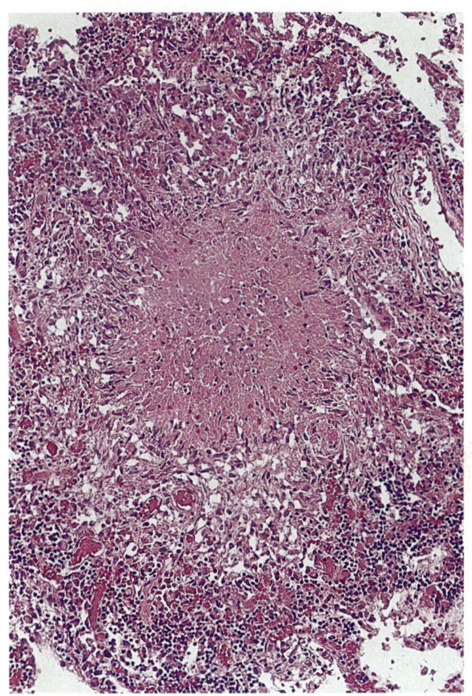

Fig. E23.   Miliary tuberculosis. This is a typical granuloma of tuberculosis, with a central zone of caseous necrosis surrounded by many epithelioid histiocytes and scattered Langhans giant cells, with an outer border of lymphocytes.   (hematoxylin-eosin)

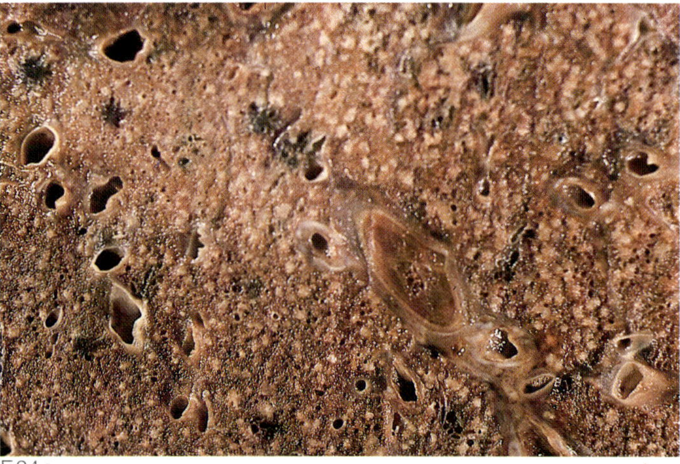

E24a

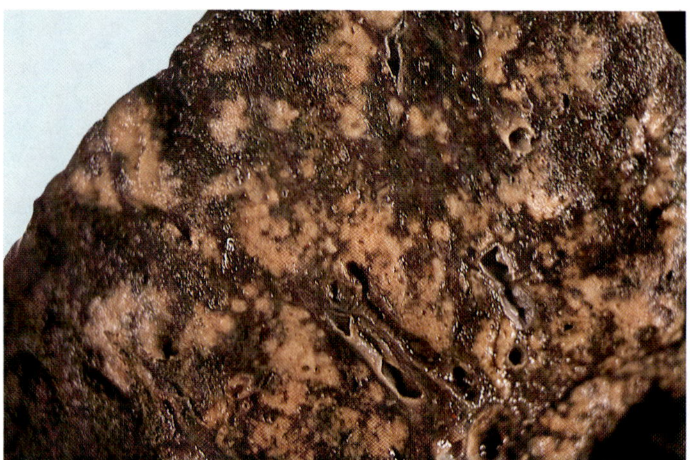

E24b

Fig. E24. Various forms of disseminated pulmonary tuberculosis.
a) Miliary tuberculosis. *b)* Nodular ("acinar-nodosa") tuberculosis.
c) Caseous pneumonia form of tuberculosis.

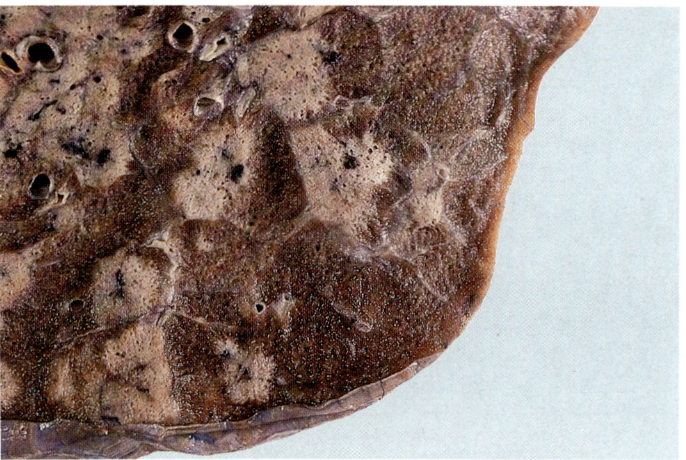

E24c

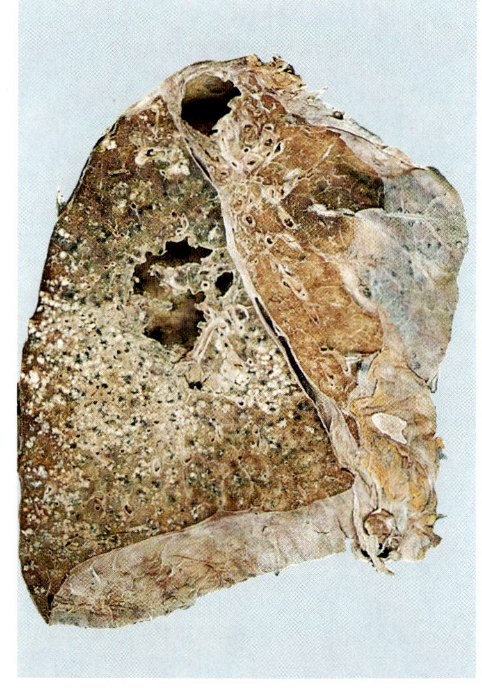

Fig. E25. Cavitary pulmonary tuberculosis with bronchogenic distribution. Sharply defined cavities are obvious at the apex of the left upper lobe and in the midportion of the left lower lobe. In the remainder of the lower lobe there are areas of nodular and caseous pneumonia forms of tuberculosis. A dark area of atelectasis is in the midportion of the upper lobe. Pleuritis is seen as thickened, adherent pleural membranes.

Sarcoidosis *(E26)*

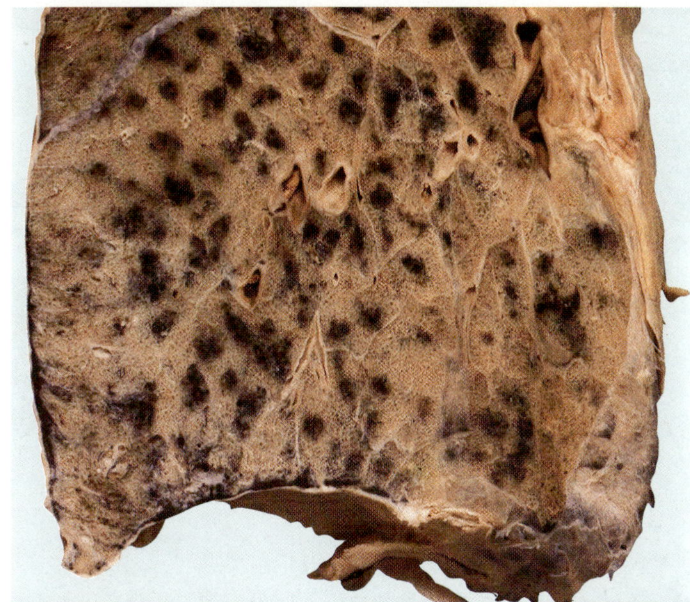

Fig. E26. Sarcoidosis. Multiple hyalinized granulomas are seen, within which there are epithelioid histiocytes, lymphocytes, and occasional Langhan's giant cells, but no necrosis. This is a relatively late stage of sarcoidosis.   (hematoxylin-eosin)

Pneumoconioses *(E27–E29)*

E27a

E27b

Fig. E27. Silicosis. The section of the lung *(a)* shows many black nodules. These are hard. The black pigmentation reflects the accumulation of environmental pigments *(see Fig. E 14 a)*. The hilar lymph nodes *(b)* of this lung are enlarged and hard, and appear slate grey on section. Histologically *(c)* the typical lesion is a hyalinized, laminated nodule within which there are only a few lymphocytes and histiocytes, with a thin mantle of environmental pigment. The lymph nodes show similar changes. Study with polarized light will disclose doubly refractile silica particles in the fine cleft-like spaces within the dense collagenous tissue.   (hematoxylin-eosin)

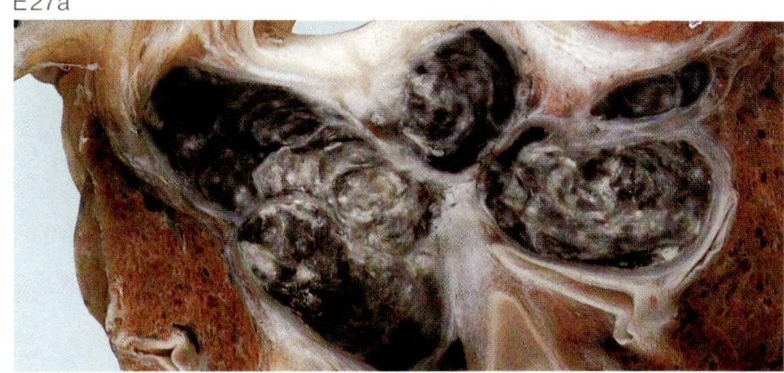

E27c

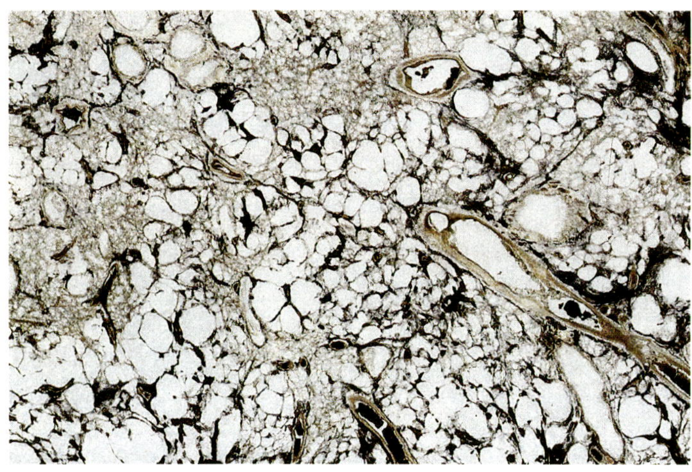

Fig. E28. Extensive emphysema in a patient with silicosis. The dilated air spaces surround black pigmented nodules of silicosis.

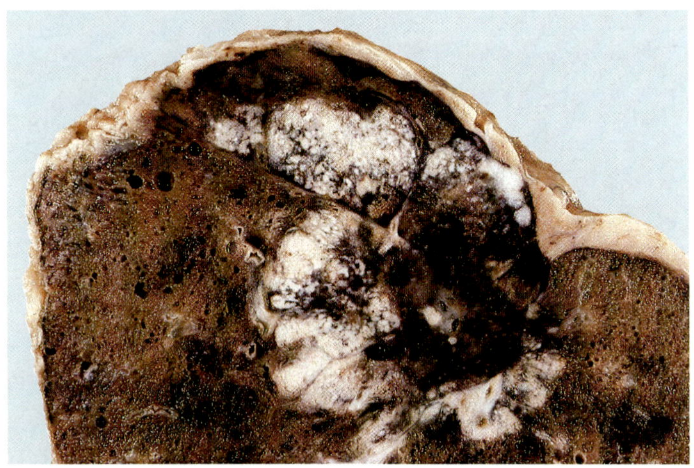

Fig. E29. Bronchogenic (squamous cell) carcinoma surrounds a large black silicotic nodule. The pleura is thickened because of prior pleuritis.

Neoplasia   *(E30–E33)*

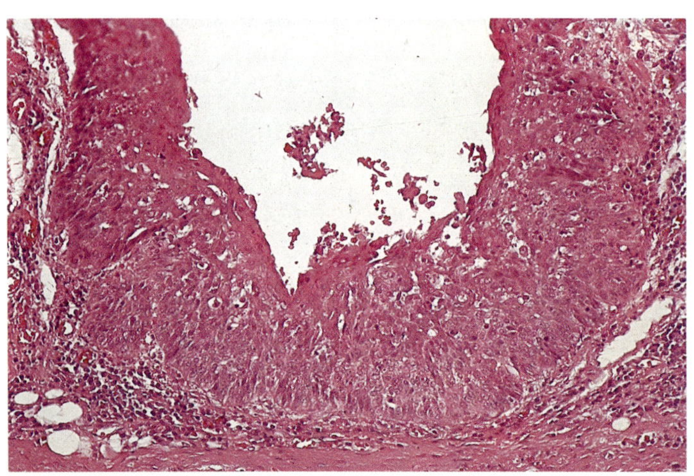

Fig. E30. Intraepithelial ("in situ") carcinoma in a bronchus. The squamous epithelium shows marked proliferation without orderly maturation from basal layer to surface, and parakeratosis. There are many atypical forms and scattered mitoses. There is no evidence of infiltration.   (hematoxylin-eosin)

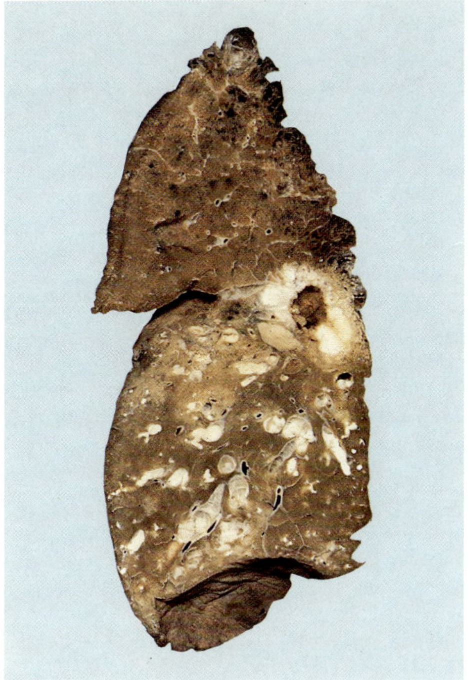

E31

Fig. E31. Bronchogenic carcinoma (middle-right). These tumors usually arise centrally in a large bronchus. The carcinoma infiltrates the surrounding tissues. Areas of bronchopneumonia are present in the lower lobe. These are a sequel to central bronchial obstruction with stasis of secretions and subsequent infection.

Fig. E32a. High magnification photomicrograph of keratinizing squamous cell carcinoma of a bronchus. This "epithelial pearl" is characteristically seen in keratinizing squamous cell carcinomas arising from various sites *(see Fig. G9)* and is not specific to the lung. (hematoxylin-eosin)

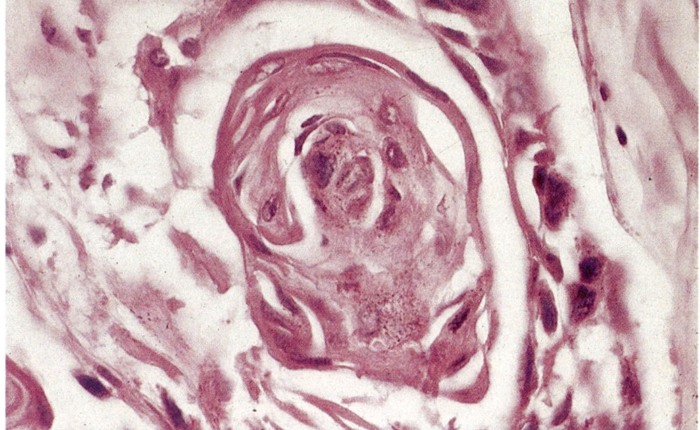

Fig. E32b. Small cell, anaplastic ("oat-cell") carcinoma of the lung. This tumor typically arises as an endobronchial lesion and consists of small round and elongated cells with indistinct cytoplasm. There may be many mitoses.   (hematoxylin-eosin)

Fig. E32c. Pulmonary adenocarcinoma. These tumors typically arise at the periphery of the lung, contain accumulated environmental pigment, and have overlying pleural puckering. This tumor consists of highly disordered glandular structures lined by malignant cells.   (hematoxylin-eosin)

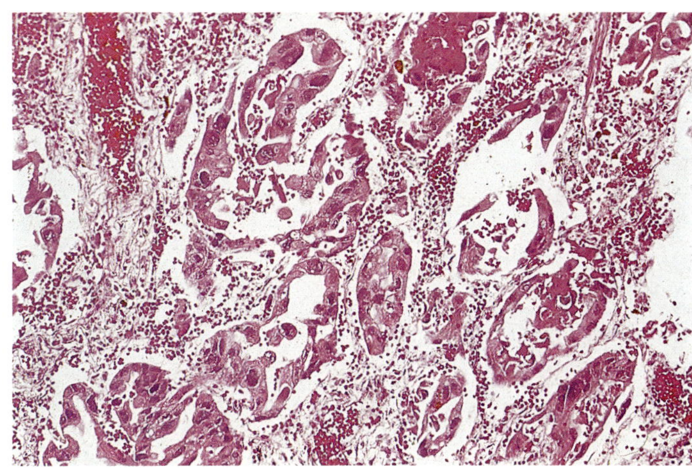

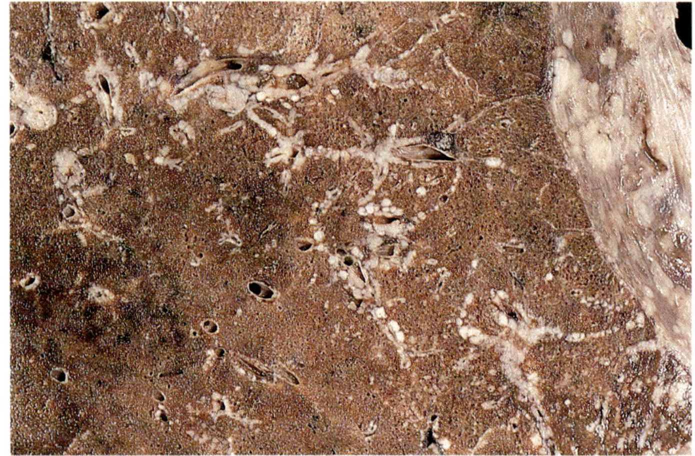

Fig. E33a. Lymphangitic spread of carcinoma. This is most often seen in metastasis to the lungs. The lymphatic network is filled with tumor. In this photograph lymphangitic spread is best seen at the lower right. The pleura is to the right and is partially covered by tumorous plaques. Connecting chains of tumor nodules are seen distending lymphatic spaces and extending from the pleura into the parenchyma.

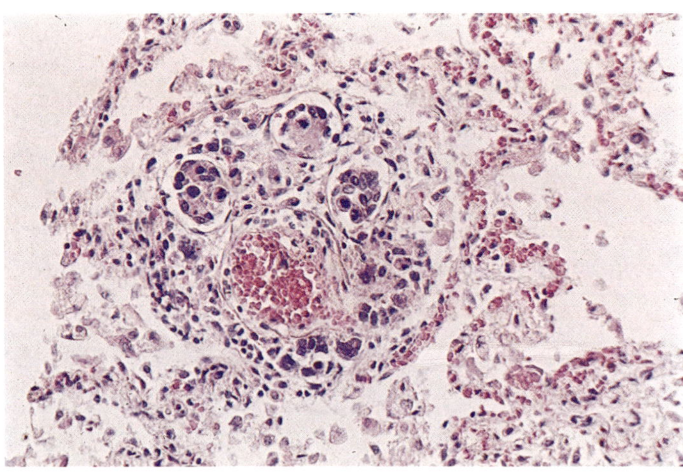

Fig. E33b. Clusters of carcinoma cells are seen in perivascular lymphatic spaces in this photomicrograph of a histologic section from the lung above.   (hematoxylin-eosin)

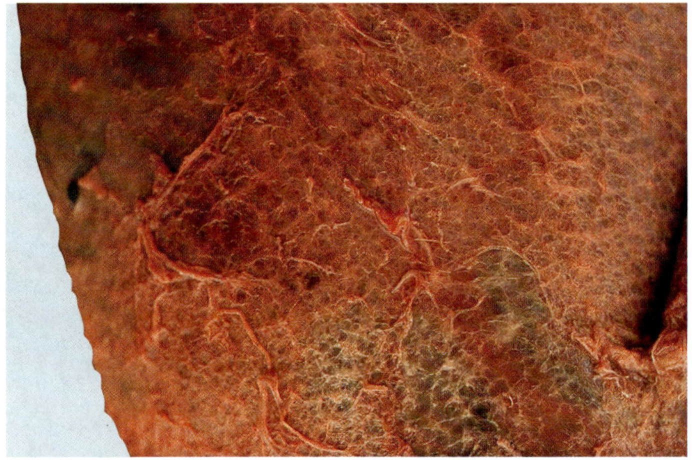

Pleural Disorders   *(E34–E35)*

Fig. E34. Uremic pleuritis. Delicate, easily removed strands of fibrin cover the pleural surface. A "friction rub" can be heard when auscultating the chest of a patient with this condition. This is the same process as seen in *Fig. A51.*

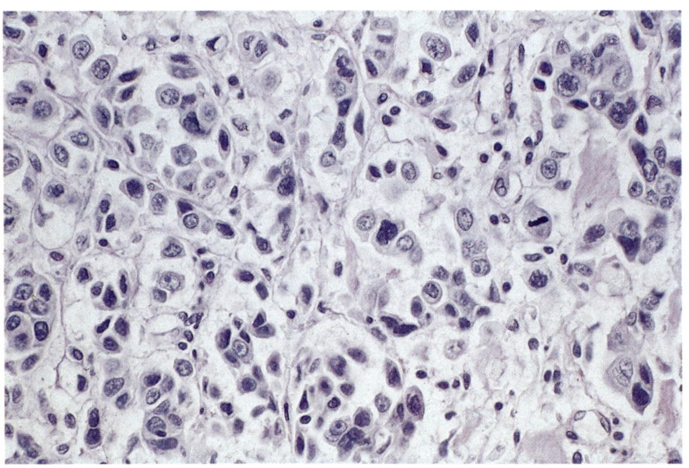

Fig. E35. Mesothelioma. This uncommon malignant neoplasm of the pleura has been well associated with exposure to asbestos, generally as an occupational hazard. Mesotheliomas may be epithelial, (as is the one in this illustration), fibroblastic, or mixed. In this photomicrograph, nuclear pleomorphism with marked atypia is evident and there are numerous mitoses.   (hematoxylin-eosin)

F. Oral Cavity

L. Bianchi, H.-E. Schaefer, W. Schilli

A variety of disorders of the tooth enamel can be seen in children. In adults dental caries and periodontal inflammation occur frequently. A variety of imflammations can affect the oral mucosa. These can be local or systemic. Inflammatory disorders of the oral mucosa reflect a variety of systemic conditions. Histologic study is necessary for the evaluation of hyperplastic mucosal changes. Preneoplastic lesions occur and squamous cell carcinoma is not uncommon.

Most of the diseases of the jaws are related to dental conditions. There may be a variety of odontogenic cysts and tumors. Osteomyelitis, due to a variety of infectious agents, can occur. Although most of the tumors of the jaw are of odontogenic origin, any bone tumor potentially can affect the jaw.

The salivary glands can show nonspecific inflammation, often due to the effects of retrograde infection via the excretory ducts. There might also be specific inflammations as components of systemic disease. The most common salivary gland tumor is the pleomorphic adenoma, which is almost always benign.

Teeth and Gums *(F1–F3)*

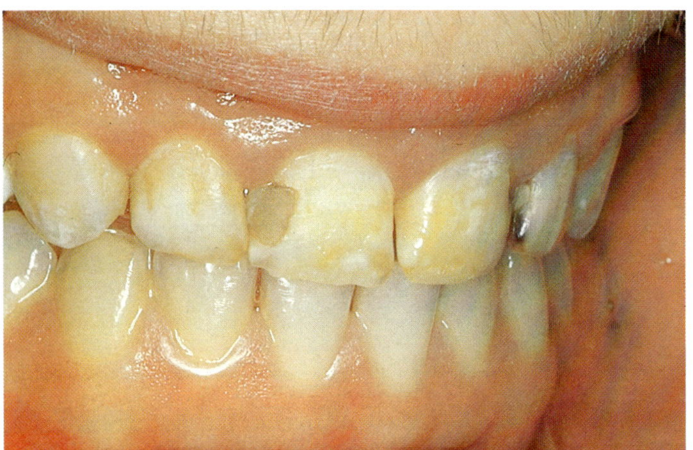

Fig. F1. Tetracycline staining of the upper incisors. This child was treated with tetracycline during infancy.

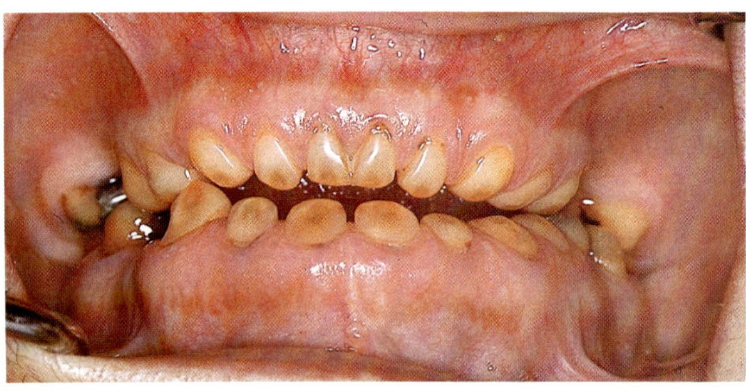

Fig. F2. Dentinogenesis imperfecta. The absence of the enamel has contributed to loss of most of the tooth structure because of relative lack of resistance to abrasions.

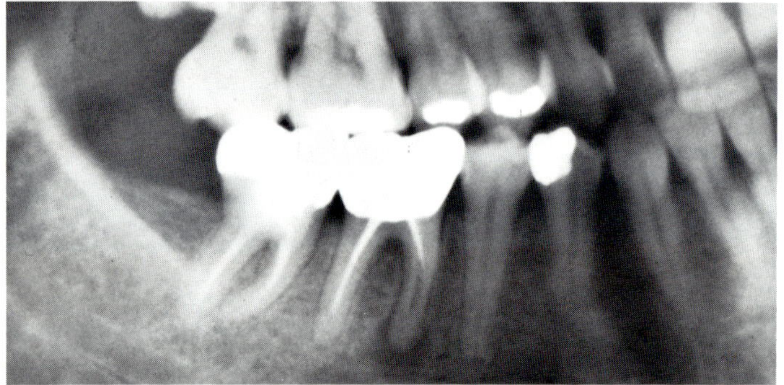

Fig. F3. Apical periodontitis. Spherical zones of bone absorption are seen at the tooth root area in this X-ray.

Oral Mucous Membranes *(F4–F12)*

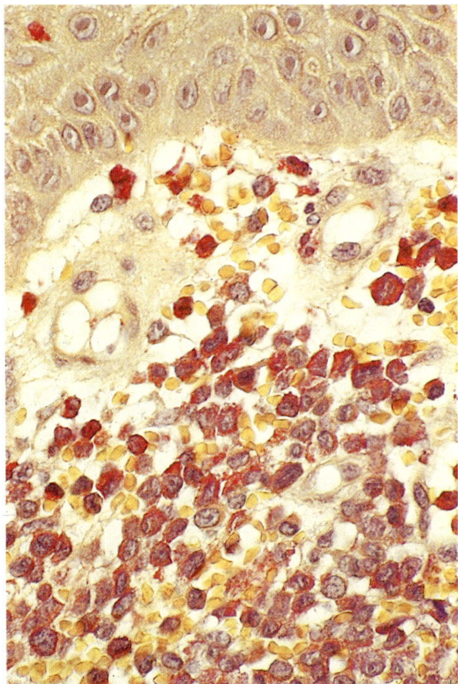

Fig. F4. Leukemic infiltration of the gingiva in a patient with acute myelogenous (granulocytic) leukemia. Many immature granulocytes, with round nonsegmented nuclei and prominent nucleoli, and containing cytoplasmic granules stained red by the chloroacetate-esterase reaction, are seen.

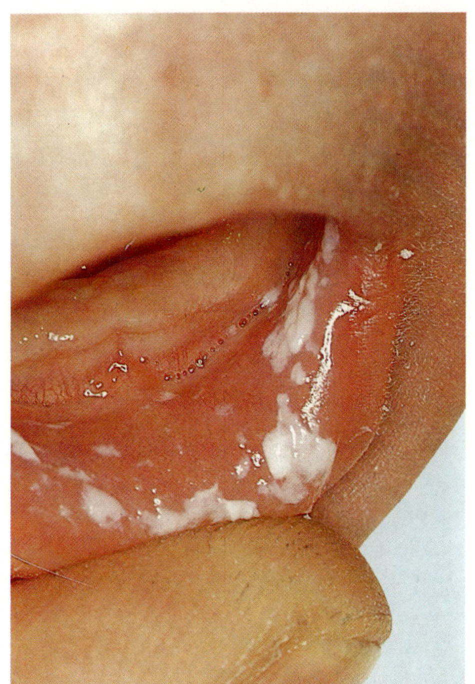

Fig. F5a. Thrush (candidiasis). The mucous membranes of this infant are covered by white, soft, friable patches which can be scraped off easily.

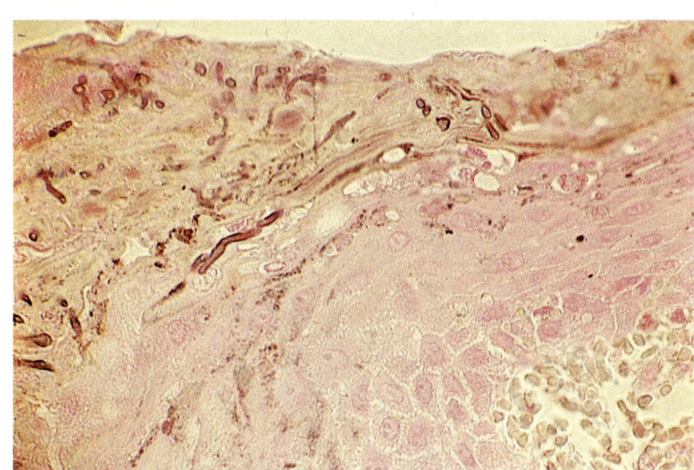

Fig. F5b. Superficial invasion of the mucous membrane epithelial cells by *Candida albicans.* The fungal hyphae stain brown-black with the silver impregnation method.

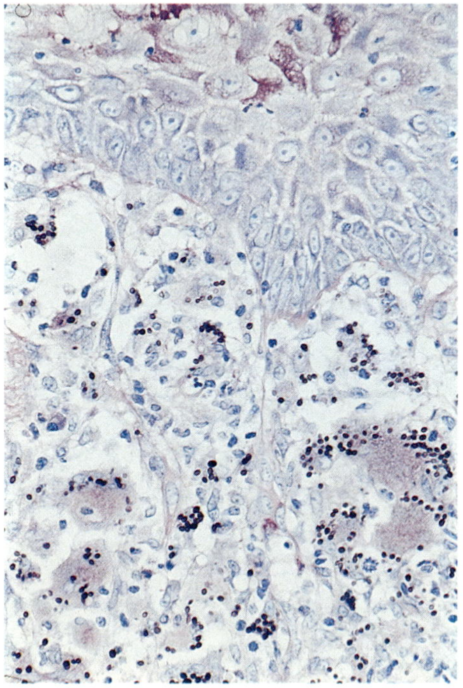

Fig. F5c. Histoplasmosis. The subepithelial tissues are extensively infiltrated by multinucleated giant cells containing masses of black staining yeast forms of *Histoplasma capsulatum.* (Grocott's silver methenamine)

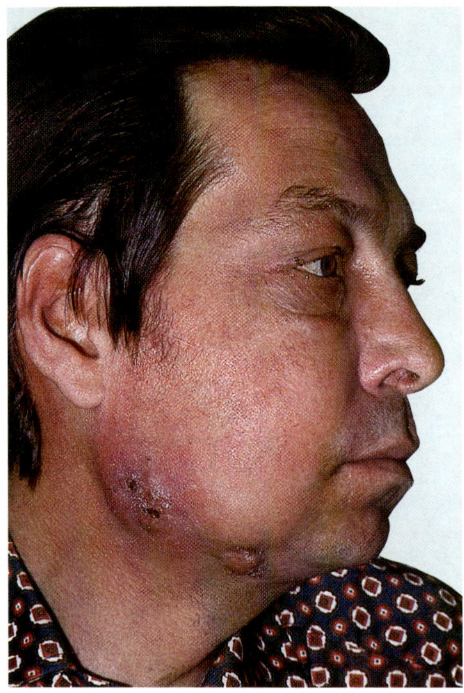

Fig. F6a. Cervicofacial actinomycosis. Multiple draining sinuses with scab formation are seen, surrounded by reddish induration and swelling.

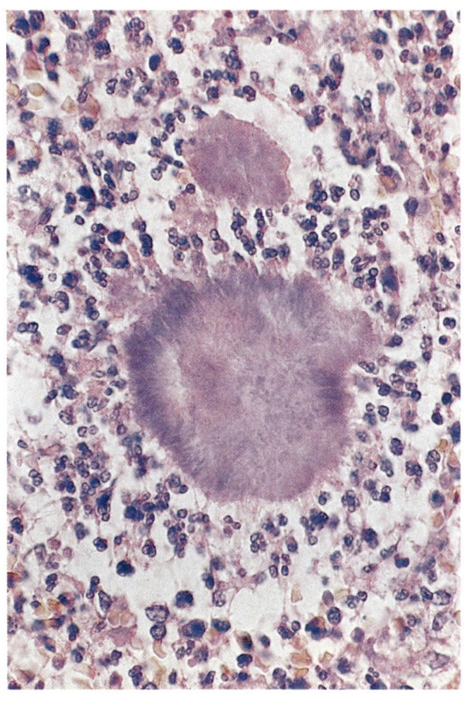

Fig. F6b. An actinomycosis granule consisting of organized aggregates of bacterial filaments of *Actinomyces israeli* surrounded by polymorphonuclear neutrophilic granulocytes and histiocytes.

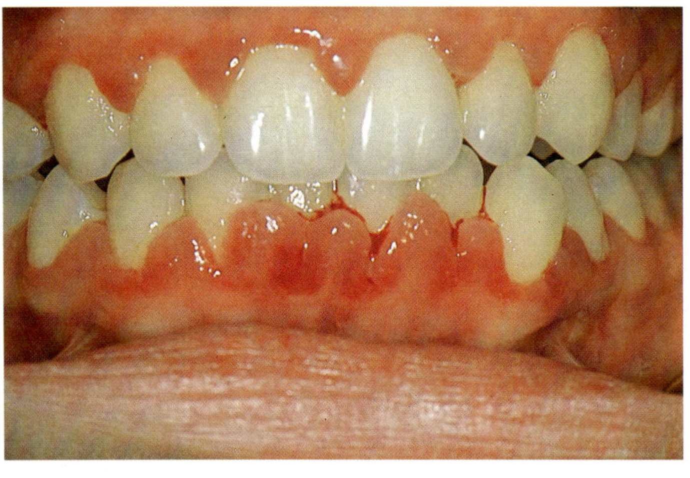

Fig. F7. Gingival hyperplasia and gingivitis of pregnancy. Bright red areas of hyperplastic gingiva, with slight bleeding, seen in the gum papilla.

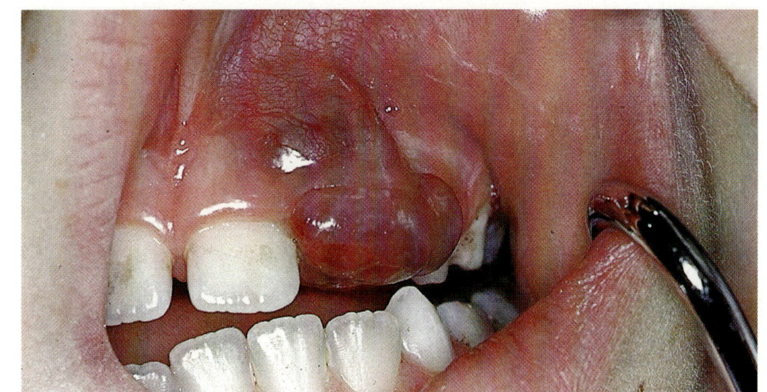

Fig. F8a. Giant cell epulis. A dark red, sharply delineated tumor fills the gum.

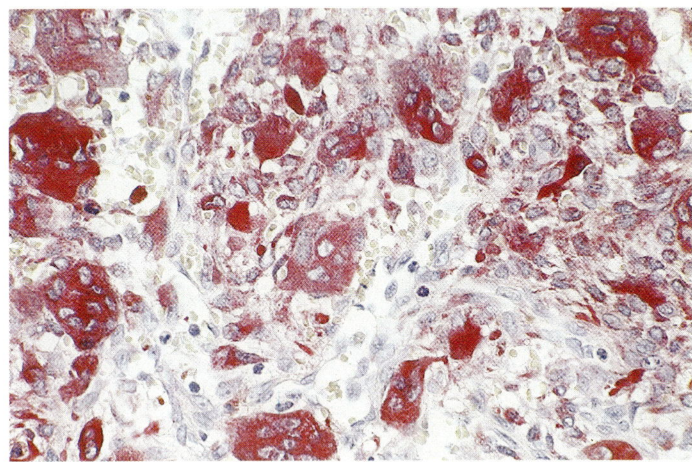

Fig. F8b. Giant cell epulis. The growth is characterized by dilated vascular spaces, a cellular component of fibroblastic cells, and multinucleated giant cells that are shown to be osteoclasts by the presence of tartrate resistant acid phosphatase (red staining).

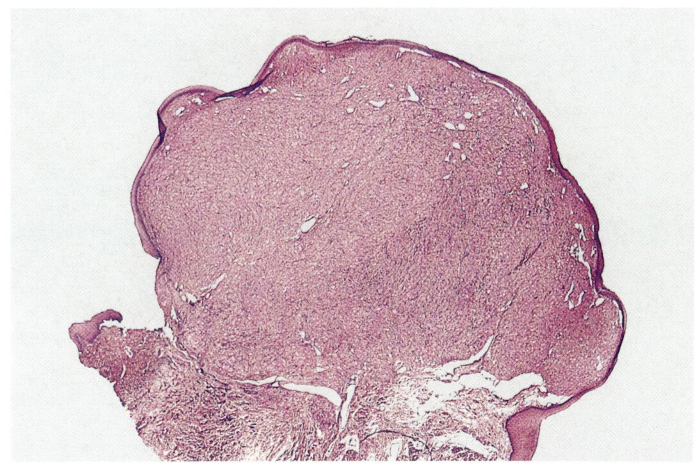

Fig. F9a. Granular cell tumor. This tumor resembled an epulis, and arose as a polypoid tumor from the alveolar ridge of the mandible.

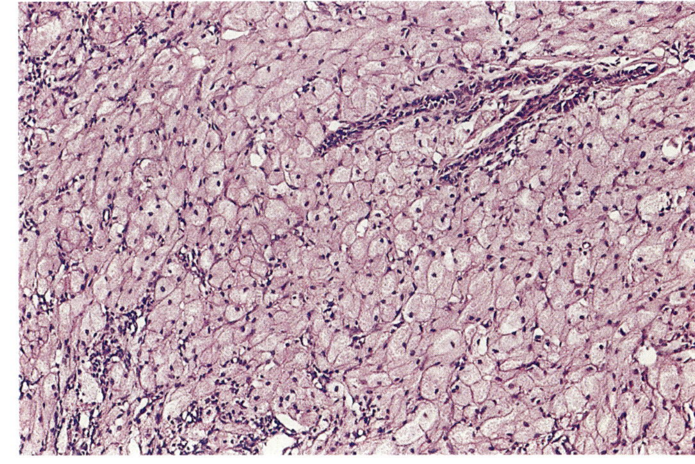

Fig. F9b. Granular cell tumor. High magnification photomicrograph of the tumor shown in *Fig. F9a*. The tumor consists of uniform, large, polyhedral tumor cells filled with granular, eosinophilic cytoplasm. At the upper right of the photomicrograph are two linear islands of residual odontogenic epithelium.

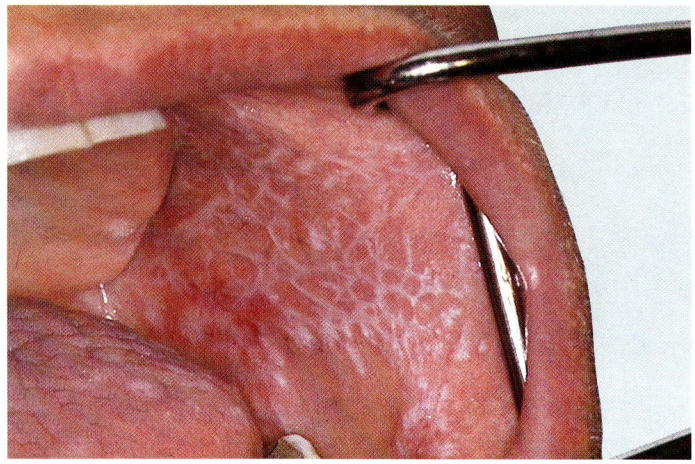

Fig. F 10a.   Lichen planus. There is an irregular, lacelike whitening of the buccal mucosa (Wickham's striae).

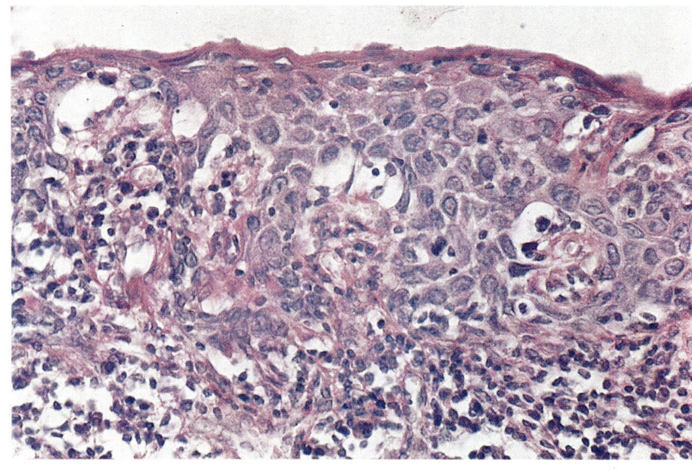

Fig. F 10b.   Lichen planus. There is liquifactive degeneration of the basal epithelial layer and a prominent subepithelial lymphocytic infiltrate.

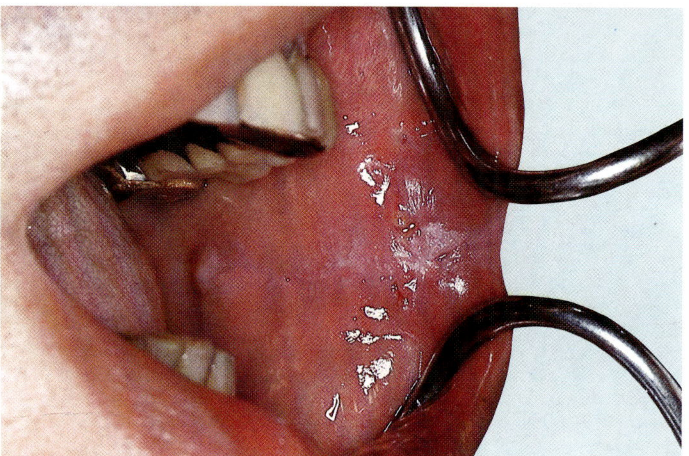

Fig. F 11a.   Leukoplakia of the mucosal aspect of the angle of the mouth. A sharply defined, elevated white lesion of the mucous membrane. Leukoplakia is a clinical, rather than a pathologic, term and does not signify a specific diagnosis.

Fig. F 11b.   Biopsy from a patient with a leukoplakia lesion showing epithelial hyperplasia and orthokeratosis with intra- and subepithelial chronic inflammatory cell infiltration, and without atypia.

Fig. F 11c.   Biopsy from another patient with a leukoplakia lesion. In this case, however, there is dysplastic epithelium with disordered squamous maturation, many atypical cells, and scattered mitoses, as well as overlying parakeratosis. Many subepithelial chronic inflammatory cells are present.

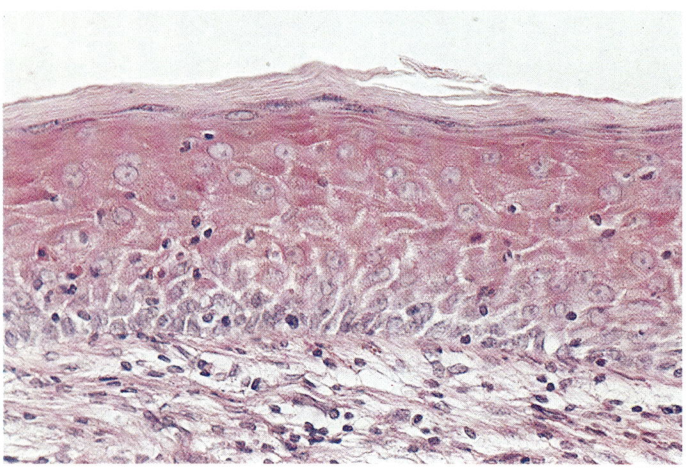

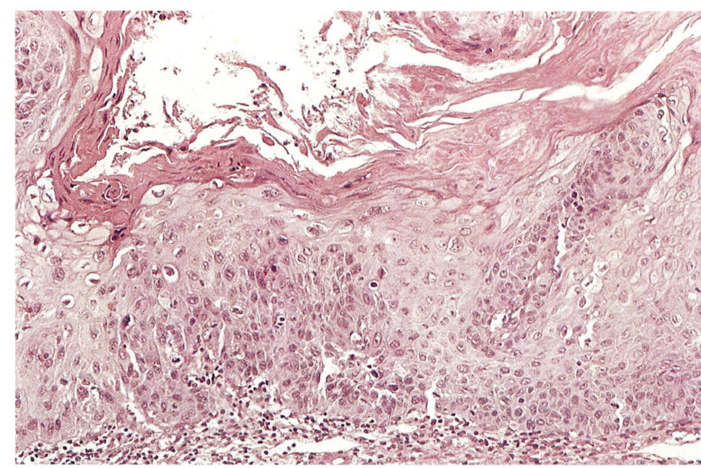

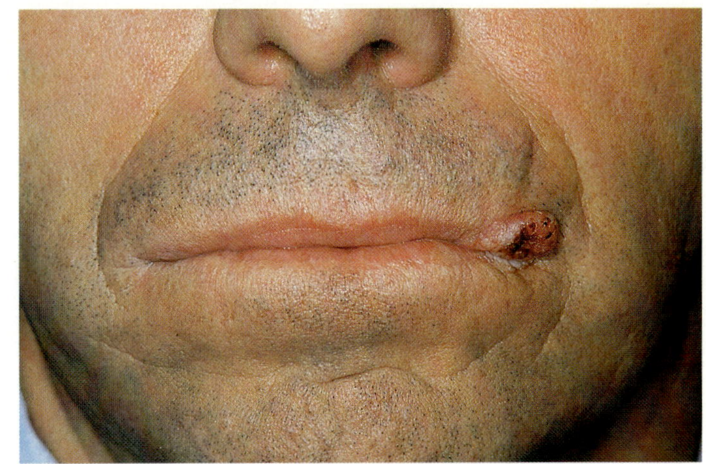

Fig. F 12 a. Squamous cell carcinoma of the lip, originating as an area of leukoplakia at the angle of the mouth.

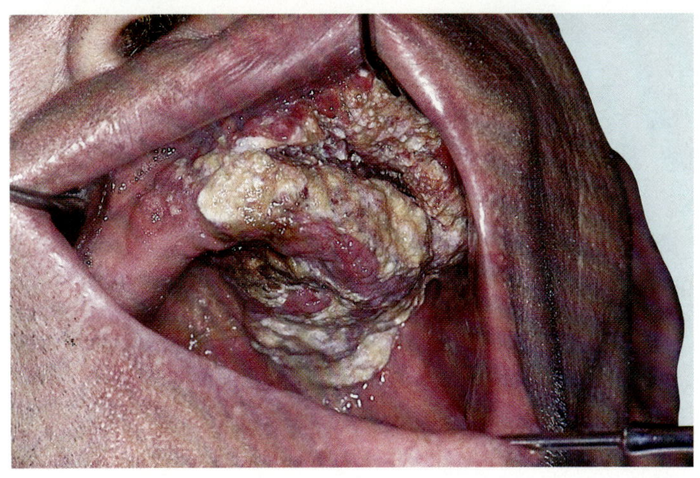

Fig. F 12 b. Extensively spreading squamous cell carcinoma of the maxillary buccal mucosa.

Fig. F 12 c. Well differentiated, but deeply infiltrating, squamous cell carcinoma. Masses of almost completely acellular keratin are obvious.

Fig. F 12 d. Poorly differentiated, non-keratinizing, invasive squamous cell carcinoma. Innumerable mitoses are seen, consistent with the rapid proliferation of this tumor. At the lower portion of the photomicrograph, tumor is seen within a blood vessel. The tumor cells are partially surrounded by red thrombus formation.

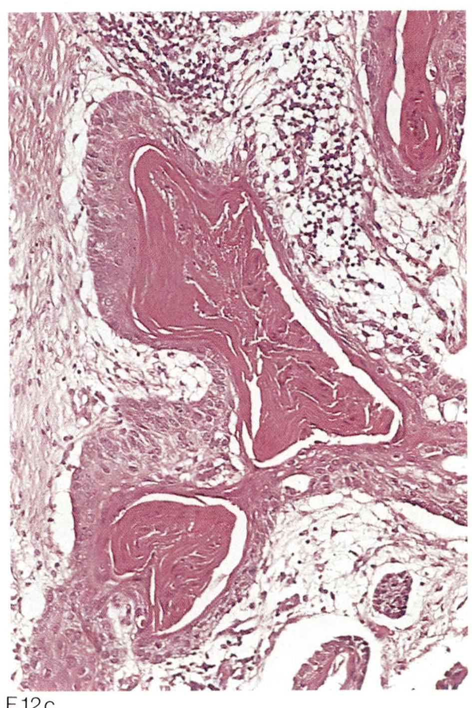

F 12 c

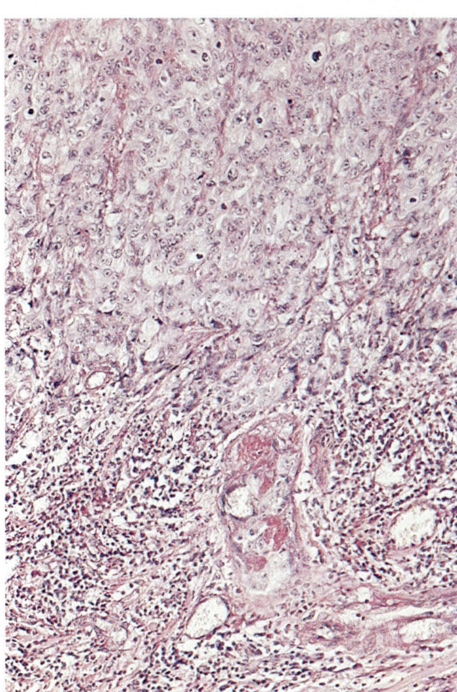

F 12 d

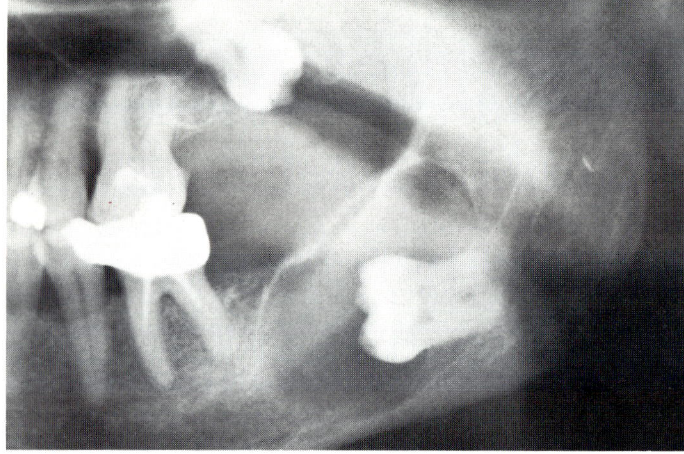

F 13

Fig. F 13. Odontogenic cyst with associated impacted wisdom tooth. The cyst is sharply delineated from the surrounding tissue and has almost broken through the mandibular bone.

Fig. F 14. Multiple odontogenic cysts in a patient with Gorlin-Goltz syndrome (odontogenic cysts, hypertelorism, anomalous ribs, ovarian fibromas, and other features). A large right mandibular cyst has displaced a tooth anlage. A medium sized cyst is at the mandibular midline. A large cyst, without clearly defined borders, in the right maxilla, has markedly displaced the tooth. There is also a wide cyst in the interdental space between teeth number three and four in the left mandible.
Note: The right side of the jaw is to the left in this X-ray.

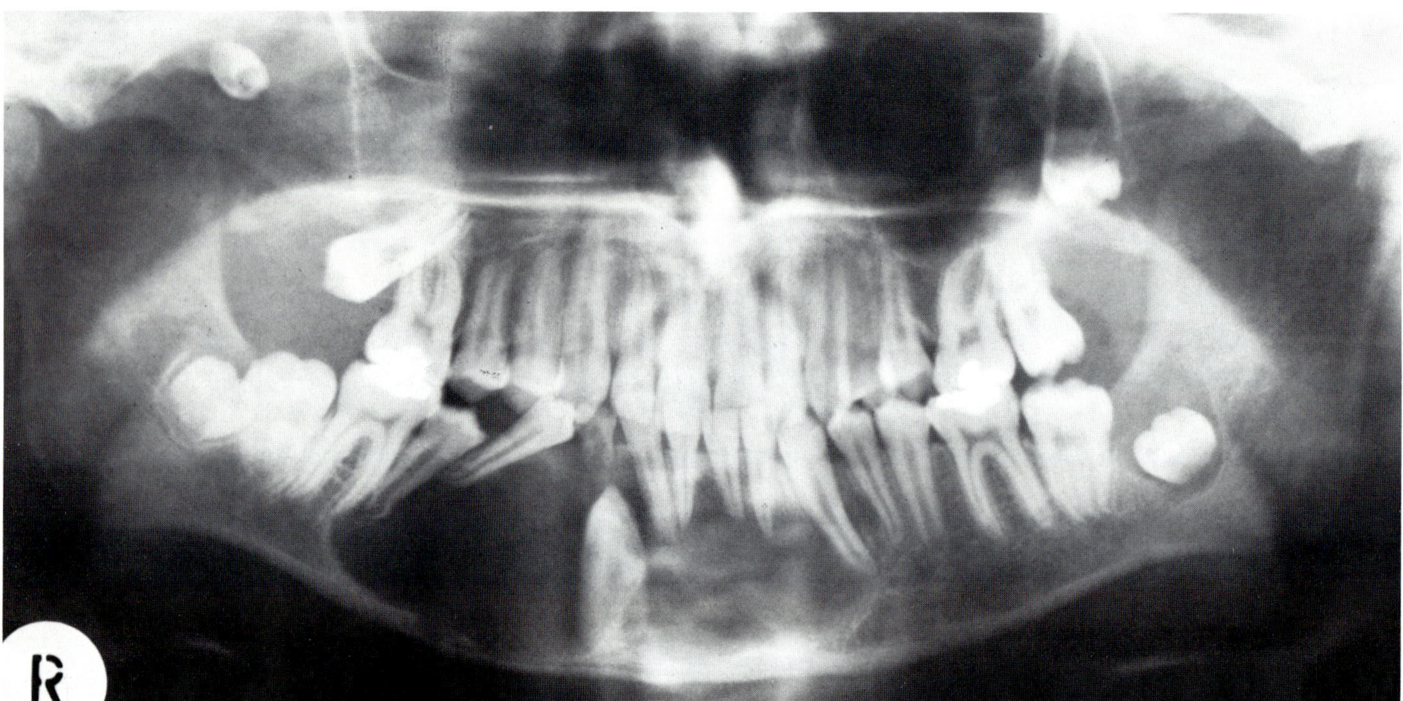

F 14

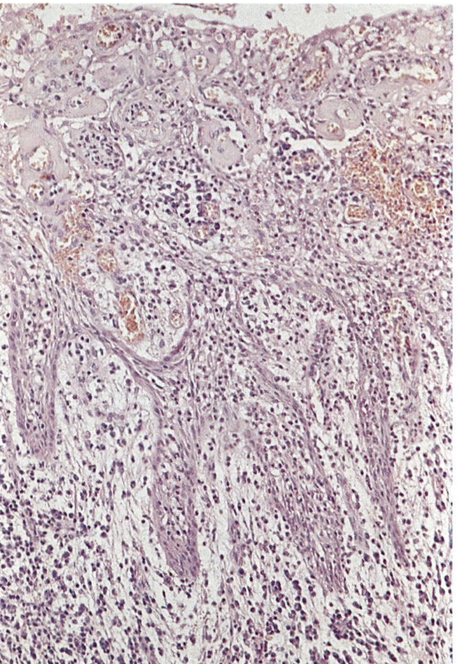

F 15

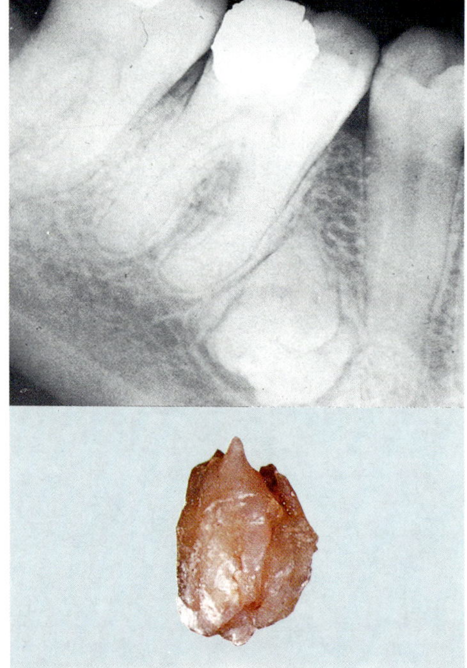

F 16

Fig. F 15. Histologic section of the wall of radicular cysts, presenting at the apex of an erupted tooth. There is intense infiltration by lymphocytes and plasma cells, in both the stratified squamous epithelium and the subepithelial tissues.

Fig. F 16. Odontoma. An interdental, radiologically visible (upper photograph) tumor with the corresponding surgical specimen (lower photograph).

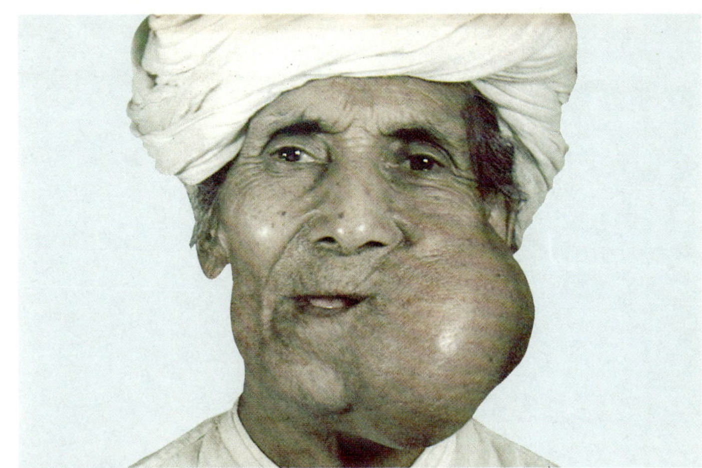

Fig. F17a. Ameloblastoma. This large, slowly growing tumor has been present for a long time.

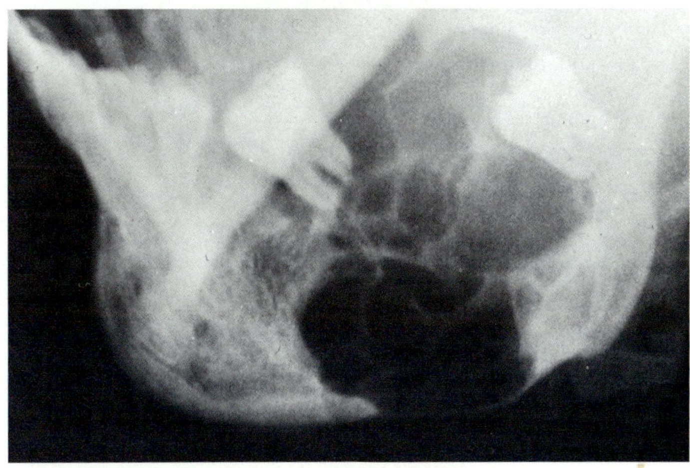

Fig. F17b. Ameloblastoma. The radiograph shows a multiloculated cystic lesion with extensive destruction of the mandible.

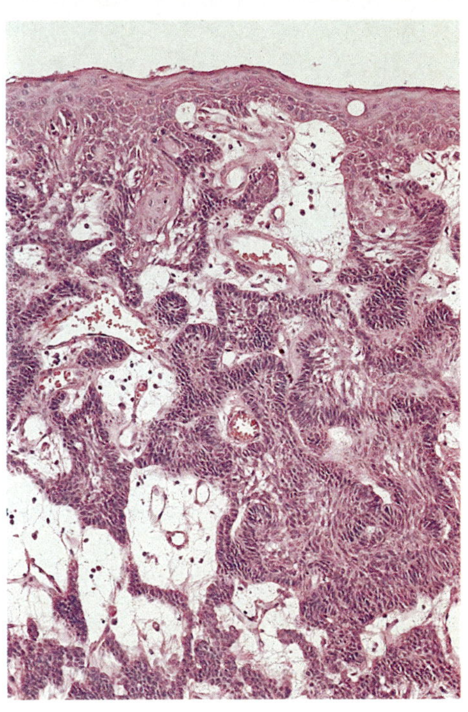

Fig. F17c. Ameloblastoma. The gingival membrane overlies the tumor which consists of islands and connecting cords of odontogenic epithelium in a connective tissue stroma.

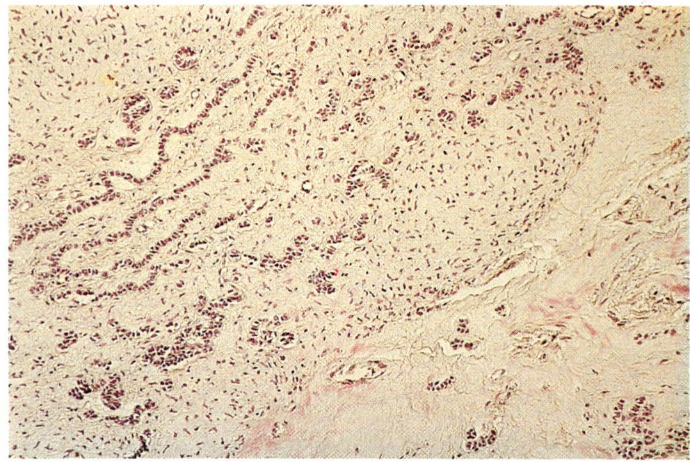

Fig. F18. Ameloblastic fibroma. Strands and small clusters of cuboid epithelial cells are enmeshed in a cellular tissue stroma. This tumor is not aggressive, in contrast to ameloblastoma, and can usually be treated by curettage, rather than resection.

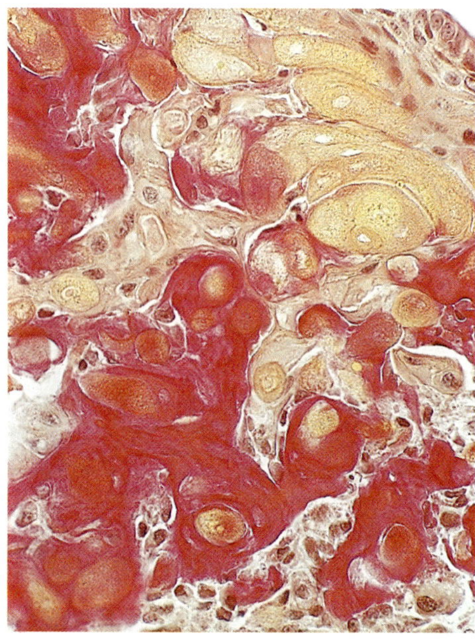

Fig. F19. Calcifying epithelium odontogenic tumor. This relatively rare tumor can be invasive and can recur locally. Degeneration of the polyhedral epithelical cells leads to numerous spherical spaces which are filled with eosinophilic homogenous material that ultimately becomes calcified and ossified. Osteoid is seen as red staining material.   (van Gieson)

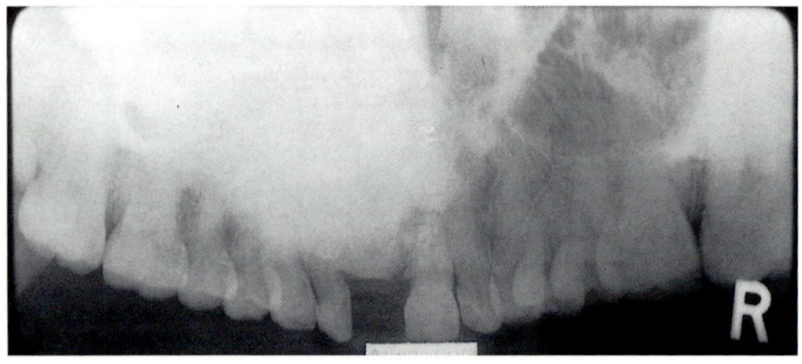

Fig. F20a. Ossifying fibroma of the maxilla seen, in this radiograph, as a compact, sharply outlined structure. The osteolytic zone is marked by radioopaque flecks of bone formation.

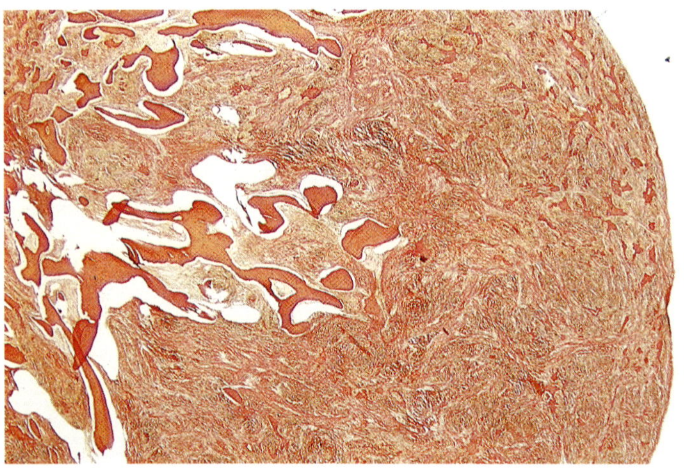

Fig. F20b. Ossifying fibroma with beginning bone formation in the fibrous tissue component at the periphery of the tumor, and mature spongy bone at the center of the tumor.

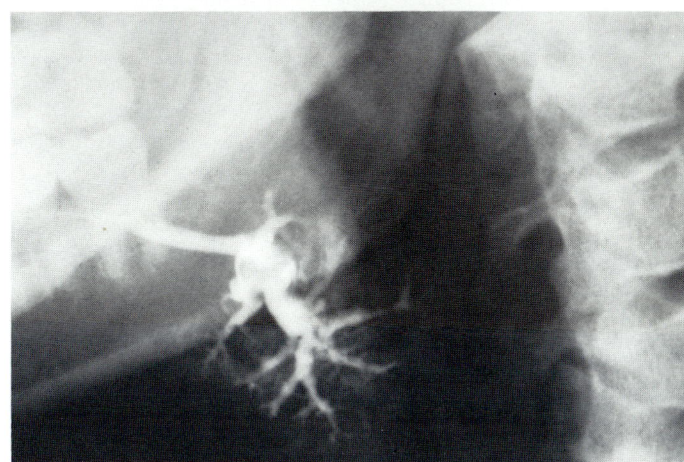

Fig. F21a.   Subacute sialadenitis of the submandibular gland. The sialogram shows an intact, finely ramifying duct system with fluffy opacities filling multiple lobules of the gland.

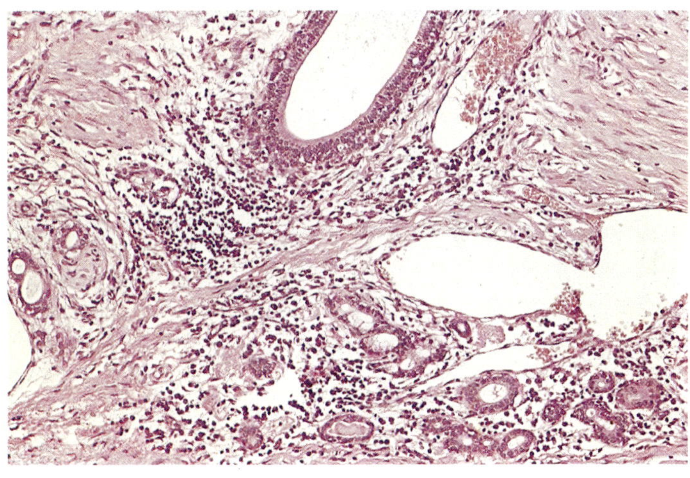

Fig. F21b.   Chronic atrophic sialadenitis of the submandibular gland, with sialolithiasis. The sialogram shows an irregularly dilated duct system, with no filling of the peripheral portions of the gland. At the upper pole a stone fills the primary duct and is seen as a relatively clear zone which displaces contrast material. The peripheral portions of the gland are not visualized.

Fig. F21c.   Nonspecific chronic sialadenitis with marked dilatation of ducts, extensive glandular atrophy, and chronic inflammatory cell infiltration, consisting mostly of lymphocytes and plasma cells. In addition, there is diffuse interstitial fibrosis.

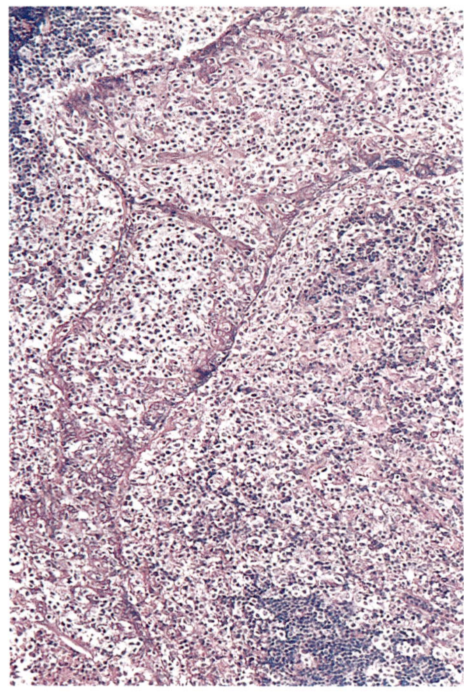

Fig. F22. Benign lymphoepithelial lesion (Mikulicz's disease). The acinar tissue is replaced by sheets of lymphocytes and histiocytes, with epimyoepithelial islands, arising from ductal proliferation, scattered throughout.

Salivary Gland Tumors *(F23–F28)*

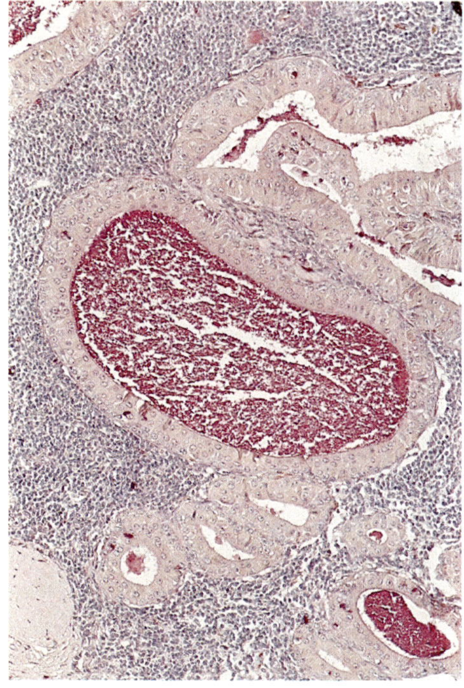

Fig. F23. Papillary cystadenoma lymphomatosum (Warthin's tumor). This benign tumor is well encapsulated and consists of tubular and cystic spaces lined with tall, nonciliated, columnar cells with oxyphilic granular cytoplasm and intervening lymphoid tissue. The spaces usually contain amorphous, granular debris, most likely derived from the epithelial cells. In this case the gland spaces are filled with granulocytes, stained red with the chloroacetate esterase reaction, perhaps as a sequel to infection.

Fig. F24 a. Pleomorphic adenoma (mixed tumor) of the parotid gland. This tumor is seen as a swelling of the face at the anterior aspect of the lower portion of the ear. The ear lobe is deflected outward. The patient did not complain of pain.

Fig. F24 b. Pleomorphic adenoma of the parotid gland. Epithelial cells are present individually, in clusters, and forming acini and cystic structures. The stroma consist of mucopolysaccharides with foci of cartilaginous transformation.

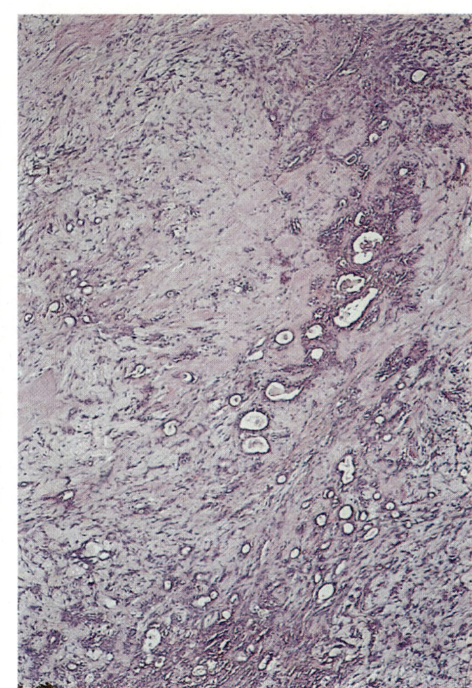

F24a

F24b

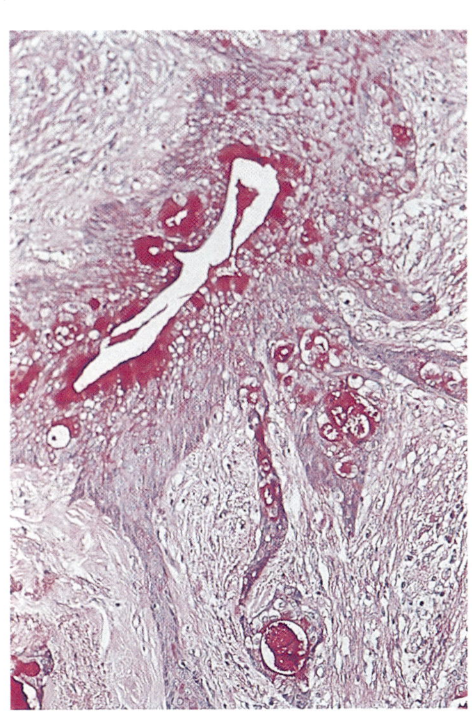

Fig. F25. Mucoepidermoid carcinoma with a mixture of squamous epithelial cells and mucous secreting glandular structures. The mucous secreting cells stain intensely red with the PAS reaction.

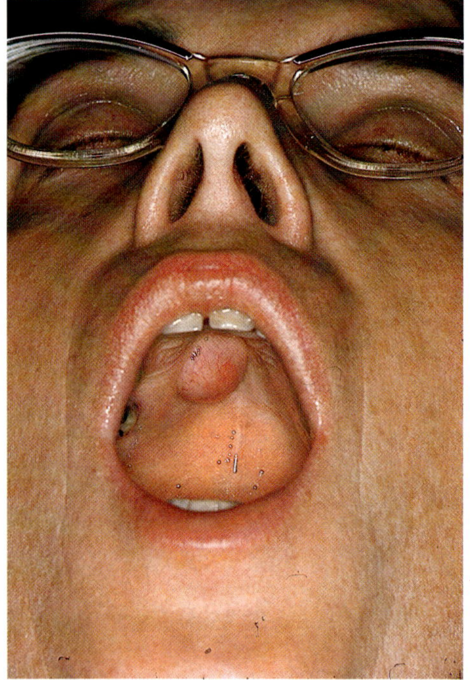

Fig. F26a. Adenoid cystic carcinoma (cylindroma) of the palate. The tumor arises from minor salivary glands in the palate.

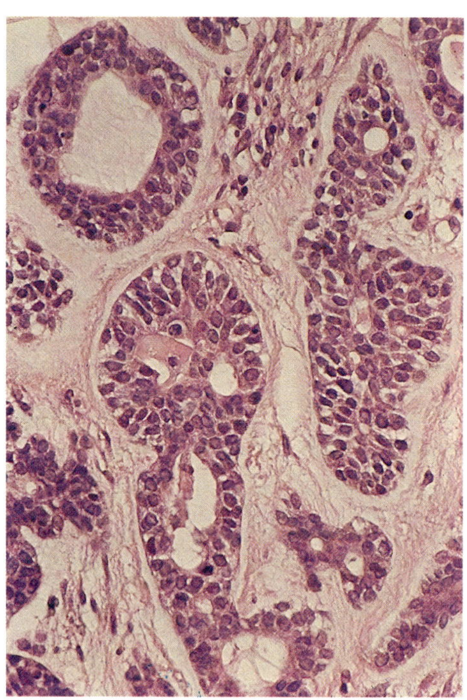

Fig. F26b. Adenoid cystic carcinoma (cylindroma) with typical cribriform and solid glandular patterns.

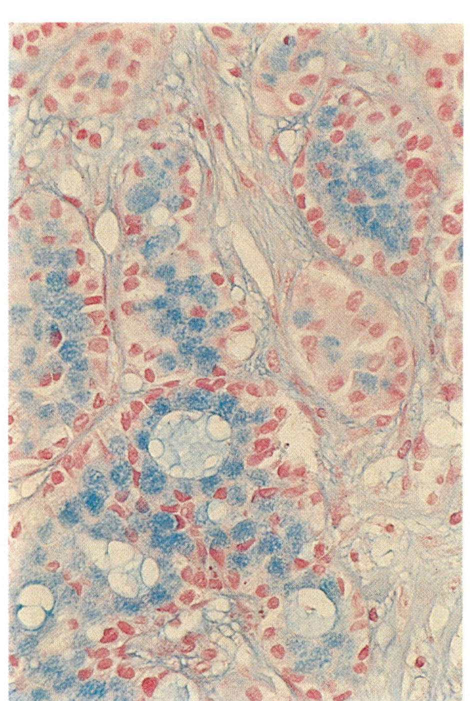

Fig. F27. Acinic cell tumor arising in the submandibular gland. Metastases were seen, in spite of the fact the tumor appears well differentiated. Mucous-secreting cells stain blue with the alcian blue method.

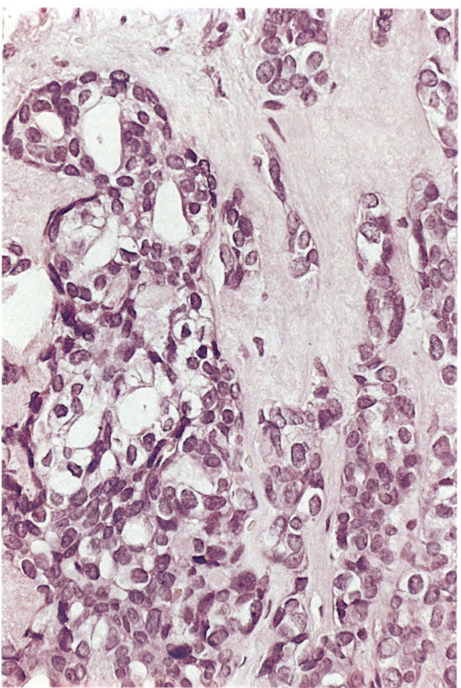

Fig. F28. Adenocarcinoma arising from the parotid gland. This malignancy arose from a pleomorphic adenoma. Atypical epithelial cells form distorted glandular structures. Mitotic activity is increased.

G. Gastrointestinal Tract

W. Oehlert

Diseases of the esophagus are unique. Despite the fact that the epithelium is the same as that of the oral cavity, most of the conditions that affect the intestinal tract do not occur in the mouth. Because the esophagus is a narrow tube, many of the disorders, both benign and malignant, cause obstruction to the transport of food and may be painful. Inflammations of the esophagus occur because of the ingestion of corrosive materials or because of the reflux of acid stomach contents. Carcinomas are not uncommon and tend to occur at the areas of constriction of the lumen. Virtually all of the malignancies of the esophagus are squamous cell carcinomas with varying degrees of differentiation. Adenocarcinoma can occur in the esophagus as a complication of the reparative re-epithelialization of the inflamed esophagus with columnar epithelium (Barrett's esophagus).

Gastric mucosa is also sensitive to exogenous corrosive agents. More common, however, are erosions and ulcers, which are thought to be related to endogenous factors. Gastritis is particularly common and can be evaluated, in terms of intensity of inflammation, by biopsy. Gastritis, if prolonged, can lead to mucosal atrophy and, in some cases, hypertrophy. Carcinoma of the stomach, which is more prevalent in the Orient, has a variety of presentations. Early carcinoma of the stomach is limited to the mucosa or submucosa and does not infiltrate the muscular coat. Patients with early gastric carcinoma can recover well and survive for years after diagnosis. In general, however, gastric carcinoma is highly malignant.

The stomach can also be affected by a variety of benign tumors.

The small intestine is less frequently the site of tumor formation. Carcinoid tumors, which are uncommon, are seen most often in the appendix and small intestine. A variety of infectious agents can cause small intestinal inflammation. Crohn's disease, the etiology of which is unknown, is particularly important and has characteristic gross and histologic features. Malabsorption can be due to severe mucosal inflammation and atrophy secondary to gluten sensitivity, or can be due to Whipple's disease.

Similarly, the large intestine can show a variety of inflammatory conditions. Appendiceal inflammation, of course, is most common. Ulcerative colitis, which is a diffuse inflammation of the entire large bowel, is an uncommon but important condition. One of the complications of chronic inflammation is the development of premalignant, and ultimately malignant, changes. The development of colon carcinoma, in these patients, might be preceded by recognizable dysplasia. Colonic polyps are common in the population at large and are the precursor lesion for colonic adenocarcinoma. Congenital disorders of the colon are relatively uncommon and generally manifest early in childhood.

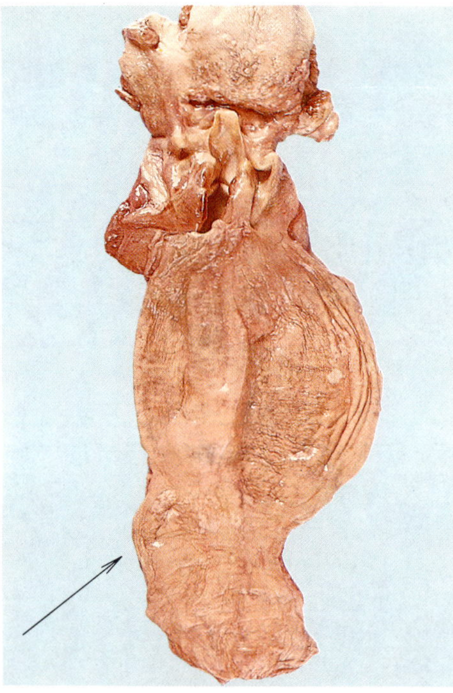

Fig. G1.   Achalasia. The upper two-thirds of the esophagus is dilated markedly and there is an area of stenosis in the lower portion *(arrow)*. Microscopically, there are no ganglion cells in the smooth muscle portion of the esophageal wall. The loss of ganglion cells in Auerbach's plexus is a consistent finding in achalasia, although the etiology of this, in most cases, is not known. A similar condition occurs as a complication of Chaga's disease. Achalasia is associated with long-term, chronic inflammation, and can be complicated further by irregular squamous hyperplasia and dysplasia, seen as leukoplakia-like white patches.

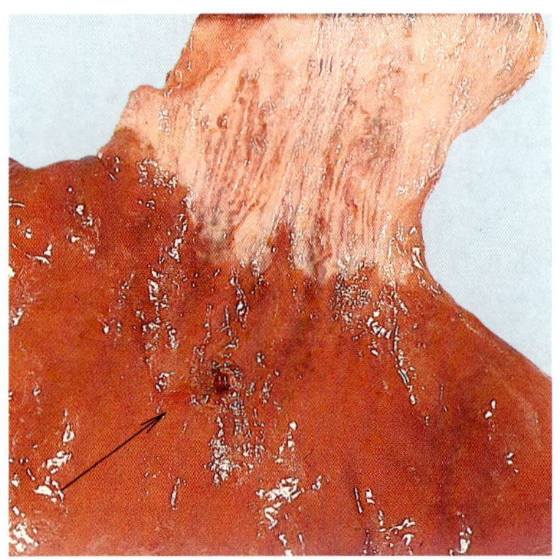

Fig. G2.   Esophageal varices with ulceration into a dilated vein *(arrow)*. Longitudinal, parallel venous varicosities are present at the cardioesophageal junction. When the mucosa is eroded, as at the area of ulceration, varices can bleed copiously. Esophageal varices occur most often as a complication of portal hypertension in the setting of hepatic cirrhosis.

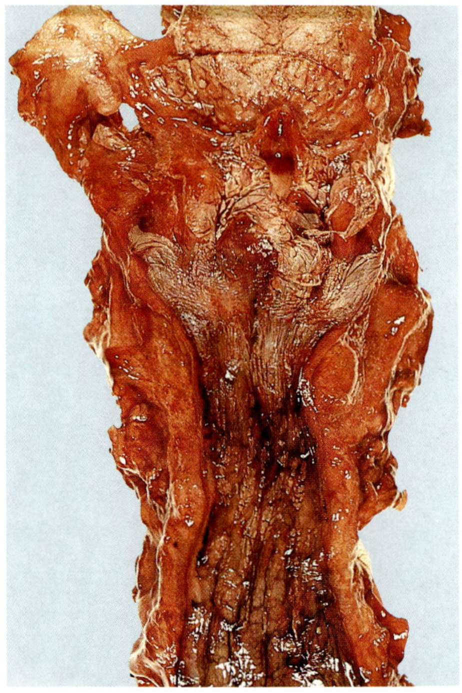

Fig. G3.   Erosive esophagitis following suicidal ingestion of hydrochloric acid. The usual white stratified squamous mucosa is almost completely absent and the esophageal lumen is irregularly and extensively ulcerated and hemorrhagic.

Fig. G4. Chronic reflux esophagitis. The surface epithelium is irregular, infiltrated by clusters of granulocytes, with small collections of necrotic debris and fibrin in areas. The epithelium is thickened and there is orderly proliferation of the basal and parabasal epithelial layers. Compare this photomicrograph with *Fig. G7a,* where the proliferation is disorderly.

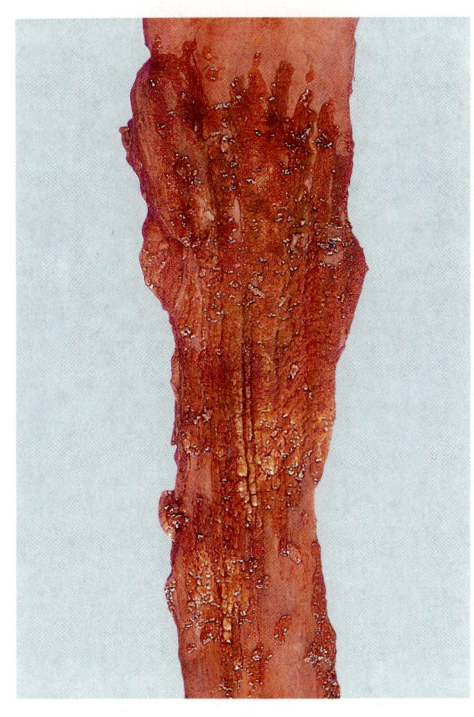

Fig. G5. Esophageal candidiasis. The usual white stratified squamous mucosa is seen only at the upper and lower portions of the esophagus. Most of the mucosa is eroded and hemorrhagic, with scattered pink and grey islands in which hyphae of Candida are admixed with necrotic debris and inflammatory cells.

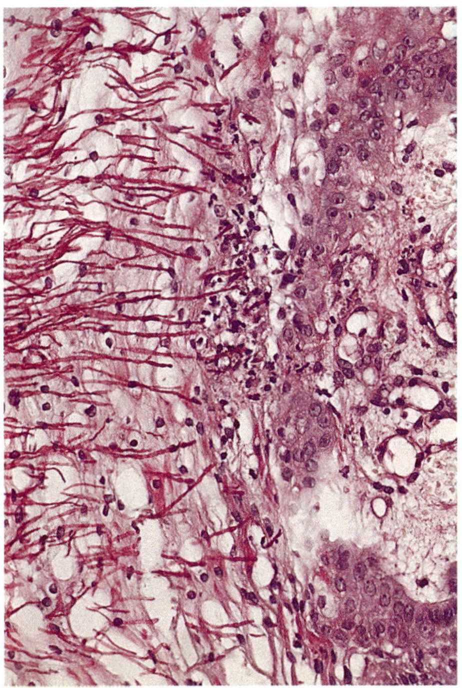

Fig. G6. Esophageal candidiasis. The histologic section has been stained with the periodic acid-Schiff reagent. Within the background of necrotic debris and pale pink fibrin the dark red invasive elongated chains of Candida hyphae are evident. A remnant of the basal layer of the esophageal epithelium is seen as a curved band of squamous cells extending, in this photomicrograph, from the right upper to the right lower corner. The extension of the fungi into the submucosa can lead to vascular invasion and subsequent dissemination.

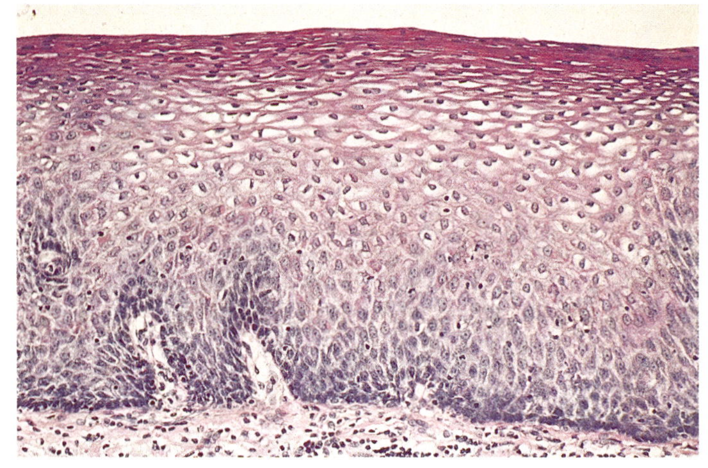

Fig. G7a. Normal esophageal mucosa. The stratified squamous epithelium is noncornified and there is an orderly pattern of maturation from the basal to the superficial cells. As the cells mature to the surface they gain more cytoplasm and the nuclei become less prominent. In addition the nuclear axis shifts so that the nuclei lie parallel to the basement membrane rather than in the perpendicular orientation seen in the parabasal and prickle cell layers. At the surface the cells have considerable glycogen, seen as red cytoplasmic material in this PAS reaction.

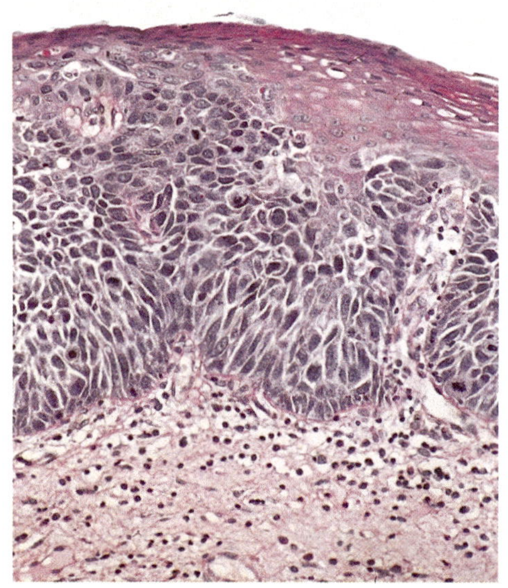

Fig. G7b. Severe esophageal dysplasia. Compare this photomicrograph with the normal *(Fig. G7a)* and with the reactive epithelium of chronic esophagitis *(Fig. G4)*. The orderly maturation of the normal epithelium is not seen. Instead the epithelium has an irregular arrangement of large atypical cells with nuclear hyperchromatism and pleomorphism, and increased nuclear-cytoplasmic ratio. The large cells extend to the surface, at the upper left of the photomicrograph. There are scattered mitoses. These are the changes of severe dysplasia and, when the epithelium is completely replaced, carcinoma in situ. In most of these cases, carcinoma will follow.

Esophageal Carcinoma   *(G8–G10)*

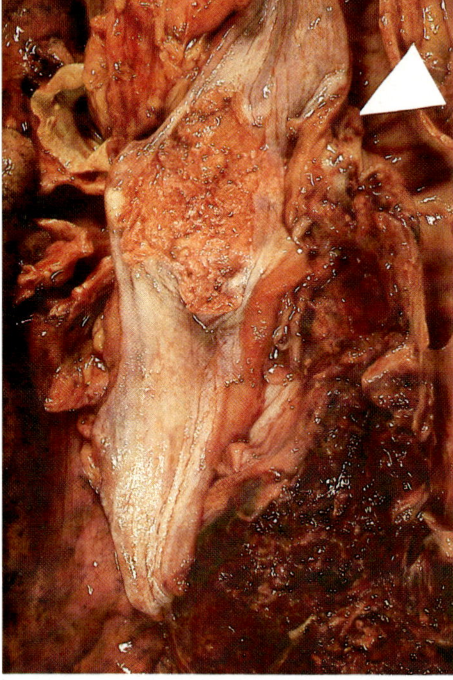

Fig. G8. Exophytic esophageal carcinoma occurring in the middle third. The mucosa is intact above and below the tumor, but completely destroyed in the area of the tumor, which is centrally ulcerated with polypoid excrescences at its periphery. The esophageal wall can be seen in cross-section in the area of the large arrow and is completely infiltrated by tumor, which extends to the adventitia of the esophagus. This patient presented with progressive dysphagia.

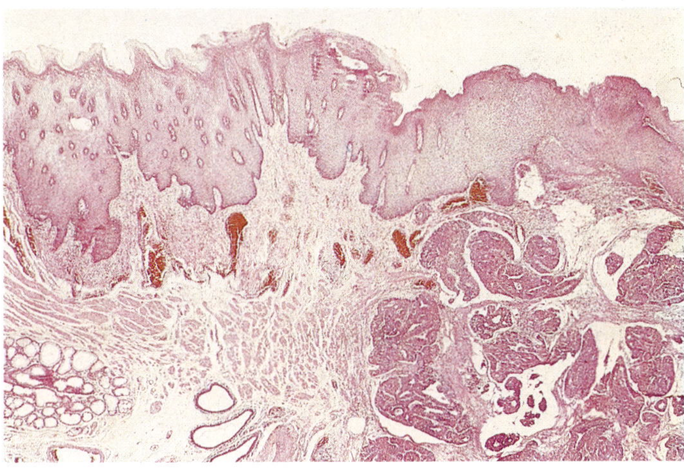

Fig. G9. Poorly differentiated squamous cell carcinoma of the esophagus. There is extensive infiltration by irregular nests of malignant cells which have an increased nuclear-cytoplasmic ratio, along with hyperchromatic and pleomorphic nuclei. In the center of these malignant islands there is some maturation, and a keratin pearl *(see Fig. E32a)* is present at the lower left, stained red with PAS reaction. Below this is a bizarre, multipolar mitotic figure.

Fig. G10. Adenocarcinoma at the distal esophagus. The stratified squamous epithelium of the esophagus is intact but, at the right, there is submucosal extension of nests of moderately well differentiated adenocarcinoma. This carcinoma arises in the gastrocardiac mucosa but presents, with progressive dysphagia, as a lower esophageal carcinoma. Adenocarcinoma is a more common cause of dysphagia at this site than is squamous cell carcinoma. Higher in the esophagus, adenocarcinoma can develop as a consequence of longstanding chronic esophagitis in which the mucosa is replaced by columnar epithelium (Barrett's esophagus).

Disorders of the Stomach *(G11–G20)*

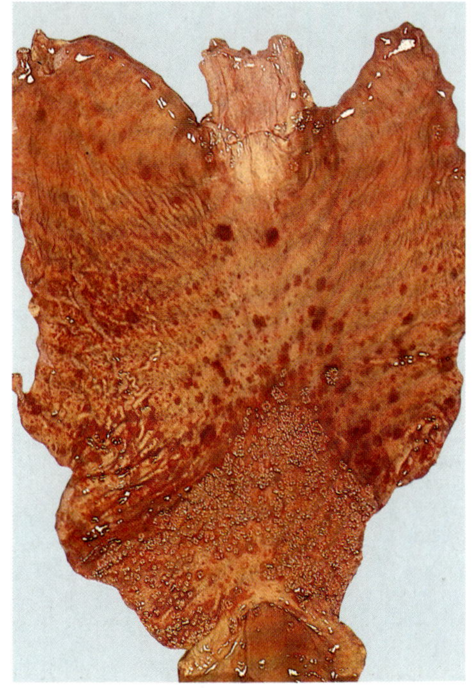

Fig. G11. Multiple gastric erosions. The gastric mucosa is marked by dark red areas. The color is due to the acid digestion of blood. The erosions are typically found on the rugal folds. The number of erosions is variable and there can be considerable acute bleeding when the erosions progress to ulceration and affect blood vessels. This pattern of erosion has been ascribed to stress and is sometimes seen in patients treated for prolonged periods of time with relatively high doses of corticosteroids.

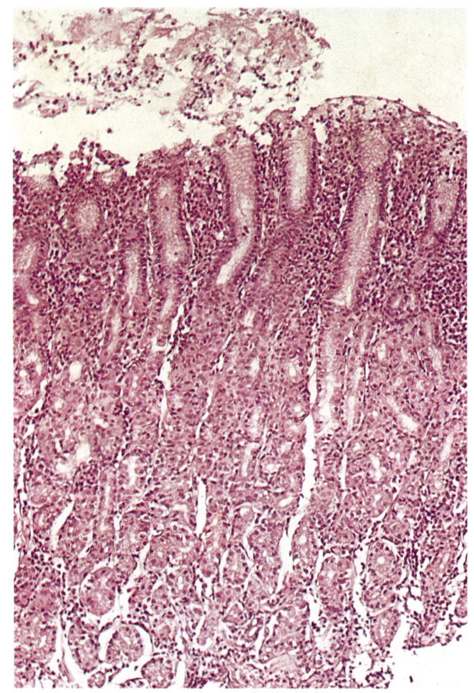

Fig. G 12. Acute gastritis with superficial erosion. An inflammatory exudate, consisting of acute inflammatory cells and fibrin, is on the surface and inflammatory cells infiltrate the superficial gastric mucosa. The covering epithelial layers are lost. This can progress to frank ulcer formation. Acute gastritis can follow ingestion of various substances (alcohol, salicylates, corrosive agents) or irradiation, can be due to viral or bacterial infections, or, in most individuals, can be associated with stress and subsequent excess gastric acid secretions.   (hematoxylin-eosin)

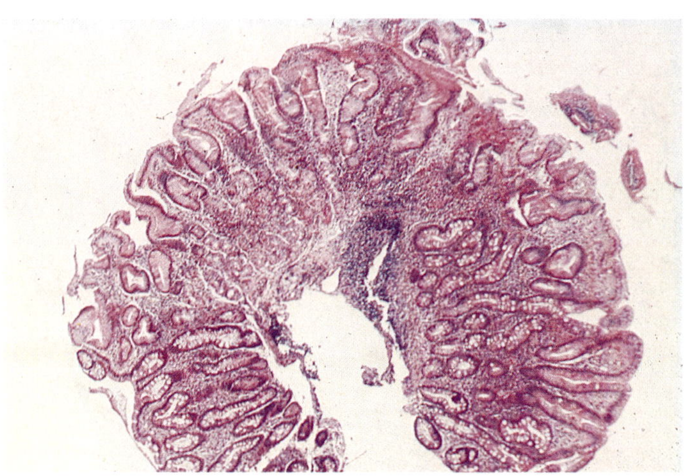

Fig. G 13. Chronic gastritis with moderate glandular atrophy and intestinal metaplasia. The entire mucosa is infiltrated by chronic inflammatory cells and there is a lymphoid aggregate at the lower central portion of the gastric biopsy specimen. The gastric body glands are reduced markedly in number and the pits are shortened. To the right and left, many goblet cells can be seen as indications of intestinal metaplasia. Individuals with intestinal metaplasia as a consequence of chronic gastritis are at increased risk for the development of gastric carcinoma.   (hematoxylin-eosin)

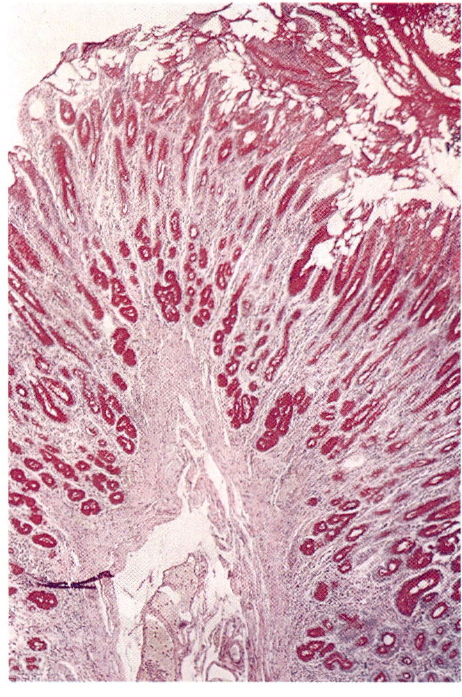

Fig. G 14. Hypertrophic gastritis (Ménétrier's disease). The gastric mucosa is markedly hyperplastic with proliferation of the surface epithelium and lengthening of the gastric pits. The macroscopic appearance is that of marked prominence of the gastric rugae, often having a cerebriform appearance. Because of the elaborate mucosal surface, there can be considerable loss of proteins and electrolytes.   (PAS)

Fig. G 15. Intestinal metaplasia of gastric mucosa. After loss of the usual gastric epithelium, the mucosa is repopulated by intestinal types of cells. The gastric pits are elongated and a villus pattern (upper right) is seen. There are many goblet cells containing neutral mucin, which stains red with the PAS reaction. Intestinal metaplasia frequently follows chronic gastritis *(see Fig. G 13)* and is a precursor for the development of gastric adenocarcinoma.

Fig. G 16. Acute erosion of the gastric body mucosa. The surface epithelium is missing and the superficial capillaries are markedly ectatic and filled with red blood cells. The area of mucosal defect is covered partially by a layer of pale eosinophilic fibrin. The basis for this type of erosion is often hard to determine. In the experimental setting, this can be induced by aspirin, taurocholic acid, and histamine. Erosion can be prevented by the use of prostaglandins. (hematoxylin-eosin)

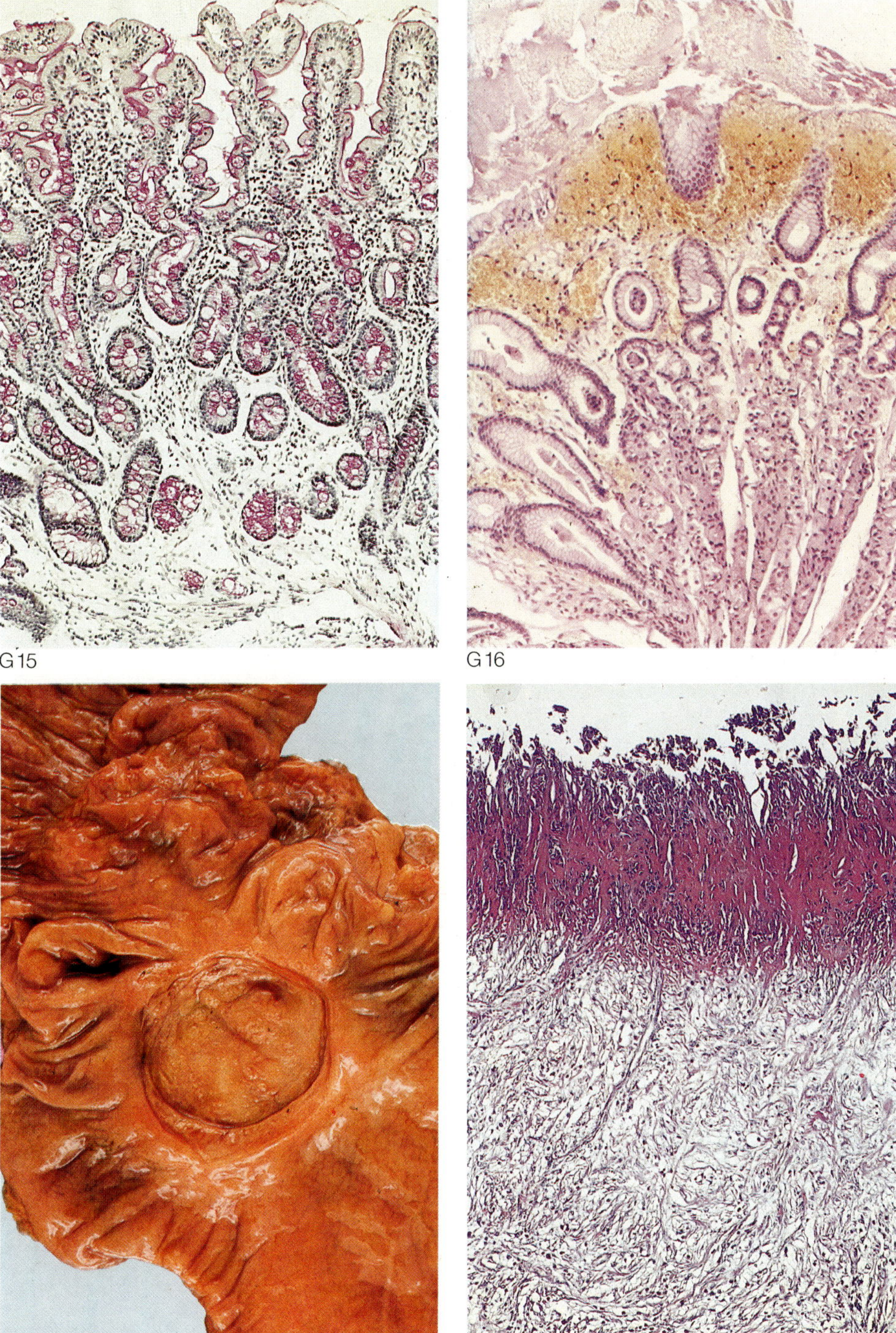

G 15

G 16

G 17

G 18

Fig. G 17. Chronic ulcer of the gastric antrum. The pyloric ring is just above the ulcer and duodenum is to the upper left. The ulcer is round with a sharply delineated border and a flat ulcer base (compare to *Fig. G 21*). There is considerable fibrosis of the ulcer base, not easily appreciated in this view, indicative of chronicity. A bleeding vessel is at the upper right portion of the ulcer. This stomach was obtained at autopsy from a patient who died of massive gastrointestinal hemorrhage from this ulcer.

Fig. G 18. Typical appearance of the base of a gastric ulcer. The surface consists of amorphous material, nuclear fragments, fibrin, and inflammatory cells. The red band consists mostly of fibrin and results from the direct necrotizing effects of acid gastric juice on the epithelium. Beneath this layer there is abundant granulation tissue, consisting of capillaries and fibroblasts, from which mature fibrous tissue, forming a scar, will develop. (PAS)

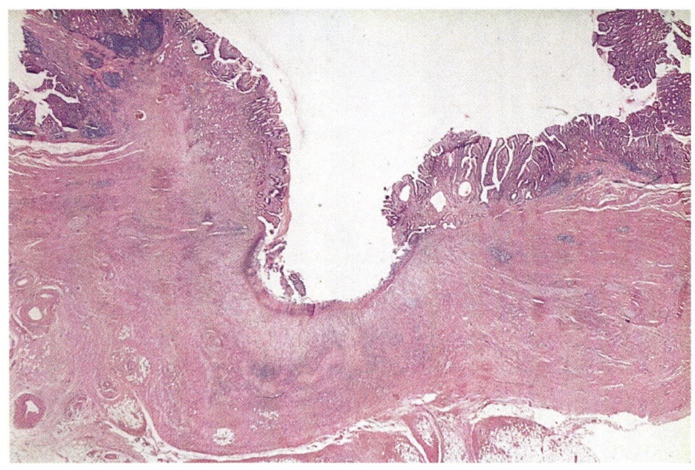

Fig. G 19. Chronic gastric ulcer with sharply delineated margins and scar formation at the base. The surface of the ulcer bed is better seen in *Fig. G 18.* The margin of the ulcer is accentuated by hyperplasia of the bordering epithelium. A cluster of lymphoid nodules, with germinal centers, is at the upper left. (hematoxylin-eosin)

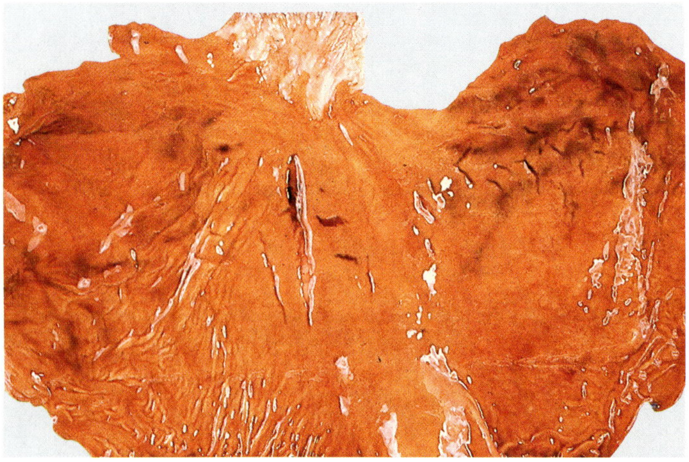

Fig. G20. Mallory-Weiss syndrome. The gastric mucosa is marked by a linear ulceration along the lesser curvature, beneath the cardioesophageal junction. This is the typical location fo this type of ulceration, which occurs in alcoholics, but can sometimes be seen in other patients.

Gastric Carcinoma *(G21–G24)*

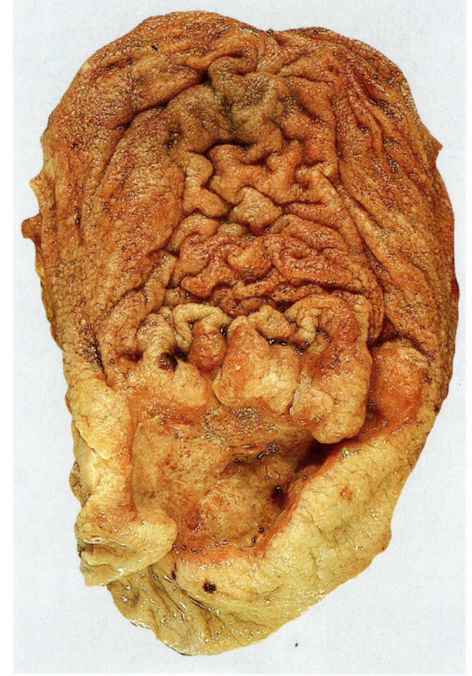

Fig. G21. Gastric adenocarcinoma with peripheral polypoid areas and central deep infiltration, with ulceration. In contrast to the benign ulcer *(Fig. G 17),* this ulcer is irregular in shape with nodular, partially overhanging edges. The cut edge of the stomach can be seen at sides of the ulcer. The carcinoma is grey-white and extends completely through the wall. The upper portion of the stomach has markedly accentuated rugal folds. These folds are prominent because of extensive mucosal infiltration.

Fig. G22. Well differentiated gastric adenocarcinoma of the intestinal type. The mucosa, to the left of the photomicrograph, is replaced by the proliferation of malignant glands. The mucosa, to the right, shows gastric metaplasia, due to chronic atrophic gastritis, as already shown in *Fig. G 13.* (hematoxylin-eosin)

Fig. G23a. Signet ring carcinoma of the stomach. Relatively large cells, with eccentric large hyperchromatic nuclei and foamy cytoplasm, can be seen between the gastric glands. (hematoxylin-eosin)

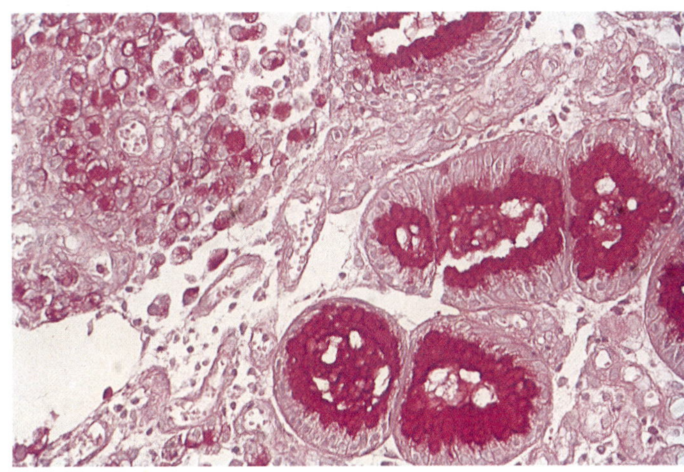

Fig. G23b. Signet ring carcinoma of the stomach showing intracytoplasmic accumulation of mucin in the tumor cells (upper left), as well as the abundant mucous in the normal gastric gland epithelium (lower right). (PAS)

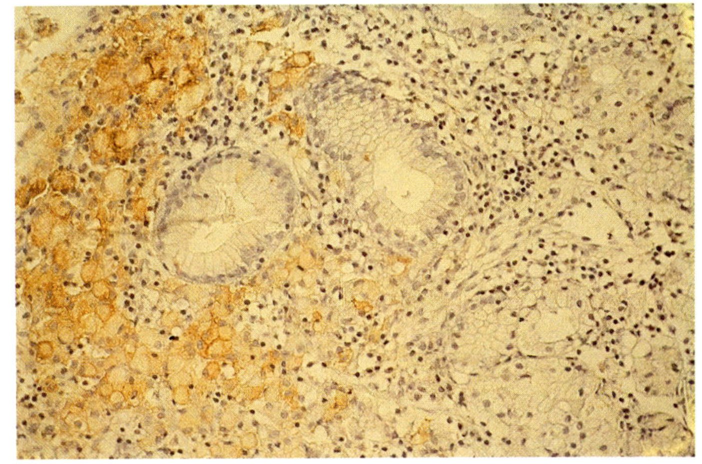

Fig. G23c. Signet ring cell carcinoma of the stomach showing the presence of carcinoembryonic antigen (CEA). The demonstration of CEA, using immunohistochemical methods, might be useful in the identification of poorly differentiated gastrointestinal tract carcinomas.

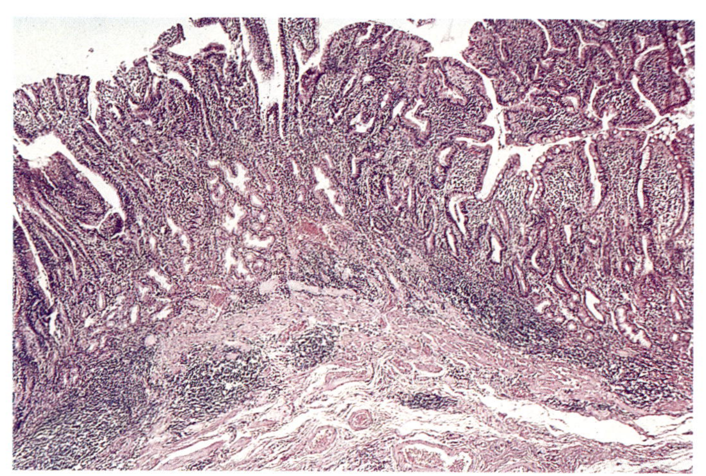

Fig. G24. Early gastric adenocarcinoma. The mucosa has a polypoid appearance. Many of the epithelial cells (at the middle of this photomicrograph) have dark nuclei with an increased nuclear-cytoplasmic ratio. In this area there is transition from a marked dysplasia to a well differentiated adenocarcinoma. The carcinoma is completely limited to the lamina propria and does not penetrate to muscularis mucosa. The diagnosis of early carcinoma could not be unequivocally made in this biopsy, but was confirmed in the gastric resection.   (hematoxylin-eosin)

Cystic Lesions and Benign Gastric Tumors   *(G25–G28)*

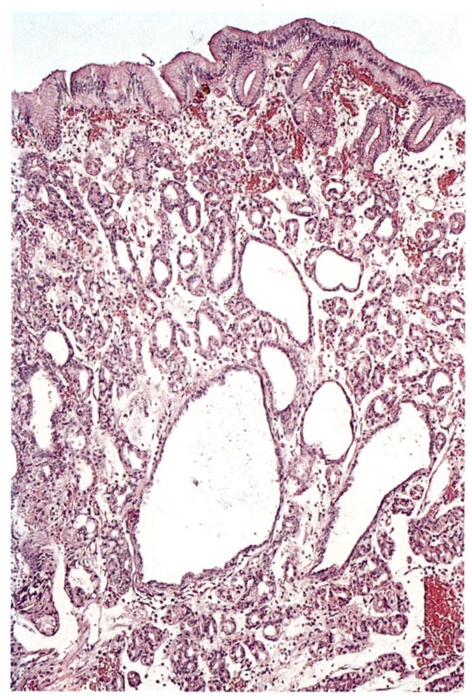

Fig. G25. Gastric body cystic change. Cystically dilated glands are evident in the middle part of this gastric body mucosa section. The numbers of parietal and chief cells are reduced, indicative of glandular atrophy. The stroma is edematous. The cystic glands contribute to prominence of the gastric mucosa, visible with the fiberoptic gastroscope. In order to establish the correct diagnosis of this polypoid process, histologic examination is necessary. The basis of this change is unclear, but it might be the early stage of hyperplastic polyp *(see Fig. G26).*   (hematoxylin-eosin)

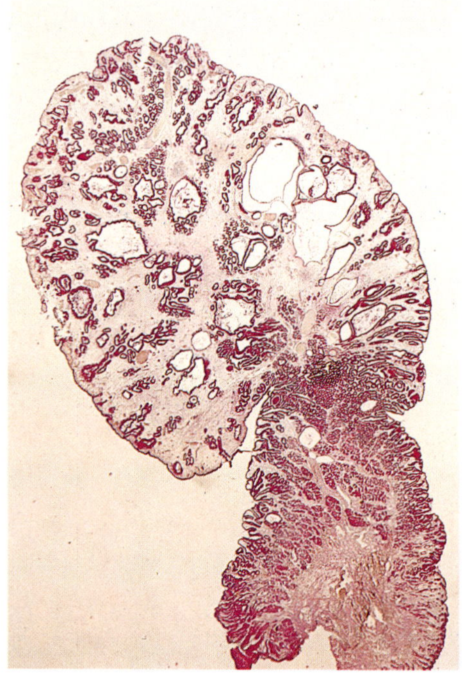

Fig. G26. Hyperplastic gastric polyp. The polyp sits on a stalklike protrusion of the gastric mucosa. At the lower area of the section a small portion of muscularis mucosae is present. The body of the polyp is marked by many cystic spaces lined by a fundic-type of epithelium similar to that of the surface epithelium. These polyps can also include gastric body-type epithelial cells. They may be single or multiple and do not have a high potential for malignant change.   (PAS)

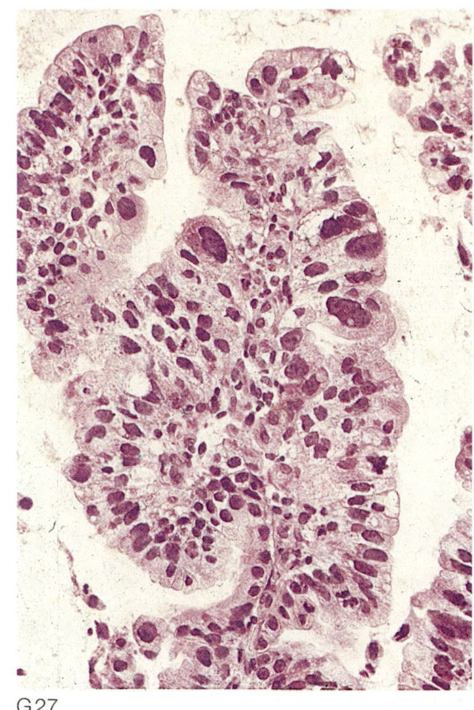

G27

Fig. G27. Malignant change in a tubulovillous adenoma of the stomach. A villus projection fills the field. The entire stomach contained similar villus structures as well as glandular forms. Relatively normal epithelial cells are seen at the upper and lower right. These tall columnar cells have small, uniform, basally situated nuclei. Scattered among the more normal appearing cells, most prominently in the middle of the photomicrograph, are larger cells with hyperchromatic pleomorphic nuclei. This localized ("in situ") malignant change can be effectively treated by polypectomy but, if left unattended, would progress to become an infiltrating adenocarcinoma.   (hematoxylin-eosin)

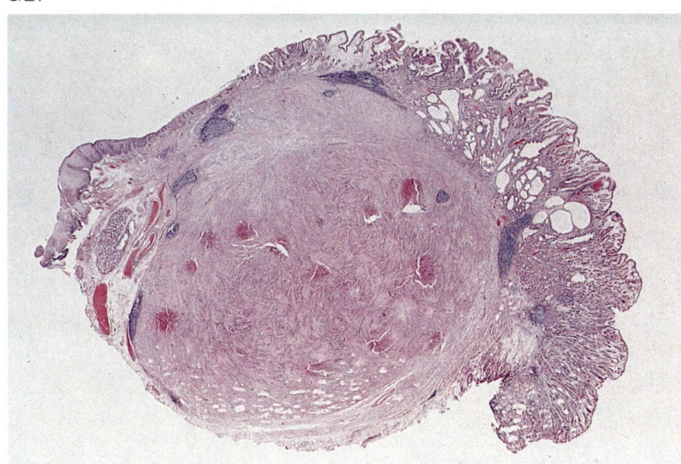

G28

Fig. G28. Leiomyoma at the cardioesophageal junction. This low magnification photomicrograph shows a well circumscribed tumor with overlying esophageal stratified squamous mucosa (left upper portion of specimen) and gastric mucosa (upper middle and right). Immediately beneath the mucosa, surrounding the spherical tumor, are blue patches of lymphoid tissue. This predominantly submucosal tumor consists of interlacing bundles of smooth muscle cells. As the tumor increases in size it may protrude onto the serosal or mucosal surfaces, or sometimes both. When the mucosa becomes stretched over the tumor it secondarily ulcerates and bleeds. Other predominantly submucosal tumors include lipomas, granular cell tumors *(see Fig. F9a),* and carcinoids. In this case there is a well differentiated adenocarinoma in the hyperplastic gastric mucosa to the right. (hematoxylin-eosin)

Small Intestine   *(G29–G35)*

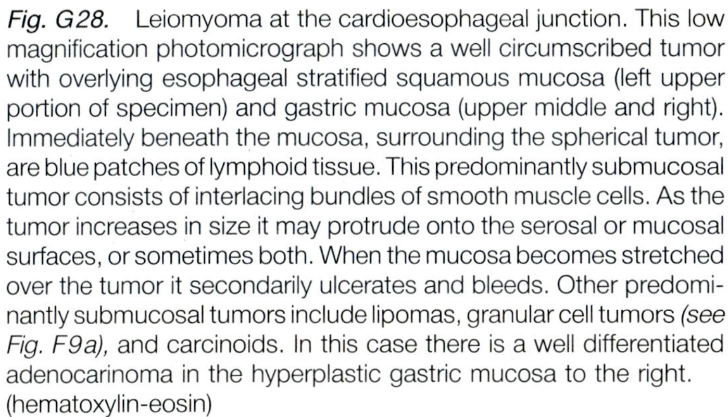

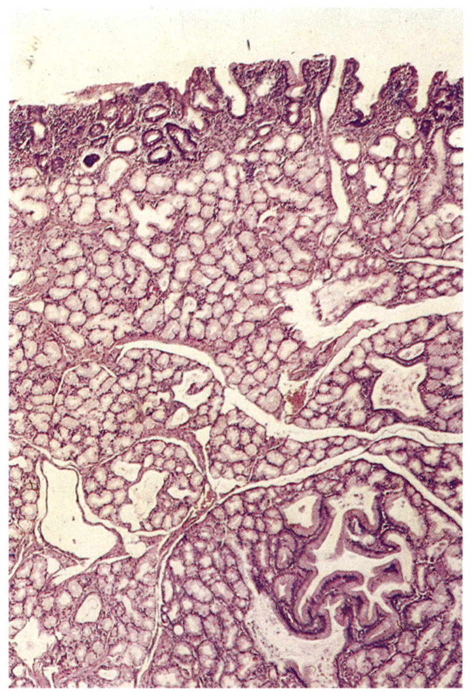

Fig. G29. Brunner gland adenoma arising in the duodenal bulb. The overlying duodenal mucosa is somewhat atrophic because of the expanding mass of Brunner gland acini. It is not completely clear that these proliferations are truly neoplastic. Many regard this lesion as Brunner gland hyperplasia rather than adenoma. There may be multiple areas in the duodenum. Endoscopically they appear as small, broad-based polypoid excrescences.   (hematoxylin-eosin)

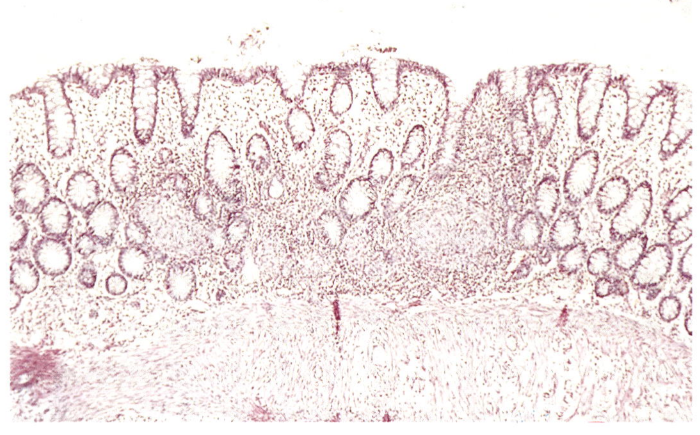

Fig. G30. Crohn's disease. Multiple noncaseating epithelioid and giant cell granulomata are seen in the lamina propria of this small intestinal section. These granulomas are seen in only 30–40% of Crohn's disease specimens and are probably most prevalent in the early stages of the disease. (hematoxylin-eosin)

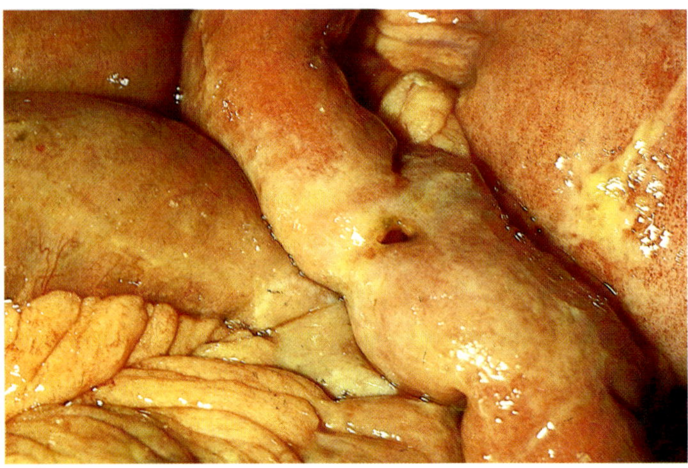

Fig. G31. Crohn's disease. This intraoperative photograph shows the serosal surfaces of small bowel loops with a portion of mesentary to the lower left. The serosal surfaces are partially covered with a yellow exudate and the central loop, which is distal ileum, has a small perforation. This perforation is a result of the inflammatory fissures which extend through the wall in Crohn's disease and which can lead to the formation of fistulous tracts, characteristic of this condition.

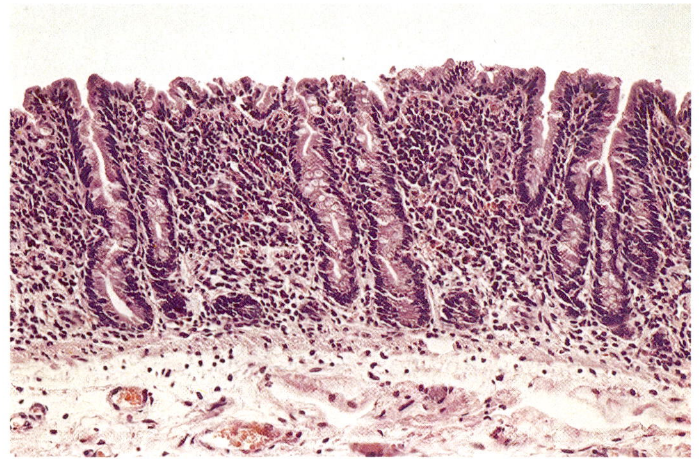

Fig. G32. Partial villus atrophy in gluten sensitive ("nontropical") sprue.
a) The small intestinal mucosa has the characteristic appearance of sprue with almost complete loss of villous structure, and marked lamina propria infiltration by lymphocytes, plasma cells, and other monocytes. A few stunted villi remain to the right of the photograph. The crypts are shortened and some epithelial cells are atypical. The number of mitotic figures is increased. The process does not extend beyond the muscularis mucosae. (hematoxylin-eosin)
b) Scanning electron micrograph of sprue. The epithelial surface is relatively flat with no villus projections and prominent crypts.

Fig. G33. Epithelial repair after dietary restriction of gluten in a sprue patient.

a) In contrast to *Fig. 32a,* the surface of the mucosa is raised and there is some evidence of villus formation to the right of center. The inflammatory cell component is less prominent, and there is less epithelial cell atypia. Mitoses might still be plentiful in this reparative stage. Eventually the mucosa will return to a normal appearance. (hematoxylin-eosin)

b) Scanning electron micrograph. The crypts cannot be seen directly, as they were in *Fig. G32b,* because of the prominent villus projections.

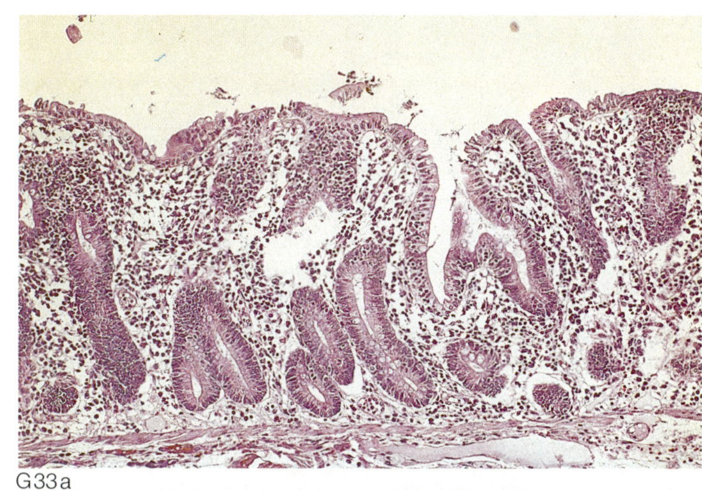

G33a

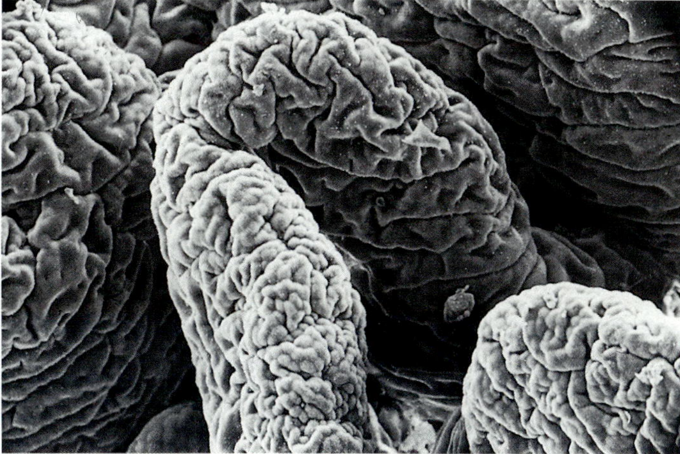

G33b

Fig. G34. Whipple's disease.

a) The villi are distorted markedly. There are oval or spherical spaces lined by a single layer endothelial cell. These are markedly dilated lymphatics ("lymphangiectasia"). In addition there are multiple aggregates of large, pale-staining, eosinophilic, granular histiocytes, among which there is a sparse scattering of lymphocytes and plasma cells.   (hematoxylin-eosin)

b) The histiocytes are characteristically reactive with periodic acid-Schiff (PAS) reagent, and are filled with PAS-positive material. The lymphangiectatic spaces are seen easily.

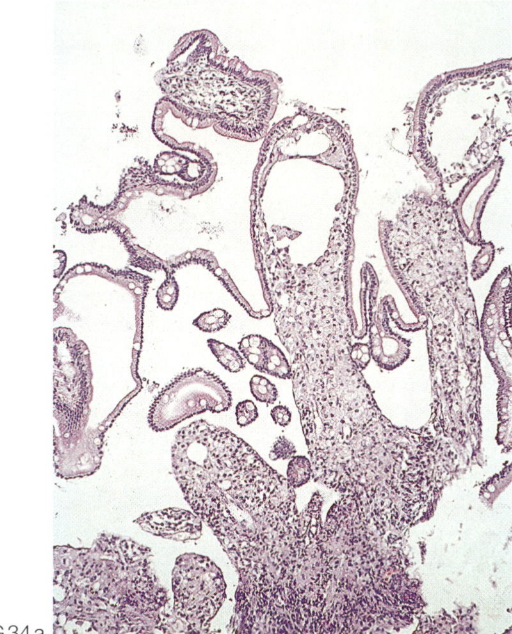

G34a

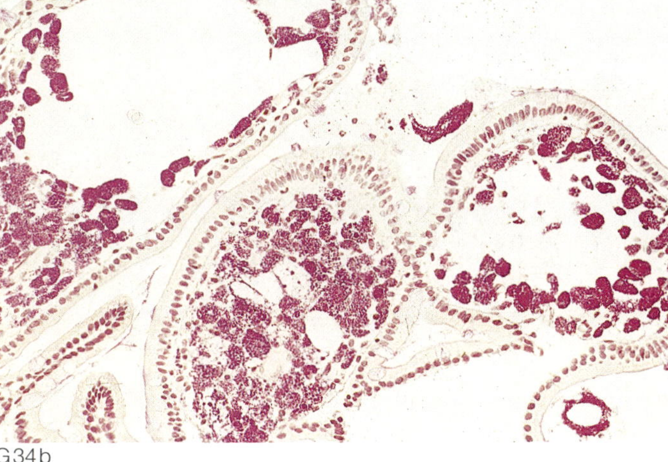

G34b

Fig. G35. Transmission electron micrograph of a typical Whipple's disease histiocyte, in which the causative agent of Whipple's disease can be seen. The bacterial fragments are Corynebacteria. Whipple's disease can be treated effectively with antibiotics, which results in the restoration of the morphologic and functional integrity of the small intestinal mucosa.

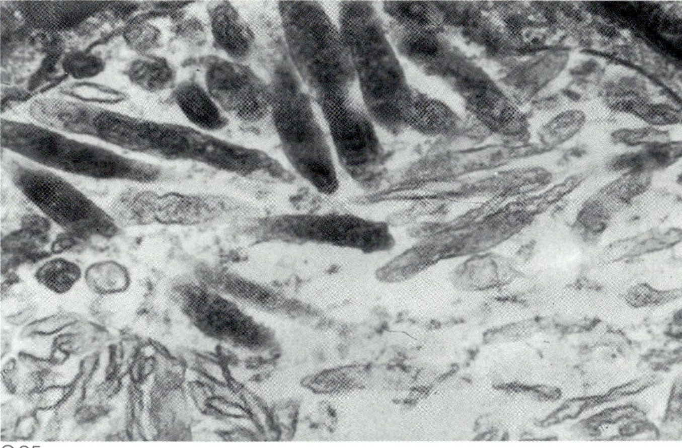

G35

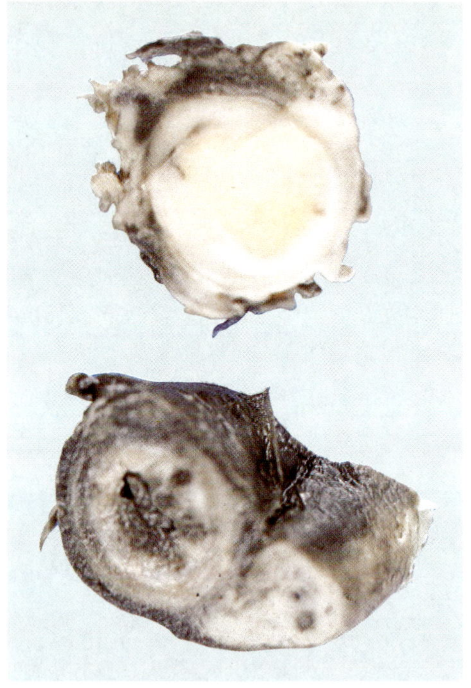

Fig. G36.   Appendiceal carcinoid. The appendix has been cut transversely. The lower segment shows a dark, irregular lumen rimmed by white submucosal tissue. The upper segment has only a slitlike lumen that is compressed by the tan and yellow homogeneous nonencapsulated tumor. The yellow hue is typical of carcinoids.

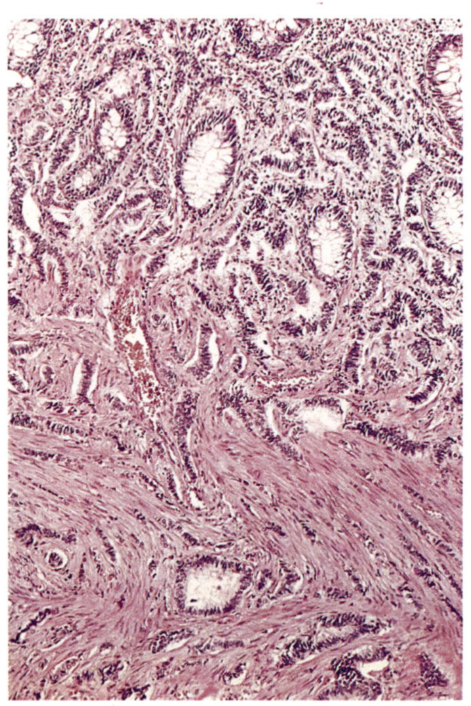

Fig. G37.   Appendiceal carcinoid. The mucosa (above) is replaced by glands and cords of fairly uniform tumor cells which infiltrate the muscularis (below). Although they infiltrate the wall, appendiceal carcinoids almost never metastasize, in contrast to ileal carcinoids which can be quite aggressive.   (hematoxylin-eosin)

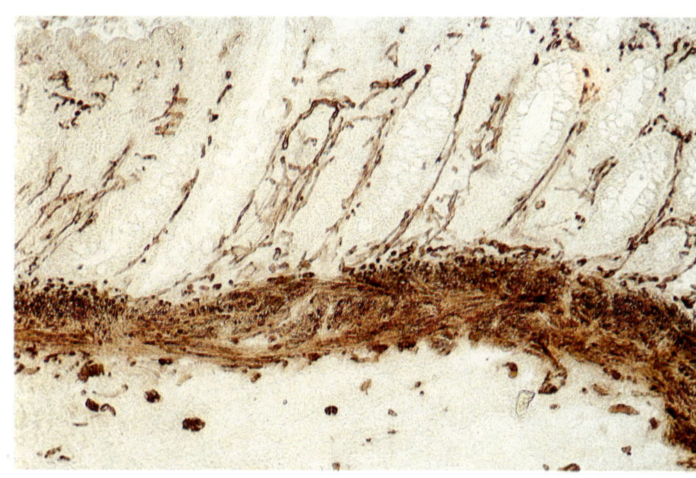

Fig. G38. Hirschsprung's disease. Histologic reaction for acetyl cholinesterase in a frozen section preparation. The brown-reacting nerve bundles are seen easily in the region of the muscularis mucosae, and positive cells are also between crypts in the lamina propria. The normal mucosa does not show acetyl cholinesterase-positive nerve cells.

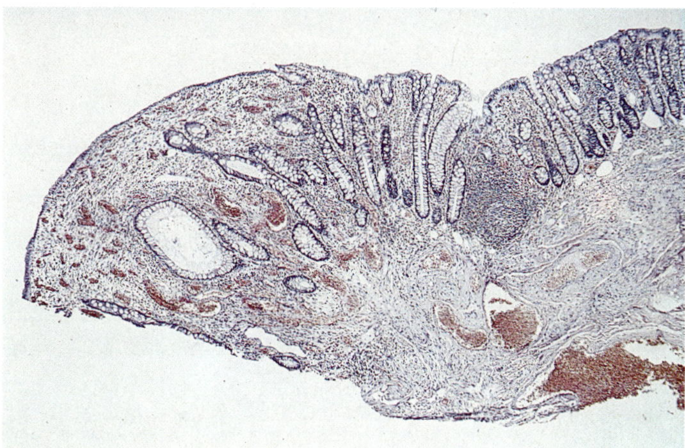

G39a

Fig. G39. Intestinal angiodysplasia.
a) Blood-filled ectatic thin-walled vessels are seen, in this colonic biopsy, in the submucosa, penetrating the muscularis mucosae, and in the lamina propria. Injury to the relatively delicate mucosa can cause bleeding.
b) High magnification photomicrograph of angiodysplasia showing many iron-laden macrophages in the lamina propria. In addition, the stroma, in this view, consists mostly of dilated thin-walled vessels filled with red blood cells.   (Prussian blue)

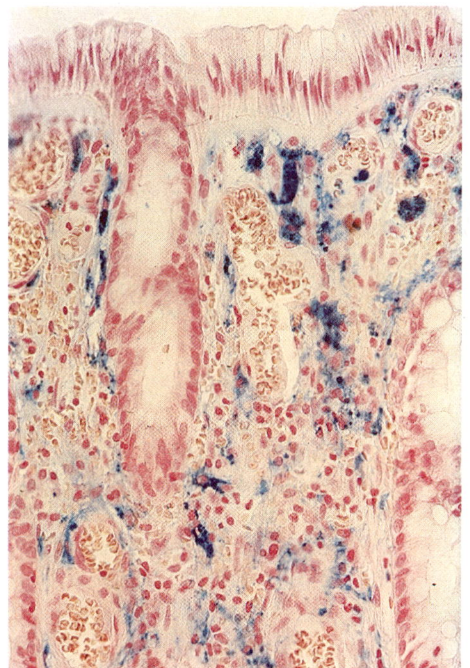

G39b

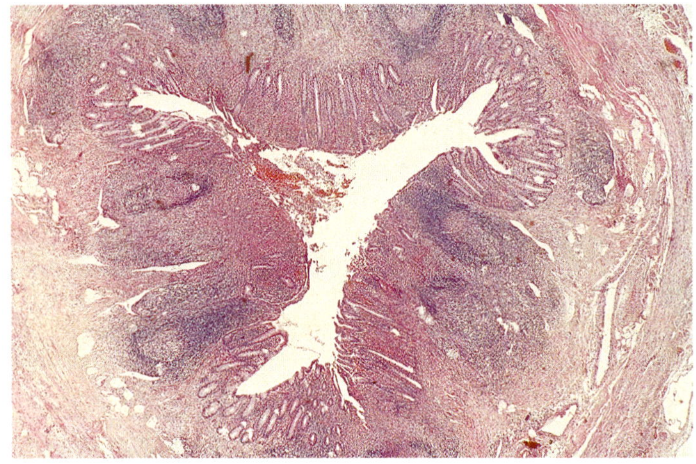

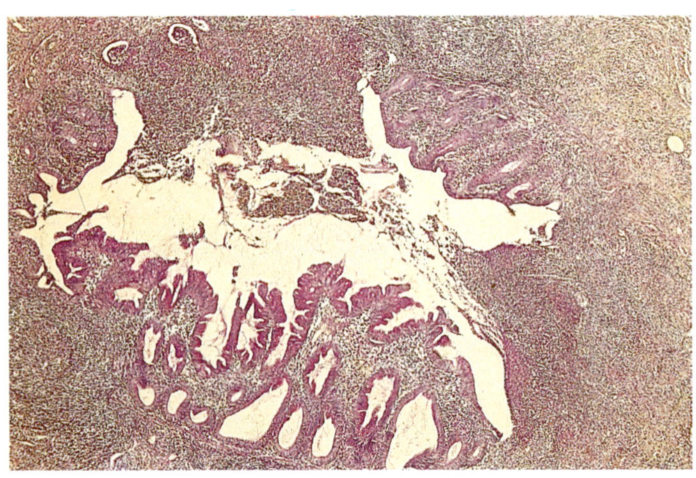

Fig. G40a. Acute appendicitis, early stage. The mucosa is irregularly hyperemic, particularly in the portion immediately to the left of the lumen. An acute inflammatory cell infiltration, consisting primarily of polymorphonuclear leukocytes, is present. These inflammatory cells are also seen as a hemorrhagic exudate in the lumen, overlying an area of surface epithelial loss. The usual appendiceal lymphoid nodules are easily seen.   (hematoxylin-eosin)

Fig. G40b. Severe appendicitis. The mucosa is ulcerated, at the upper portion of the photomicrograph and to the left, and there is a dense infiltration of polymorphonuclear leukocytes in the mucosa and submucosa. The serosa is not seen in this picture, but was partially covered by an acute inflammatory exudate.   (PAS)

Fig. G41. Amebiasis.
a) The colonic mucosa is eroded focally and there is an overlying membrane of debris and fibrin in which there are many *Entamoeba histolytica* trophozoites (PAS). Typically the bowel has flasklike undermining ulcerations which are not seen in this photomicrograph.
b) *Entameoba histolytica* trophozoites filled with erythrocytes. By close examination one can see eccentric nuclei within the cytoplasm between the phagocytosed erythrocytes.   (PAS)

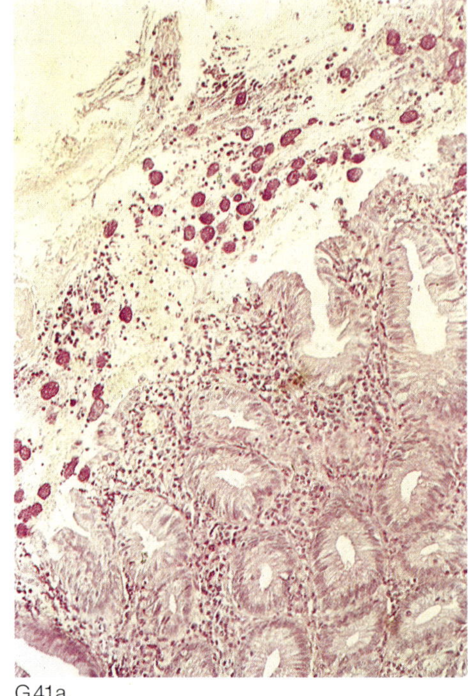

G41a

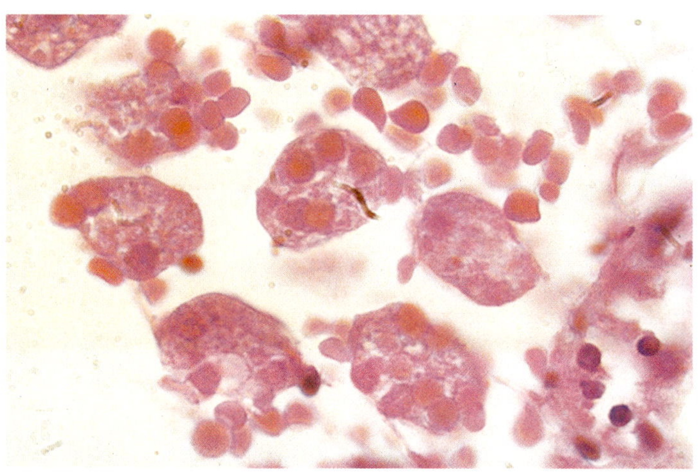

G41b

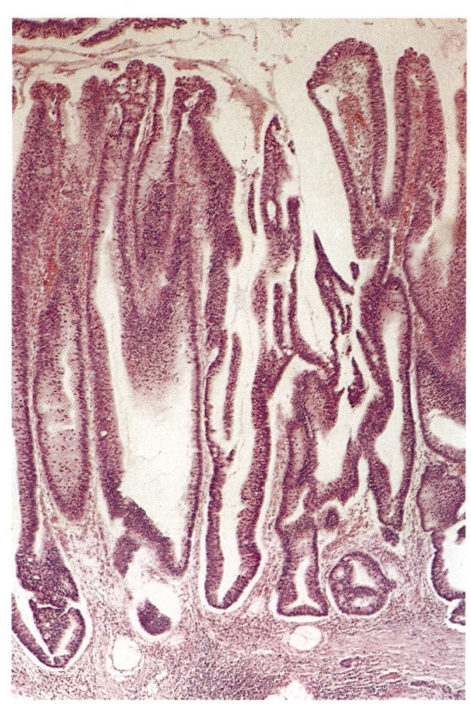

Fig. G42. Ulcerative colitis. This colonic biopsy shows the typical appearance of ulcerative colitis. The overlying epithelium is lost and the glandular pattern is distorted. Many of the crypts are dilated, with necrosis of their epithelial cells, and contain polymorphonuclear leukocytes ("crypt abscess"). The stroma is densely infiltrated by predominantly chronic inflammatory cells, including lymphocytes and plasma cells, as well as eosinophils. Some of the epithelial cells show regenerative change. At the lower right the intact muscularis mucosae is seen. Typically, in ulcerative colitis, the inflammation remains limited to the lamina propria.   (PAS)

Fig. G43. Dysplasia in ulcerative colitis. The usual mucosa pattern, in this patient with ulcerative colitis, is lost and there is a villiform epithelial proliferation. The epithelial cells are atypical and are stratified and, at the lower right, a gland shows bridging of epithelial cells, without stroma, across its lumen ("cribriform"). This is a form of severe dysplasia and, if untreated, frank adenocarcinoma will develop in this area.   (hematoxylin-eosin)

Fig. G44. Multiple foci of colonic adenocarcinoma in a patient with chronic ulcerative colitis. This patient had active colitis for 14 years. The longstanding inflammation caused the mucosa to be generally flat and atrophic. There are four separate sites of adenocarcinoma *(arrows),* the largest of which is seen to the right at the ileocecal valve. As can be appreciated at the second area from the left, colonic adenocarcinoma can be relatively flat and subtle in patients with ulcerative colitis and might not be seen readily by the endoscopist.

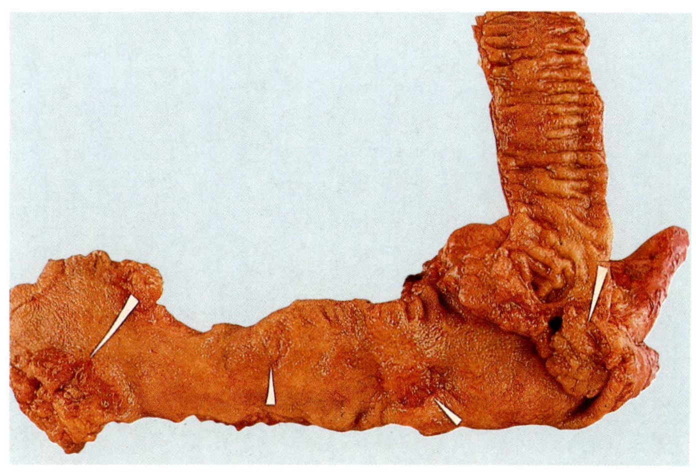

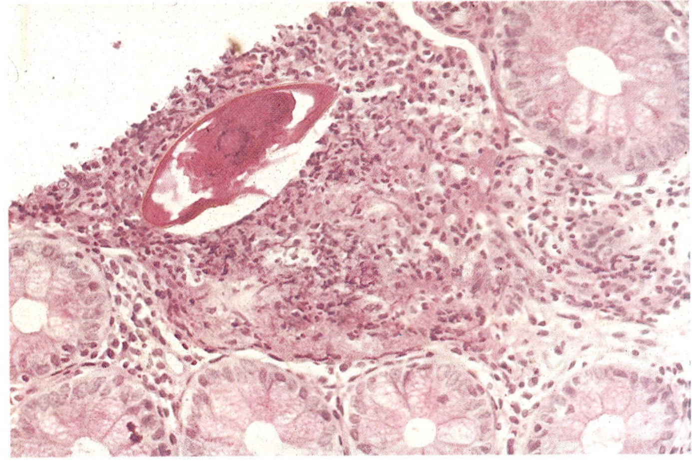

Fig. G45.   Schistosomiasis. In this high-magnification photomicrograph, an epithelioid-cell granuloma, with many eosinophils, is seen between the crypts. Within the granuloma there is a typical *Schistosoma mansoni* egg.   (PAS)

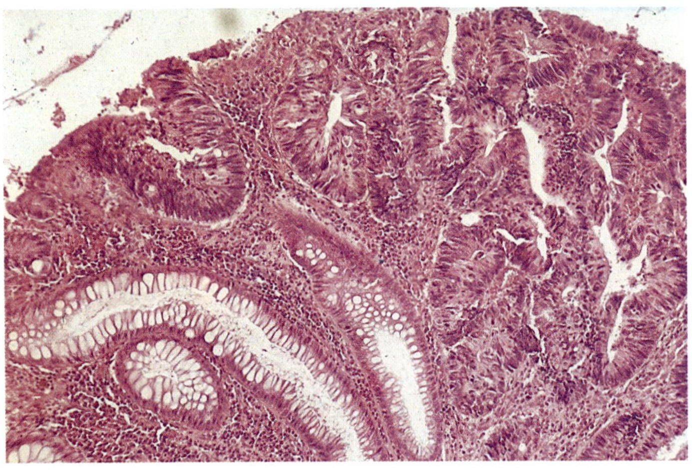

Fig. G46.   Well differentiated colonic adenocarcinoma. To the left are benign glands of an underlying adenoma. The glands are lined by tall columnar mucous-secreting epithelial cells with basally oriented round uniform nuclei. To the right are the irregular malignant glands lined by highly variable, non-mucous-producing cells which have large, pleomorphic, hyperchromatic nuclei that are stratified in a disorderly fashion.   (hematoxylin-eoson)

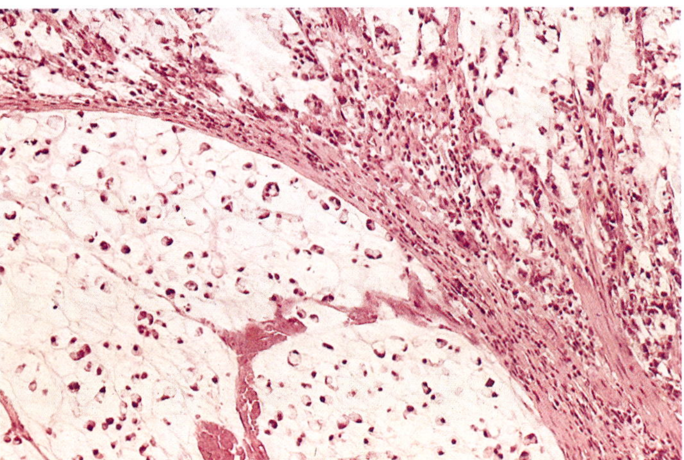

G 47

Fig. G47.   Poorly differentiated carcinoma of the rectum with abundant mucous production ("colloid carcinoma"). A large mucous-filled space is at the lower left, within which there are single, or small clusters of, tumor cells. Many of these malignant cells are "signet ring" in form. At the upper the pattern of the malignancy is glandular and there is relatively little mucous production. (hematoxylin-eosin)

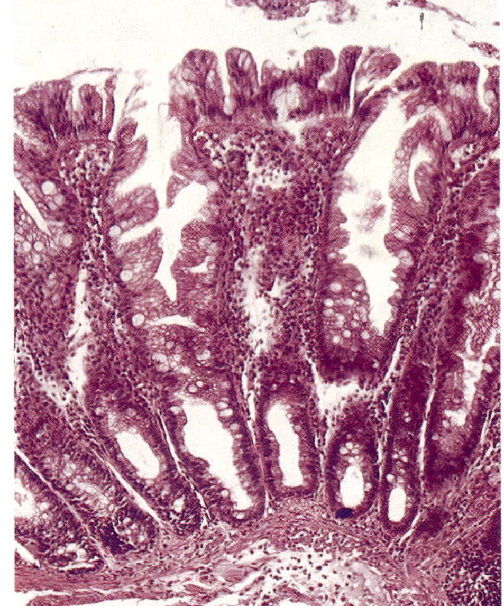

G 48

Fig. G48.   Hyperplastic polyp. This polyp is characterized by proliferation of epithelial cells to form papillary infoldings within the crypt space. Although this polyp is generally regarded as non-neoplastic, there is some suggestion that this pattern precedes the development of the usual adenomatous polyp and is obliterated as the polyp grows. (PAS)

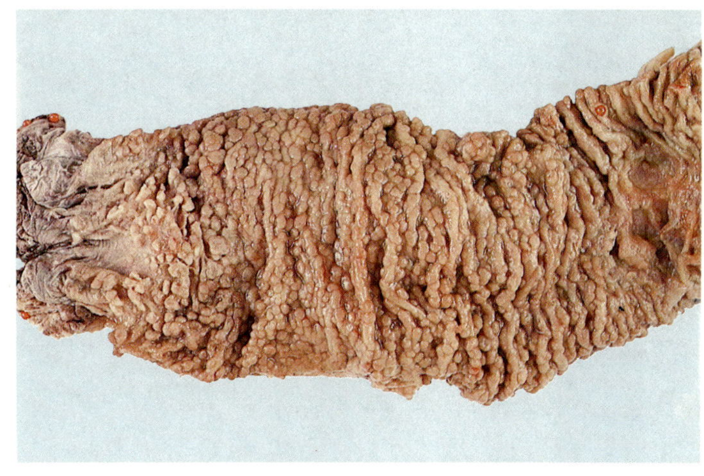

Fig. G49. Familial (multiple) polyposis of the colon. This specimen of the sigmoid, rectum, and anus (left, with grey-white stratified squamous mucosa) was resected from a 22-year-old man. The mucosa is covered almost completely by innumerable, fairly uniform, polypoid excrescences. Polyps become clinically manifest, in this condition, at the end of adolescence. If left unresected, virtually all of these patients will develop adenocarcinoma. Histologically these polyps are indistinguishable from the usual form of adenomatous polyp.

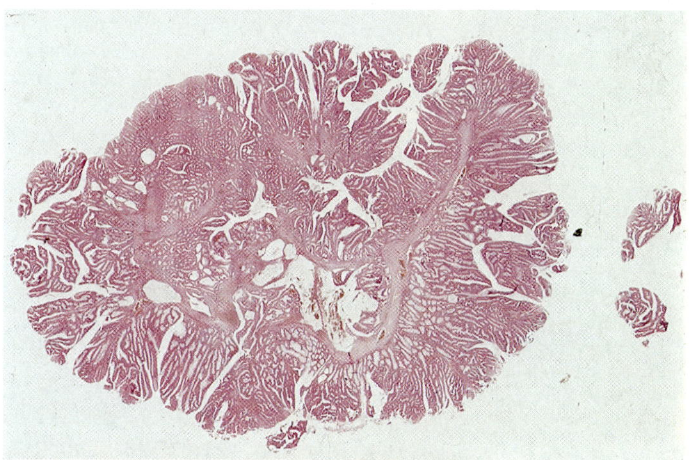

Fig. G50. Villous adenoma of the large intestine. As adenomatous polyps increase in size they are more likely to take on a villous pattern. In this resected polyp the surface consists almost entirely of delicate fingerlike projections with an almost imperceptible supporting stroma. The villous pattern of adenomatous polyp has a greater likelihood of malignant change than the tubular pattern. (hematoxylin-eosin)

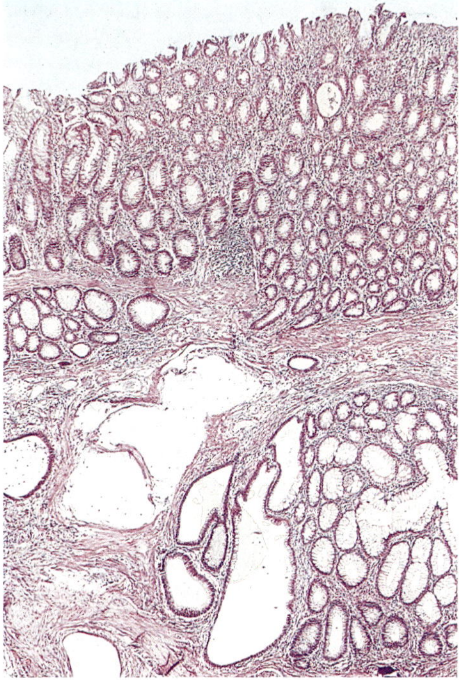

Fig. G51. Colitis cystica profunda. In this benign condition, colonic glands can be found beneath the lamina propria. In this photomicrograph deformed glands are present within the muscularis mucosae and in the submucosa, lined by tall mucous-secreting columnar cells with basally oriented nuclei. This lesion can follow various inflammatory conditions.   (PAS)

H. Liver

H.-W. Altmann, O. Klinge

The liver is the largest and most compact human organ. It is composed principally of one cell type, the hepatocyte. Because of the relative uniformity of the liver, it has proven to be a particularly valuable object of study in the elucidation of the mechanisms of disease. In addition to hepatocytes, the liver contains a major component of the reticuloendothelial system, the Kupffer cells. Liver architecture is distinct and consists of a liver lobule that includes, at its center, the portal tract, and, at its periphery, the terminal hepatic vein. The portal tract contains the tributaries of the portal vein, the hepatic artery branches, and the bile ducts. The bile ducts carry the bile produced by the liver cell. Bile is emptied into the canaliculi, then into the bile ducts and, eventually, out into the biliary tree to the duodenum.

The organelles of the hepatocyte have been particularly well studied in various disease states. The various cytoplasmic components can be altered significantly, in terms of both numbers and distribution. Some of the alterations are characteristic.

The liver is subject to major morphologic changes in blood circulatory disorders. Obstructions to the hepatic outflow, whether caused by cardiac congestion (as in right heart failure) or by hepatic vein thrombosis, contribute to morphologic, and eventually functional, changes. Since the liver has a dual blood supply, with contributions from both the hepatic artery and, principally, the portal vein, infarcts are distinctly unusal unless there is significant reduction in systemic and splanchnic pressures, as might occur in protracted shock. Microinfarcts also can occur in disseminated intravascular coagulopathies, such as eclampsia, in which there is diffuse fibrin thrombosis of the sinusoids.

A full range of metabolic disorders can affect the liver. Glycogen storage diseases often cause hepatic alteration. The liver can undergo significant fatty change because of inherent metabolic defects or from anoxia. A number of exogenous and endogenous pigments affect the liver. Idiopathic hemochromatosis leads to iron deposition in the hepatocytes, with relatively little Kupffer cell deposition, whereas the secondary hemosideroses, following transfusion or hemolytic anemia, usually cause Kupffer cell iron storage initially.

In recent years, toxic hepatitis, especially caused by therapeutic agents, has become increasingly recognized. One of the best studied toxins, of course, is alcohol. Alcohol-associated changes in the liver can be acute or, with prolonged ingestion, chronic, with the ultimate development of cirrhosis.

Bile secretion can be affected by a variety of conditions. The hepatocytes themselves can be injured with alterations of the bile secretory mechanism. Jaundice can follow hemolytic anemias, in which the amount of bilirubin brought to the liver cell might be great. In addition, of course, obstruction of the extrahepatic biliary tree can lead to jaundice and, if severe and prolonged, necrosis of liver cells.

The most important hepatic inflammation is hepatitis. The common forms of hepatitis – A, B, non-A, non-B – might, in the acute stage, be histologically indistinguishable. Hepatitis can progress to at least two chronic forms: chronic persistent hepatitis and chronic active hepatitis. The other viruses that can cause hepatitis are often recognizable because of distinct morphologic or clinical features. Similarly, other inflammations that affect the liver, such as tuberculosis and sarcoidosis, as well as amebiasis, are also usually recognizable.

The bile ducts can be deficient because of congenital anomalies or because of immunologically mediated injury, as in primary biliary cirrhosis.

Hepatic cirrhosis is well known. Cirrhosis must be thought of as a pathophysiologic condition in which there is both significant nodular regneration of hepatocytes after injury and highly vascular fibrous septae which serve to shunt the blood through the liver without necessarily exposing it to hepatocytes. Cirrhosis is an end-stage condition and the etiology of the injury may not be apparent at the time cirrhosis becomes manifest. The regeneratory nodules might be small and approximately equal in size (micronodular, Laennec's) or large and varied (macronodular).

Tumor metastasis to the liver is most common. The liver can also be the site of primary tumor development. Benign tumors are relatively uncommon. Hepatocellular carcinoma (hepatoma) may develop in the setting of cirrhosis or may, less commonly, develop spontaneously.

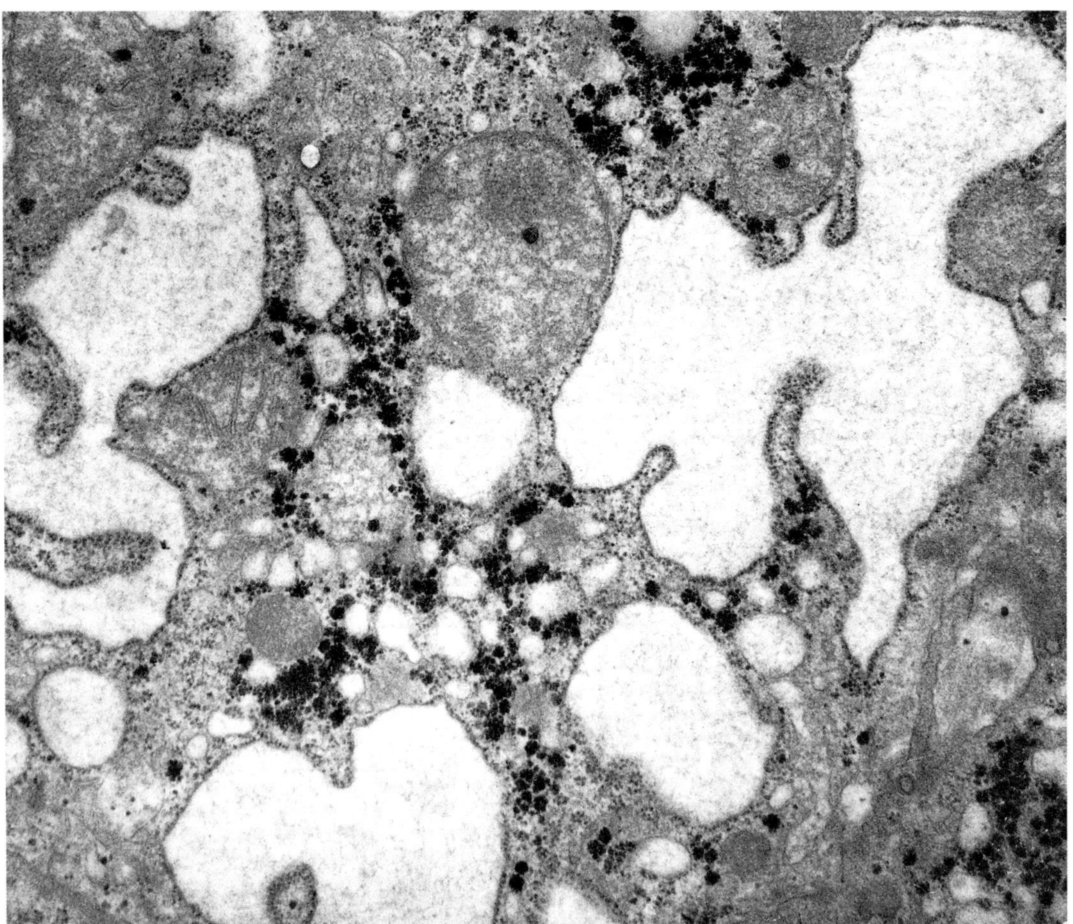

Fig. H1. Hydropic change appears on light microscopy as a pale swollen hepatocyte. Ultrastructurally, the endoplasmic reticulum is markedly dilated and filled with water.

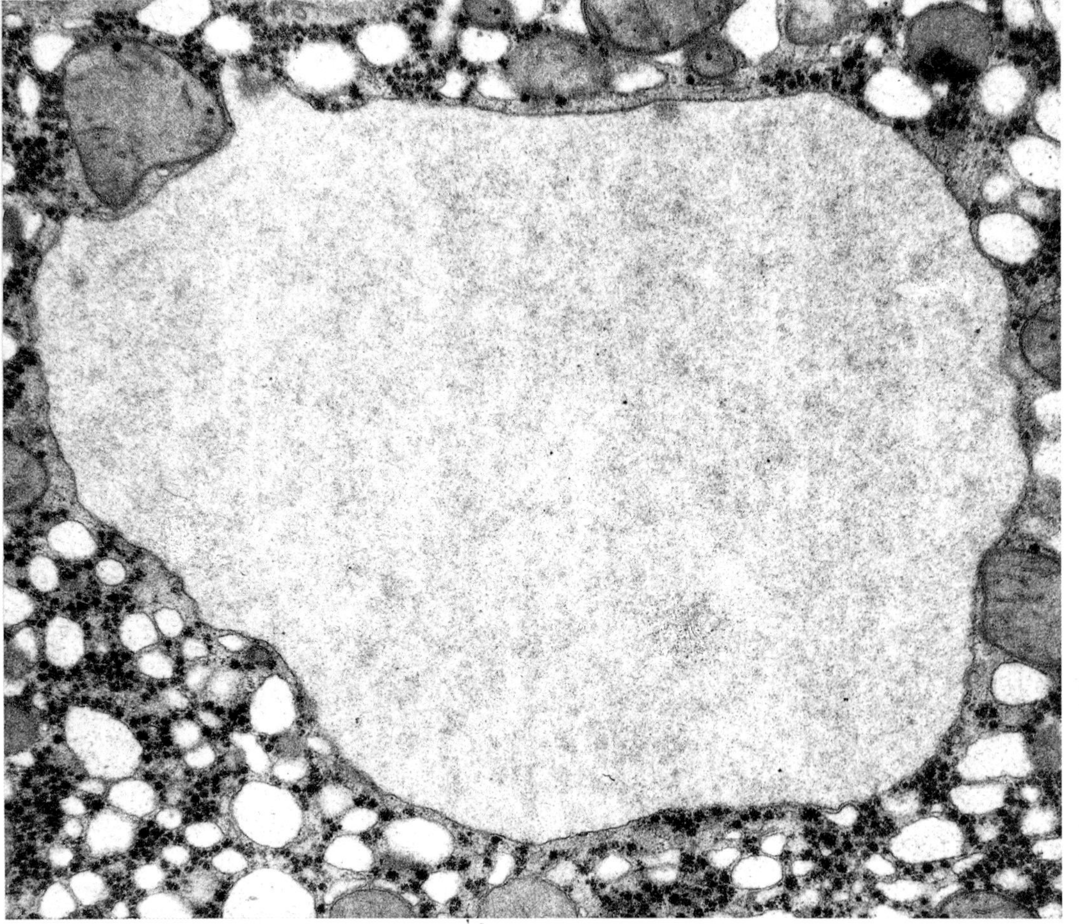

Fig. H2. Intracisternal protein storage. A markedly dilated portion of the rough endoplasmic reticulum is filled with a granular protein secretory product. This is the ultrastructural appearance of the alpha-1-antitrypsin deficiency inclusion body.

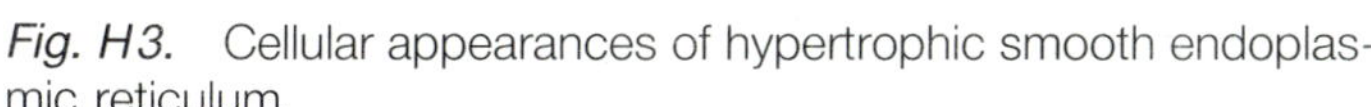

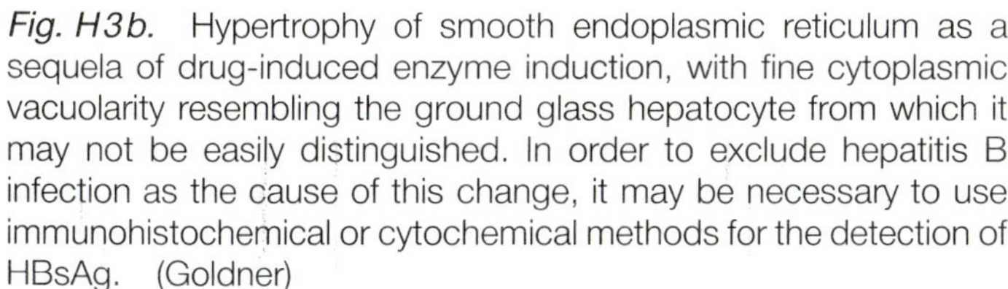

Fig. H3. Cellular appearances of hypertrophic smooth endoplasmic reticulum.

Fig. H3a. Ground glass hepatocyte. The homogenous finely granular cytoplasm is a reflection of the accumulation of hepatitis B surface antigen (HBsAg) in the smooth endoplasmic reticulum. (Ladewig)

Fig. H3b. Hypertrophy of smooth endoplasmic reticulum as a sequela of drug-induced enzyme induction, with fine cytoplasmic vacuolarity resembling the ground glass hepatocyte from which it may not be easily distinguished. In order to exclude hepatitis B infection as the cause of this change, it may be necessary to use immunohistochemical or cytochemical methods for the detection of HBsAg. (Goldner)

Fig. H4. Hepatitis B surface antigen in the smooth endoplasmic reticulum. This is an electron micrograph of a ground-glass cell from a patient with hepatitis B. The smooth endoplasmic reticulum is filled with fibrillar and tubular structures of the virus.

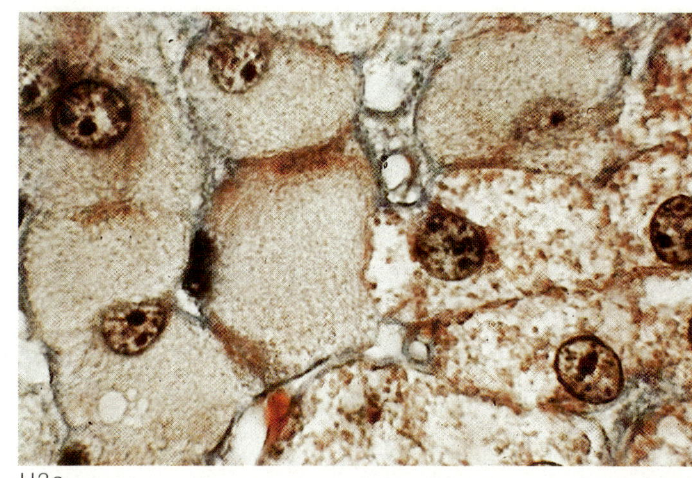

H3a

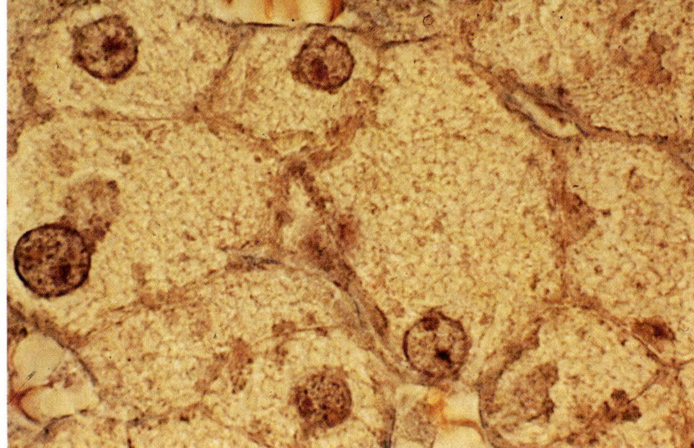

H3b

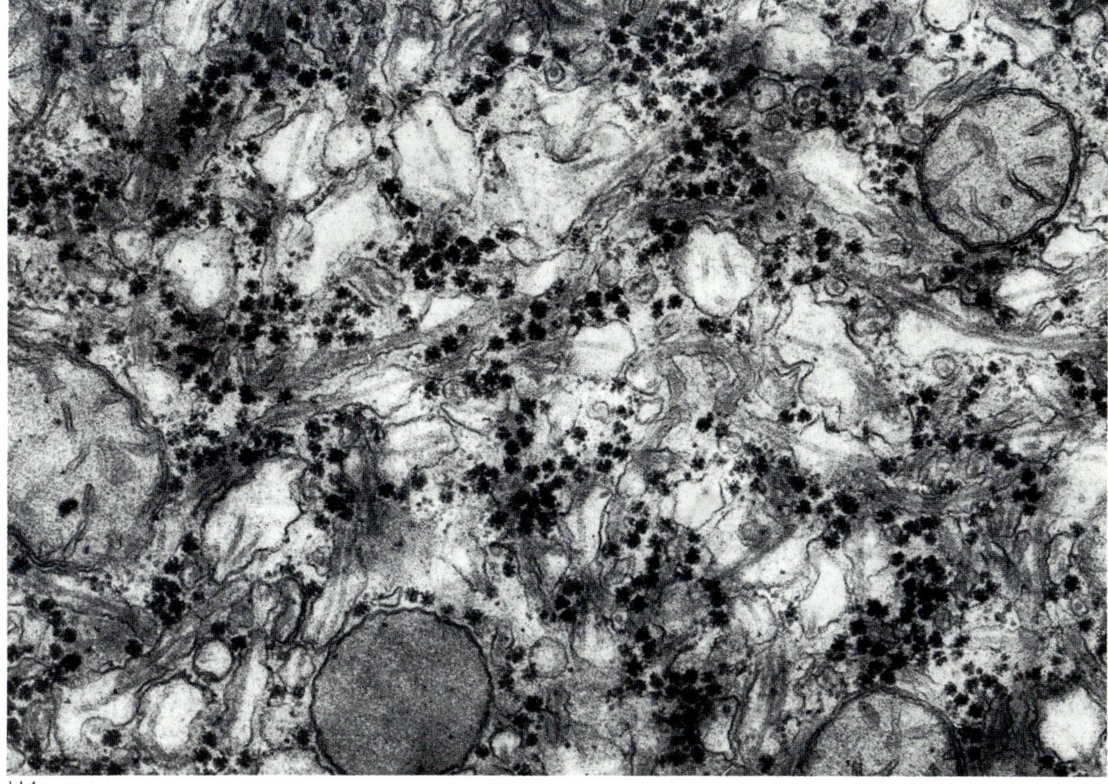

H4

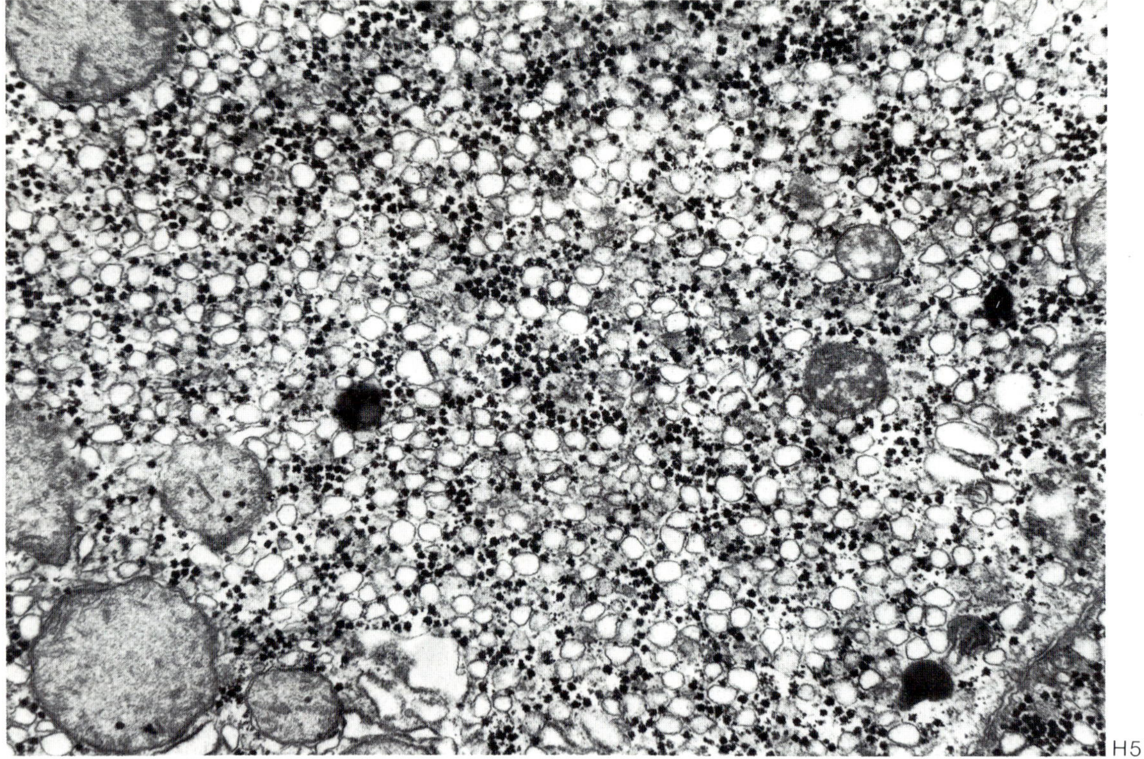

H5

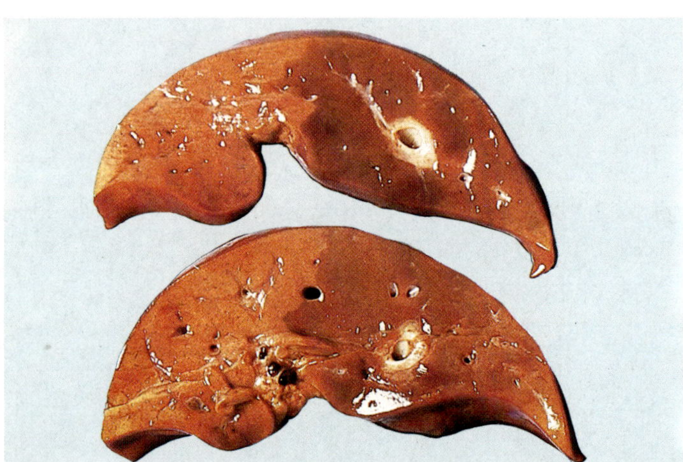

H6a

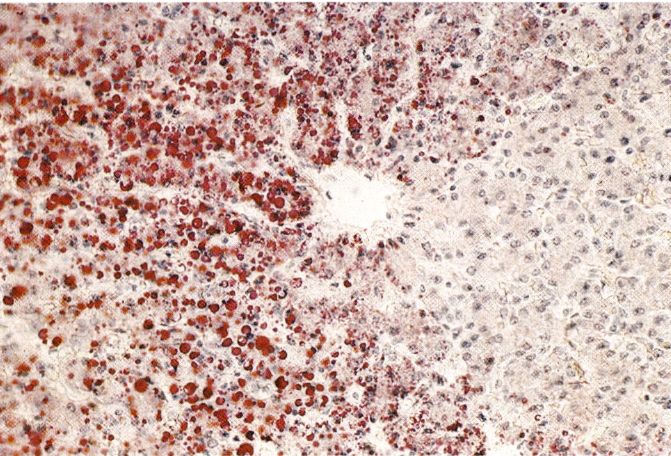

H6b

Fig. H5. Drug-induced hypertrophy of the smooth endoplasmic reticulum. In this electron micrograph there is a vesicular transformation of the endoplasmic reticulum. The mitochondria (upper and lower right) and other organelles are pushed aside and darkly staining glycogen rosettes are between the membrane system vesicles.

Fig. H6. Fatty change of the right half of the liver. This change is due to intrauterine anoxia following partial obstruction to the fetal umbilical vein. *a)* A sharp line delineates the pale right half from the more normal appearing left half. Note that this delineation does not correspond to the line between the anatomic lobes. In the photomicrograph *(b)* the fat vacuoles (steatosis) are stained red with the Sudan method. This histologic section is from the line between the two liver lobes.

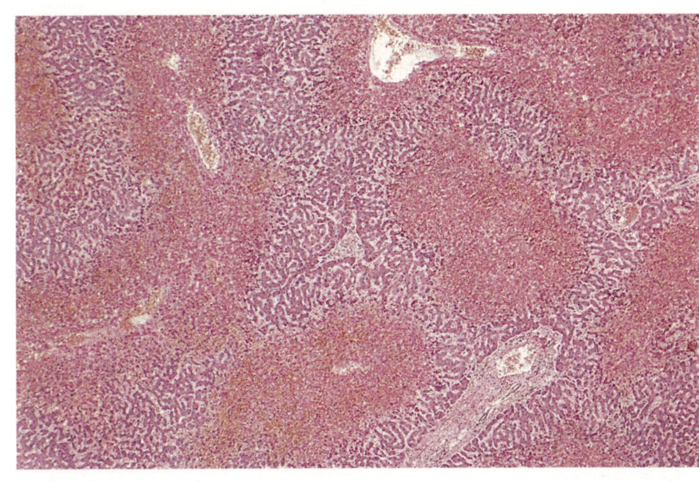

Fig. H7.   Hepatic congestion.

Fig. H7a.   Heart failure. The liver is acutely and severely congested. The portion of the lobule around the terminal hepatic venule ("central vein") is markedly hyperemic because of the congested sinusoids.   (hematoxylin-eosin)

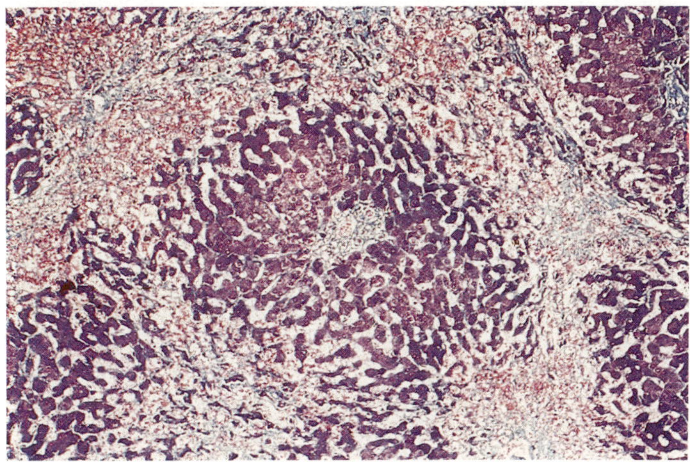

Fig. H7b.   Longstanding congestion of the liver. The hepatocytes around the terminal hepatic venule ("central vein") have become atrophic and the venules themselves are barely seen. A venule at the upper left has increased collagen (blue) which extends into the sinusoids. A portal tract is in the center. Longstanding congestion leads to a picture of reversal of lobular architecture.
(Masson trichrome)

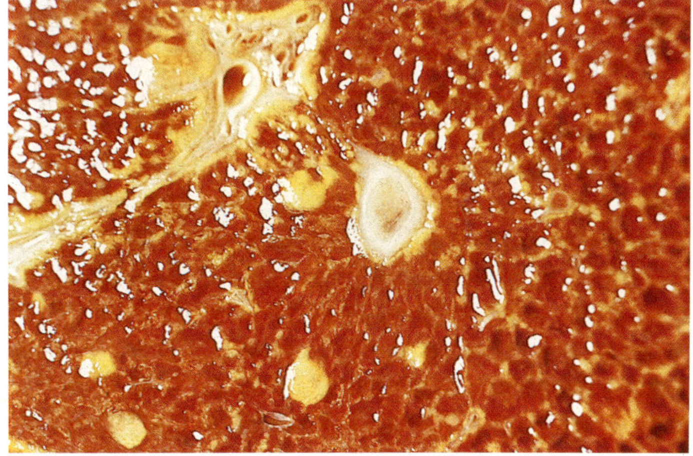

Fig. H7c.   Budd-Chiari syndrome. The hepatic vein is thrombosed at its juncture with the inferior vena cava. In the photograph the intrahepatic vein (center) is completely thrombosed and the liver is markedly congested. Much of the parenchyma shows acute hemorrhagic necrosis. A large portal tract is at the upper left and residual, still viable, periportal areas are seen throughout as yellow, slightly raised zones.

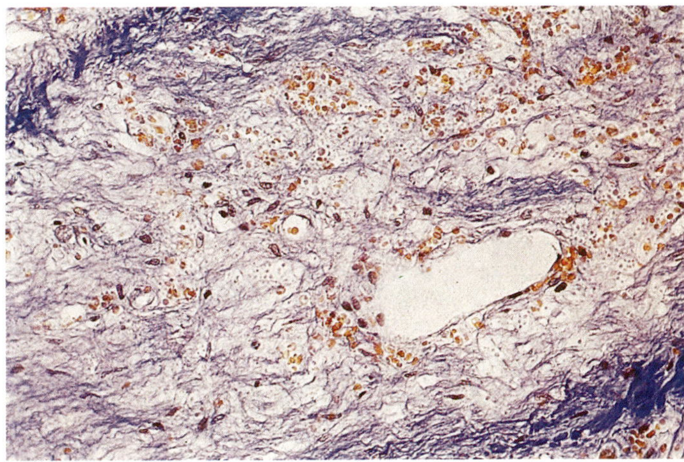

Fig. H7d.   This photomicrograph shows an almost completely obliterated vein, as a result of an endophlebitis. The vein wall is seen at the upper left and lower right. The lumen is filled with a loose connective tissue stroma within which recanalized channels, containing red blood cells, are seen.   (Ladewig)

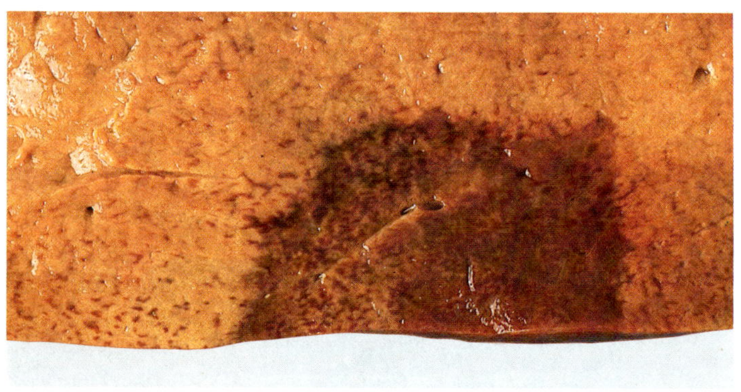

Fig. H8.   Zahn's infarct of the liver. This is not a true infarct. This sharply outlined, dark lesion is a reflection of marked sinusoidal congestion and hepatocyte atrophy, due to a reduction of portal flow without compromise of hepatic artery circulation. This change is often seen at the periphery of metastatic tumors.

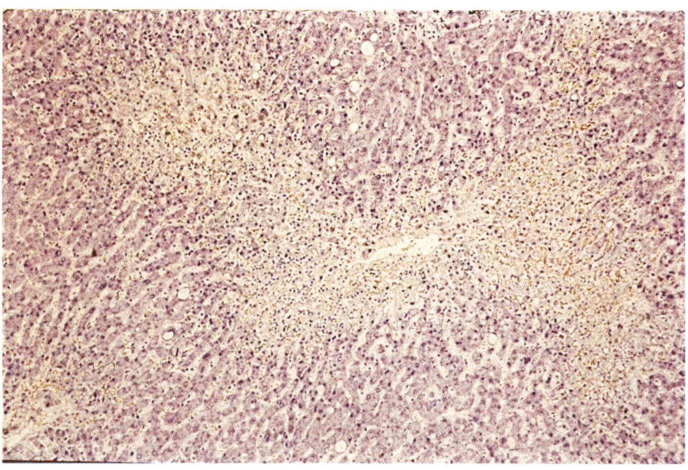

Fig. H9.   Hepatic necrosis following shock.

Fig. H9a.   This is the classic picture of centrolobular (zone 3) necrosis due to prolonged shock. The nuclear staining (basophilia) of the hepatocytes around the terminal hepatic venules is lost and the hepatocytes are fragmented. The sinusoidal lining cells remain. (Cresyl violet)

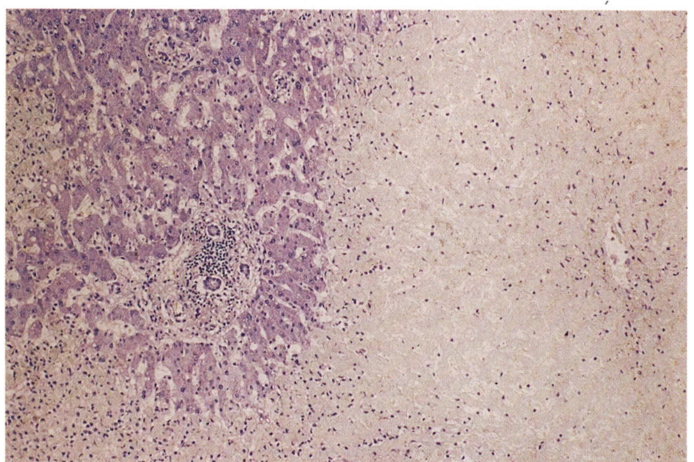

Fig. H9b.   Patients with longstanding shock can be sustained with modern intensive care methods. This can lead to complete necrosis of the hepatocytes around the terminal hepatic vein and in the midzonal region. In this photomicrograph, only the hepatocytes surrounding the portal tract appear viable.   (hematoxylin-eosin)

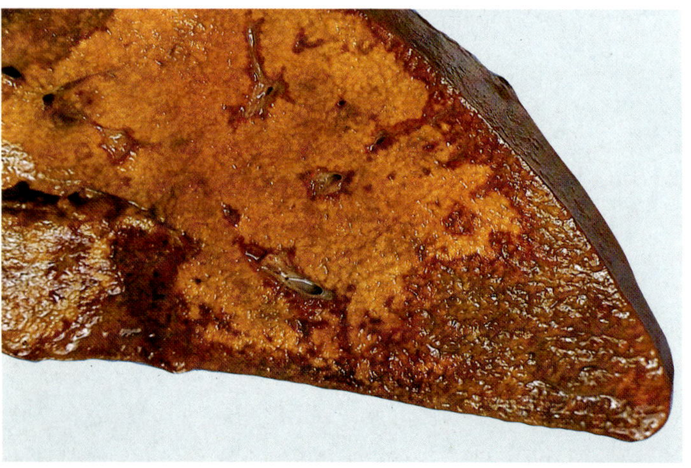

Fig. H10.   Hepatic infarct following protracted shock. There is a large irregular zone of yellow necrosis. Hepatic infarcts are uncommon and are rarely due to vascular obstruction since the liver has a dual circulation of both portal vein and hepatic artery. In shock, however, the hepatic circulation can be compromised and infarct can occur. The darkly staining hepatic parenchyma around the infarct shows accentuated lobular architecture *(see Fig. H7d)*. This is the same liver as in *Fig. H9b.*

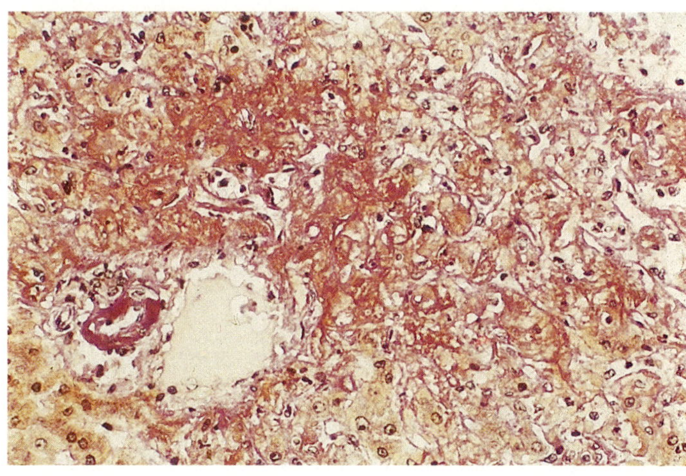

Fig. H11.   Conditions leading to sinusoidal dilatation.

Fig. H11a.   Intravascular fibrin deposition in eclampsia. This form of disseminated intravascular coagulation syndrome (DIC) is characterized by the formation of fibrin thrombi in the periportal sinusoidal spaces. In this photomicrograph the portal tract artery also shows fibrinoid necrosis.   (Trichrome-PAS)

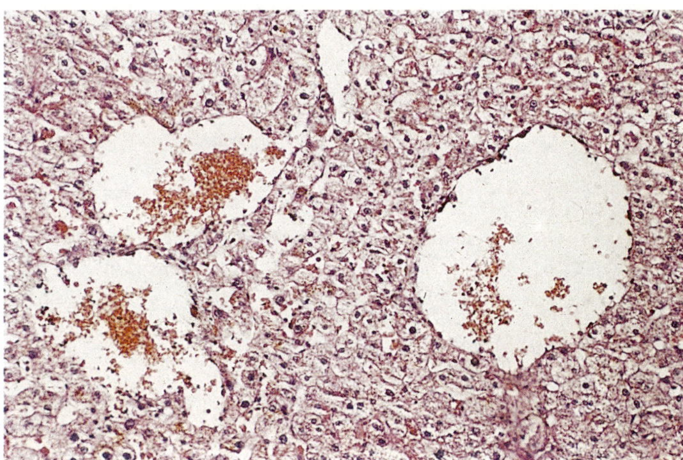

Fig. H11b.   Peliosis hepatis. Sinusoidal spaces are markedly ectatic and contain red blood cells. The lining of the space is of endothelial cells. Peliosis hepatis has been associated with the use of oral contraceptives and anabolic steroids.   (hematoxylin-eosin)

Metabolic Storage Diseases   *(H12–H18)*

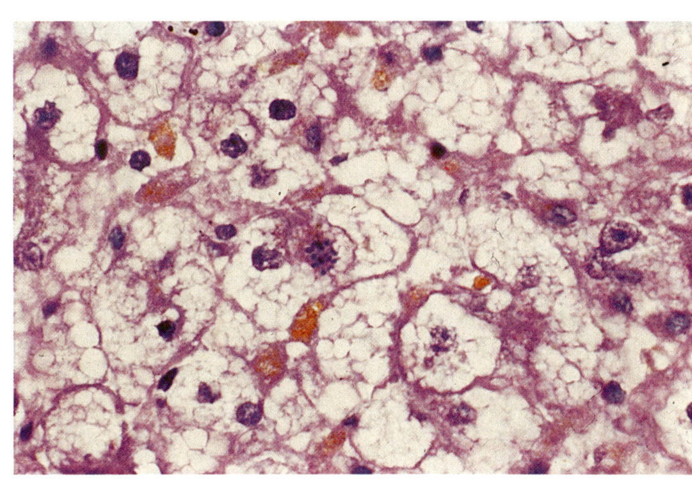

Fig. H12.   Fatty liver of pregnancy. The hepatocytes are distended by multiple microvesicles of fat which appear clear in formalin-fixed paraffin-embedded tissue. In the middle of the photomicrograph a mitotic figure is present, as a reparative response to single cell necrosis.   (hematoxylin-eosin)

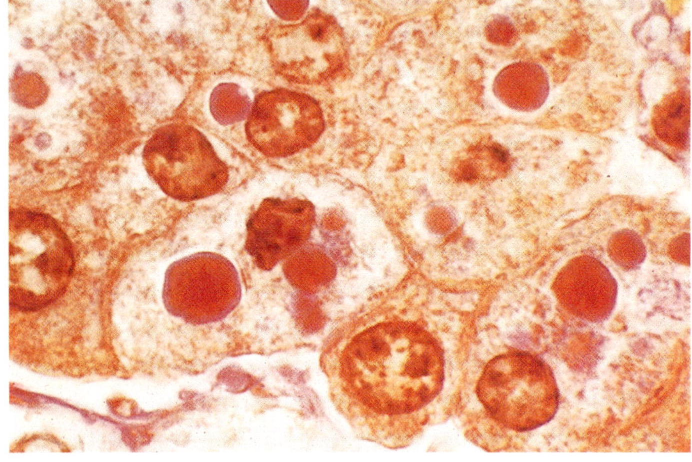

Fig. H 13.   Metabolic disorders affecting the liver.

Fig. H 13a.   Alpha-1-antitrypsin deficiency. The hepatocytes contain homogeneous, spherical, PAS-positive inclusions. These are not easily seen on hematoxylin-eosin stained sections. These inclusions are in the rough endoplasmic reticulum *(see Fig. H2)* and are pathognomonic.   (trichrome-PAS)

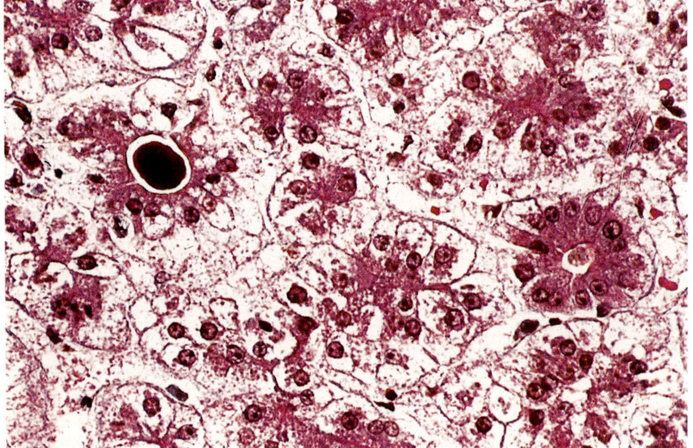

Fig. H 13b.   Glycogen storage type I (von Gierke's disease). This autosomal recessive disorder is due to a deficiency of glucose-6-phosphatase. Liver cells are greatly distended by glycogen stores. The cells appear optically clear in this preparation, with nuclei generally pushed to the cell membrane. Chronic liver disease is not seen in type I glycogen storage disease.   (Ladewig)

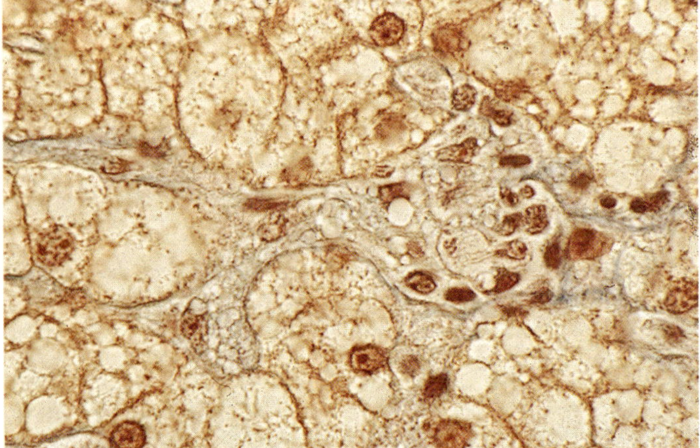

Fig. H 13c.   Galactosemia. Many of the liver cells contain microvesicular fat droplets. The liver cells are in rosette-like arrangements, often surrounding bile canaliculi. A dilated canaliculus, filled with bilirubin, is at the upper left. This autosomal recessive disorder is due to congenital deficiency of galactose-1-phosphate uridyl-transferase. The ocular nerves and brain might be affected also. (hematoxylin-eosin)

Fig. H 13d.   Cholesterol ester storage disease (Wolman's disease). This fatal autosomal recessive disorder affects nearly all organs. In this photomicrograph the liver cells are greatly enlarged and filled with fine droplet fat. Lipid accumulation is due to deficiency of acid esterase.   (Ladewig)

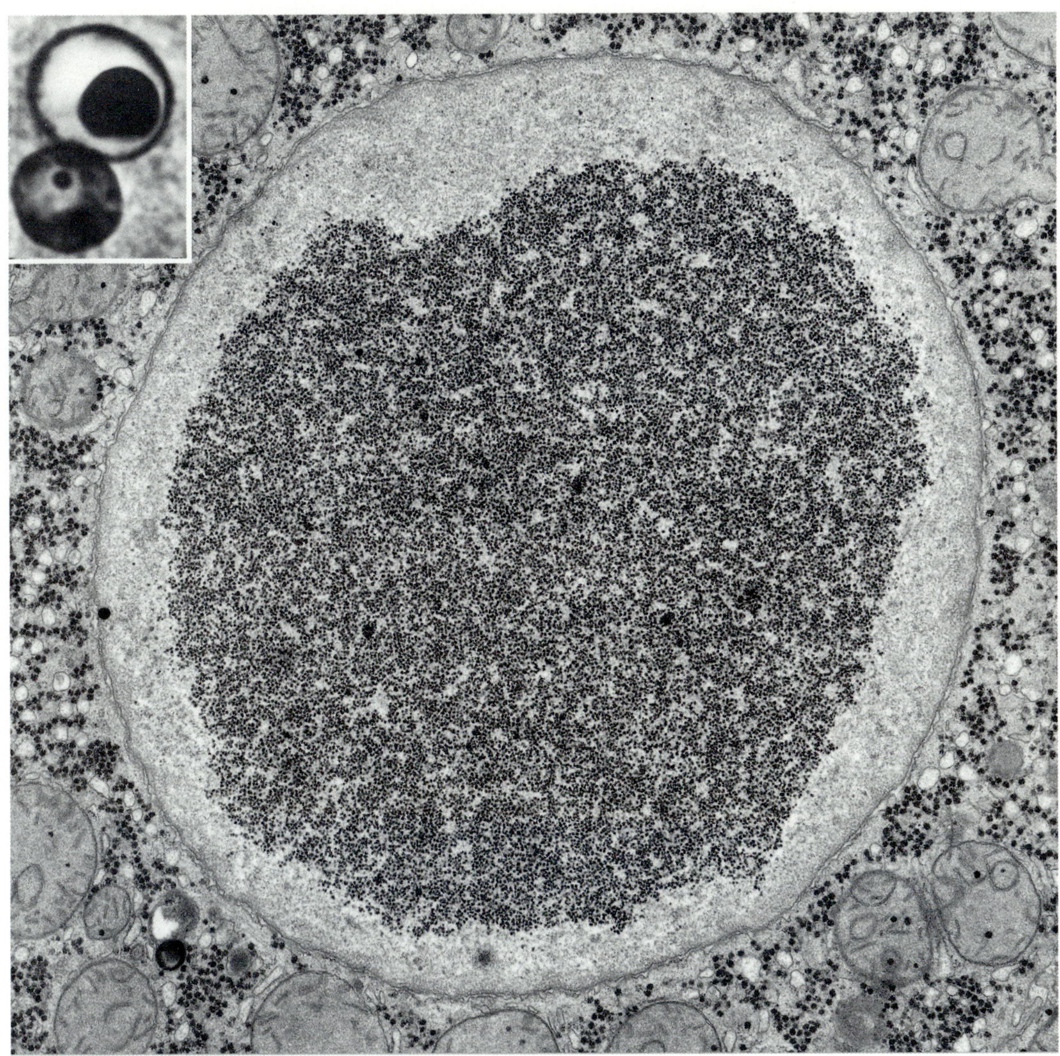

Fig. H14. Glycogen nucleus. The inset shows the light microscopic appearance of glycogen nuclei. The nucleus appears generally clear with margination and clumping of chromatin. In the electron micrograph the individual glycogen granules can be appreciated. In addition, the nuclear membrane appears to be doubled. This is because this process is, in reality, cytoplasmic and not nuclear. The nucleus becomes stretched over a spherical glycogen aggregate and, when sectioned, the aggregate appears to be intranuclear. Glycogen nuclei are increased in number in diabetes mellitus *(see Fig. H 18 a)*, but also can occur as a normal phenomenon during adolescence and in the aged.

Fig. H15. Amyloidosis. In this case the pattern of amyloid deposition is perisinusoidal in the space of Disse, between hepatocytes and endothelial cells. Amyloid is seen in this Congo red preparation as smudgy eosinophilic material. The Congo red-stained amyloid has a characteristic applegreen fluorescence after polarization. The hepatocytes become atrophic as the amount of amyloid increases; they might eventually disappear.   (Congo red)

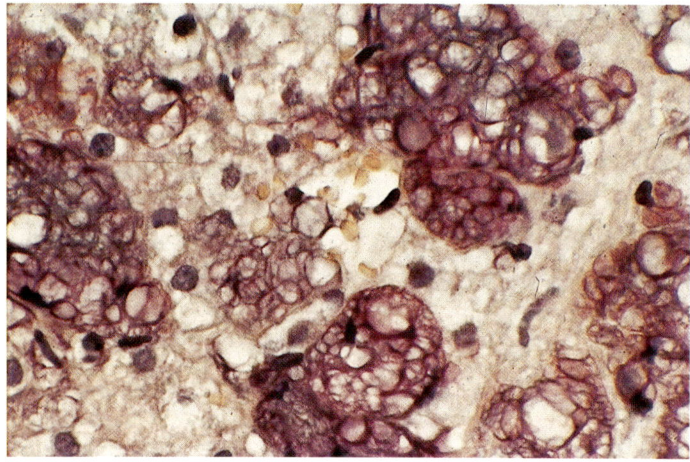

Fig. H 16.   Exogenous materials in the liver.

Fig. H 16a.   Storage of Periston (a plasma expander used in Europe) in Kupffer cells. This material stains with PAS and Congo red and is avidly phagocytosed by the hepatic reticulendothelial cells.   (PAS-diastase)

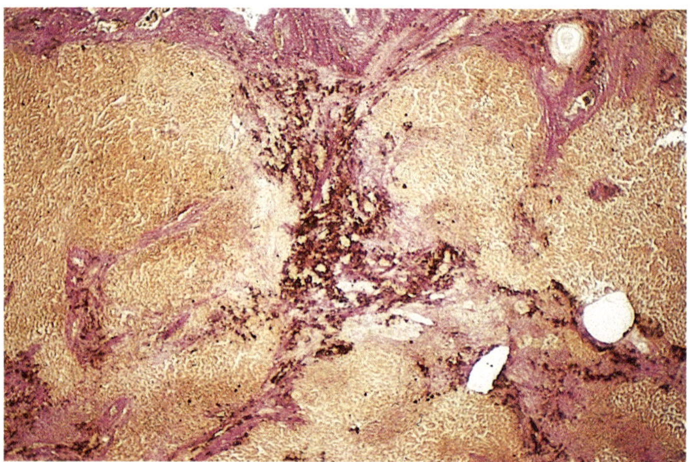

Fig. H 16b.   Thorotrast. A brown refractile granular material is in the portal tract macrophages. This is from the utilization of thorium dioxide as a radiocontrast material, a technique used particularly in the 1940s and 1950s for angiographic studies. The material continues to emit alpha radiation for as long as 50 years and can lead to the development of angiosarcoma and, less often, hepatocellular carcinoma.   (van Gieson)

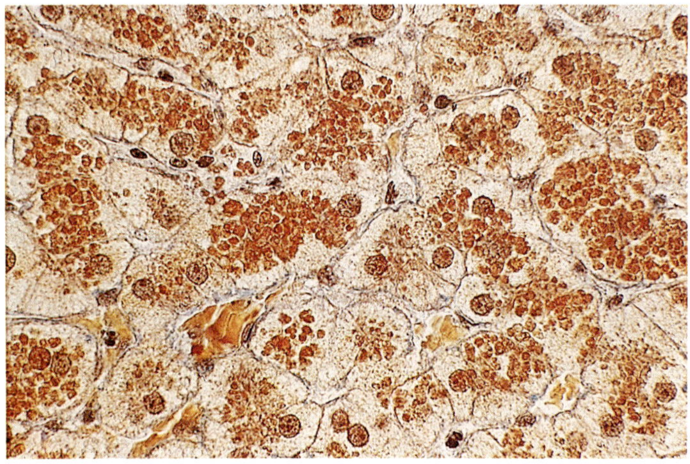

Fig. H 17.   Noniron deposits.

Fig. H 17a.   Lipofuscin granules. In this biopsy (from a patient who ingested excess phenacetin) there are many large, round, brown granules in hepatocytes. Lipofuscin increases normally with aging, but also occurs in many conditions which cause nonspecific hepatocyte injury. Rarely, the liver will atrophy ("brown atrophy"). (Ladewig)

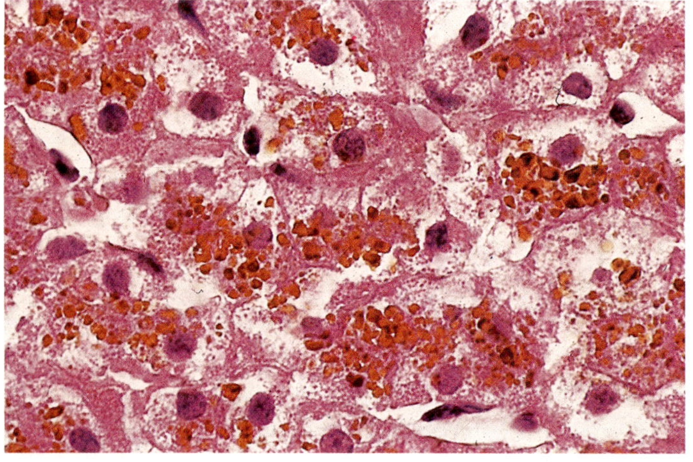

Fig. H 17b.   Dubin-Johnson syndrome. In this syndrome, patients have nonhemolytic jaundice associated with an increase in conjugated and, to a lesser degree, unconjugated bilirubin. Onset occurs usually, in young adulthood, and the condition persists through life. Grossly, the liver is dark brown. Histologically, there are dark brown or black granules in hepatocytes.   (hematoxylin-eosin)

Fig. H 18. Iron accumulations.

Fig. H 18a. Idiopathic (primary) hemochromatosis. Liver cells contain many hemosiderin granules in a patient with idiopathic hemochromatosis. This autosomal recessive disorder is due to excessive iron absorption from the intestinal tract. Associated phenomena are parenchymal deposition of iron and eventual tissue damage, especially affecting the liver, pancreas, and heart. Cirrhosis and hepatocellular carcinoma sometimes develop. Many affected patients develop diabetes mellitus because of the pancreatic involvement. The glycogen nuclei *(see Fig. H 14)* are evidence of diabetes in this patient.   (Prussian blue)

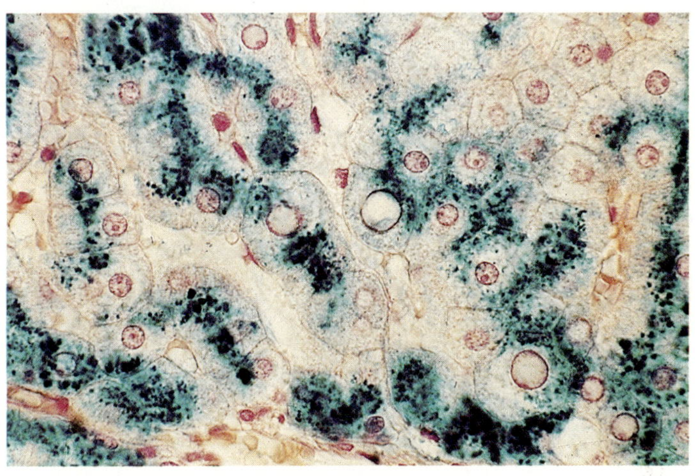

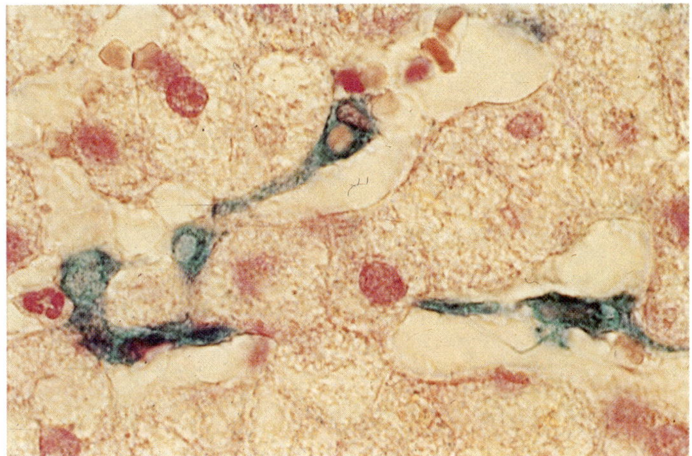

Fig. H 18b. Secondary hemosiderosis. Kupffer cells contain hemosiderin granules, whereas the hepatocytes, in contrast to *Fig. H 18a,* are free of stainable iron. Secondary hemosiderosis may be due to erythrophagocytosis (upper portion of photomicrograph), hemolytic anemias, or the effects of transfusion.   (Prussian blue)

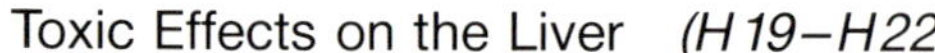

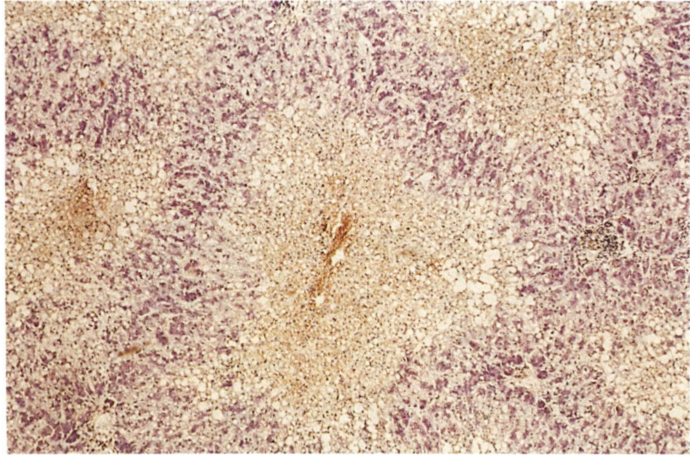

Fig. H19.   Toxic necrosis of the liver.

Fig. H19a.   Carbon tetrachloride. There is necrosis of the centrolobular (zone 3) hepatocytes. The periportal hepatocytes are still viable, but the injury may, at this stage, be lethal. The endothelial cells might still be present.   (hematoxylin-eosin)

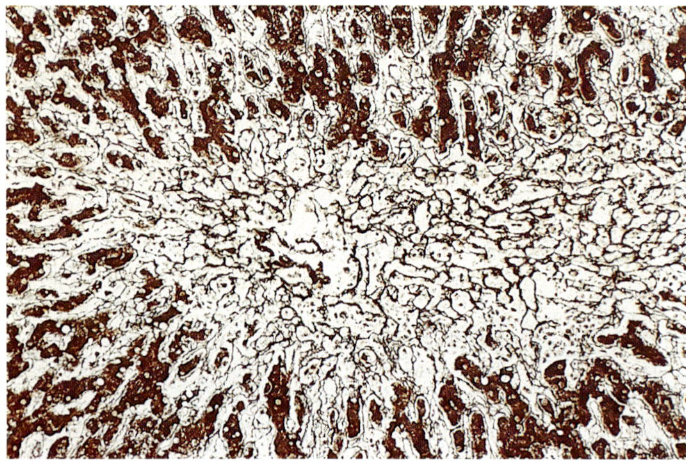

Fig. H19b.   Mushroom poisoning. This specimen is from a patient who ingested *Amanita phalloides.* Histologically this sample is similar to *Fig. H19a.* In this preparation, stained with a silver impregnation method to demonstrate reticulin fibers, the hepatocytes surrounding the terminal hepatic vein are absent and only the reticulin framework of the liver remains.

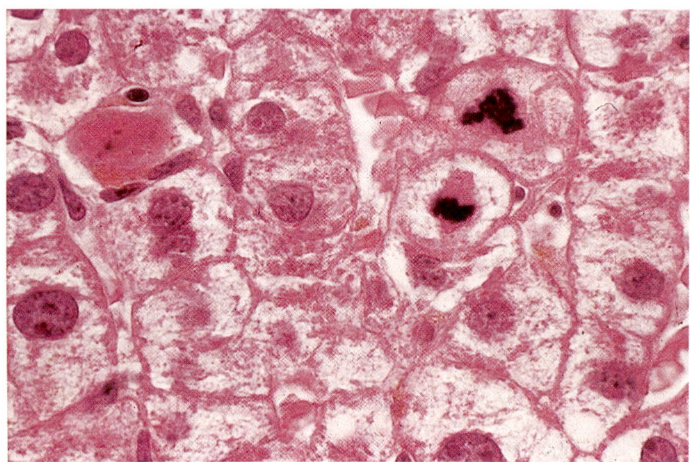

Fig. H20.   Drug-induced hepatic necrosis.

Fig. H20a.   A necrotic liver cell ("acidophilic body") is seen as a homogenous pink structure at the upper left of the photomicrograph. The mitotic figures are evidence of reparative activity. The histologic picture is nonspecific.   (hematoxylin-eosin)

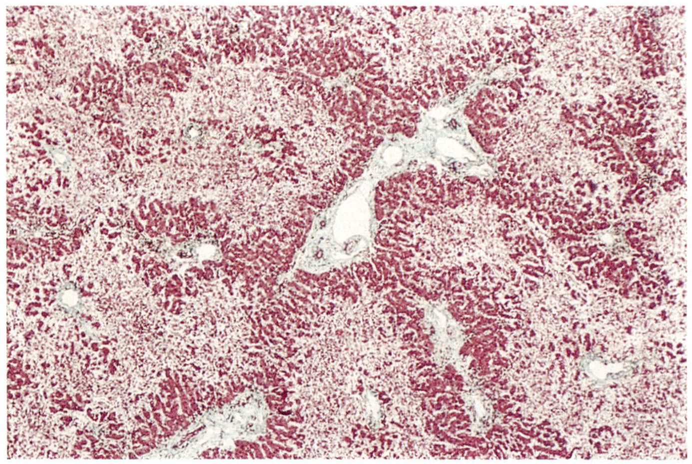

Fig. H20b.   In this severe injury the central (zone 3) and mid-(zone 2) portions of the hepatic lobule are completely necrotic and only a narrow periportal zone of hepatocytes persists. The reticulin framework is still present *(see Fig. H19b).*   (hematoxylin-eosin)

Fig. H21.   Alcoholic liver disease.

Fig. H21a.   Diffusely fatty liver with an anucleate necrotic liver cell (center).   (hematoxylin-eosin)

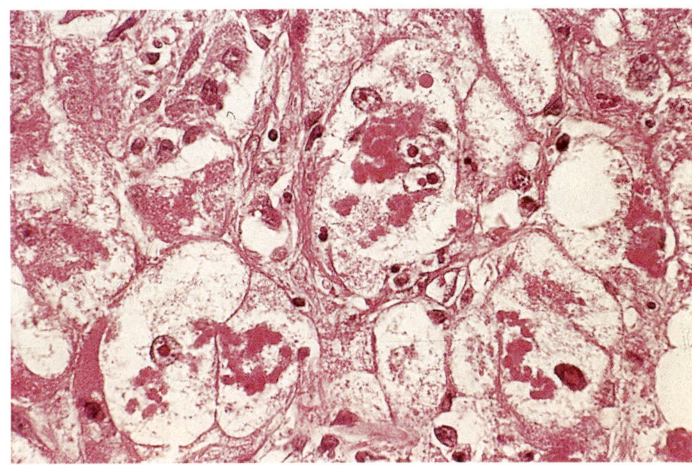

Fig. H21b.   Swollen liver cells containing brightly eosinophilic alcoholic hyalin (Mallory bodies). These structures are due to increased, clumped intermediate filaments.   *(see Fig. H22)* (hematoxylin-eosin)

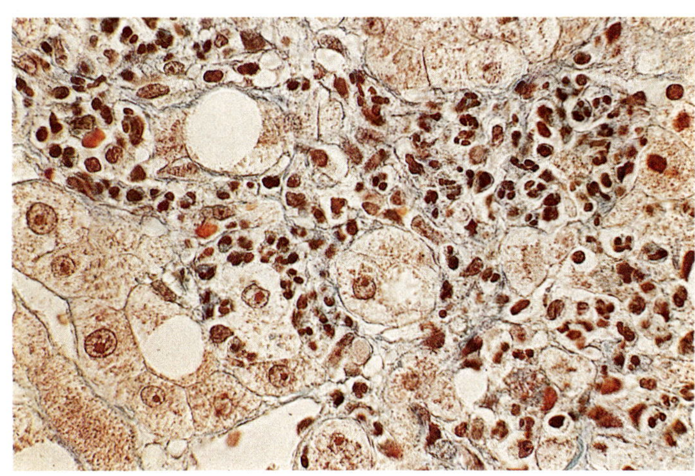

Fig. H21c.   Alcoholic hepatitis. Groups of polymorphonuclear leukocytes are between swollen liver cells and are removing dead hepatocytes.   (hematoxylin-eosin)

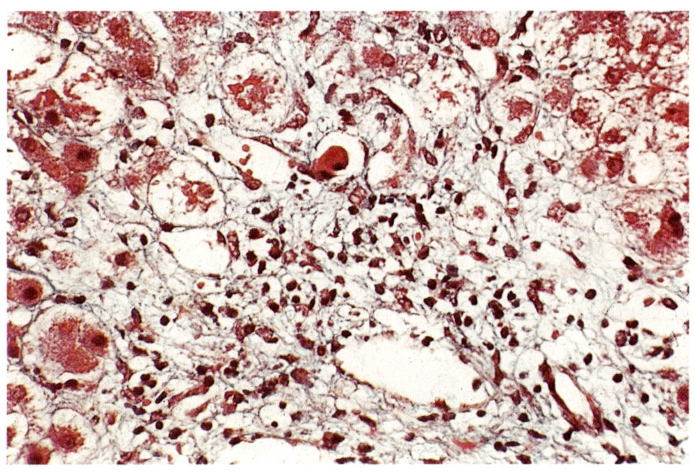

Fig. H21d.   Sclerosing hyaline necrosis, after heavy alcohol intake. Mallory bodies are seen. In addition, there is an increase of perivenular collagen, seen here as pale green material around the terminal hepatic vein and extending into the parenchyma.   (Ladewig)

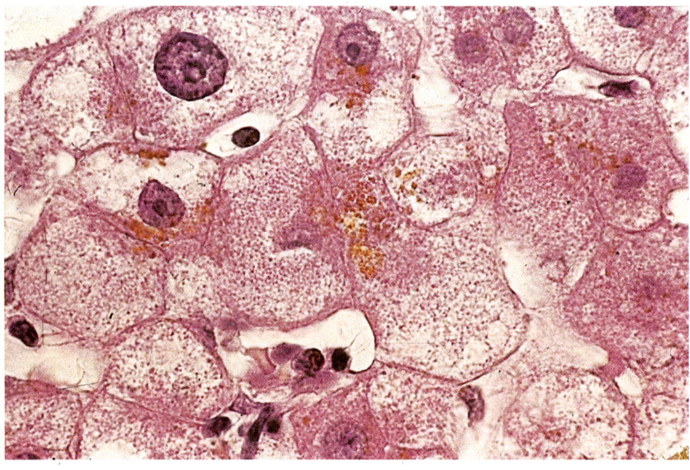

Fig. H21e. Granular swelling of liver cells. In some cases the injury might not manifest as fatty liver or hydropic swelling. Instead there might be a diffuse increase of mitochondria, seen as closely packed, delicate granules in the cytoplasm.   (hematoxylin-eosin)

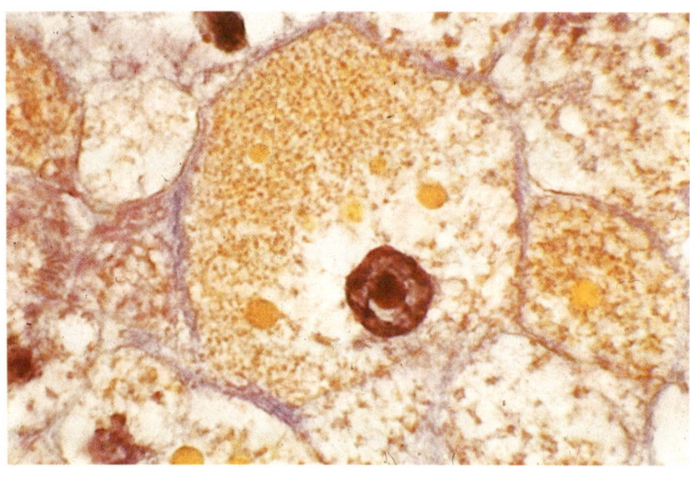

Fig. H21f. Giant mitochondria. In this case of granular swelling of the liver cell distinct hyalinlike bodies are seen. These are giant mitochondria which develop as a nonspecific response to injury. (Ladewig)

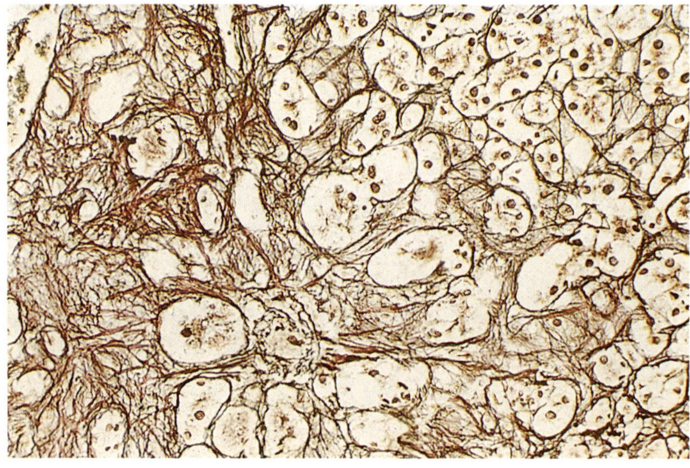

Fig. H21g. Centrolobular sclerosis. Reticulin fibers are markedly increased in the area surrounding the central vein. Many of the hepatocytes show hydropic change. The fibers are coalescing in areas to form fibrous bands.   (silver impregnation)

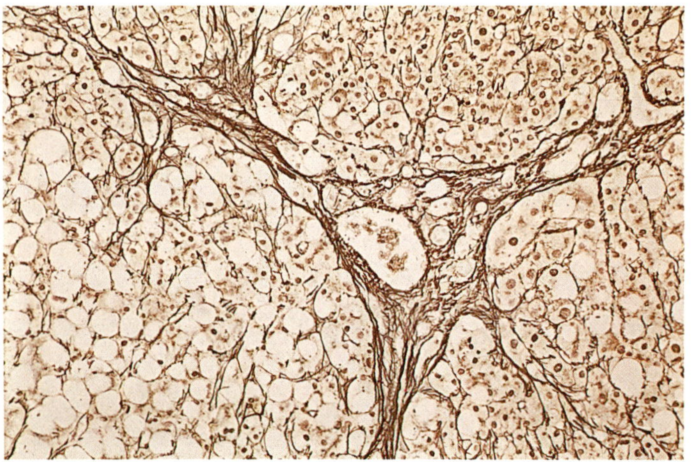

Fig. H21h. Portal fibrosis. A portal tract is seen slightly to the right of center. Reticulin fibers, as a part of fibrosing bands, are seen radiating from the portal tract to a neighboring central vein (upper right) as well as into the lobule.   (silver impregnation)

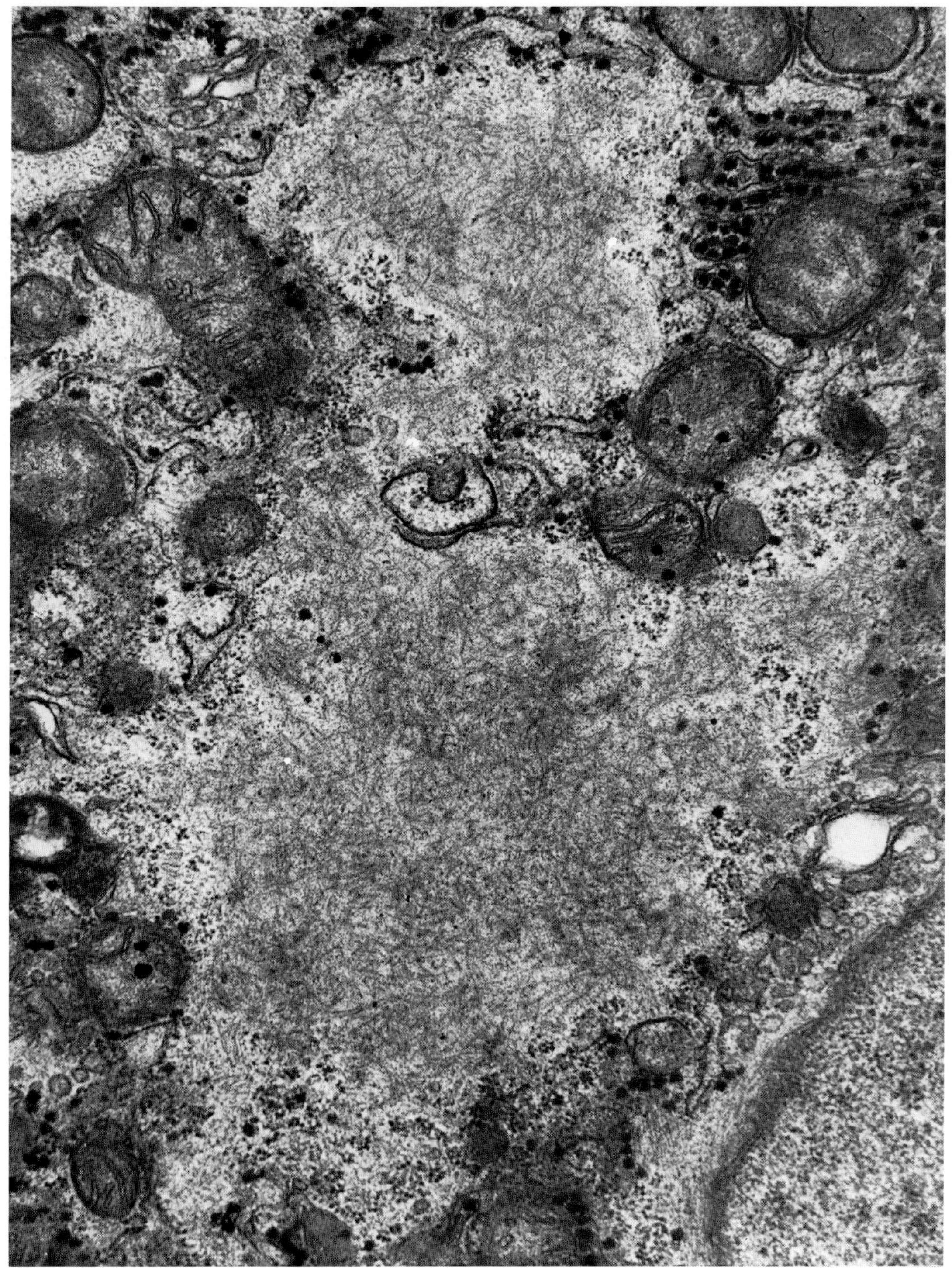

Fig. H22. Alcoholic hyalin (Mallory body). The light microscopic appearance of the Mallory body is shown in *Fig. H21b*. In this electron micrograph, tangles of intermediate filaments are concentrated in the lower portion of the cell. A few, less clumped filaments are at the upper portion of the cell.

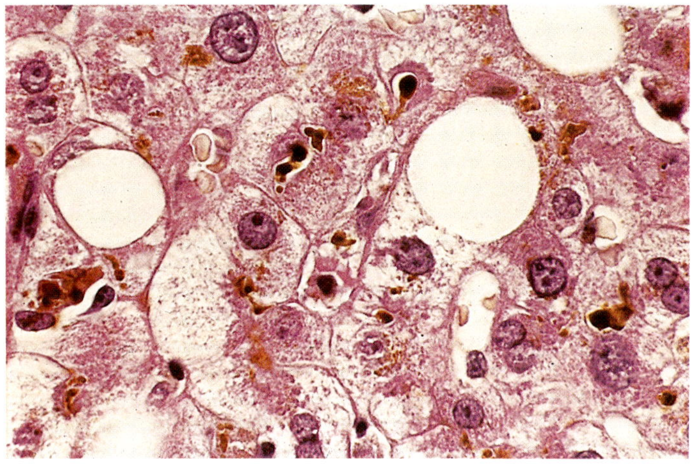

Fig. H23.   Intrahepatic cholestasis. This form of icterus sometimes follows treatment with various drugs. Bile plugs are seen, to the left of center, in dilated canaliculi. Immediately surrounding the canaliculi, the cytoplasm is concentrated whereas, at the periphery of the cell, it is relatively clear. This change is often seen in intrahepatic cholestasis.   (hematoxylin-eosin)

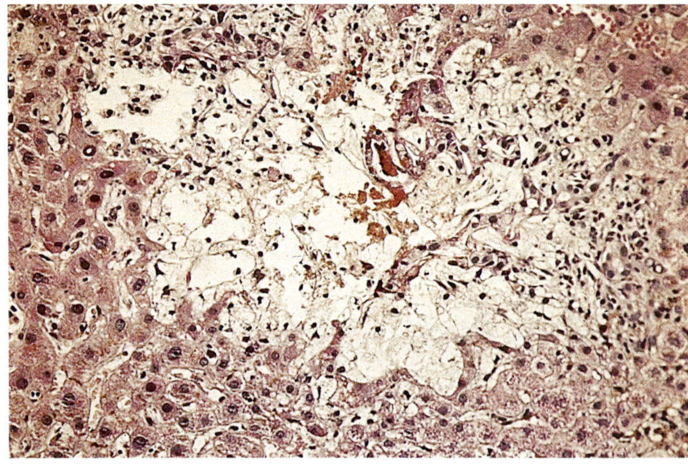

Fig. H24.   Bile infarct associated with extrahepatic biliary obstruction. A bile duct was obstructed in this patient. The patient was jaundiced and the liver biopsy shows "feathery degeneration" of hepatocytes. This change is typical of cholestatic conditions. This is not a true infarct.   (hematoxylin-eosin)

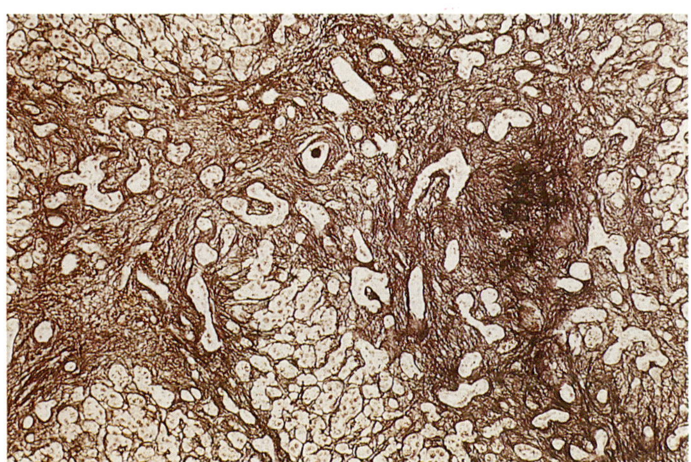

Fig. H25.   Biliary atresia in a newborn.

Fig. H25a.   Extrahepatic biliary atresia. The silver impregnation shows considerable fibrosis of the liver in this two-month-old infant. The fibrosis distorts the hepatic architecture markedly and individual portal tracts cannot be defined. Left untreated this condition leads to secondary biliary cirrhosis.

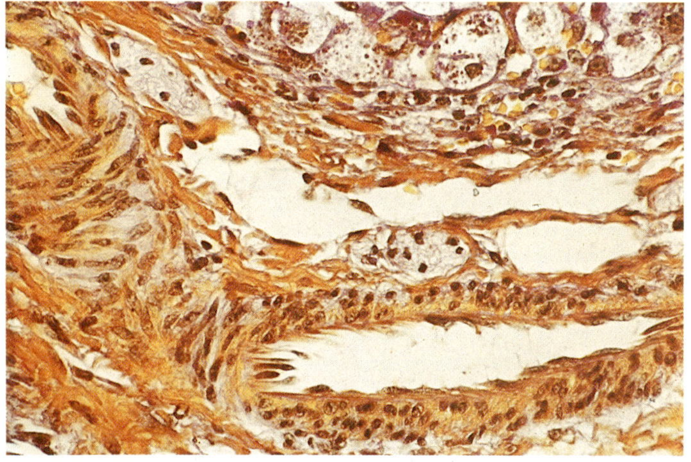

Fig. H25b.   Intrahepatic biliary atresia. The muscular wall of the hepatic artery is seen at the lower right of this photomicrograph, and above it are portal vein tributaries. This portal tract lacks bile ducts and ductules.   (van Gieson)

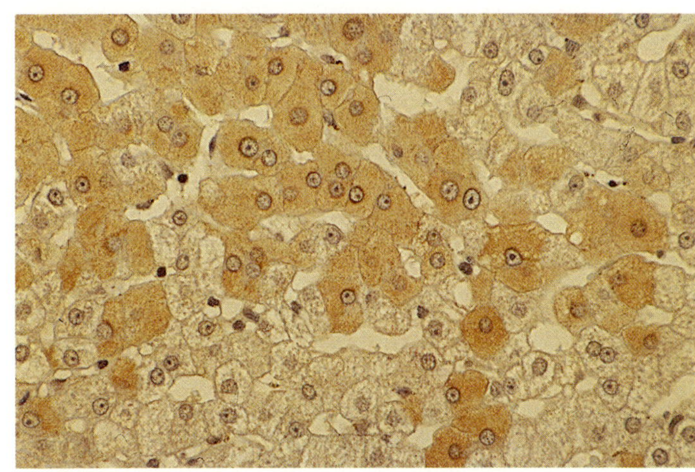

Fig. H26.   Immunohistochemical demonstration of hepatitis B virus.

Fig. H26a.   HBsAg within the hepatocytes, demonstrated with the immunoperoxidase technique. By light microscopy these cells appear as ground-glass hepatocytes.   *(see Fig. H3a)*

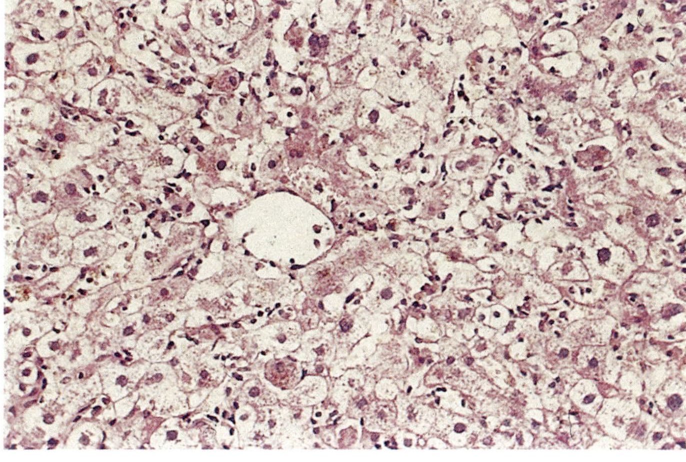

Fig. H26b.   The nuclei of these hepatocytes contain hepatitis B core antigen, as seen in this immunoperoxidase preparation. Some of the hepatocytes can be seen to have a ground-glass appearance.

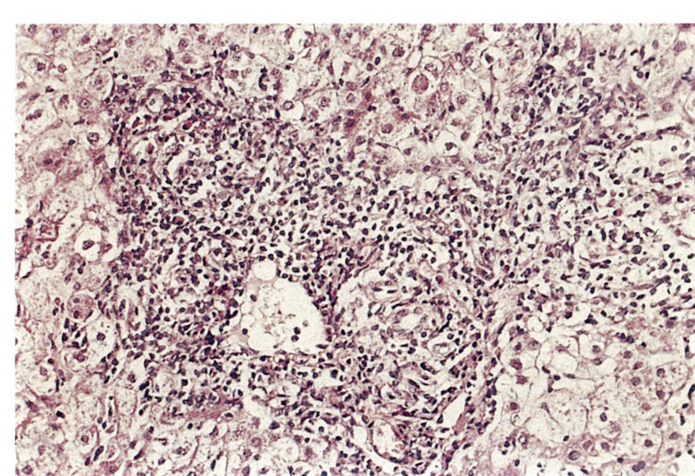

Fig. H27.   Acute viral hepatitis.

Fig. H27a.   This is the typical picture of acute viral hepatitis. The hepatic lobules appear disordered. One sees a variety of alterations of liver cells. There are swollen liver cells, binucleate forms, and acidophilic bodies scattered throughout without a recognizable pattern. Some of the liver cells have a delicate brown pigmentation, evidence of cholestasis. A terminal hepatic venule is seen near the center.   (hematoxylin-eosin)

Fig. H27b.   Inflammatory cells fill the portal tract and spill over into the surrounding parenchyma.   (hematoxylin-eosin)

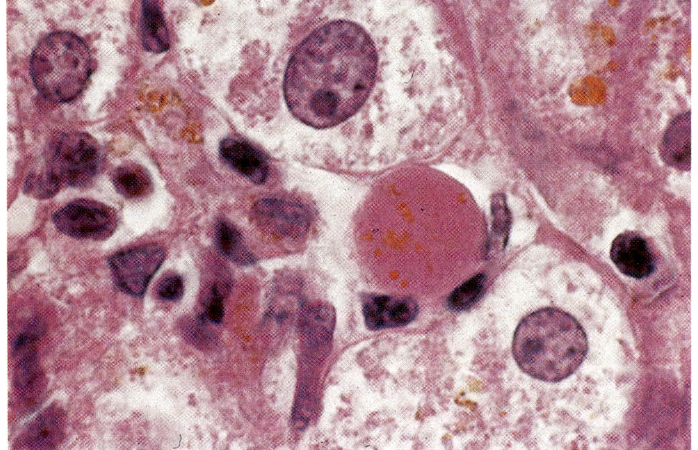

H27c

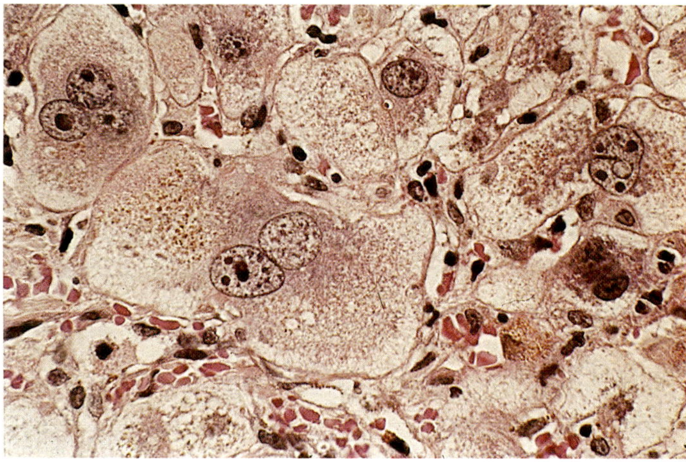

H27d

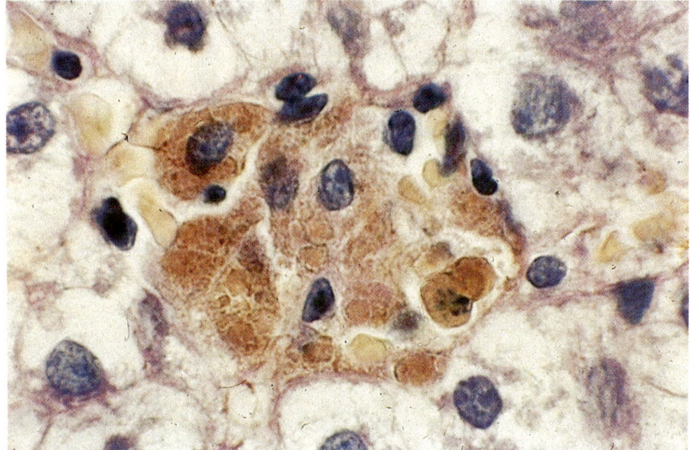

H27e

Fig. H27c.   Single cell necrosis with formation of an acidophilic body (Councilman-like body). These changes are seen throughout the lobule. They are due to the loss of water and the coagulation of protein. They are not specific for viral hepatitis, but they are characteristic. In addition to this homogenous, eosinophilic, anucleate body, lymphocytes and monocytes also infiltrate the liver in this case of viral hepatitis.   (hematoxylin-eosin)

Fig. H27d.   Markedly swollen cells in viral hepatitis. These "balloon" cells appear after cellular insult and reflect cell membrane injury, allowing inflow of water, and failure of the sodium pump to expel the water. If the insult continues, the water will be completely lost and an acidophilic body will result. The cells also contain some cholestatic pigment, and there are surrounding inflammatory cells. (hematoxylin-eosin)

Fig. H27e.   Accumulation of macrophages, containing ceroid pigment, in an area of hepatocyte necrosis. This change can be seen throughout the lobule.   (hematoxylin-eosin)

Fig. H27f.   In some cases of acute hepatitis there is also a hemolytic anemia with foci of erythrophagocytosis in the liver. The iron-laden Kupffer cells sometimes persist beyond the stage of hepatitis and might be the only evidence of the preceding illness. (Prussian blue)

Fig. H27g.   In this fulminant acute hepatitis here are large areas in which the hepatocytes have been lost completely.   (Ladewig)

Fig. H27h.   In this case almost all of the hepatocytes were necrotic and were lost. There is bile ductular proliferation.   (hematoxylin-eosin)

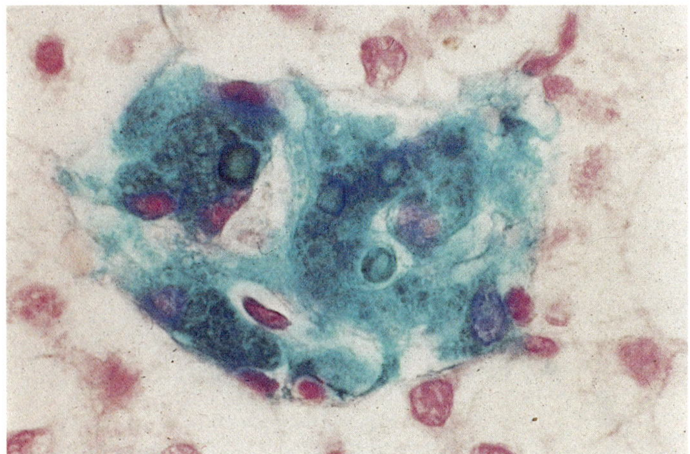

H27f

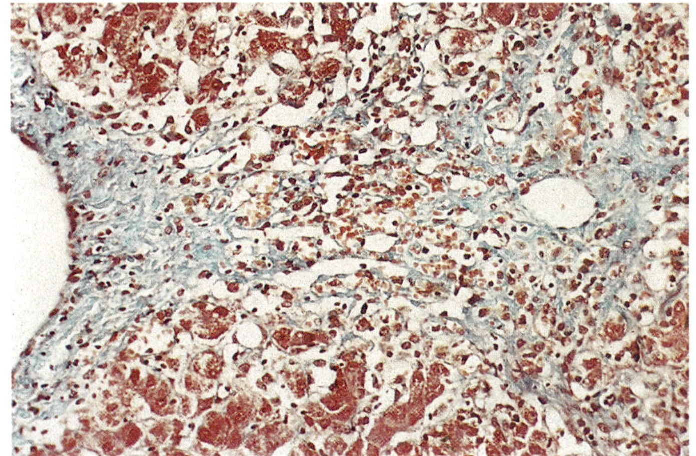

H27g

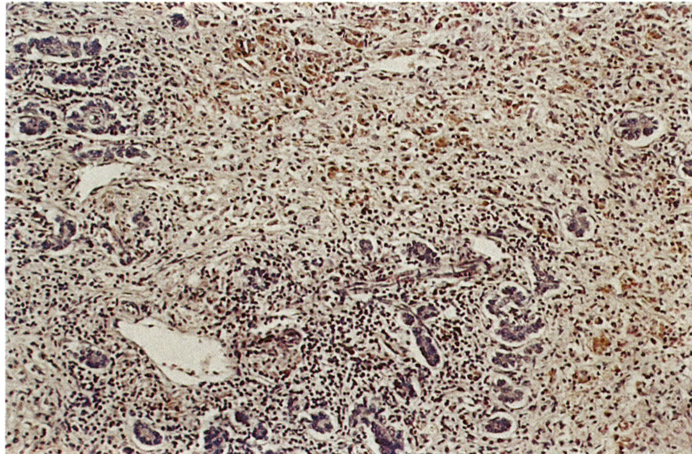

H27h

Fig. H28.   Chronic hepatitis B.

Fig. H28a.   Persistent hepatitis. Many of the hepatocytes contain hepatitis B surface antigen, demonstrated with the orcein (Shikata) method. This finding can be seen in the carrier state as well as in minimal hepatitis.

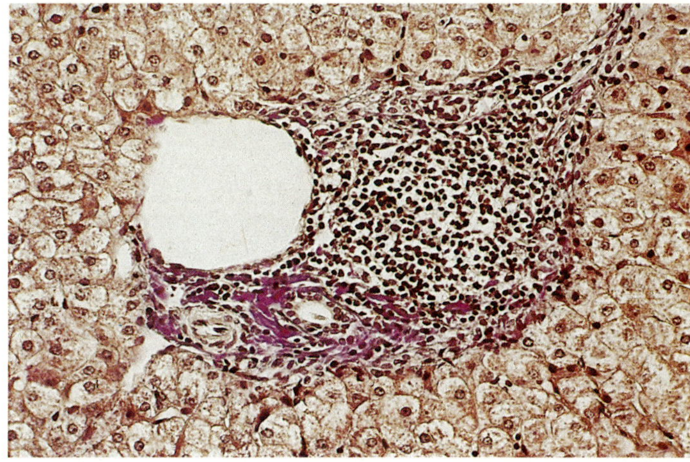

Fig. H28b.   Persistent hepatitis. A portal field is filled with lymphocytes. The surrounding hepatocytes are unremarkable and the limiting plate (the collection of hepatocytes immediately bordering the portal tract) is intact.   (Ladewig)

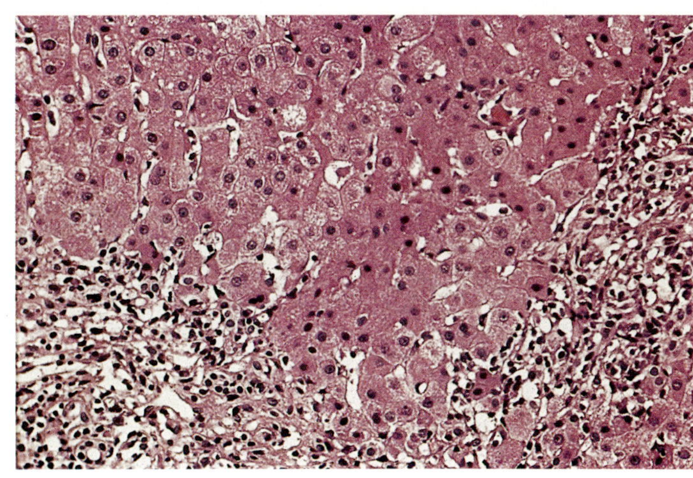

Fig. H28c.   Chronic active hepatitis. This more aggressive form of chronic hepatitis is characterized by a lymphocytic and plasmacytic infiltrate in the portal tracts, with inflammatory necrosis of the cells of the limiting plate ("piecemeal necrosis"). In addition, as in this case, there might be some lobular involvement. A few swollen hepatocytes are present and an acidophilic body is near the upper right. (hematoxylin-eosin)

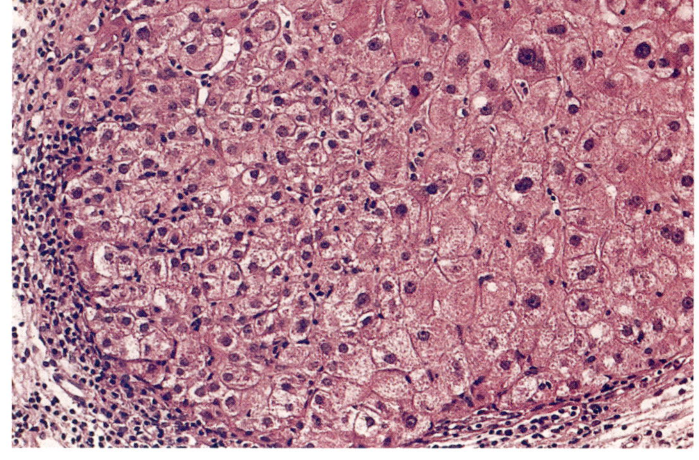

Fig. H28d.   Chronic active hepatitis. In this case the portal tract is seen to the lower left, with its increased numbers of inflammatory cells and piecemeal necrosis of the limiting plate. The hepatocytes in this portion of the lobule also show inflammatory changes with scattered lymphocytes in sinusoids. To the right the hepatocytes are enlarged; this is an area of regeneratory activity. (hematoxylin-eosin)

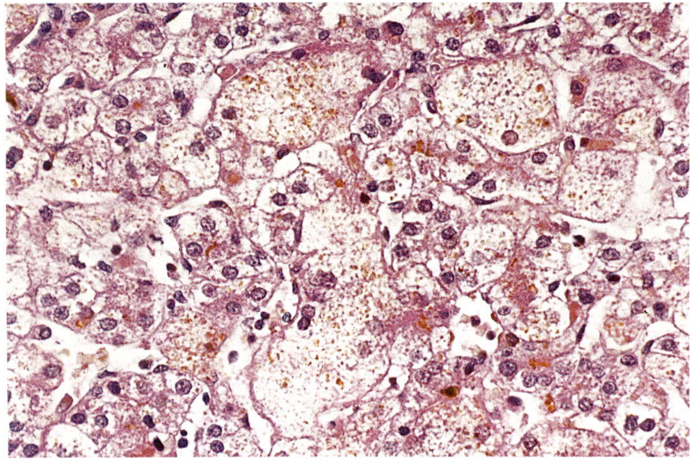

Fig. H29. Giant cell hepatitis from an infant. In this photomicrograph there are a number of confluent hepatocytes forming giant cells. The cytoplasm of these cells contains accumulated bilirubin. This change is not specific but is a characteristic reaction of the infant's liver to a number of injurious agents, including viruses. (hematoxylin-eosin)

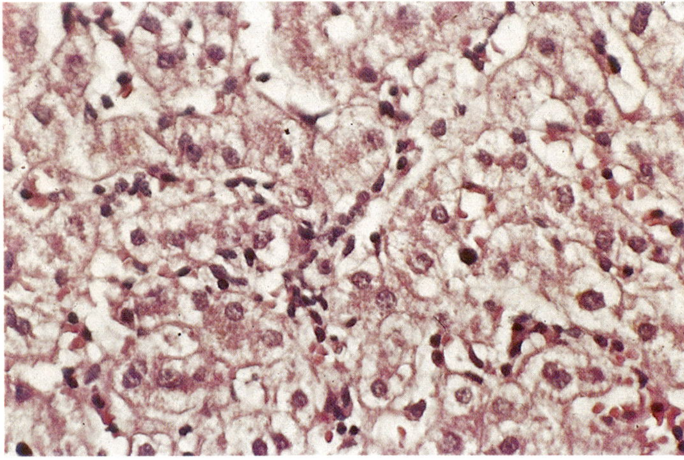

Fig. H30. Infectious mononucleosis. The sinusoids contain atypical lymphocytes and monocytes. This is a relatively benign form of viral hepatitis. The portal tract, which is not seen in this photomicrograph, usually contains a moderate lymphoid infiltrate. (hematoxylin-eosin)

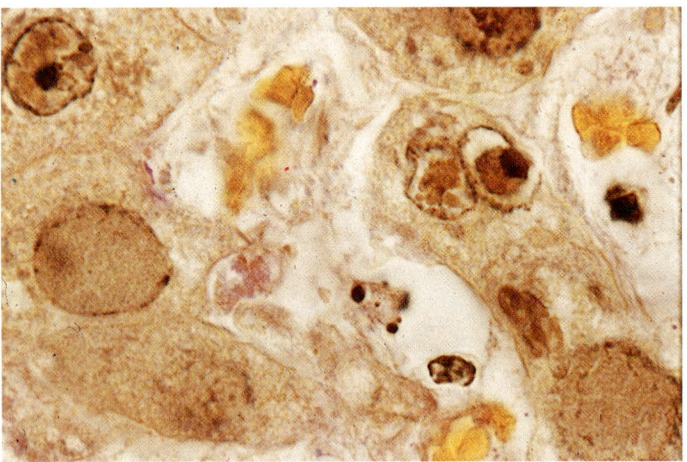

Fig. H31. Other forms of viral hepatitis.

Fig. H31a. This is a case of herpesvirus hepatitis, from a newborn. The hepatocytes have characteristic intranuclear inclusions. These consist of virus material and appear as finely granular pale material within the nucleus, often surrounded by a clear zone (seen to the right of center). (van Gieson)

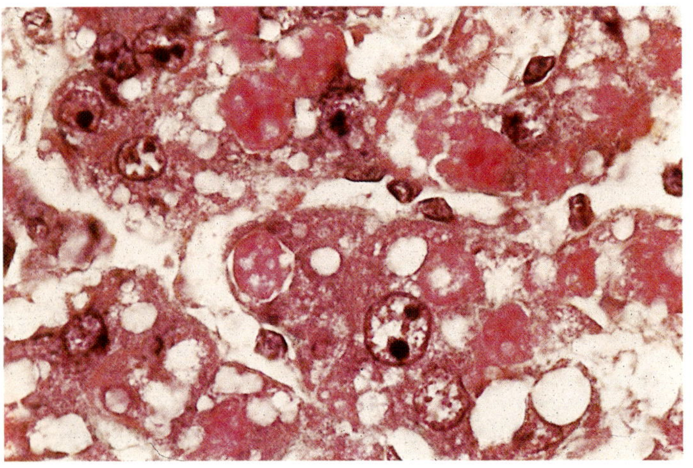

Fig. H31b. Yellow fever with extensive hepatocyte necrosis and accumulation of fat in zone 2 of the hepatic lobule. These coagulated, brightly eosinophilic, anucleate bodies are true Councilman cells. (hematoxylin-eosin)

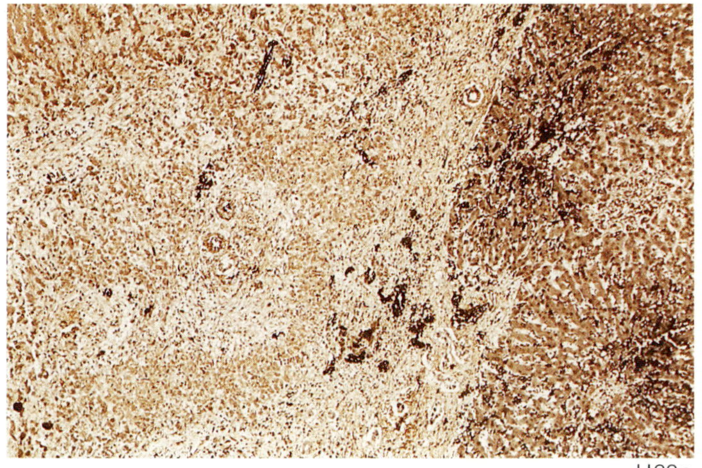

H32a

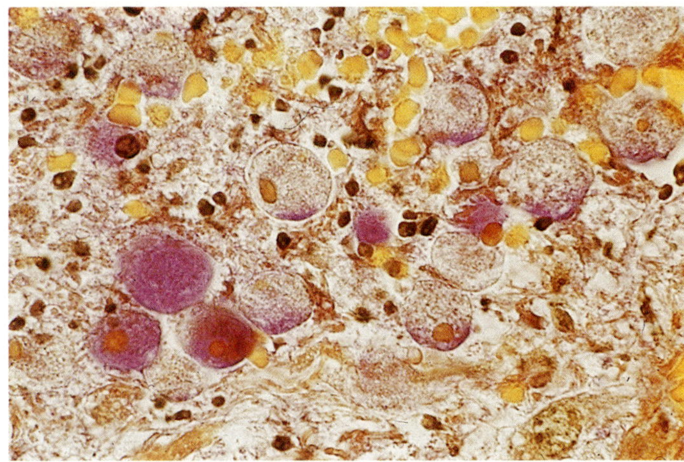

H32b

Other Infectious Disorders   *(H32–H37)*

Fig. H32.   Amoebic abscess. There is a discrete area of necrosis due to growth of *Entamoeba histolytica*. The organisms reach the liver via the portal vein, generally from a site in the cecum, and then spread through the sinusoids.
a) To the left is the area of necrosis with barely perceptible residual parenchyma. To the right is the relatively uninvolved parenchyma. (hematoxylin-eosin)
b) Discrete trophozoites of *Entamoeba histolytica* are seen in a background of necrotic debris and red blood cells. Some of the trophozoites are glycogen rich and, in others, phagocytosed red blood cells can be seen.   (Trichrome-PAS)

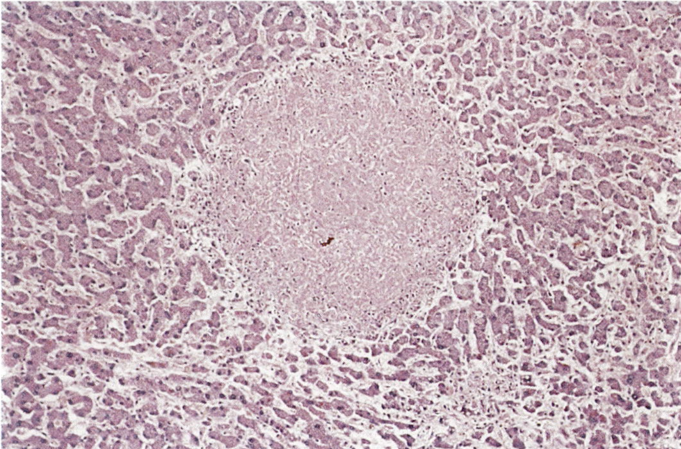

H33

Fig. H33.   Tuberculosis. A caseous granuloma in the liver is seen as a distinct round area of necrosis with a narrow surrounding rim of mononuclear cells and fibroblasts. Within this necrosis, tubercle bacilli were demonstrable. This is a case of reactivated tuberculosis. (hematoxylin-eosin)

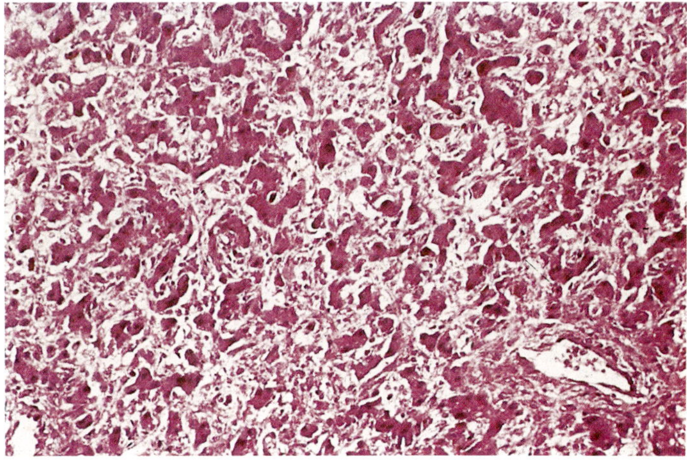

Fig. H34.   Congenital syphilis. In this case there is a diffuse interstitial hepatitis. The normal pattern of liver plates is markedly disturbed. Between the hepatocytes there are many fibroblasts and isolated leukocytes.   (Masson)

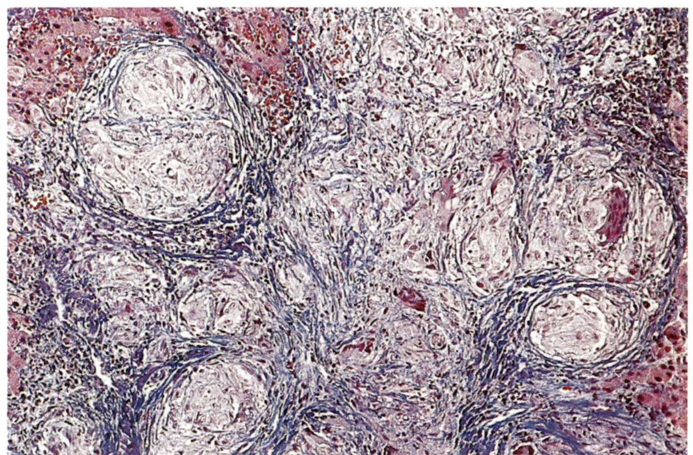

Fig. H35.   Sarcoidosis. Many epithelioid and giant cell granulomata are seen in this portal area of the liver. The granulomata also include Langhans'-type giant cells, but there is no necrosis. The granulomata remain discrete with surrounding sclerosis.   (Ladewig)

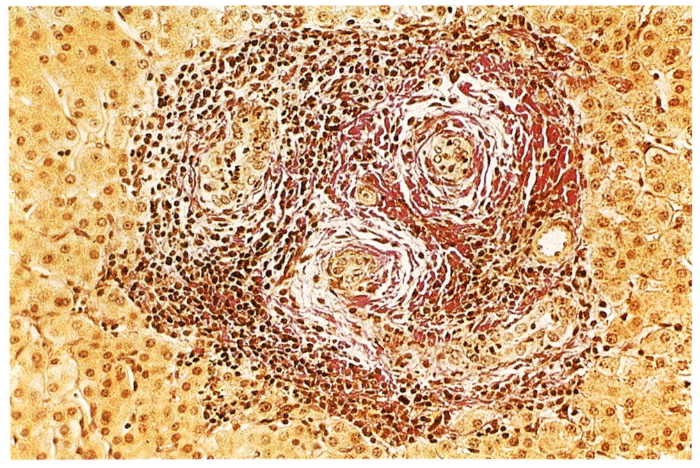

Fig. H36. Purulent cholangitis. A portal tract fills the photomicrograph field. It is greatly enlarged and distorted because of the marked accumulation of polymorphonuclear leukocytes. The bile ducts contain accumulations of bilirubin. This followed biliary obstruction due to gallstones. There is increased fibrosis, evidence that this acute episode was preceded by prior obstruction. (van Gieson)

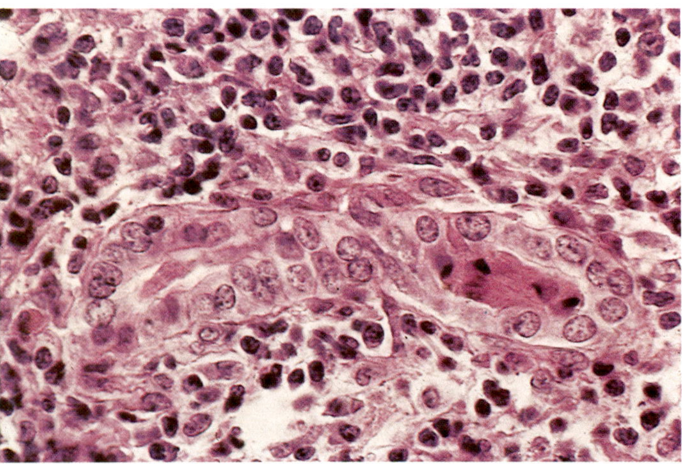

H37a

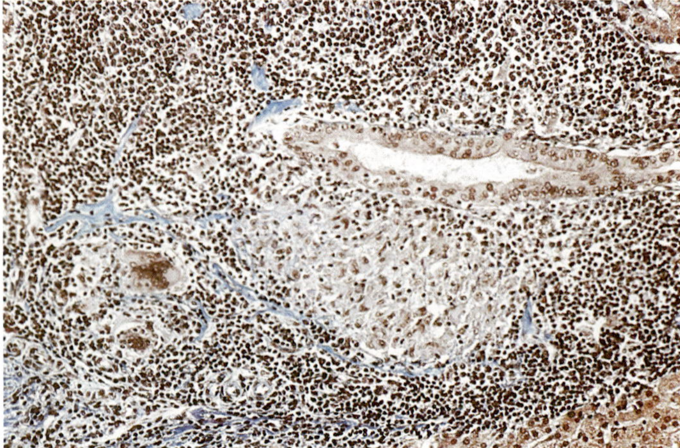

H37b

Fig. H37. Destructive cholangitis.
a) A small bile duct is surrounded by a lymphocytic and plasmacytic infiltrate. A few lymphocytes extend into the epithelial layer and are associated with single cell necrosis. The basement membrane is still intact.   (hematoxylin-eosin)
b) In many cases the portal tracts contain noncaseating epithelioid and giant cell granulomata.   (Ladewig)
c) The granulomata can be found adjacent to small bile ducts. (Ladewig)
d) In longstanding inflammation the biliary structures can be obliterated completely by the fibrosis.   (Ladewig)

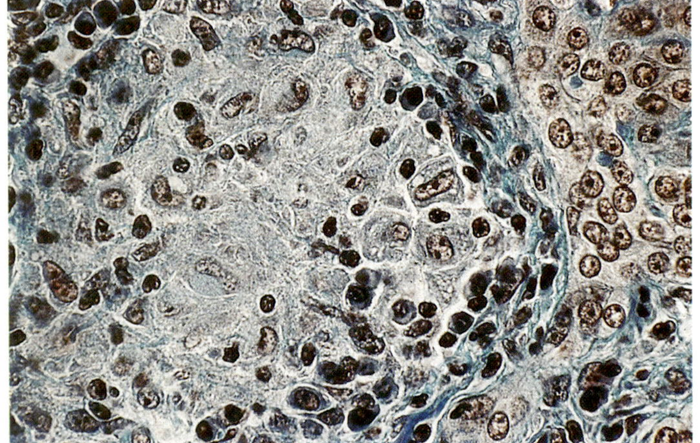

H37c

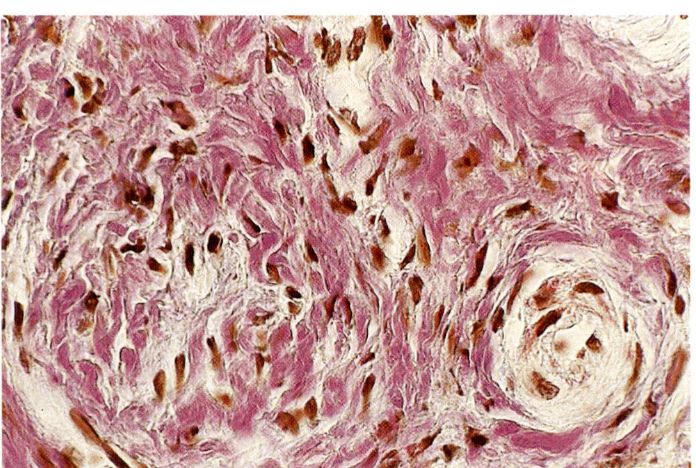

H37d

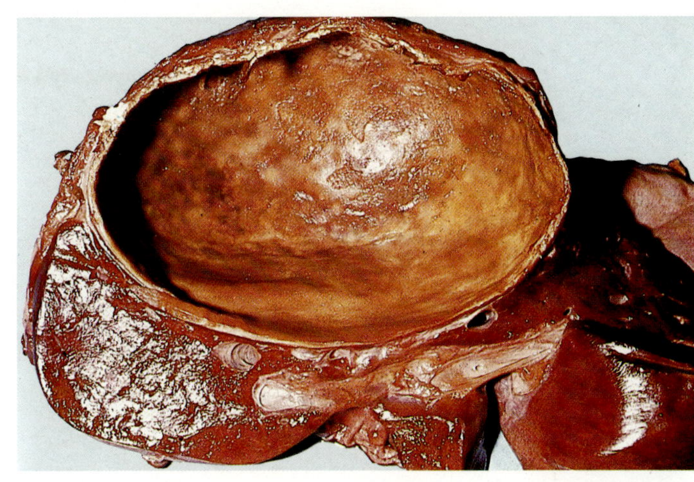

Fig. H38a.   Chronic echinococcal cyst. The wall of this "pseudo-cyst" consists of dense hyalinized fibrous tissue. The parasitic contents are not easily recognized macroscopically. The cyst contains clear fluid but, microscopically, one can still identify residual scolices and hooklets.

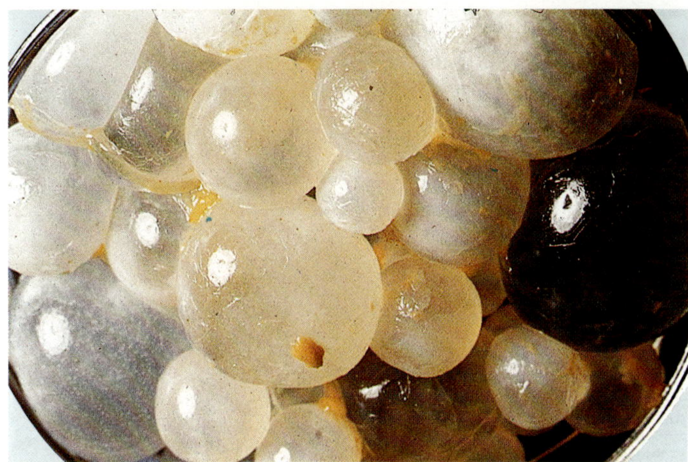

Fig. H38b.   Multiple daughter cysts from an active echinococcal cyst.

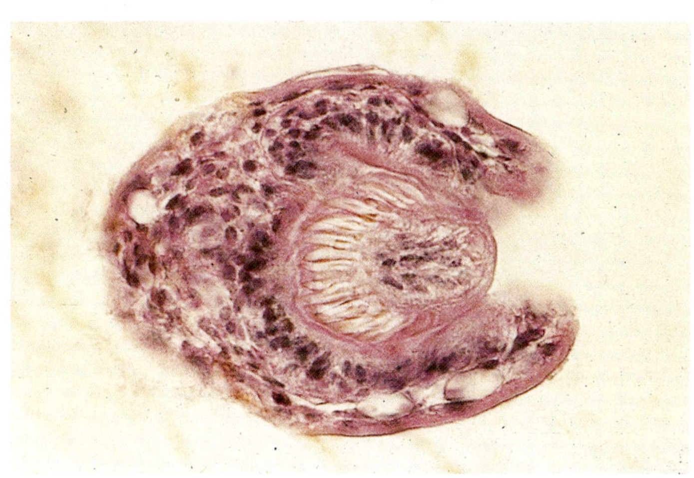

Fig. H38c.   This is a typical scolex with distinct hooklets. (hematoxylin-eosin)

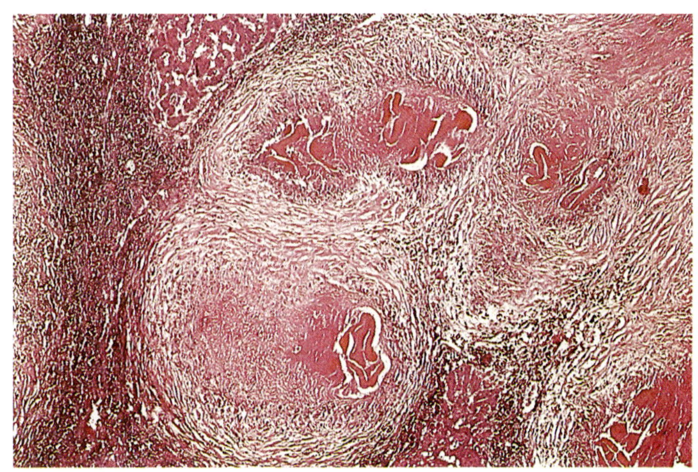

Fig. H38d.   Multiple echinococcal abscesses in the liver. Scolices are not present. There is a bright zone of necrosis with surrounding granulation tissue.   (hematoxylin-eosin)

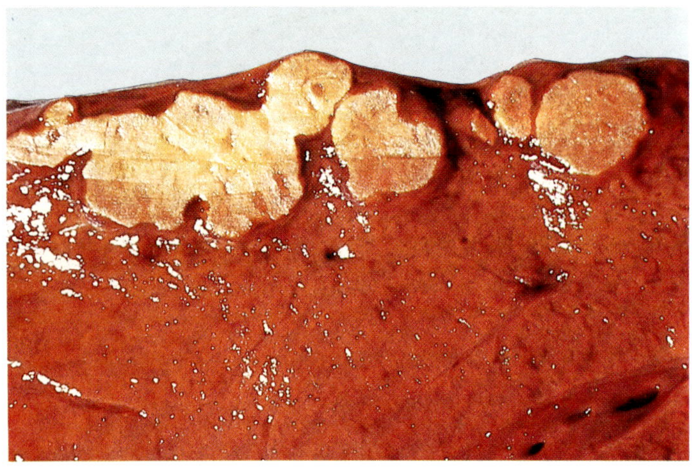

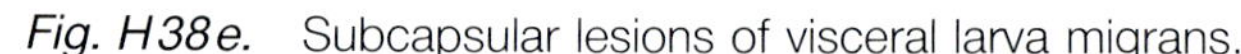

Fig. H38e. Subcapsular lesions of visceral larva migrans.

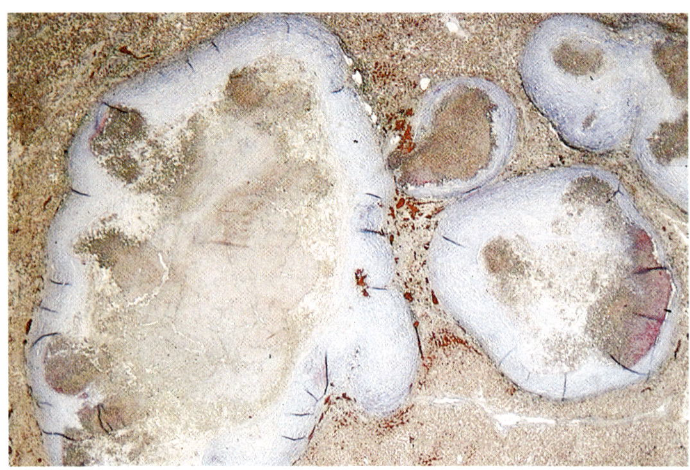

Fig. H38f. Photomicrograph of the lesions caused by *Toxocara* from dogs or cats. In man the lesions are typically subcapsular and consist of poorly circumscribed necrotic lesions within which there are eosinophilic granulocytes in large numbers. This lesion is often mistaken, macroscopically, for metastatic tumor.   (Ladewig)

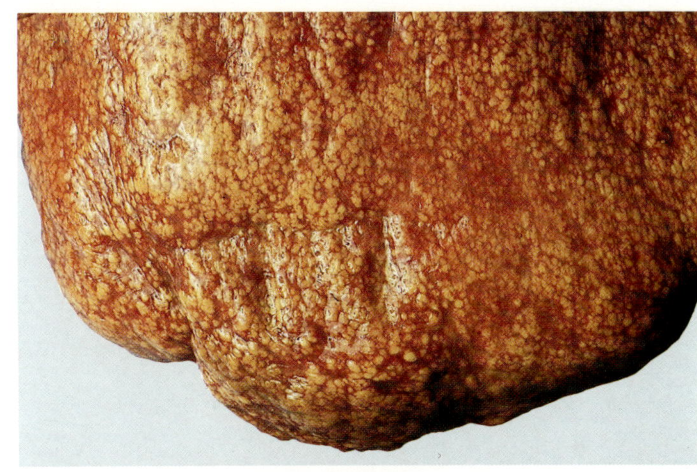

Fig. H39a.   Micronodular (Laennec's) cirrhosis. The liver capsule is granular. The individual nodules are approximately 3 mm in size and are diffusely distributed. These represent areas of regeneration. The somewhat depressed areas, between the yellow nodules, are areas of scarring.

Fig. H39b.   Micronodular cirrhosis. The regeneratory nodules are clearly seen as fairly uniform nodules with intervening fibrous bands. To the right are compressed hepatic veins and portal veins are seen to the left. This is the pattern of cirrhosis usually seen in alcoholic liver injury, but is not specific for that etiology.

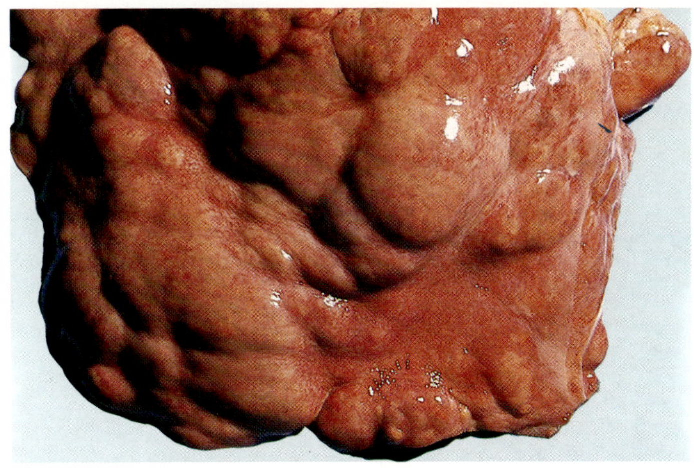

Fig. H39c.   Macronodular cirrhosis. The liver is markedly distorted, as seen from this capsular view, by small and large nodules. At this stage there is usually considerable portal hypertension.

Fig. H39d.   Macronodular cirrhosis. In this section of the liver the variation in the size of the nodules is easily appreciated. Small nodules, similar to those seen in *Fig. H 39b,* are to the right and scattered throughout the rest of the liver, but most of the liver consists of very large irregular regeneratory masses. There are broad bands of fibrous tissue separating clusters of nodules. This type of pattern is often seen following viral hepatitis or after toxic injury to the liver, but is not pathognomonic.

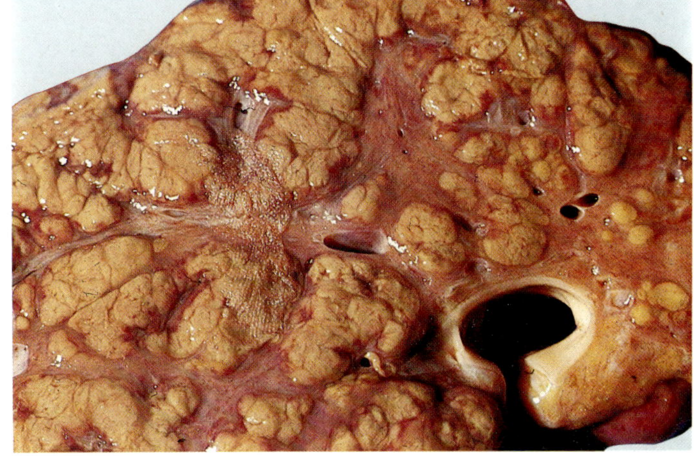

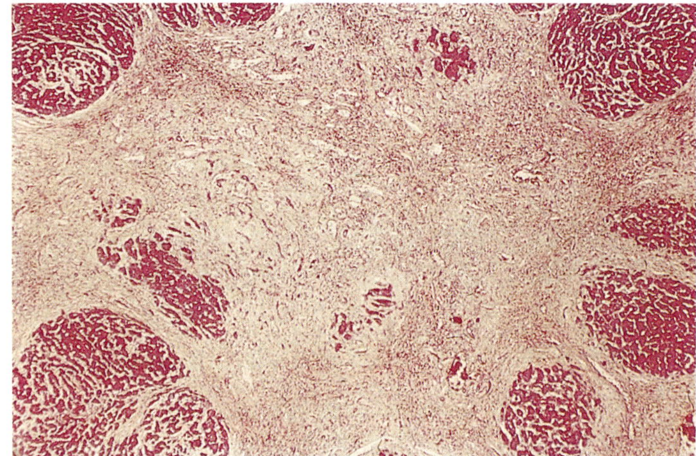

Fig. H40.   Advanced alcoholic cirrhosis.

Fig. H40a.   Although alcoholic cirrhosis tends to be micronodular *(Figs. H39a, b),* with relatively narrow bands of fibrous tissue separating nodules, it can progress to a more irregular form in which there are broad areas of fibrosis as a sequel to ongoing injury and necrosis.   (hematoxylin-eosin)

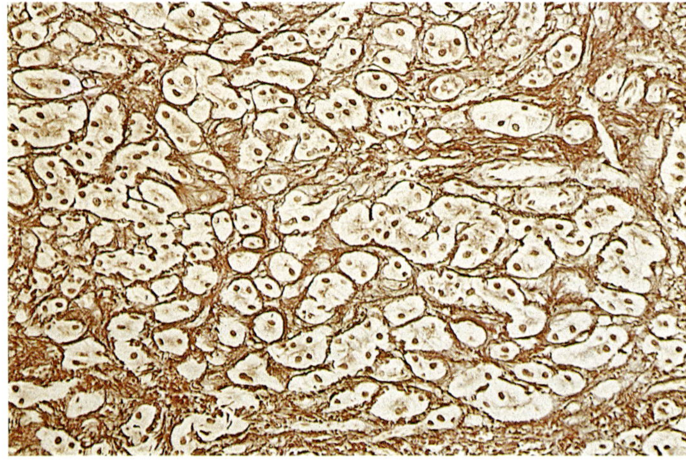

Fig. H40b.   Diffuse hepatic cirrhosis following toxic injury, in this case from alcohol, without the formation of regeneratory nodules. Instead the interstitium is marked by fibrosis. The liver cords do show some regeneratory activity, in the form of two cell thick liver plates, but there is no nodule formation.   (silver impregnation)

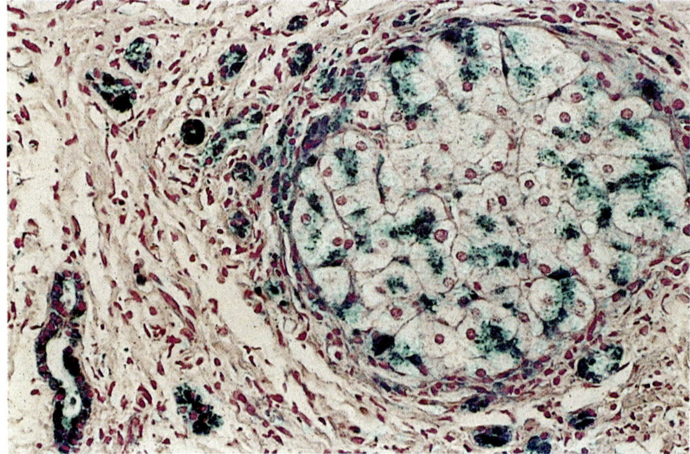

Fig. H41.   Other forms of cirrhosis.

Fig. H41a.   Idiopathic hemochromatosis. The hepatocytes, present as a regeneratory nodule, and the bile duct epithelial cells contain abundant iron pigment. Hepatocyte iron deposition is not pathognomonic, and similar changes can be seen in alcoholic liver injury, for example. The marked iron deposition in bile ducts and ductules, however, is strongly suggestive of primary hemochromatosis.   (Prussian blue)

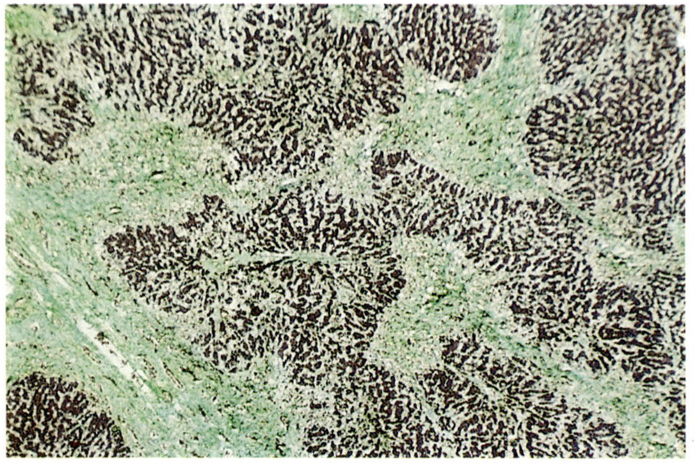

Fig. H41b.   Secondary biliary cirrhosis from biliary atresia. The liver has a "jigsaw" pattern of fibrosis. This is not a cirrhosis in the usual sense, since there is little or no regeneratory activity. Instead there is extensive fibrosis, with distortion and interruption of the usual lobular pattern.   (Goldner)

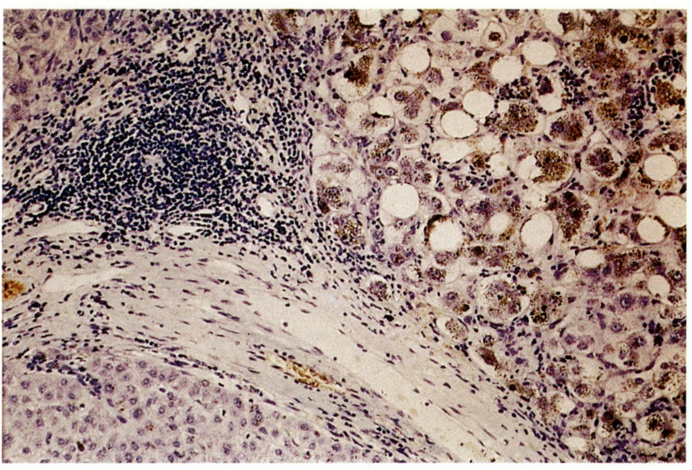

Fig. H42.   Primary biliary cirrhosis.

Fig. H42a.   In the early stages of this disorder there is no cirrhosis, and the alternative name of primary nonsuppurative cholangitis is more descriptive. Here we see a portal tract filled with lymphocytes. Bile duct structures are not visible, since they have been destroyed by this immunologic disorder. Surrounding hepatocytes contain golden brown pigment of intracellular cholestatis.   (Cresyl violet)

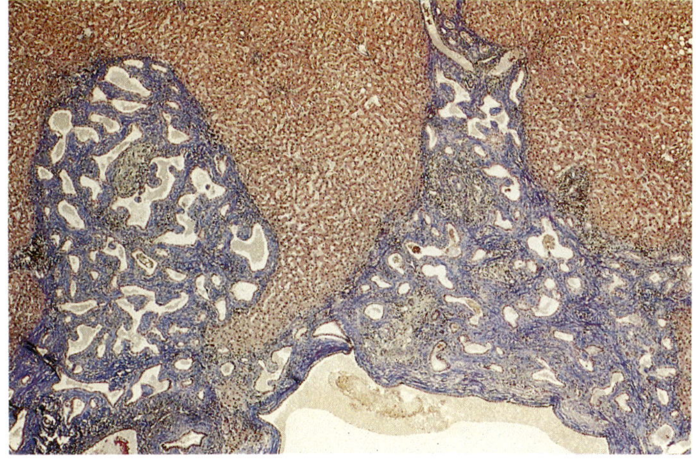

Fig. H42b.   End-stage primary biliary cirrhosis. There is still a marked inflammatory cell component in this liver, but the portal tracts also have considerable fibrosis. There is relatively little regeneratory activity and the nodular pattern is predominantly caused by the bands of fibrous tissue distorting the lobule. (Ladewig)

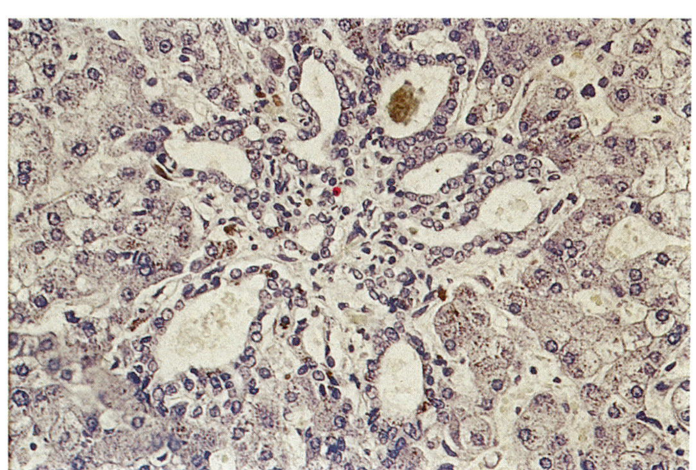

Fig. H43.   Developmental abnormalities of the small intrahepatic bile ducts.

Fig. H43a.   Multiple bile duct hamartomas (von Meyenburg complexes). These small aggregates of bile ducts can be seen, in some cases, macroscopically as cystlike lesions, often just beneath the liver capsule. They do not have any particular clinical significance in most cases, except that they might appear macroscopically as metastatic tumor and, in addition, might occasionally be misinterpreted as metastatic carcinoma in liver biopsy specimen. (Ladewig)

Fig. H43b.   Congenital hepatic fibrosis. Congenital hepatic fibrosis is a rare, autosomal recessive disorder which is characterized by the development of portal hypertension. The liver is interrupted by bands of collagenous fibrous tissue, not well delineated in this photomicrograph, in which there are numbers of microscopic, well formed bile ducts, some of which contain bile, as seen here. The fibrous tracts might contain small arterial branches, but veins are usually indistinct. (hematoxylin-eosin)

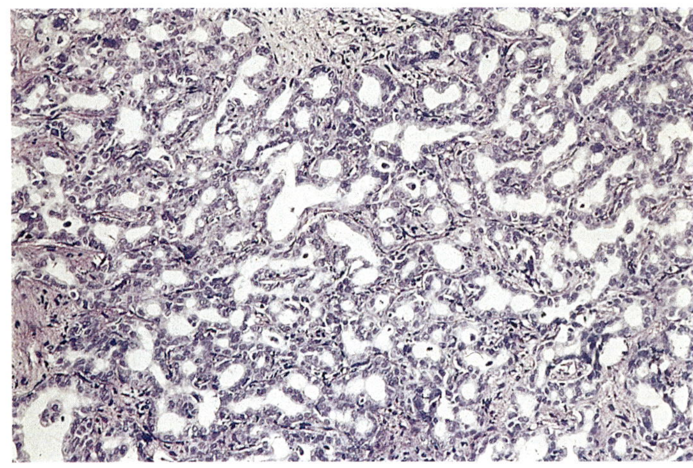

Fig. H44a.   Cholangiocarcinoma. Histologically this is a glandular tumor arising from intrahepatic bile ducts. The tumor cells arrange themselves in tubules, mimicking normal bile ducts. There is no bile secretion. Etiologic factors include *Clonorchis sinensis* infestation, thorotrast *(Fig. H16b),* anabolic steroids, and congenital fibrocystic diseases of the liver.   (hematoxylin-eosin)

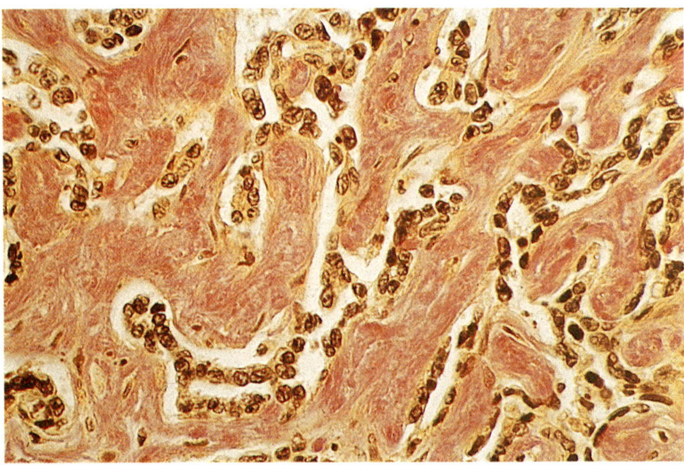

Fig. H44b.   Cholangiocarcinoma. In this high magnification photomicrograph the infiltrating carcinoma can be seen to consist of small ductlike structures separated by fibrous tissue, with little or no capillary formation. The cells are cuboidal and infiltrate periportal lymphatics. This is generally a tumor of older persons and jaundice can be prominent.   (van Gieson)

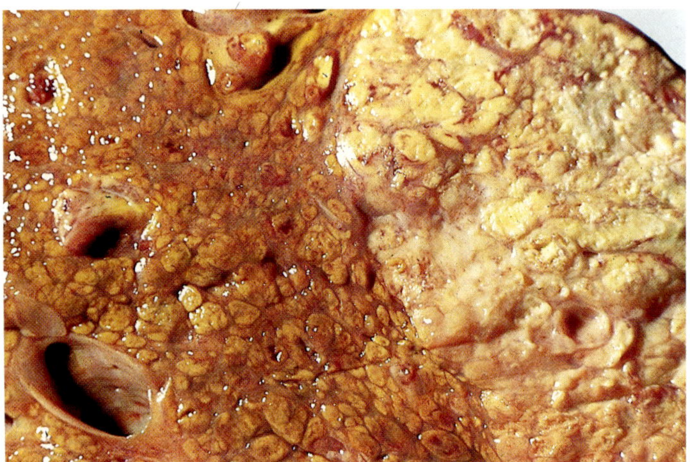

Fig. H45.   Hepatocellular carcinoma in cirrhosis.

Fig. H45a.   Cirrhosis is obvious to the left, and a dominant malignant mass is seen occupying the right portion of this section.

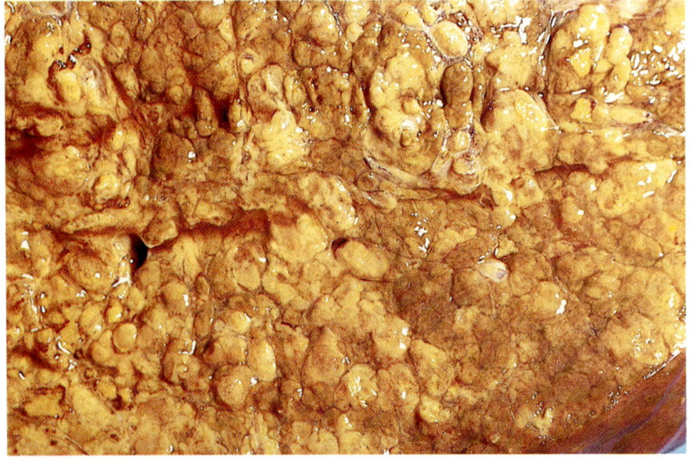

Fig. H45b.   In this cirrhotic liver, there are foci of malignant change affecting regeneratory nodules. The malignant areas are seen as prominent, bulging, yellow nodules. Hepatocellular carcinoma can be multifocal in cirrhosis or can arise in one site as in the previous photograph.

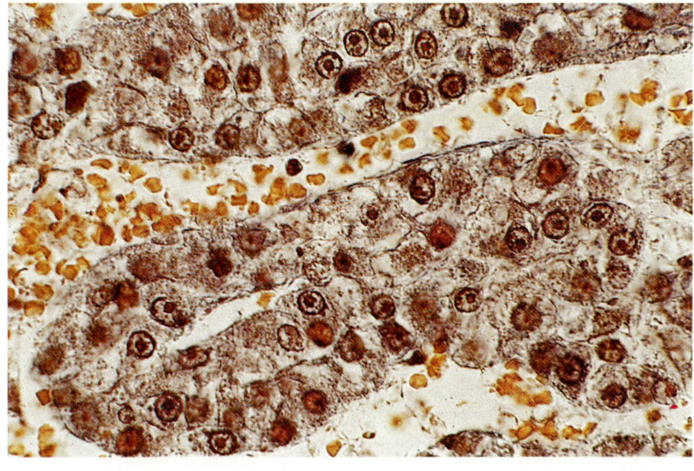

Fig. H46.   Histopathology of hepatocellular carcinoma.

Fig. H46a.   Hepatocellular carcinoma can vary considerably in the pattern of tumor differentiation. The cells, however, tend to resemble liver cells. In this example sinusoids are readily seen traversing broad trabeculae of liver cells which are not cytologically bizarre. Instead the cells are generally regular, with evenly sized nuclei, some of which have prominent nucleoli, and abundant granular cytoplasm. (Ladewig)

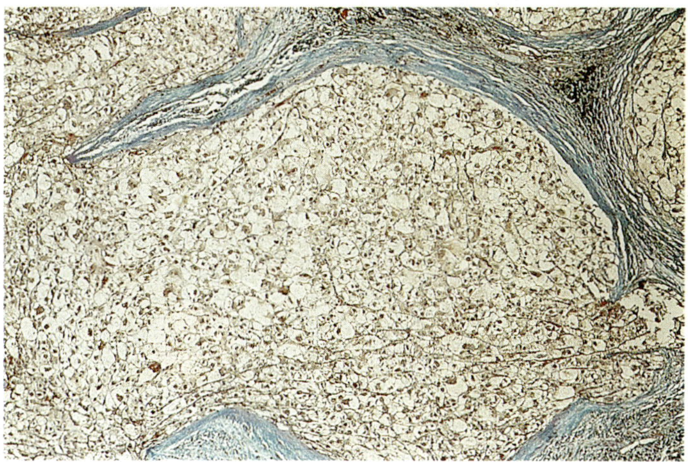

Fig. H46b.   In this pattern of hepatocellular carcinoma, the tumor cells appear as broad sheets as well as trabecular forms, and there are distinct acinar arrangements.   (hematoxylin-eosin)

Fig. H46c.   In this photomicrograph, the trabecular pattern of the tumor is barely discernible. The tumor grows as an expansile mass with compression of surrounding structures imparting an almost encapsulated appearance. Because of the lack of sinusoidal structure there is little or no blood circulation in contact with individual cells. A frequent pattern of spread, for hepatocellular carcinoma, is invasion of portal veins.   (Ladewig)

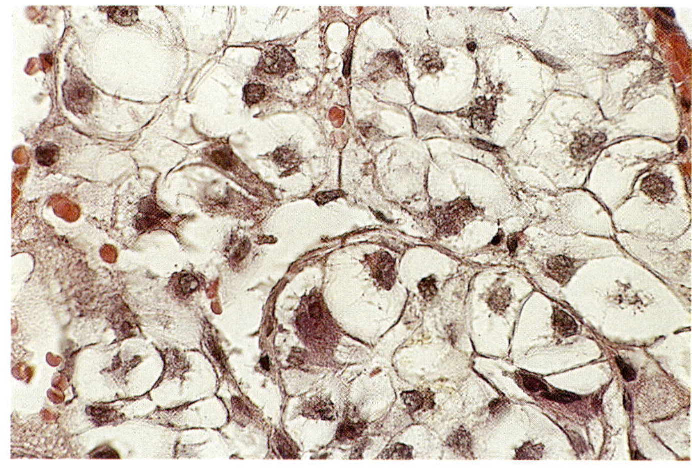

Fig. H46d.   Clear cell hepatocellular carcinoma. This is a rare variation of hepatocellular carcinoma in which tumor cells appear optically clear. The tumor cells contain abundant glycogen. This form of hepatocellular carcinoma can be difficult to distinguish from adrenocortical carcinoma and renal cell carcinoma. This form of hepatocellular carcinoma is often associated with hypoglycemia and hypercholesterolemia.   (hematoxylin-eosin)

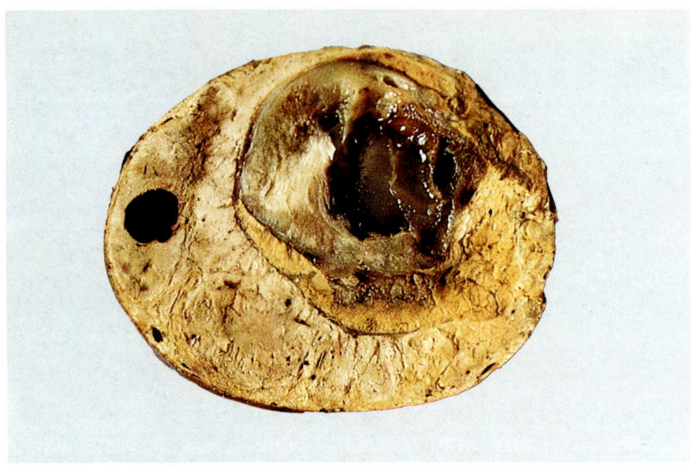

Fig. H47.   Hepatic adenoma.

Fig. H47a.   Surgically resected hepatic adenoma showing a well-formed capsule. There is a large zone of necrosis with secondary cyst formation. Hepatic adenomas were among the rarest of tumors until the advent of oral contraceptives. They are still distinctly unusual. They can also occur during pregnancy.

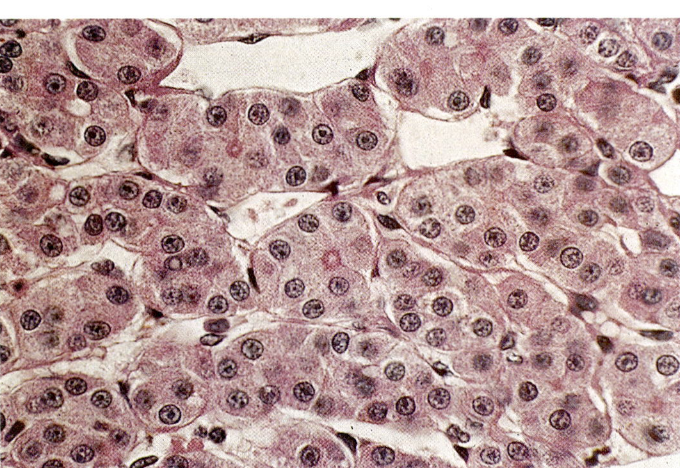

Fig. H47b.   Hepatic adenoma tends to have a trabecular arrangement of cells which distinctly resemble normal liver cells. Canaliculi are easily seen, in contrast to hepatocellular carcinoma, in which there is no canaliculus formation. The sinusoidal structure is retained but distorted somewhat.   (hematoxylin-eosin)

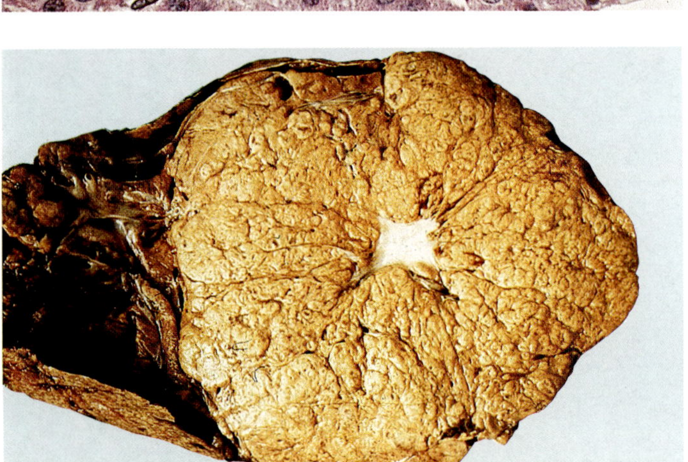

Fig. H48.   Focal nodular hyperplasia.

Fig. H48a.   This well circumscribed, nonencapsulated lesion presents as a nodular mass in an otherwise normal liver. On cut section a central scar, containing an artery, is seen. Septa radiate from that scar, subdividing the mass into nodules and causing it to resemble cirrhosis.

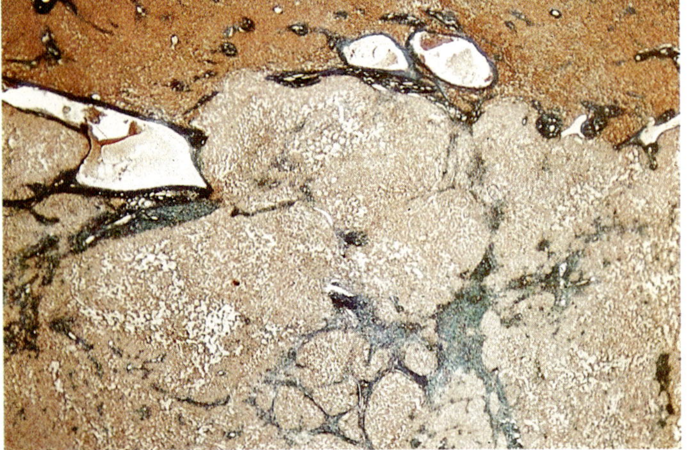

Fig. H48b.   Histologically the central core consists of fibrous tissue with proliferating bile ducts. The hepatocytes are normal. This condition has been associated with the use of oral contraceptives, but does not have as strong an association as does adenoma, since it affects both sexes, including children and women who have never taken contraceptives. Normal liver is seen at the upper portion of the photomicrograph.   (Ladewig)

I. Extrahepatic Bile Ducts

O. Klinge, H.-W. Altmann

The normal functions of the extrahepatic bile ducts and of the gallbladder can be affected by a variety of pathologic conditions. Inflammations are particularly common, and can occur either with or without gallstones. Inflammation can lead to mucosal ulceration. Healing might be complete, there might be scarring, and there might be secondary epithelial proliferation. The most important neoplasm of this system is adenocarcinoma, which can occur anywhere in the extrahepatic biliary tree. Such tumors are often detected late in the course of disease and tend to have a poor prognosis.

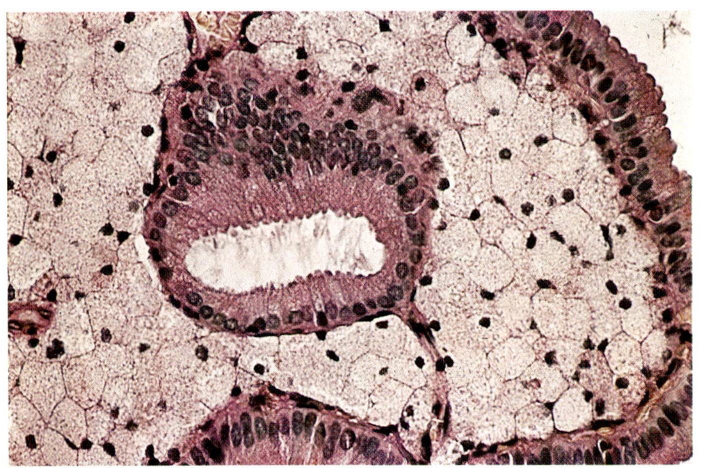

Fig. I 1.   Cholesteatosis. Large subepithelial collections of lipid-laden histiocytes are seen immediately beneath the gallbladder epithelium. These mucosal deposits appear macroscopically as bright yellow flecks. They have no clinical significance. (hematoxylin-eosin)

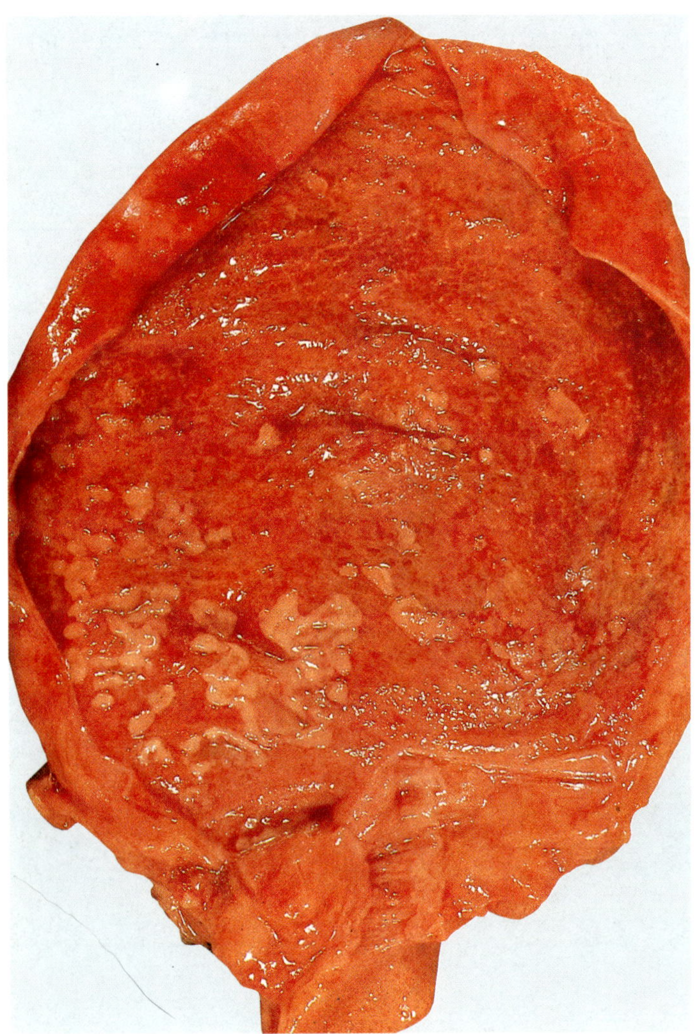

Fig. I 2.   Acute necrotizing cholecystitis. The gallbladder is markedly inflamed. It is dilated, as is the cystic duct, which can be recognized at the lower middle portion of the photograph where the spiral valves of Heister are evident. The gallbladder wall is thickened and the serosal surface, seen at the upper right and upper left, shows inflammatory change (as does the mucosa). There are irregular geographic areas of necrosis with inflammatory exudate, most visible at the lower left.

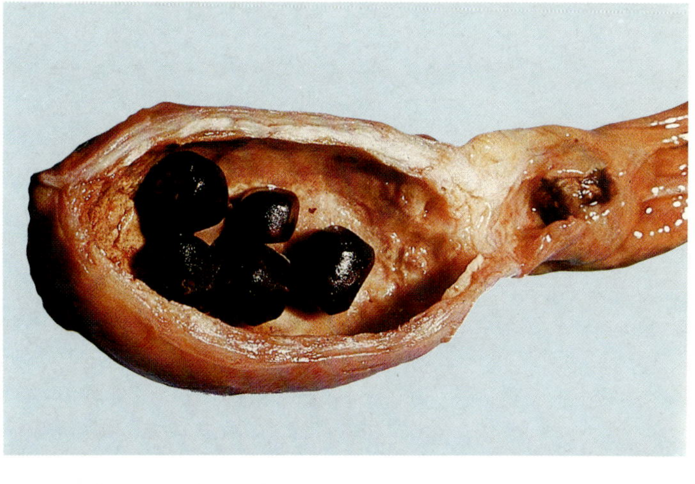

Fig. 13.   Chronic cholecystitis and cholelithiasis.

Fig. 13a.   Multifaceted gallstones in a fibrotic gallbladder. A gallstone can be seen to the right, lodged in the cystic duct. These stones are black, suggesting a high bilirubin content. Because of the obstruction to the cystic duct the gallbladder did not contain bile, but did have a clear, somewhat mucinous fluid ("hydrops").

Fig. 13b.   Histologic section of a "porcelain" gallbladder. In this condition chronic inflammation has contributed to the complete loss of the structures of the gallbladder wall and replacement by dense fibrous tissue and, eventually, diffuse deposition of calcium salts, causing a macroscopic appearance of porcelain. In the calcified state the gallbladder becomes radio-opaque.   (van Gieson)

Fig. 13c.   Chronic cholecystitis. There is accentuation and proliferation of the gallbladder epithelium. Evenly distributed small cystic glands penetrate the musculature and are present throughout the wall. These branching tubular forms all communicate with the surface and consist of the usual mucous-secreting epithelium. The gallbladder lacks a muscularis mucosae and one should not interpret this pattern of glandular inflammation as infiltrating carcinoma. These elaborate structures are known as Rokitansky-Aschoff sinuses. There is also an extensive inflammatory process consisting of lymphocytes, plasma cells, mononuclear cells, and a few eosinophils.   (van Gieson)

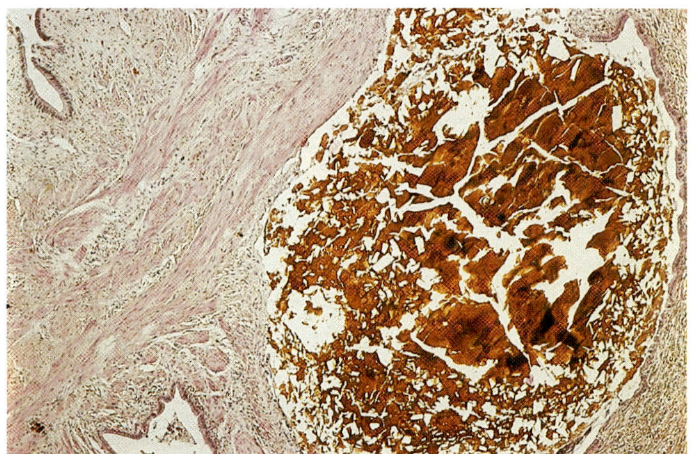

Fig. 13d.   In some of the cystically dilated Rokitansky-Aschoff sinuses one can see crystalline aggregates of bile forming small calculi.   (van Gieson)

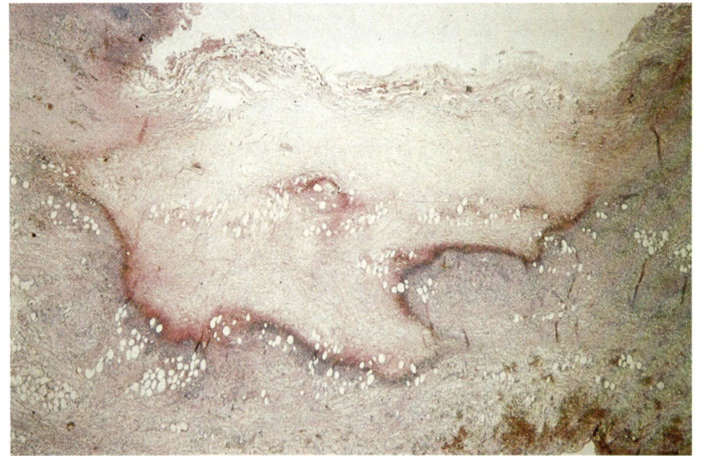

14a

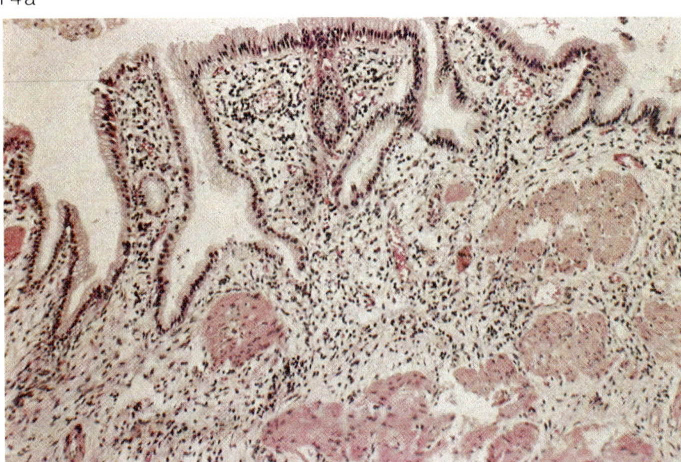

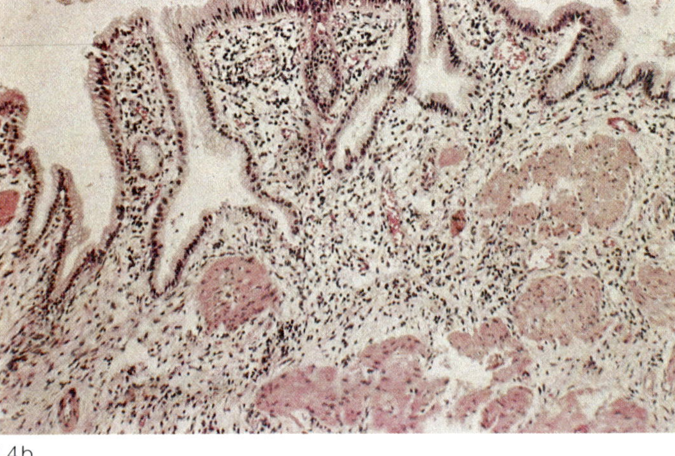

14b

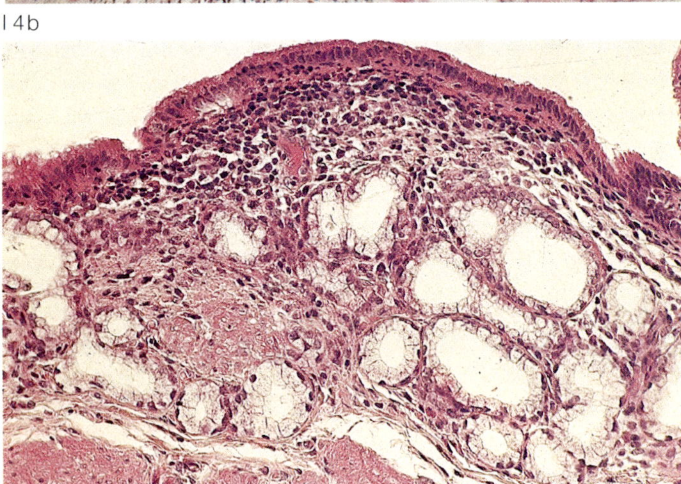

14c

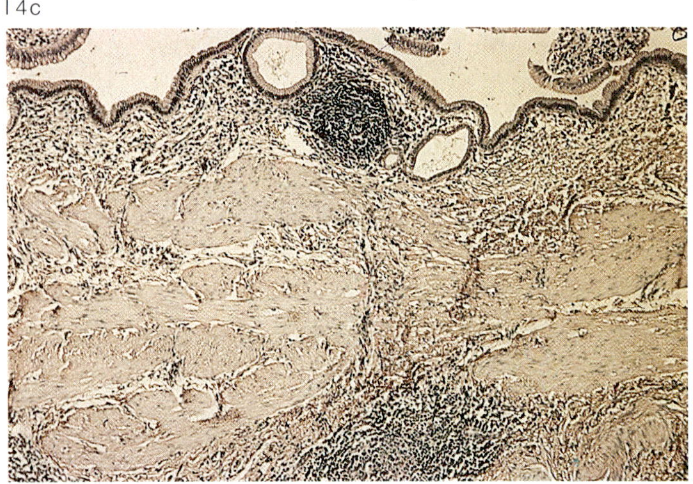

14d

Fig. I 4. Cholecystitis.
a) Acute ulcerating necrosis of the gallbladder mucosa extending into the fibromuscular layers in association with a gallstone.
b) Chronic cholecystitis, with accentuated mucosal folds due to edema, increased numbers of chronic inflammatory cells, and early subepithelial fibrosis.
c) Regenerated epithelium in a chronically inflamed gallbladder. Many goblet cells are seen.
d) Loss of mucosal pattern with atrophy of mucosa. In addition to a diffuse lymphocytic infiltrate, there is a reactive lymphoid nodule.
e) Inflammatory mucosal hyperplasia. There is proliferation of glands and villiform change of the overlying epithelium.
f) Papillary hyperplasia of the mucosa with marked goblet cell metaplasia.
(Stains a–c, e–f: hematoxylin-eosin, d: van Gieson)

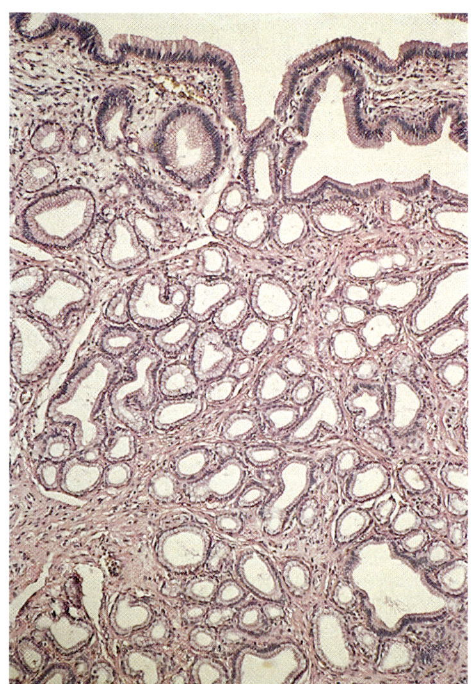

14e

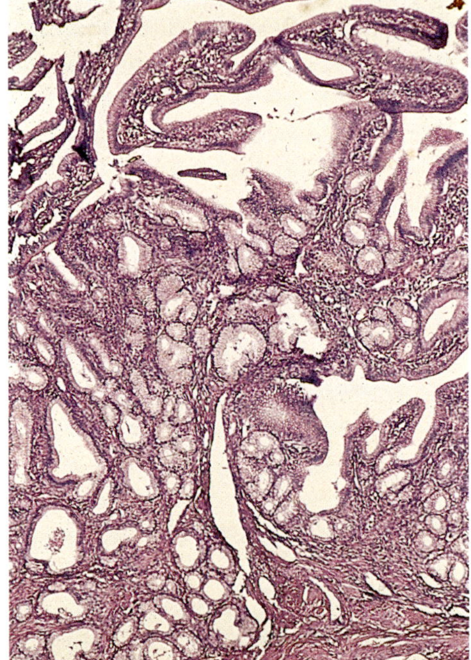

14f

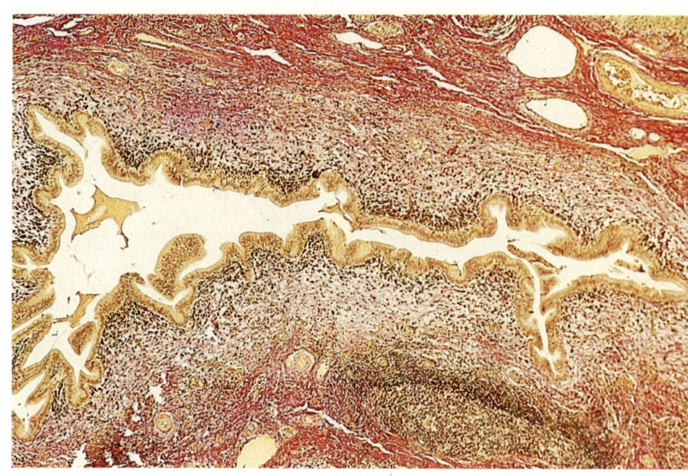

Fig. 15. Idiopathic, noninflammatory hydrops of the gallbladder as a complication of obstruction of the cystic duct by a cholesterol stone. The greatly dilated gallbladder was filled with an almost clear, mucinous fluid, and there was no biliary pigment.

Fig. 16. Chronic inflammation of the common duct from recurrent biliary obstruction due to gallstones. There is a severe chronic inflammatory cell infiltration and a lymphoid follicle, with a well formed germinal center, is seen to the lower right.   (van Gieson)

Neoplasia   *(17–19)*

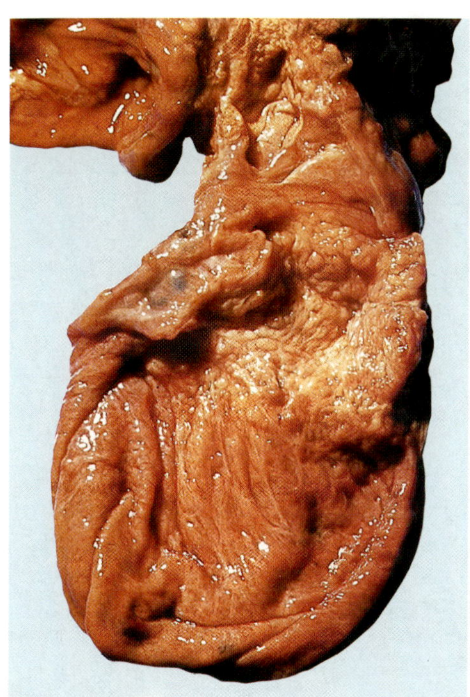

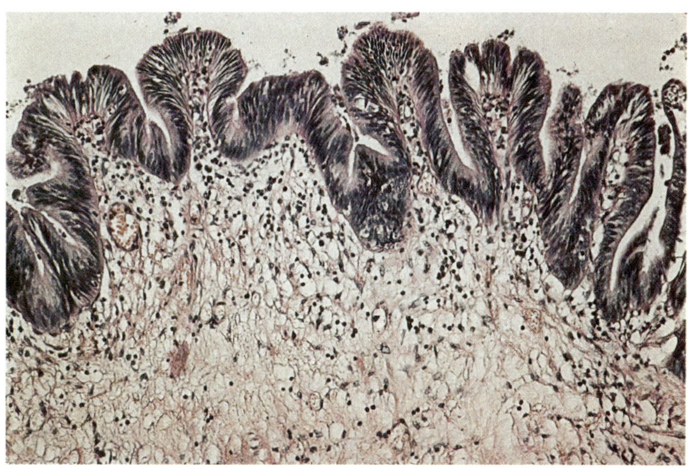

Fig. 17. Carcinoma in situ of the gallbladder epithelium. The epithelium consists of papillary formations with large irregular cells in which the nuclei have lost their usual basal orientation. In addition the nuclei are markedly hyperchromatic, pleomorphic, and there are scattered mitoses.   (hematoxylin-eosin)

Fig. 18. Gallbladder carcinoma. There is diffuse infiltration of the wall of the gallbladder by a centrally ulcerated, peripherally exophytic tumor mass. This tumor mass was stony hard. The infiltration is best seen at the right center of the photograph.

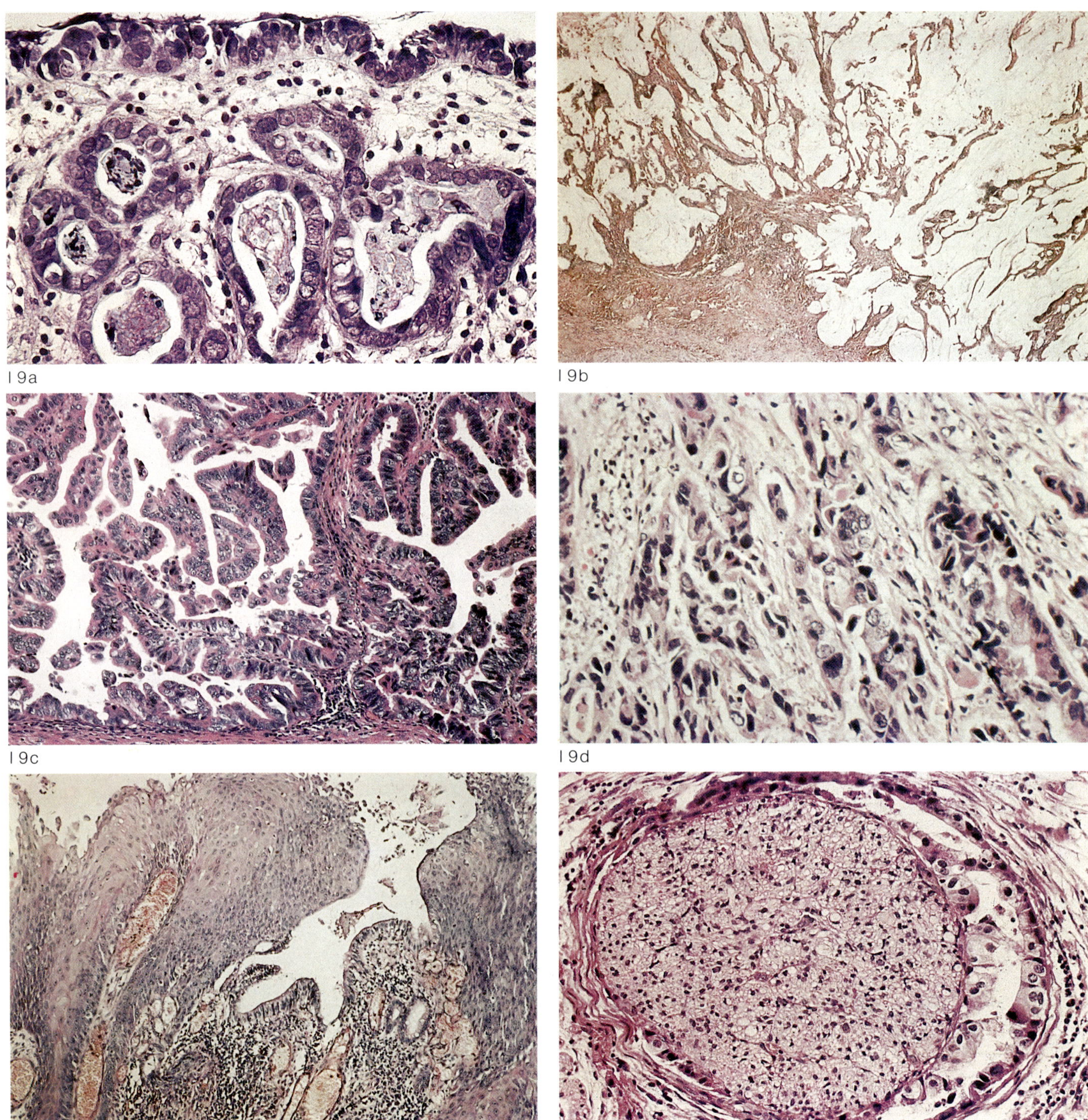

Fig. I 9. Various histologic features of gallbladder carcinoma.
a) A focus of adenocarcinoma with highly atypical epithelium. There is ample stroma with mild lymphocytic infiltrate.

b) Adenocarcinoma with abundant mucous production ("colloid"). The tumor cells are highly atypical. This tumor had spread to the peritoneal surfaces and throughout the abdomen.

c) Papillary adenocarcinoma. The usual mucosal pattern has been replaced by a papillary proliferation of bizarre epithelial cells with a markedly increased nuclear-cytoplasmic ratio, hypochromatism, pleomorphism, and many mitoses.

d) Poorly differentiated adenocarcinoma. Poorly formed glands and rows of single cells are seen infiltrating the connective tissue. This tumor resembles "linitis plastica" of the stomach and infiltrates the gallbladder wall extensively and the surrounding structures.

e) Squamous cell carcinoma of the gallbladder. This relatively rare tumor of the gallbladder follows squamous metaplasia in the face of a chronically inflamed gallbladder of the perineural lymphatics from a gallbladder adenocarcinoma.

f) The space around the nerve is almost completely filled by cuboidal and low columnar epithelial cells. This is a relatively frequent occurrence. This painless complication tends to develop early, rendering total resection of the gallbladder impossible in many cases.

(Stains a, c−f: hematoxylin-eosin, b: van Gieson)

J. Exocrine Pancreas

O. Klinge, H.-W. Altmann

The pancreas is especially susceptible to injury because of its function as an enzyme producing and enzyme secreting organ. The various pathologic processes can, of course, affect the pancreas but, superimposed on the causative injury might be the effects of release of tissue destructive enzymes. There are a number of alterations of the pancreas which do not affect significantly the functional integrity of the pancreatic parenchyma. These include degrees of fibrosis and fatty infiltration. Alterations in the composition of pancreatic secretions, as well as obstruction to flow, can cause severe damage to the pancreas. Acute hemorrhagic pancreatitis is a severe, and often fatal, disorder in which the release of pancreatic enzymes causes extensive parenchymal destruction. Chronic pancreatitis can also follow abnormalities of pancreatic secretion, but also results from nutritional and metabolic disorders (as in chronic alcoholism). In those cases, of course, the alcoholism can contribute to a primary disturbance of pancreatic excretory function. Carcinoma of the pancreas is the most important neoplasm of the pancreas and one of the most important neoplasias of man. Because of the unique anatomic position of the pancreas, carcinomas are often discovered late and the fatality rate is high.

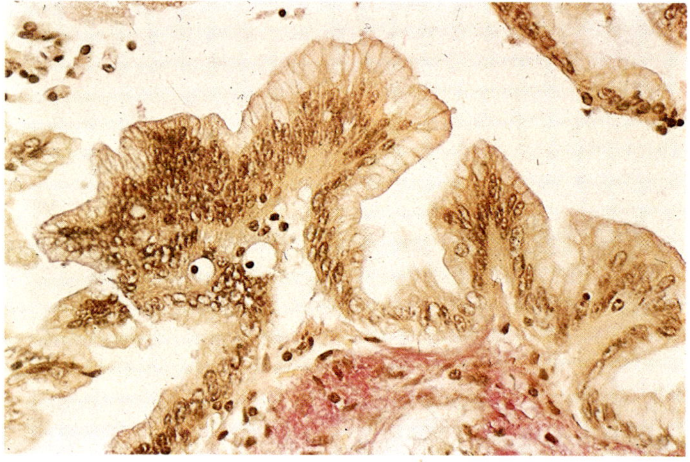

Fig. J1a.   Various injuries can lead to changes of the pancreatic duct with proliferative epithelial changes. Here the usual tall mucous-secreting columnar cells are seen as papillary proliferations. (van Gieson)

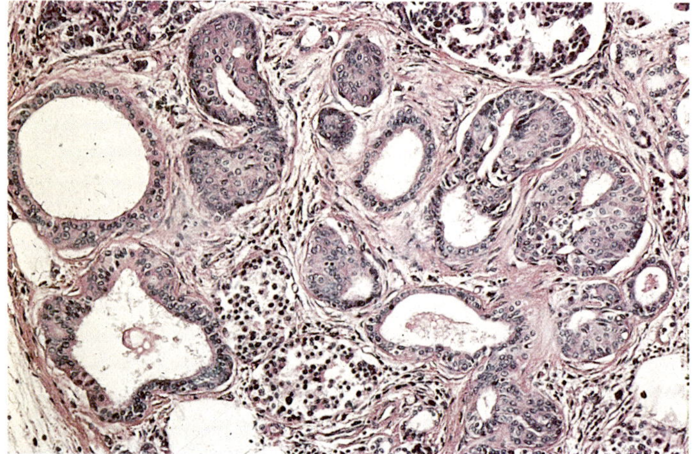

Fig. J1b.   In this case there are other nonspecific changes as a result of injury. The ductules are dilated, forming cystlike spaces, and the usual ductular columnar epithelium is replaced by cuboidal cells, as well as by areas of squamous metaplasia. There is marked periductular fibrosis.   (hematoxylin-eosin)

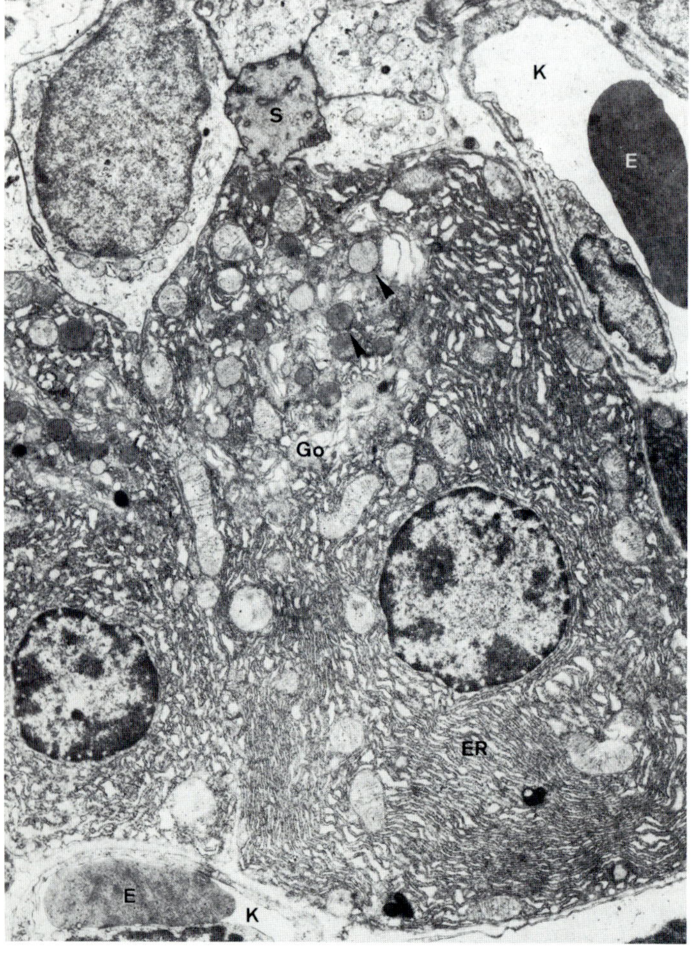

Fig. J2.   Electron micrograph of acinar cells of the rat pancreas with microvilli at the apical surface of the cell (S). The lamellar ergastoplasm (ER), with numerous ribonucleoprotein granules attached to the membranes, is at the base. The Golgi apparatus (Go) is well seen. Zymogen granules are near the apex *(arrows)*. A capillary (K) with an erythrocyte (E) is to the upper right.

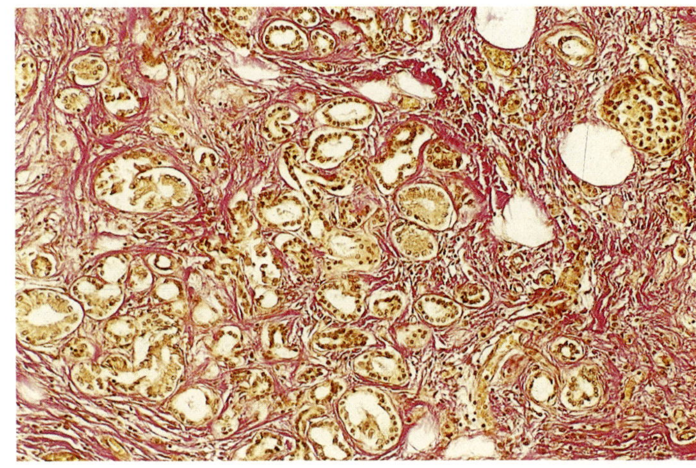

Fig. J3a.   Fatty infiltration of the pancreas. The glandular parenchyma is almost completely lost. Fatty infiltration can follow longstanding insults, such as chronic pancreatitis, which lead to chronic pancreatic destruction. This change is also seen sometimes in obesity and is nonspecific.

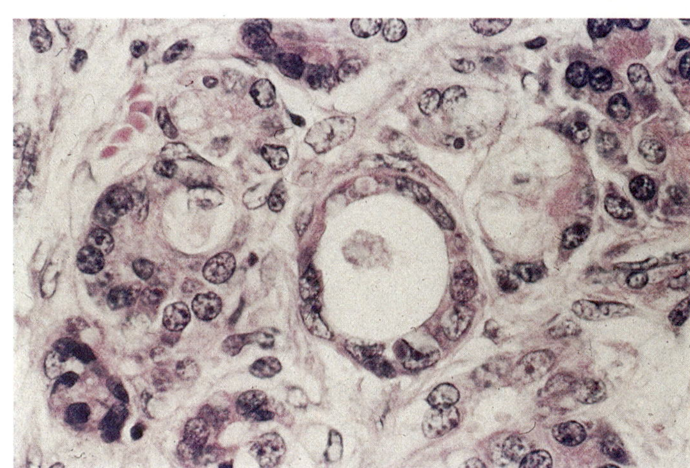

Fig. J3b.   Marked periductular fibrosis and focal parenchymal atrophy. The fibrosis can be associated with various conditions, including nutritional disorders, inflammation in the newborn, cardiac failure, atherosclerotic cardiovascular disease, and portal hypertension.   (van Gieson)

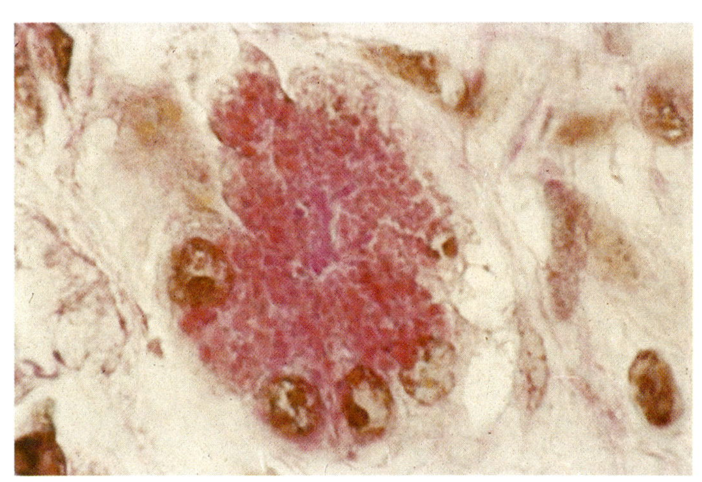

Fig. J4.   Acinar changes in uremia and dehydration.

Fig. J4a.   Vacuolization of acinar epithelial cells is seen (upper left, midright) as well as loss of cellular basophilia (i.e., reduction of ergastoplasm within the cell). The epithelial cells are low columnar and cuboidal and there are varying degrees of cystic change. This type of alteration is sometimes seen in uremia and dehydration. (hematoxylin-eosin)

Fig. J4b.   This acinus shows mucopolysaccharide-rich vacuolization of cytoplasm.   (Best's carmine)

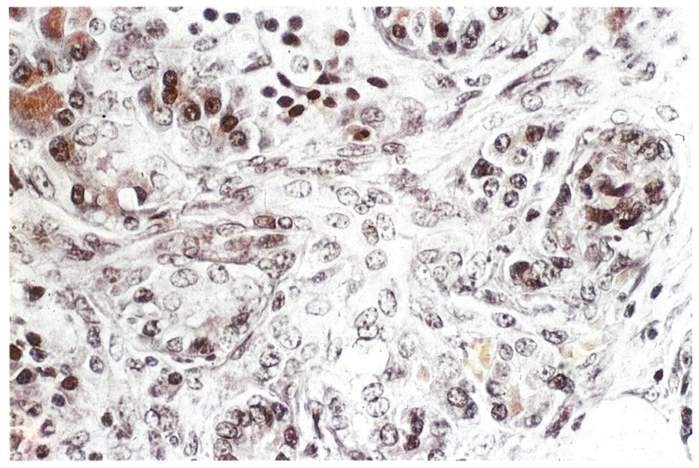

Fig. J5.   Abnormalities of ductular function.

Fig. J5a.   There is marked swelling of the area of the intercalated duct and ductules associated with chronic venous congestion. (hematoxylin-eosin)

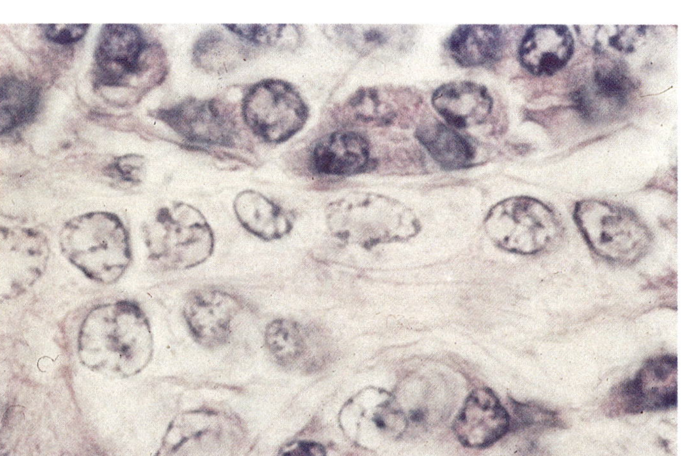

Fig. J5b.   There is nuclear enlargement and cytoplasmic swelling of the cells of the intercalated duct. A portion of an acinus is above for comparison. Normally the cells should be approximately equal in size.   (hematoxylin-eosin)

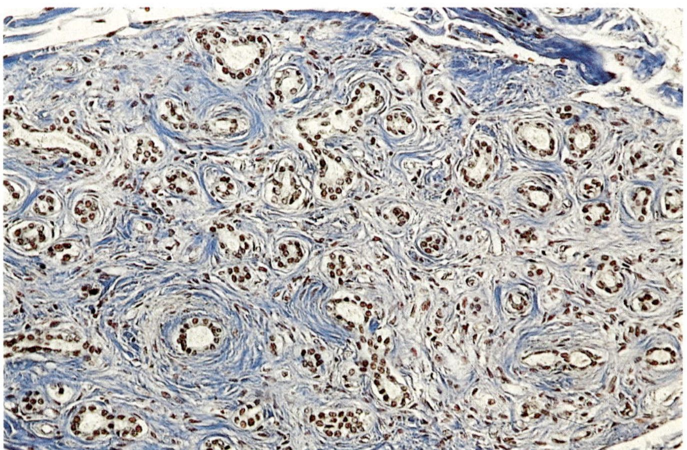

Fibrosis and Stone Formation   *(J6–J9)*

Fig. J6.   Partial duct obstruction.

Fig. J6a.   Diffuse fibrosis of pancreatic lobules following pancreatic duct obstruction, with increased retrograde pressure. The acini are completely atrophic.   (Ladewig)

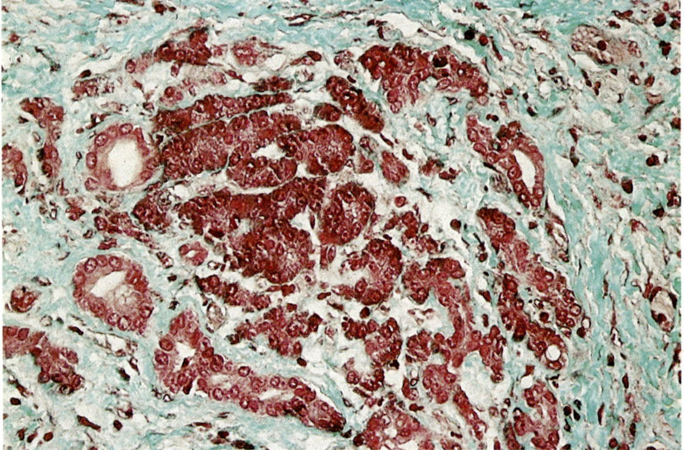

Fig. J6b.   In this photomicrograph the fibrosis is mostly perilobular, with a relatively minor intralobular component which divides the lobule. In addition there is slight atrophy and focal dilatation of acini.   (Goldner)

Fig. J6c.   Marked periductal fibrosis following duct obstruction. A small interlobular duct is surrounded completely by dense fibrous tissue. Two islets are at the upper right.   (van Gieson)

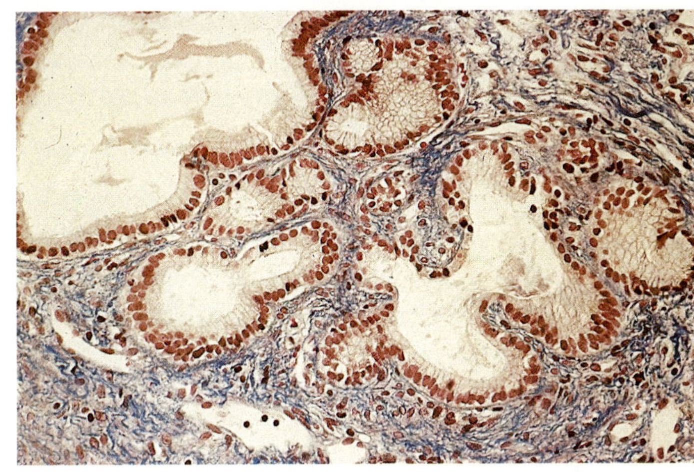

Fig. J6d.   Cystically dilated ducts with surrounding fibrosis. Mucous-secreting columnar cells line the ducts.   (Ladewig)

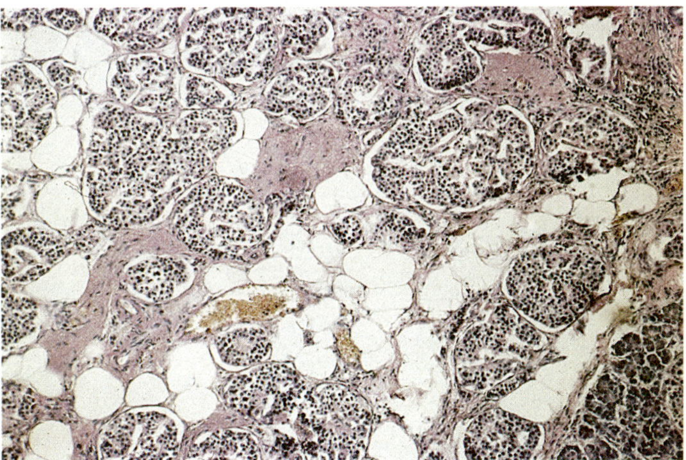

Fig. J7.   Enlarged, confluent islets of Langerhans in a case of chronic pancreatitis. There are no acini seen. Instead the islets are incompletely separated by fibrosis and fat.   (hematoxylin-eosin)

Fig. J8.   Cystic fibrosis (mucoviscidosis).
a) A group of cystically dilated, distorted ducts are filled with partially laminated concretions. Lining epithelium consists of tall columnar cells which are distended with large mucous filled vacuoles. Surrounding fibrosis is prominent. (Pearse)
b) Another area of secretion-filled dilated ducts with only a few remaining acini, in a background of fibrous tissue. The few remaining acini resemble small ducts.   (Pearse)

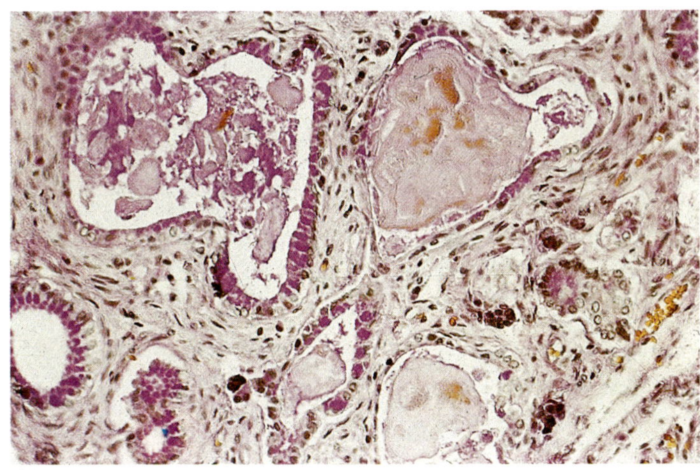

J8a

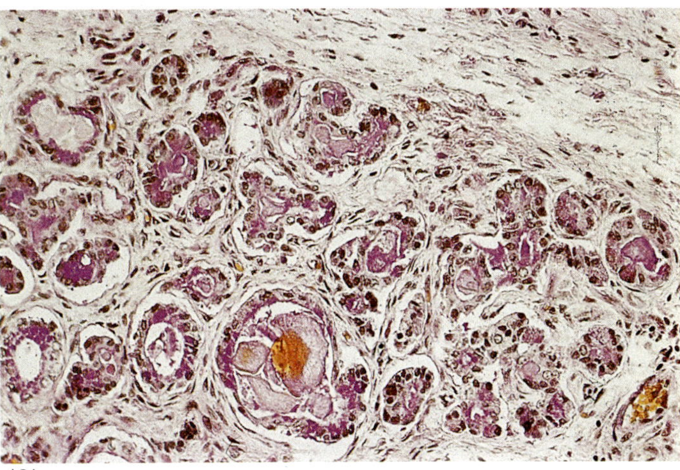

J8b

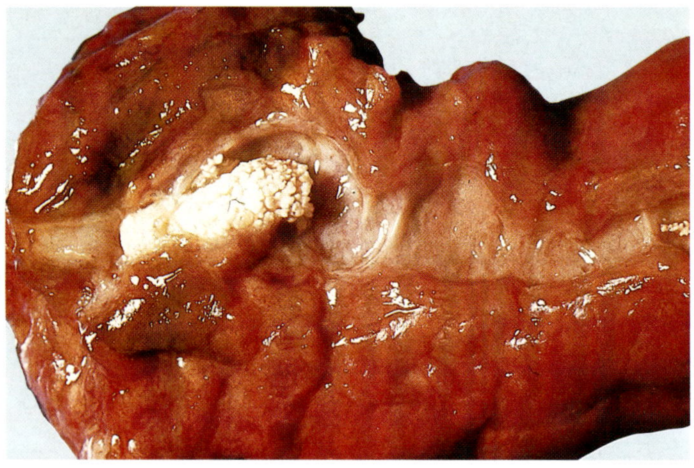

Fig. J9.   Pancreatic calculi.

Fig. J9a.   A chalky white granular calculus is lodged in the pancreatic duct at the ampulla of Vater. The distal duct, to the right of the calculus, is dilated. This stone consisted mostly of inorganic phosphates and calcium carbonate.

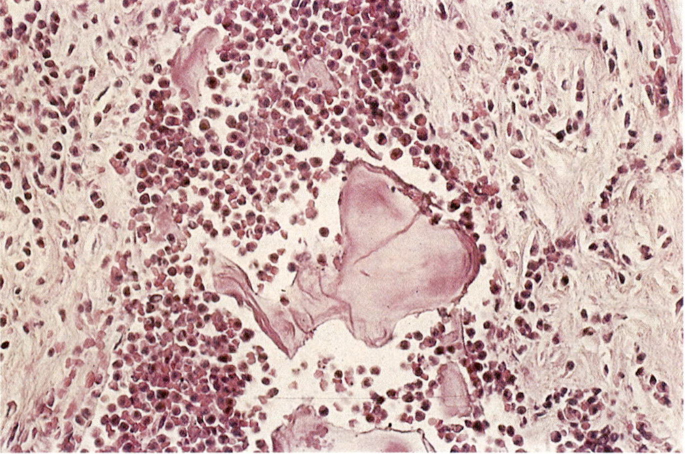

Fig. J9b.   Small pancreatic calculus ("microlithiasis"). The stone is in a small duct and formed in the setting of chronic inflammation of the duct. The partially fragmented stone is surrounded by acute inflammatory cells and fibrosis.   (hematoxylin-eosin)

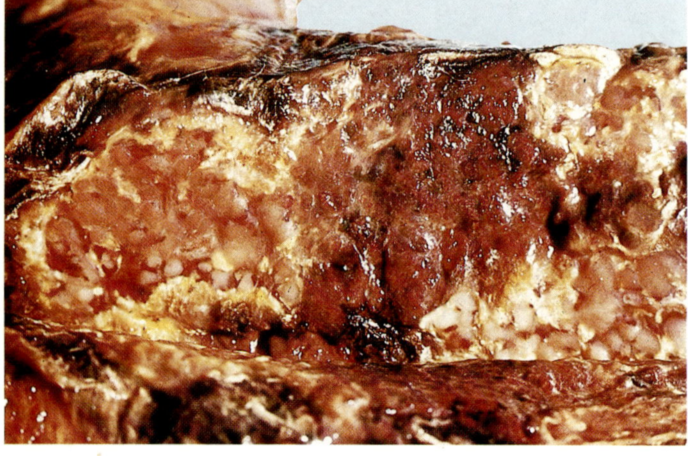

Necrosis and Inflammation   *(J 10–J 14)*

Fig. J10.   Acute hemorrhagic pancreatitis.

Fig. J10a.   The pancreas is markedly and diffusely swollen and hemorrhagic, with yellow and grey zones of coagulative and fat necrosis.

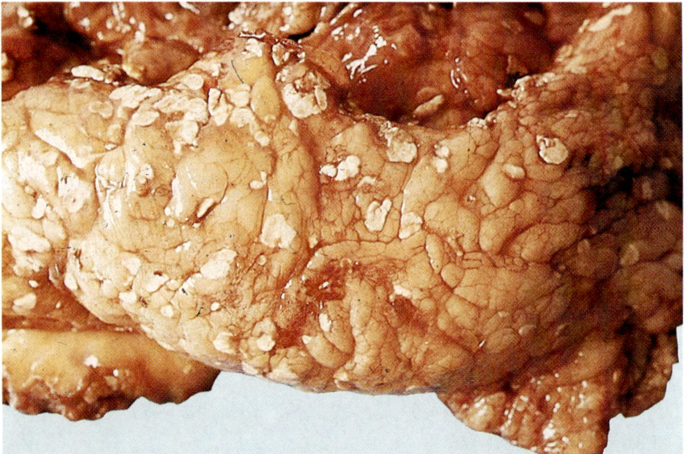

Fig. J10b.   Fat necrosis. The release of lipolytic enzymes from injured acini leads to the characteristic picture of fat necrosis. With time, saponification and, eventually, calcification, occur.

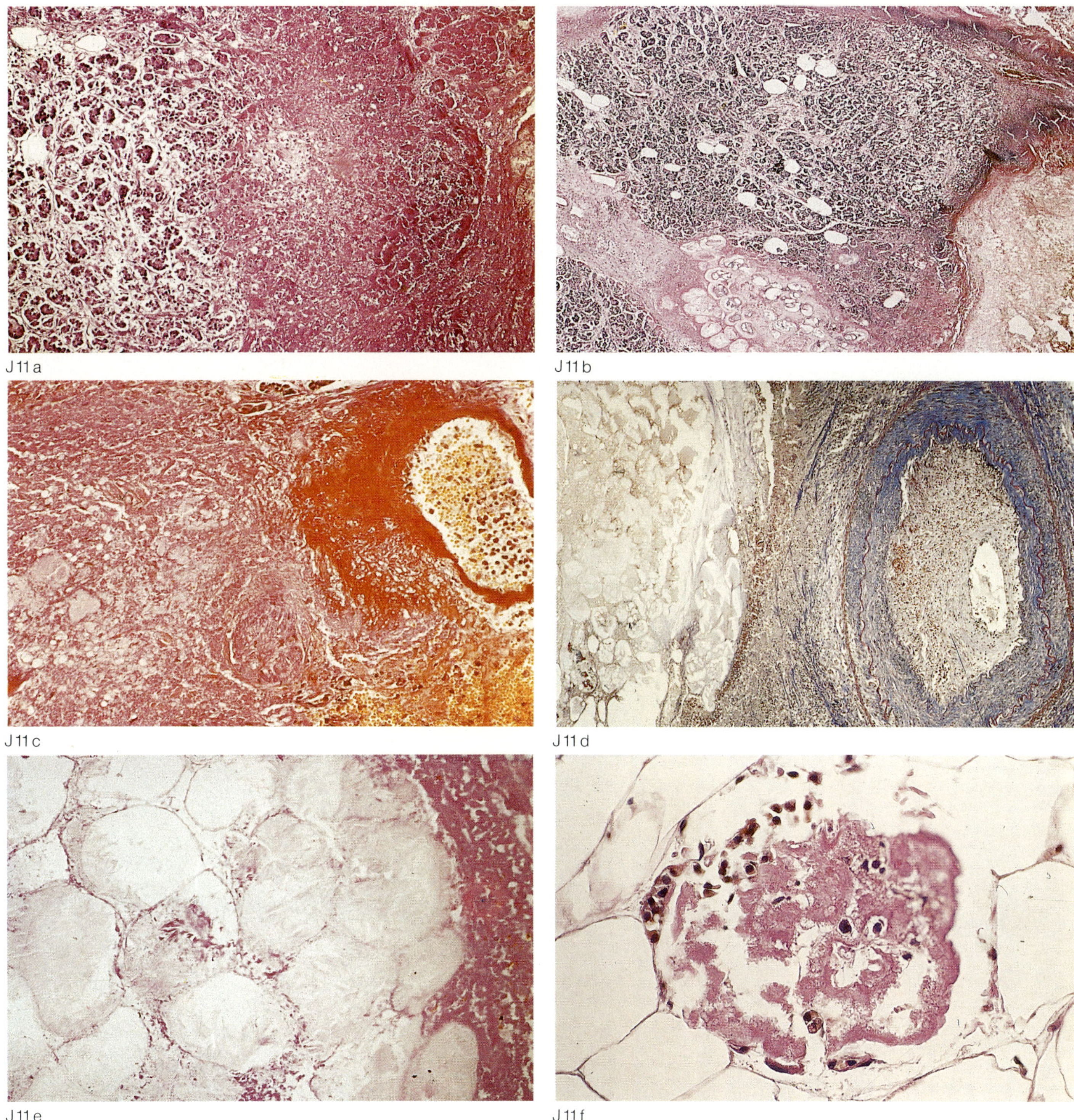

Fig. J 11.   Acute hemorrhagic pancreatitis.

a) Relatively intact acini are to the left. The central zone of this photomicrograph shows coagulative necrosis; the right shows hemorrhagic infarction.

b) Fat necrosis. At the periphery of the lobule the architecture is indistinct. Instead there are necrotic fat cells that have been hydrolyzed by pancreatic lipase into fatty acids and glycerol.

c) Necrosis of a blood vessel due to tryptic digestion. There is hemorrhage at the periphery of the vessel and the parenchyma is necrotic.

d) Secondary arterial fibrosis as a result of pancreatitis. The lumen of the artery, to the right, is almost completely obliterated, with only a small recanalized area. Fat necrosis is to the left. (Ladewig)

e) High magnification photomicrograph of fat necrosis. The fatty acids that are formed are subsequently converted to a soap (saponification) which is seen as amorphous, faintly basophilic material.

f) A microscopic focus of necrosis, consisting of a homogeneous coagulum of neutral fat with early phagocytic response.

(Stains a–c, e–f: hematoxylin-eosin, d: Ladewig)

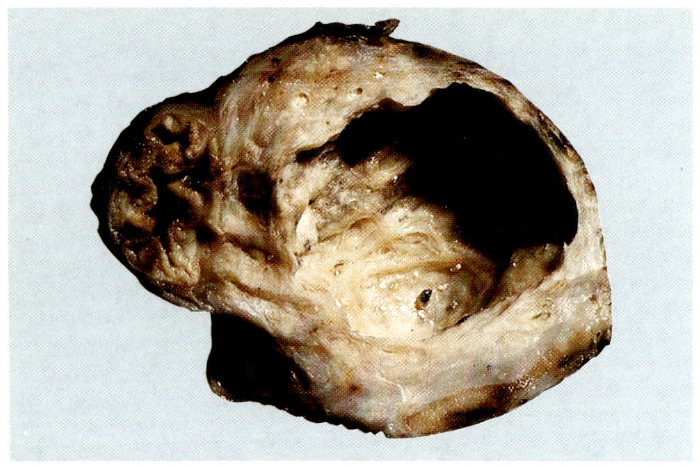

Fig. J 12. Pseudocyst of the body of the pancreas. This formed after an episode of acute pancreatic necrosis with the accumulation of enzyme-rich fluid, blood, and necrotic debris in a connective tissue capsule. This could compress neighboring organs and perforate the stomach or intestines. The compressed duodenum is to the left of the pseudocyst.

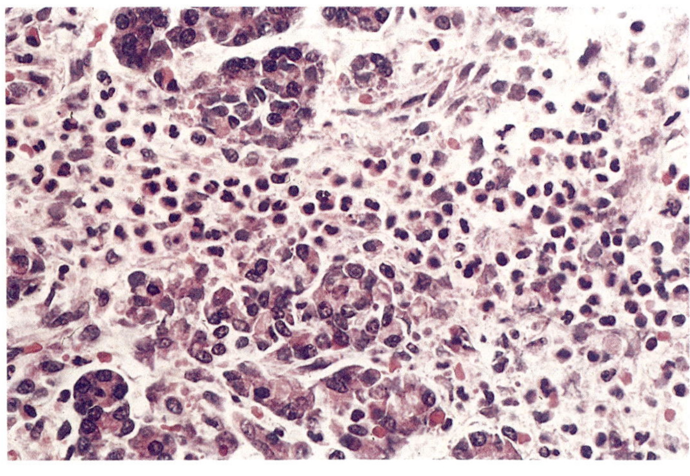

Fig. J 13. Chronic pancreatitis. The interstitium is edematous and there is an accumulation of chronic inflammatory cells with destruction of glands, but without typical features of tryptic digestion. This might be due to preceding bacterial infection or immunologically mediated pancreatitis, and may also be associated with some of the exanthematous childhood diseases, such as mumps. (hematoxylin-eosin)

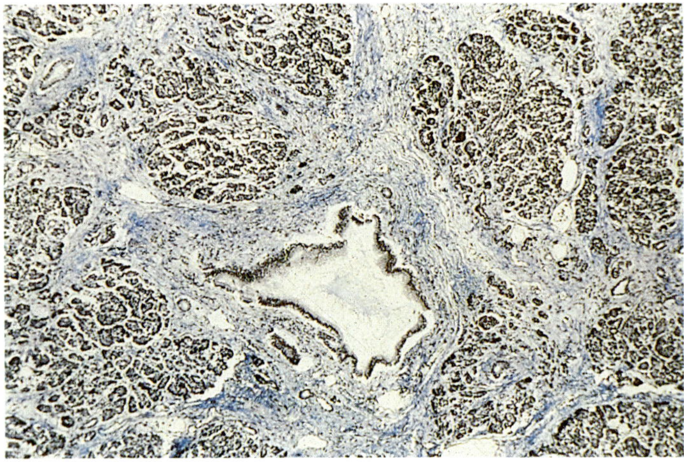

Fig. J 14. Chronic fibrosing pancreatitis.

Fig. J 14a. The interstitium is at first replaced by fibrous tissue, with retention of acinar patterns. In this case there was longstanding pancreatic duct obstruction. A centrilobular duct, at the center of the photomicrograph, is dilated and filled with mucous. (Ladewig)

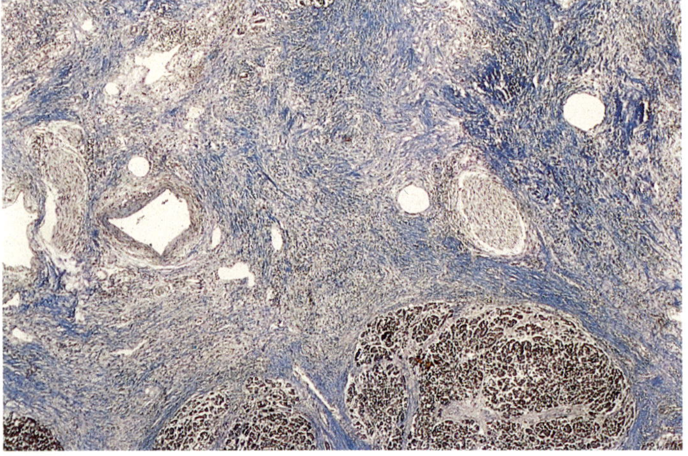

Fig. J 14b. In a later stage, much of the parenchyma is replaced by dense connective tissue within which small, distorted residual ducts can be identified. Relatively intact lobules are at the lower portion of the picture. (Ladewig)

Fig. J 14 c.   With continuing injury the parenchyma is almost completely replaced by fibrosis. A few remaining ducts show reactive epithelial changes. Islets of Langerhans are recognizable at the right and lower middle portions of the photomicrograph.   (Ladewig)

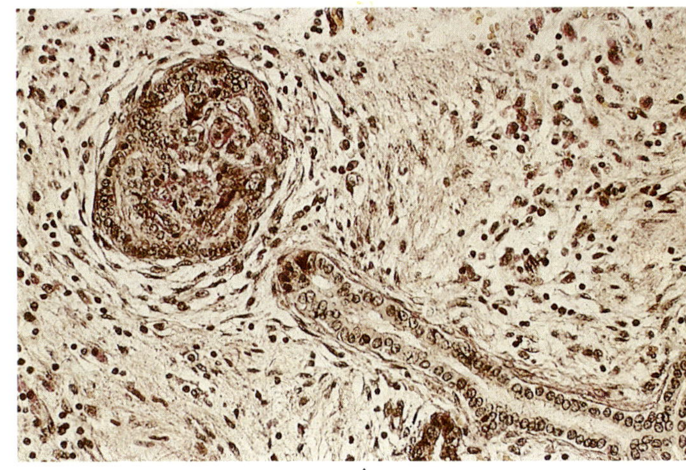

Fig. J 14 d.   In the final stages of chronic pancreatitis the organ consists almost entirely of scar tissue. Tiny islands of distorted parenchyma persist and a duct is seen. There are chronic inflammatory cells present in the connective tissue.   (van Gieson)

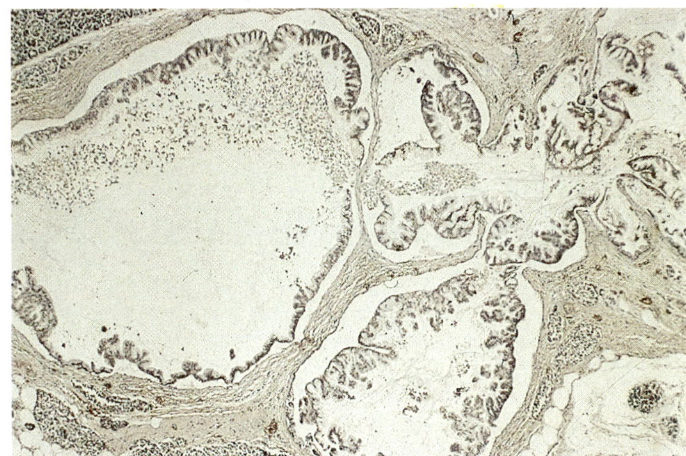

Pancreatic Cysts   *(J 15)*

Fig. J 15.   Pancreatic cysts.

Fig. J 15 a.   Pancreatic cysts can be due to pancreatic duct obstruction. The epithelium is partially flattened and there is surrounding fibrosis. The cyst contains retained secretory material. (van Gieson)

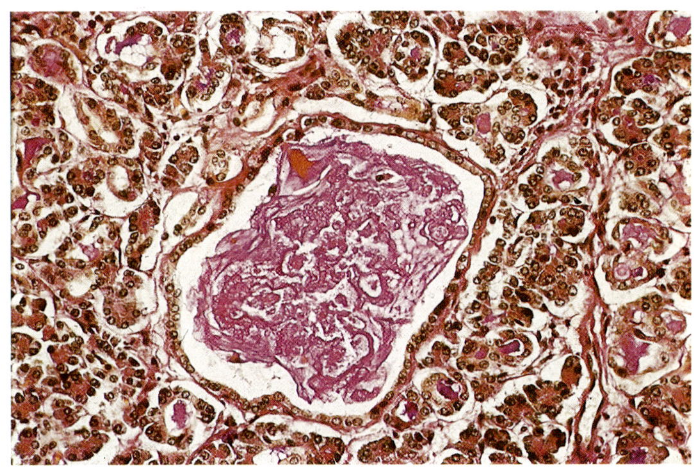

Fig. J 15 b.   Congenital cysts also can occur in the pancreas. They can be associated with hepatic and renal cysts. There may be relatively little surrounding collagen. The cysts sometimes contain dense proteinaceous material.   (Pearse)

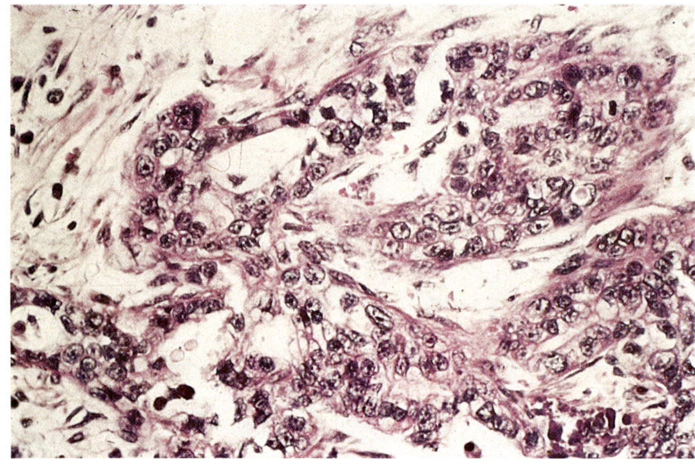

Fig. J 16.   Pancreatic adenocarcinoma.

Fig. J 16 a.   Moderately well differentiated adenocarcinoma, consisting of highly atypical epithelial cells forming ductlike structures. A rim of fibrosis is seen.   (hematoxylin-eosin)

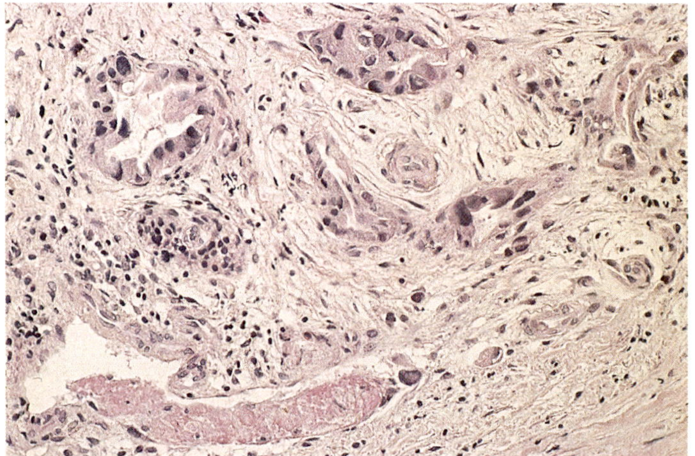

Fig. J 16 b.   In this variant of pancreatic adenocarcinoma there is marked fibrosis. This is the characteristic picture of pancreatic carcinoma. Ductlike structures are seen in the dense connective tissue along with chronic inflammatory cells. The tumor would feel stony-hard.   (hematoxylin-eosin)

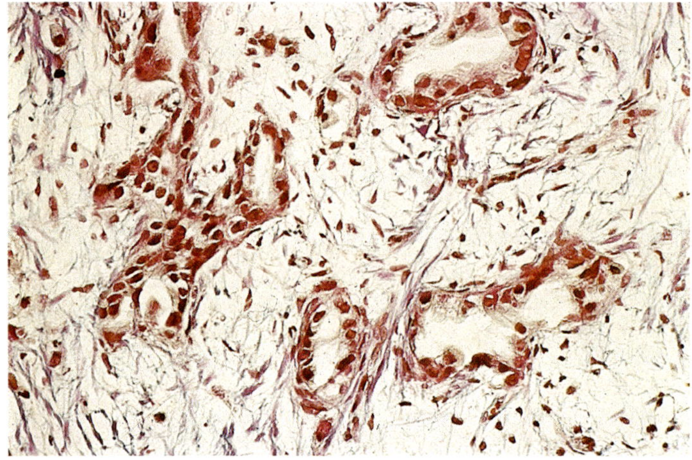

Fig. J 16 c.   Well differentiated pancreatic adenocarcinoma. The connective tissue matrix is loose and the epithelial cells are not markedly dysplastic. These cases may be difficult to distinguish from benign fibrosis *(see Fig. J 6 a).*   (Ladewig)

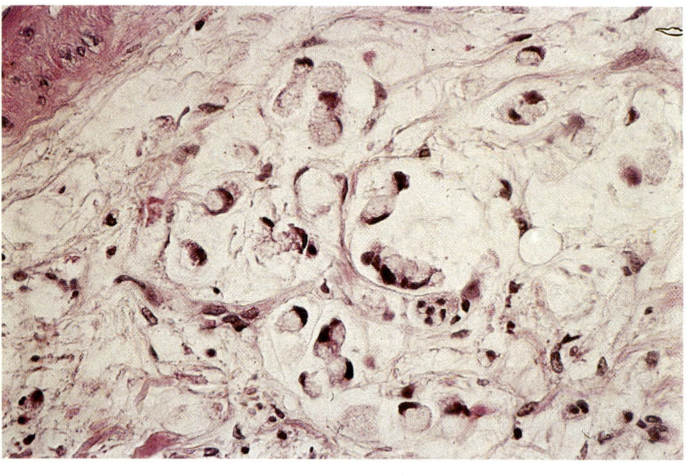

Fig. J 16 d.   Poorly differentiated pancreatic adenocarcinoma with marked mucous production. Signet ring cells are apparent within pools of mucous.   (hematoxylin-eosin)

K. Endocrine Organs

Chr. Hedinger, G. Klöppel, W. Saeger

The pituitary may be affected by such systemic conditions as circulatory disorders and inflammations. When the function of the posterior pituitary is impaired, diabetes insipidus may result.

The anterior pituitary is the center of endocrine regulation. Necrosis of the anterior pituitary, often caused by shock, may lead to pituitary insufficiency. Tumors of the anterior pituitary are almost always benign, but they may lead to considerable abnormalities of function and may be locally destructive. The histopathology of pituitary adenomas does not usually indicate function. Craniopharyngioma is one of the distinctive tumors of the pituitary which may be locally destructive because of its expansive nature.

The adrenal glands may show atrophic or hyperplastic changes due to degenerative, circulatory, and immunologically mediated phenomena. Functional deficits may follow these changes. Adenomas of the adrenal cortex are not uncommon and may manifest as a variety of functional disorders, such as Cushing's syndrome or Conn's syndrome. Adrenocortical carcinomas are often quite large and metastasize widely. The most important condition of the adrenal medulla is the pheochromocytoma. This tumor is usually benign but may cause hypertension and other manifestations because of its secretion of catecholamines.

The thyroid is affected by many conditions, and may functionally demonstrate disorders of both thyroxine and calcitonin activity. There may be a variety of inflammatory conditions of the thyroid. The thyroid may be hyperplastic, with the formation of goiter. Thyroid hyperplasia (Grave's disease) is particularly common in our society. Thyroid tumors are also frequently observed. The most common, of course, is the benign proliferation. Papillary carcinoma has distinct features as do follicular and medullary carcinomas. In older women there may be a particularly aggressive form of thyroid carcinoma.

The parathyroid glands control calcium metabolism and may themselves cause disordered calcium activity or may be secondarily hyperplastic, as in the case of chronic renal insufficiency. Primary hyperparathyroidism is most often a reflection of adenoma. The parathyroid glands may, as secondary response, be uniformly enlarged.

An important concept is the recognition of the diffuse endocrine (neuroendocrine) system in which cells with potential of endocrine activity are scattered in various organs. These cells have been designated as APUD (amine precursor uptake decarboxilase) cells and almost always contain distinct neurosecretory granules with specific enzymes. The carcinoid tumor is typical of this system. It often occurs in the gastrointestinal tract and generally is of low grade malignancy. Carcinoid tumors may produce a variety of hormones (serotonin, gastrin, somatotrophin, etc.). There may be a variety of paragangliomas, resembling pheochromocytoma, which can be found in the neck and along the aorta, following the distribution of arteries.

The endocrine portion of the pancreas also has characteristic changes. In diabetes mellitus, the islets of Langerhans may show a variety of alterations. There may be loss of B-cells, often with a surrounding lymphocytic infiltration as evidence of autoimmunity. Tumors of the endocrine pancreas resemble carcinoids but, because of their relative frequency and their special biologic characteristics, are classified independently.

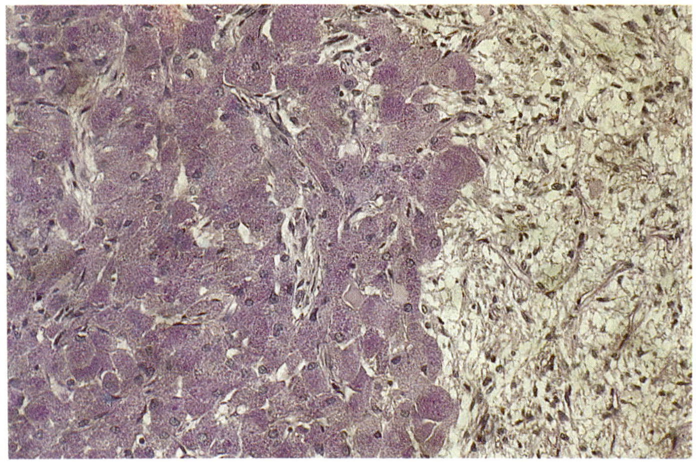

Posterior Pituitary (Neurohypophysis) *(K 1)*
W. Saeger

Fig. K1. Granular cell tumor of the posterior pituitary. A portion of uninvolved posterior pituitary is to the right. This tumor consists of large, polyhedral cells with uniformly granular cytoplasm and relatively small, bland nuclei. The granules are PAS-positive. This tumor is rare. (PAS).

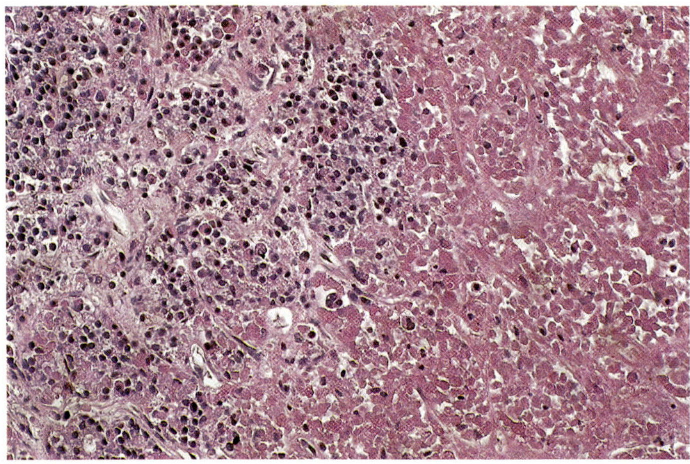

Anterior Pituitary (Adenohypophysis) *(K2–K11)*
W. Saeger

Fig. K2. Recent coagulative necrosis of the anterior pituitary is *to the right,* with residual epithelial cells *to the left.* The structure of the gland is still recognizable in the necrotic area. This patient had preceding shock.   (hematoxylin-eosin)

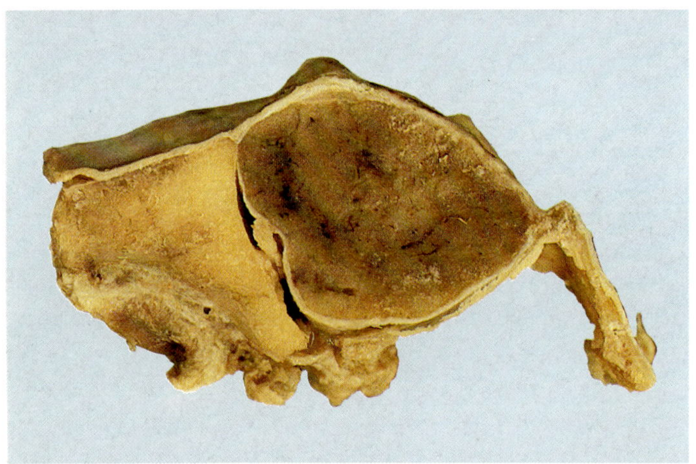

Fig. K3. Pituitary adenoma. There is massive enlargement of the sella turcica. This proved to be an oncocytic type adenoma. The clivus is *to the left* and the sphenoid cavity *to the right.* The light microscopic appearances of the common pituitary tumors do not definitively indicate functional characteristics. Some oncocytic adenomas are nonfunctional, whereas others may cause Cushing's syndrome or the amenorrhea-galactorrhea syndrome.

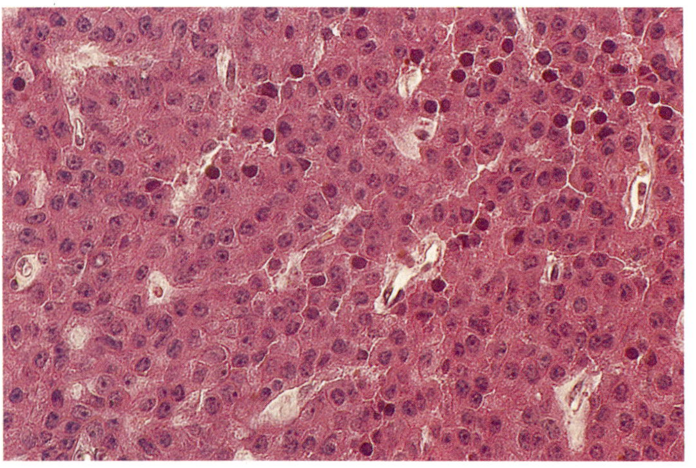

Fig. K4. Acidophilic adenoma. In this tumor there is a medullary pattern of growth consisting of uniform cells with intensely eosinophilic cytoplasm and regular, round nuclei. This histologic picture is indicative of an alpha cell proliferation which can produce either growth hormone (GH) or prolactin (PRL). In this case, somatotrophic hormone (STH) was immunocytochemically identified, evidence of its GH-producing activity.   (hematoxylin-eosin)

Fig. K5. Basophilic adenoma of the pituitary with PAS-positive granularity ("mucoid" cells). Here, as in *Fig. K4,* the growth pattern is medullary with interspersed small cells having clumped chromatin or pyknotic nuclei. In this patient the tumor elaborated ACTH (PAS).

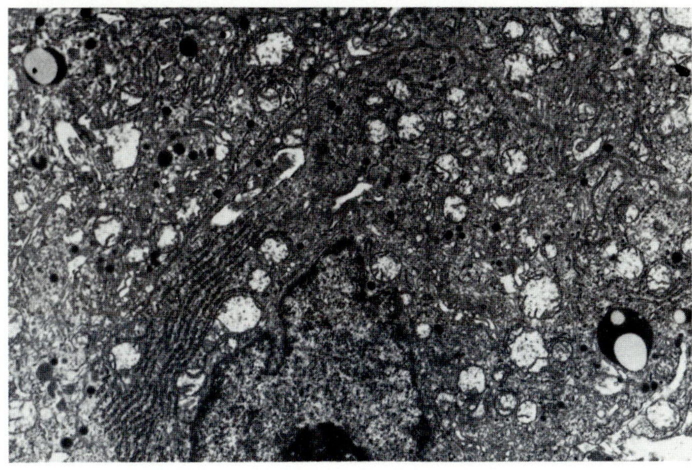

Fig. K6. Electron micrograph of a large cell chromophobe adenoma of the pituitary. There are abundant mitochondria and prominent rough endoplasmic reticulum, distinct Golgi apparatus, and an elaborate cell membrane with microvilli. The cytoplasm also contains loosely arranged granules of varying sizes and a few isolated lysosomes. The nucleus, with central nucleolus, is below. Chromophobe adenomas are not usually hormone-productive.   (magnification 6110×)

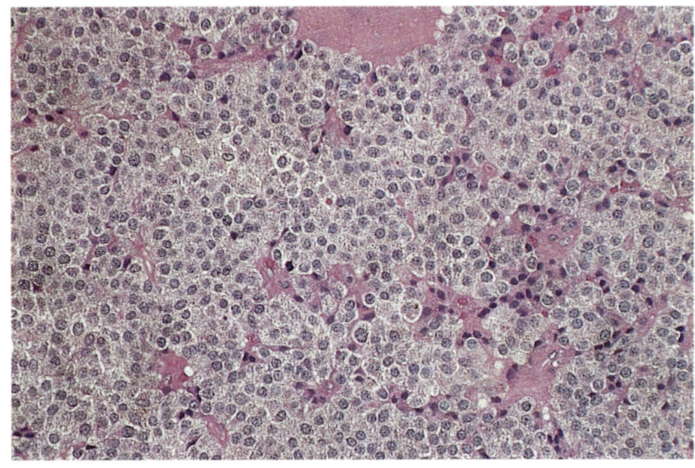

Fig. K7. Chromophobe adenoma of the pituitary, small cell type, with a medullary growth pattern consisting of small uniform cells with a moderate amount of faintly eosinophilic cytoplasm with almost indistinct granularity.   (hematoxylin-eosin)

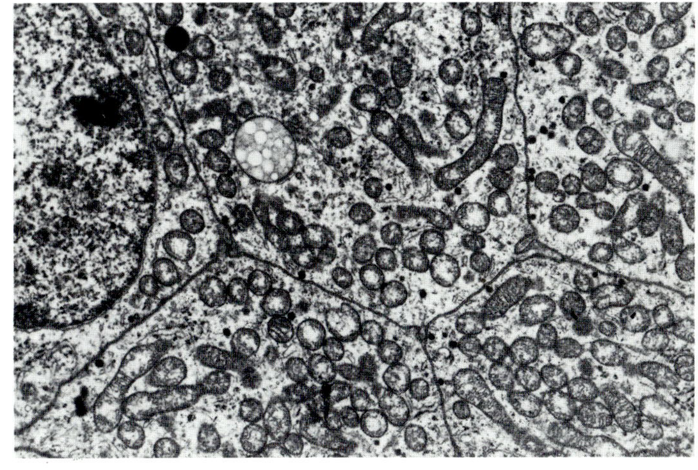

Fig. K8. Oncocytic pituitary adenoma. The five cells seen all contain many large pleomorphic mitochondria. The mitochondria impart the granularity seen on light microscopy *(see Fig. K4).* A few small neurosecretory granules are seen, as are a few small lysosomes.   (magnification 6860×)

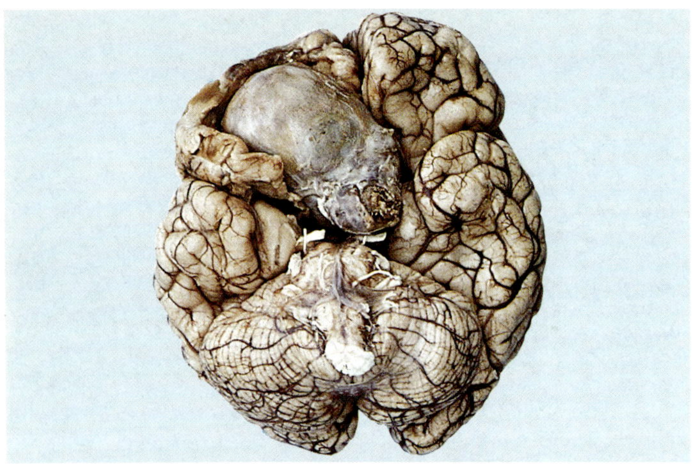

Fig. K9. Craniopharyngioma. A large, encapsulated, cystic tumor is seen at the base of the brain, growing from the region of the sella turcica with marked compression of the right frontal lobe and anterior cranial nerves, including the optic chiasm. This is a benign tumor, but may cause marked tissue destruction because of pressure of the growing mass.

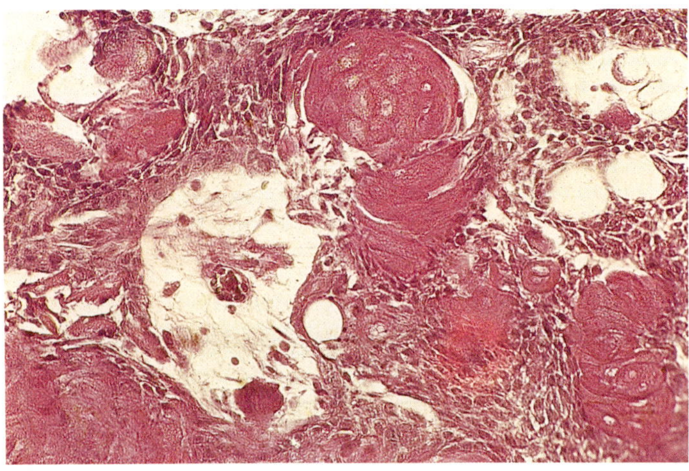

Fig. K10. Craniopharyngioma. There are nests of well-differentiated stratified squamous epithelium within bands of stellate- and spindle-shaped cells, with scattered areas of microcysts formation. (hematoxylin-eosin)

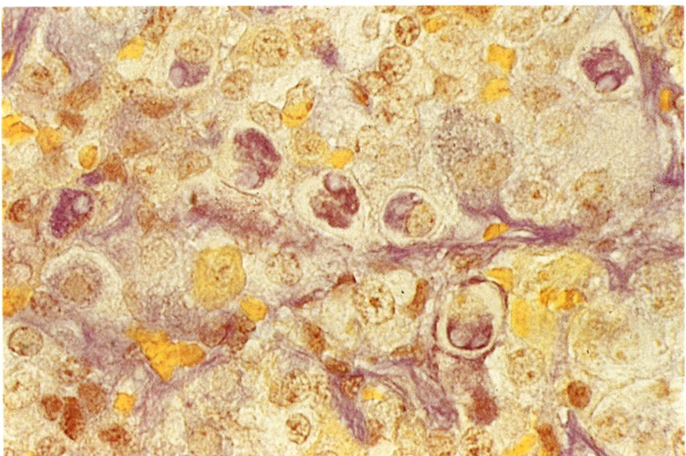

Fig. K11. Crooke's hyaline change. This is often found in the pituitary in conditions associated with excess circulating adrenocortical hormones, including the use of exogenous glucocorticoids. The ACTH-producing basophils are affected and undergo a hyalinization of the cytoplasm. The nucleus and cell body enlarge and there may be cytoplasmic vacuolization. The unchanged acidophilic cells are yellow in this preparation, and the gonadotrophic cells have fine blue granules. (Acid alcian blue-PAS-orange G)

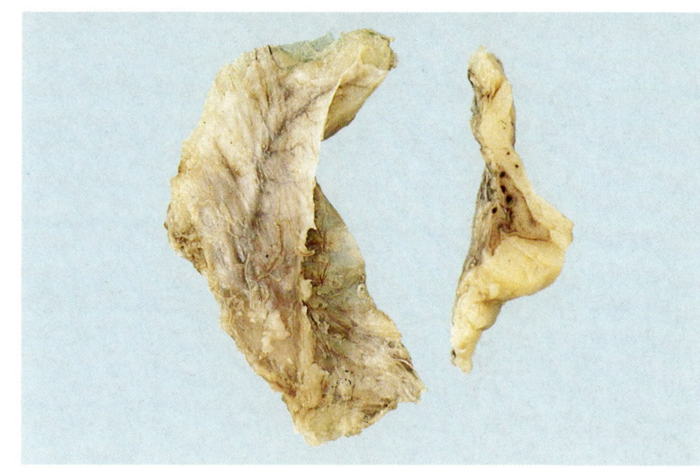

Fig. K12.   Myelolipoma. These proliferations present as tumors but may actually represent enlarged mesenchymal rests. Between the fat cells there are a few scattered degenerating cortical cells and islands of hematopoiesis.   (hematoxylin-eosin)

Fig. K13a.   Severe adrenocortical atrophy due to idiopathic adrenalitis. To the left is a normally formed adrenal gland for comparison. To the right is cross-section of the atrophic adrenal. Peri-adrenal fat is increased. The cortex is paper thin and there is mostly medullary tissue visible.

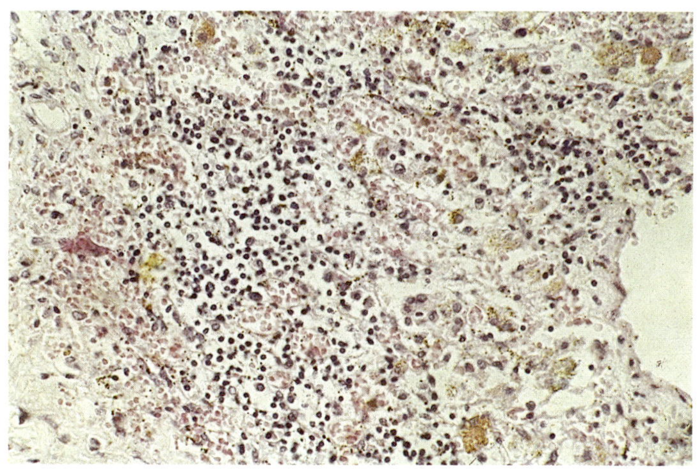

Fig. K13b.   "Autoimmune" adrenalitis with marked lymphocytic and plasmacytic infiltration, and extensive necrosis of adrenocortical cells. The capsule is to the left, and the medulla is to the right. (hematoxylin-eosin)

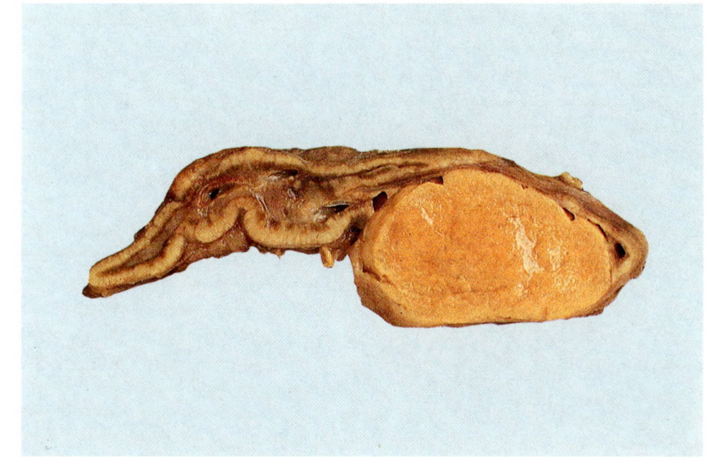

Fig. K14.   Adrenocortical adenoma with hyperaldosteronism (Conn's syndrome). The adrenal adenoma in Conn's syndrome has a distinct gross appearance. It is homogenous and distinctly orange. In other respects it resembles other adrenal adenomas, being well-encapsulated, but generally has little necrosis. The relatively normal cortex and medulla, to the left, are particularly well seen in this cross-section.

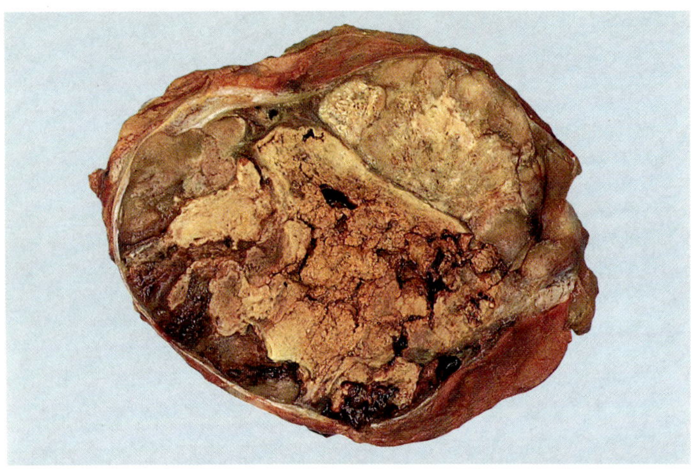

Fig. K15.   Adrenocortical carcinoma in a patient with the adreno-genital syndrome. This enormous tumor was 1,090 gms, had an extensive necrosis and hemorrhage, and many areas of capsular infiltration. As many as 50% of adrenal carcinomas are functional.

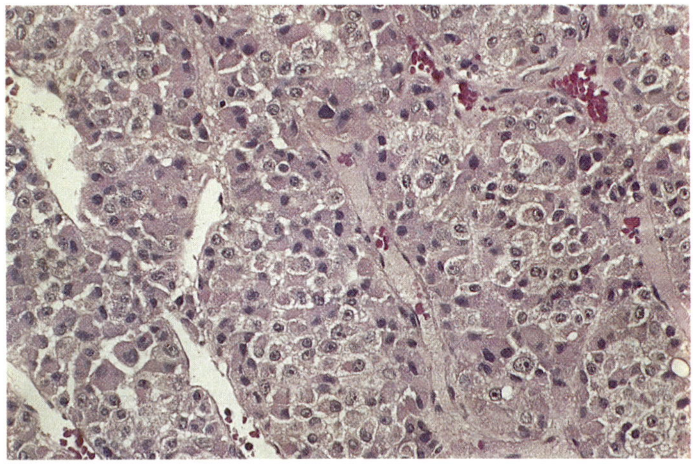

Fig. K16.   Adrenocortical carcinoma in a patient with Cushing's syndrome. There is marked cellular pleomorphism and almost complete absence of lipids. There are distinct sinusoids between sheets of tumor cells. The functional activity cannot be accurately determined from either light or electron microscopic morphologic studies.

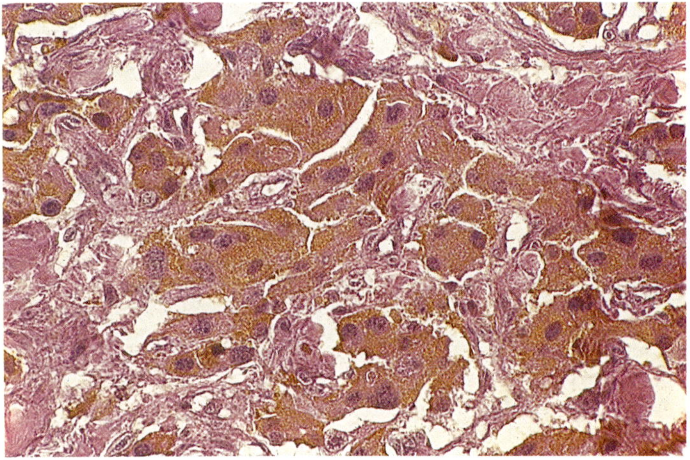

Fig. K17.   Pheochromocytoma. Large variable tumor cells show-ing positive chromaffin reaction (brown) are seen. Pheochromocy-tomas typically show marked variability of cells and nuclear size, as well as arrangement, and mitoses are rare. These tumors may secrete epinephrine, norepinephrine, or both, and usually cause paroxysmal hypertension.

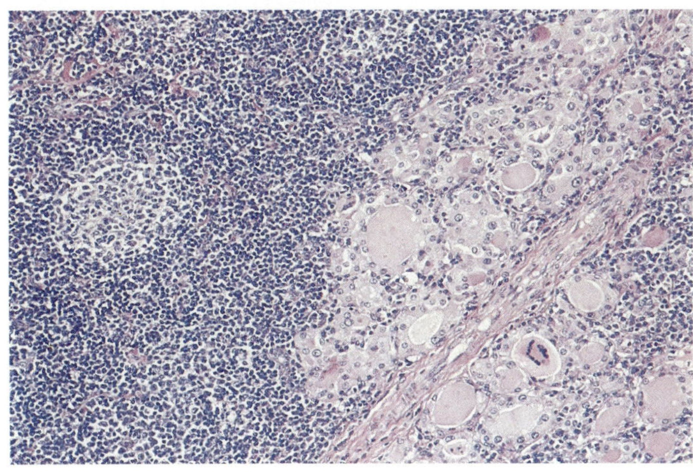

Fig. K18. Granulomatous (de Quervain's) thyroiditis. This is also known as giant cell thyroiditis and subacute thyroiditis. This disorder occurs mostly in middle-aged and young women and is clinically common, but rarely comes to surgery and, consequently, is rarely seen by the pathologist. The histologic findings vary with the stage of disease. Initially there is destruction of follicles with neutrophilic infiltration. This is replaced by lymphocytes, histiocytes, and multi-nucleated giant cells, and, eventually, granuloma formation. (hematoxylin-eosin)

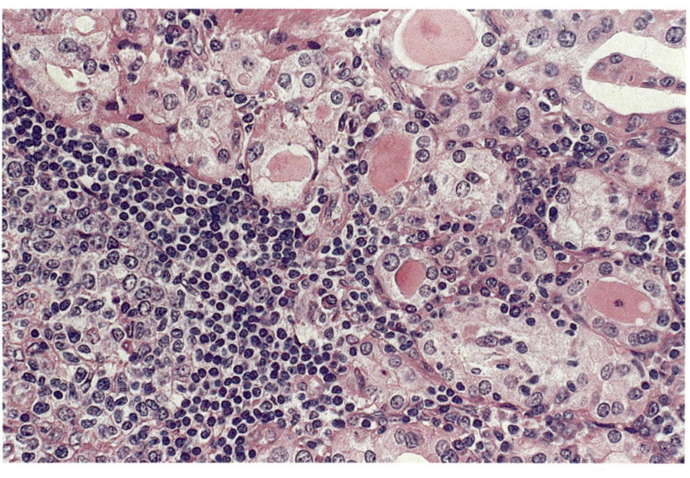

Fig. K19. Hashimoto's thyroiditis (struma lymphomatosum). There is an intense lymphocytic infiltration, with a small germinal center, to the left. To the right are small, partially destroyed thyroid follicles. This thyroid was from a 53-year-old woman with hypothyroidism. Hashimoto's thyroiditis is an autoimmune disorder and antibodies to various thyroid antigens are found in almost 100% of patients.   (hematoxylin-eosin)

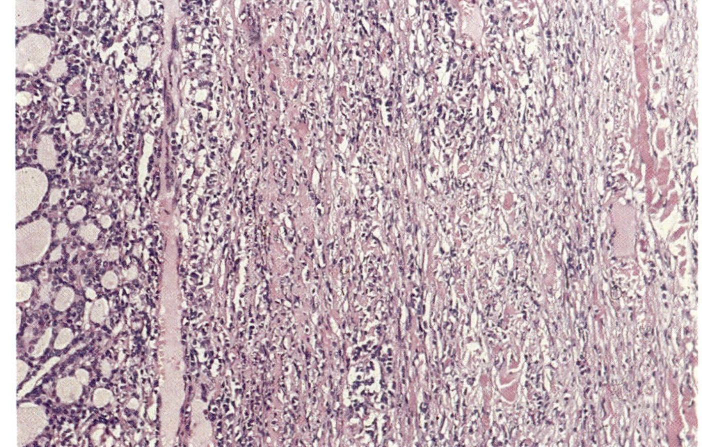

Fig. K20.   Hashimoto's thyroiditis. At the lower left is the intense lymphocytic infiltration with a germinal center. To the right are typical small follicles with many of the epithelial cells having abundant eosinophilic granular (oxyphilic) cytoplasm, enlarged hyperchromatic nucleus, and prominent nucleolus (Askanazy cells). This is the same specimen shown in *Fig. K19.*   (hematoxylin-eosin)

Fig. K21.   Riedel's thyroiditis (invasive fibrous thyroiditis). This is an extremely rare condition, and may involve the whole gland or part of the gland. In this 27-year-old man the thyroid is partially replaced by dense fibrous tissue within which chronic inflammatory cells are seen. Surrounding muscle (right) is also infiltrated. The thyroid capsule has been completely obliterated.   (hematoxylin-eosin)

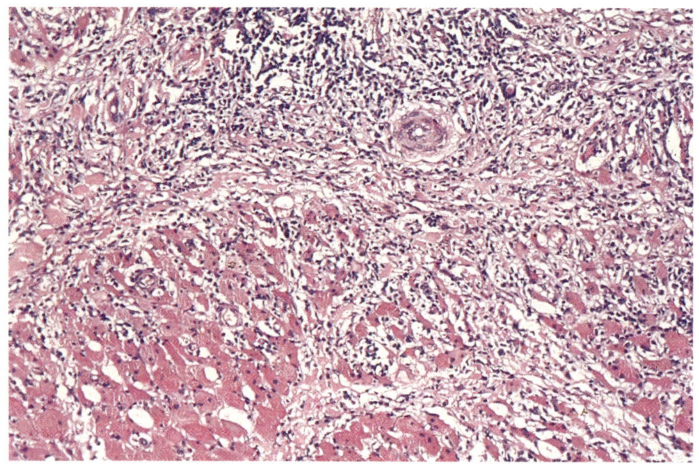

Fig. K22. Riedel's thyroiditis. In this photomicrograph, the same specimen as *Fig. K21,* the muscles of the neck surrounding the thyroid are partially replaced by the fibrous tissue and inflammatory cell infiltration. Invasion of neck structures is regarded by many as the *sine qua non* for diagnosis of this condition. (hematoxylin-eosin)

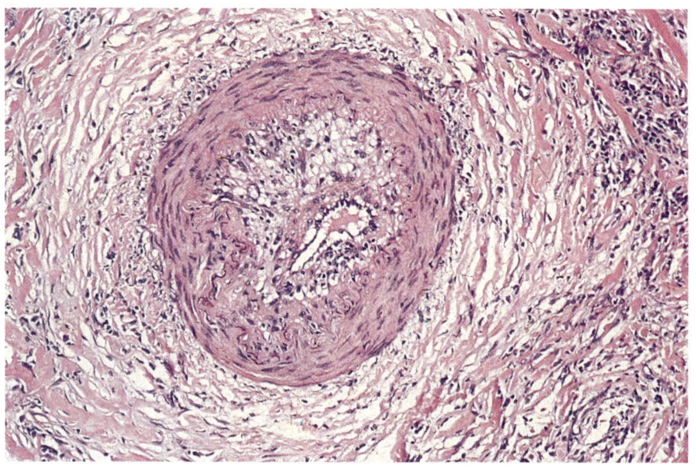

Fig. K23. Riedel's thyroiditis. The inflammatory and fibrous process surrounds a blood vessel, which demonstrates intimal proliferation with a few inflammatory cells, as a secondary angiitis. (hematoxylin-eosin)

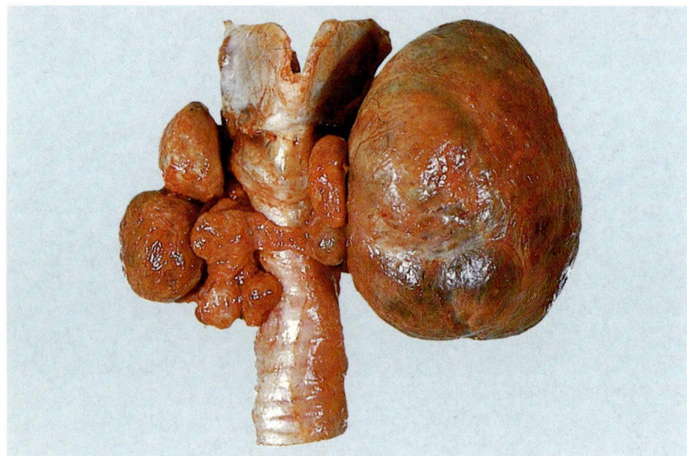

Thyroid Hyperplasias *(K24–K27)*
Chr. Hedinger

Fig. K24. Nodular goiter. The right thyroid lobe, seen to the left in this photograph, has multiple adenomatous nodules. The left lobe has a very large dominant hyperplastic nodule. Nodular goiter is most likely an end-stage of diffuse thyroid enlargement ("goiter"), resulting from alternating periods of hyperplasia and involution.

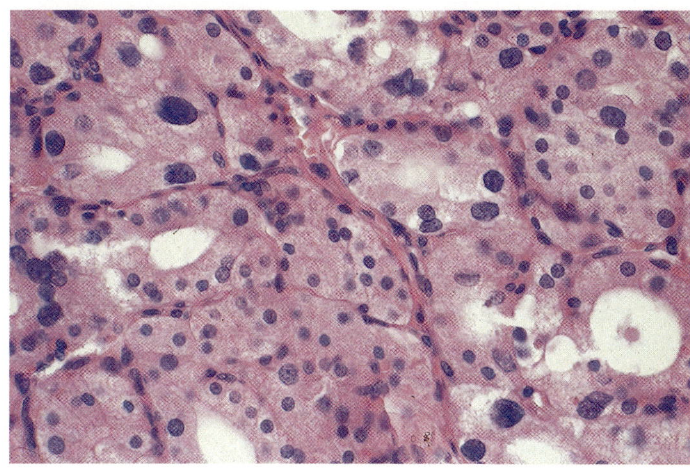

Fig. K25. Colloid nodule in a 63-year-old woman with nodular hyperplasia. There is a thin surrounding capsule. The follicles are partly distended by homogeneous colloid. The lining epithelial cells are flattened.   (hematoxylin-eosin)

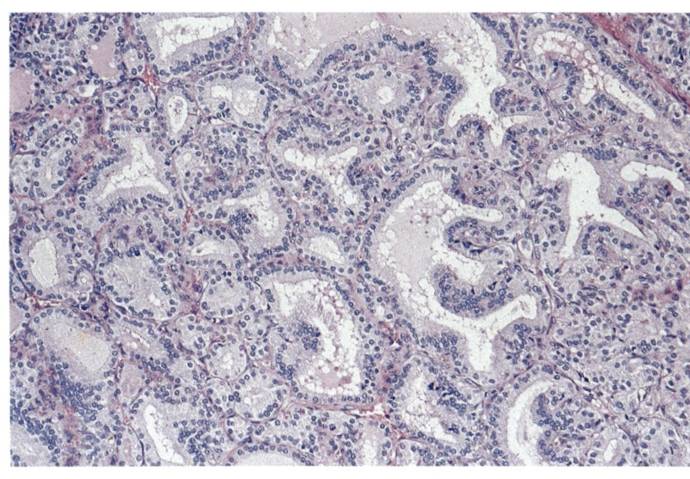

Fig. K26. Thyroid from a patient with congenital hypothyroidism. The follicles are small, lack colloid, and are lined by irregularly enlarged epithelial cells, many of which have very large nuclei. This could be misinterpreted as evidence of malignancy, although mitoses are not seen. Indeed, similar cytologic variation can be seen in other endocrine organs and the establishment of a malignant diagnosis should rest on the finding of capsular invasion or metastasis. In this type of case, malignant change is rarely found. (hematoxylin-eosin)

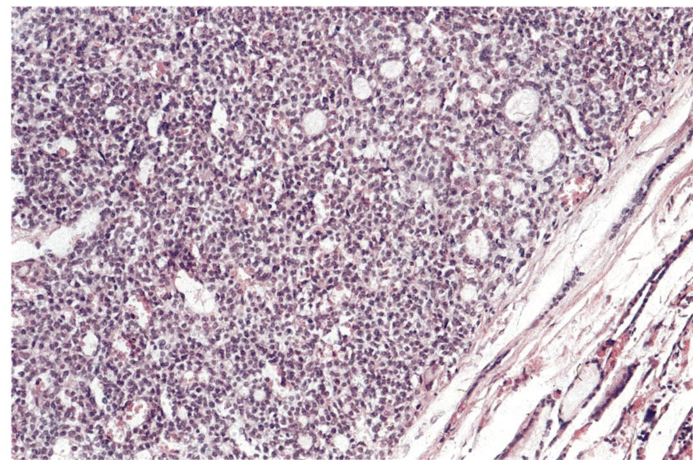

Fig. K27. Graves' disease (diffuse toxic goiter) is characterized by hyperthyroidism, ophthalmopathy, and diffuse thyroid enlargement. The follicles vary in size but are generally enlarged and filled with pale colloid which is retracted from the epithelial cells imparting a vacuole-like appearance. The tall columnar epithelial cells have papillary-like infoldings.

Thyroid Tumors   *(K28–K36)*
Chr. Hedinger

Fig. K28. Microfollicular adenoma. The tumor is encapsulated and consists of uniform small follicles devoid of colloid. The benign tumors are histologically indistinguishable from malignancies of the same histology, and the capsule must be extensively sectioned to exclude the possibility of carcinoma. In contrast, the macrofollicular adenoma is virtually always benign.   (hematoxylin-eosin)

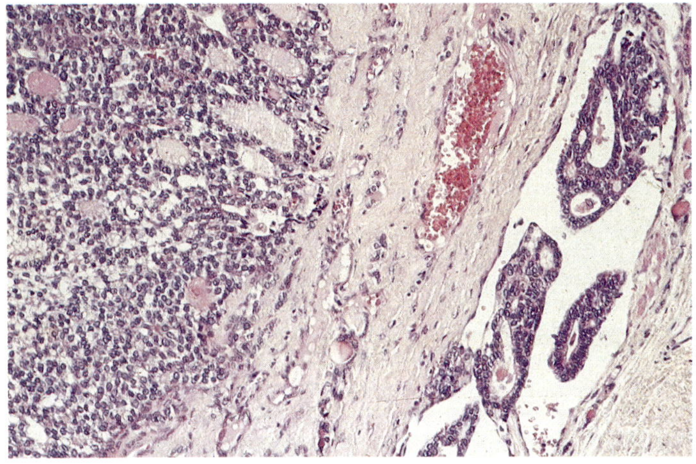

Fig. K29. Follicular carcinoma of the thyroid. This thyroid, from a 68-year-old woman, demonstrates tumor invasion of the capsule structures (right). The tumor consists of mostly small poorly-formed follicles with a few large follicular forms. Although regional lymph nodes are not generally involved in follicular carcinomas, distant metastases may be seen in as many as 25% of people at the time of diagnosis.   (hematoxylin-eosin)

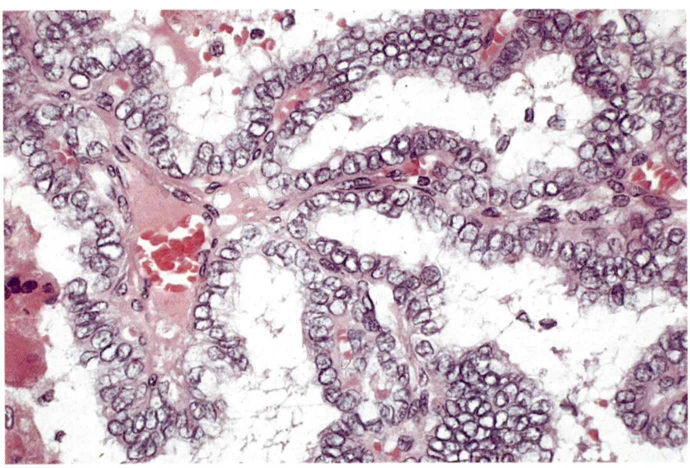

Fig. K30. Papillary carcinoma of the thyroid. This is the most common type of thyroid carcinoma. Typically the epithelial cells line slender fibrovascular structures and have large optically clear ("orphan Annie eyes") nuclei, with relatively indistinct cytoplasm. Papillary carcinoma can manifest as a predominantly follicular tumor, with little or no fibrous stroma, and correct identification can be made by the recognition of these typical cellular features. (hematoxylin-eosin)

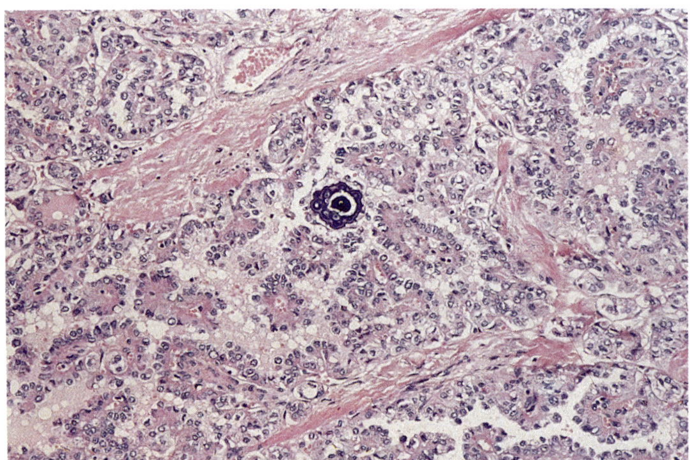

Fig. K31. Papillary carcinoma of the thyroid with a psammoma body. Psammoma bodies may occur in papillary carcinomas arising from other primary sites and are not pathognomonic of thyroid carcinoma. They may, of course, be found in lymph nodes when the tumor metastasizes, but may also be found occasionally in the absence of recognizable tumor cells.   (hematoxylin-eosin)

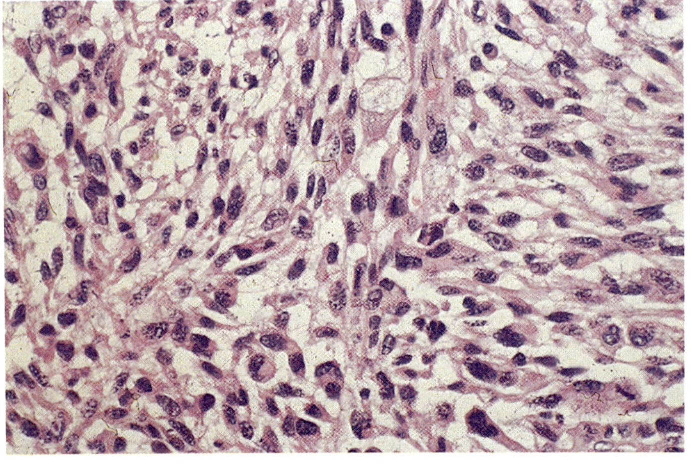

Fig. K32. Undifferentiated spindle cell carcinoma of the thyroid. This epithelial malignancy may closely resemble a sarcoma and its epithelial nature may be difficult to confirm unless epithelial structures, such as follicles, can be identified. This type of tumor generally occurs in older individuals, especially women. This thyroid was from a 74-year-old woman. There may be a giant cell component *(see Fig. K33).* This tumor, in contrast to papillary or follicular thyroid carcinoma, is highly aggressive.   (hematoxylin-eosin)

Fig. K33. Undifferentiated giant and spindle cell carcinoma of the thyroid, from an 84-year-old woman. In this field, atypical multinucleated giant cells are obvious in the background of highly pleomorphic bizarre round cells. (hematoxylin-eosin)

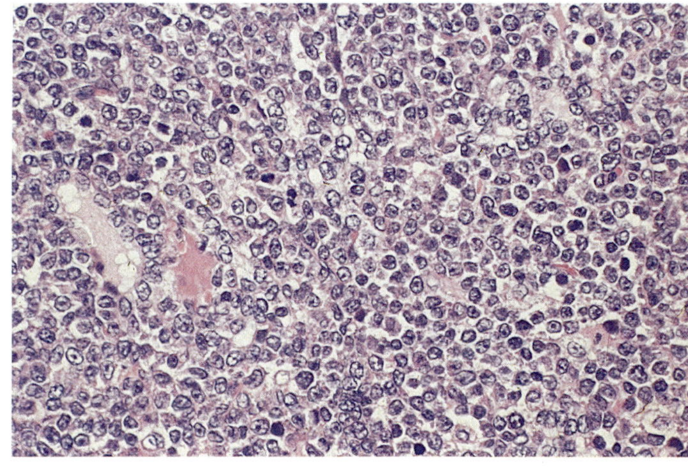

Fig. K34. Malignant lymphoma of the thyroid. This immunoblastic lymphoma presented as a thyroid mass in a 75-year-old woman and resembled an undifferentiated small cell carcinoma. Correct diagnosis was established with immunocytochemical studies. (hematoxylin-eosin)

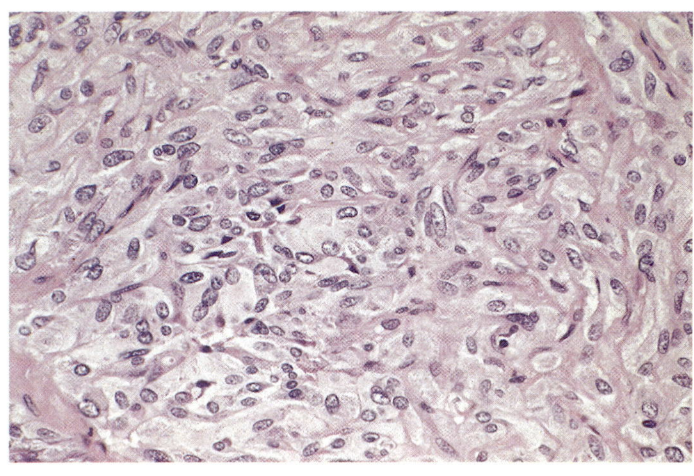

Fig. K35. Medullary carcinoma of the thyroid. This tumor arises from the parafollicular ("C") cells of the thyroid, rather than from follicular epithelial cells, and the tumor cells typically produce and secrete calcitonin, but may elaborate other hormones. Tumor cells tend to be polygonal, round, or spindle shaped, and are arranged in nests or ribbon-like structures. Characteristically, as in this tumor from a 39-year-old man with Sipple's syndrome, there is an amyloid stroma, seen, in this photomicrograph, at the lower left. (hematoxylin-eosin)

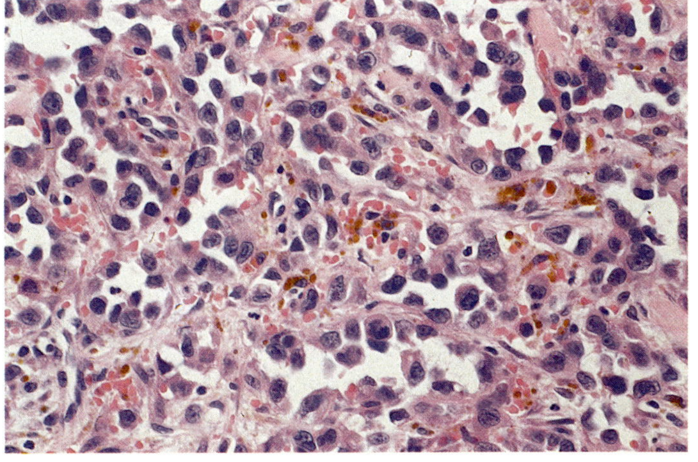

Fig. K36. Malignant hemangioendothelioma of the thyroid in an 80-year-old woman. This is an exceedingly rare tumor and is histologically similar to malignant hemangioendothelioma arising in other organs. The tumor consists of vascular spaces lined by highly atypical and pleomorphic endothelial cells. The stroma contains iron-laden histiocytes as evidence of previous focal hemorrhage. (hematoxylin-eosin)

Parathyroid Hyperplasia   (K37–K41)
Chr. Hedinger

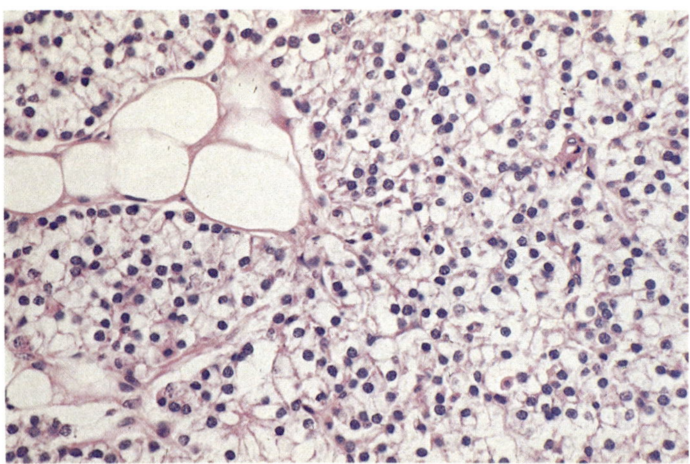

Fig. K37.   Secondary parathyroid hyperplasia with predominantly clear cell proliferation. This 42-year-old man had renal failure from malignant nephrosclerosis.   (hematoxylin-eosin)

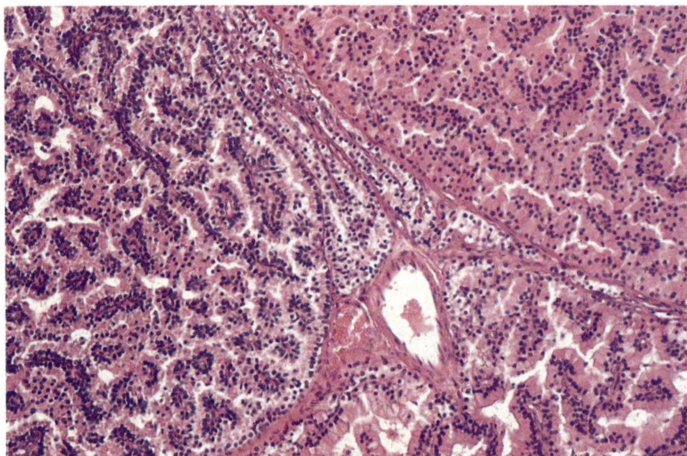

Fig. K38.   This 38-year-old woman had chronic renal insufficiency from urate nephropathy and was maintained on hemodialysis for many years. All four parathyroids show this picture with proliferation mostly of chief cells, but areas consisting entirely of oxyphilic cells (upper right).   (hematoxylin-eosin)

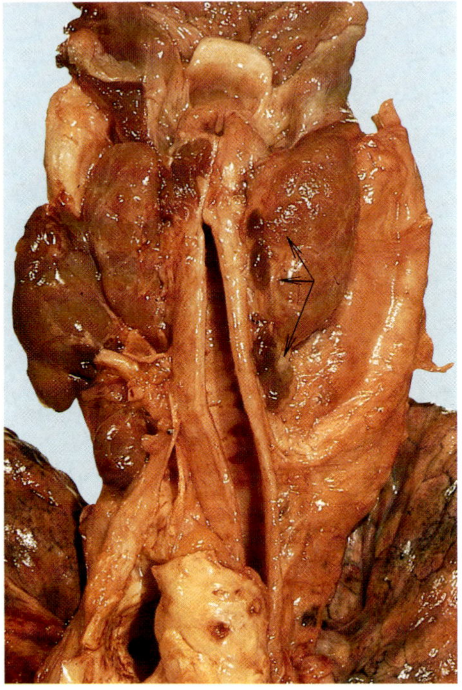

Fig. K39.   Primary water-clear-cell hyperplasia. This rare condition is probably a variant of longstanding primary chief cell hyperplasia. The parathyroids are all enlarged and typically appear dark brown *(arrows).* This is the posterior view of the neck structures. The epiglottis is above, and the trachea has been opened posteriorly.

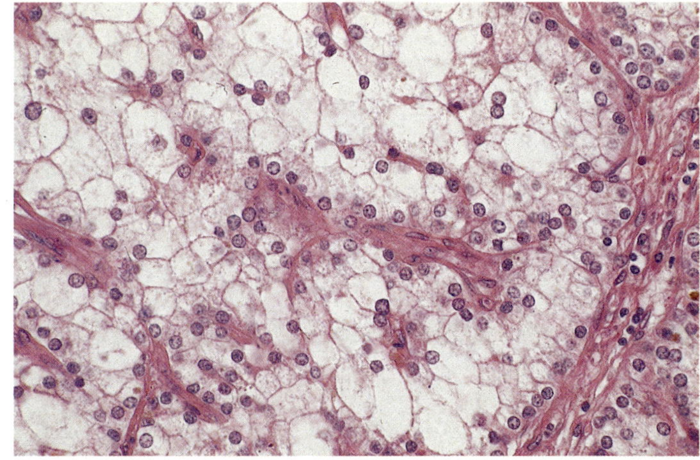

Fig. K40. Primary water-clear-cell hyperplasia. The cells are much larger than those water-clear-cells seen in secondary hyperplasia *(see Fig. K37)* with which they can be confused. (hematoxylin-eosin)

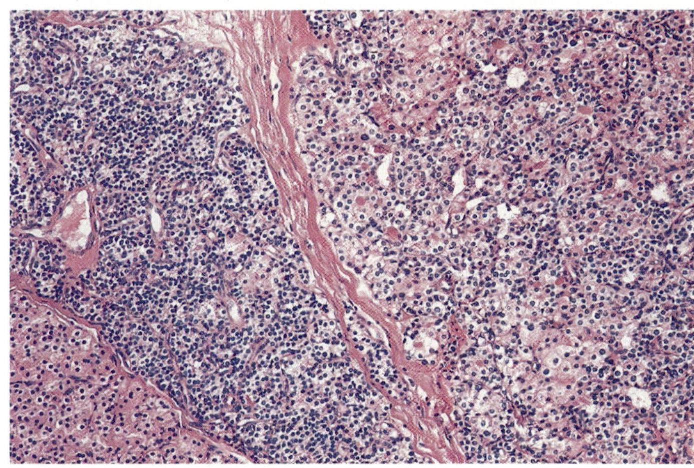

Fig. K41. Primary chief cell hyperplasia involving all four parathyroids in a 66-year-old woman. There may be uneven involvement of the glands and differentiation from adenoma may be histologically quite difficult *(see Fig. K43).* Before establishing the diagnosis for an enlarged parathyroid, it is important to examine all of the parathyroids grossly and to histologically examine at least one other parathyroid.   (hematoxylin-eosin)

Parathyroid Adenomas   *(K42–K43)*
Chr. Hedinger

Fig. K42. Parathyroid adenoma. This 61-year-old woman had generalized osteitis fibrosa cystica, and a 12.5 gm parathyroid was found at autopsy *(arrow).*

Fig. K43. Parathyroid adenoma. The majority of adenomas are composed of chief cells, as in this case.   (hematoxylin-eosin)

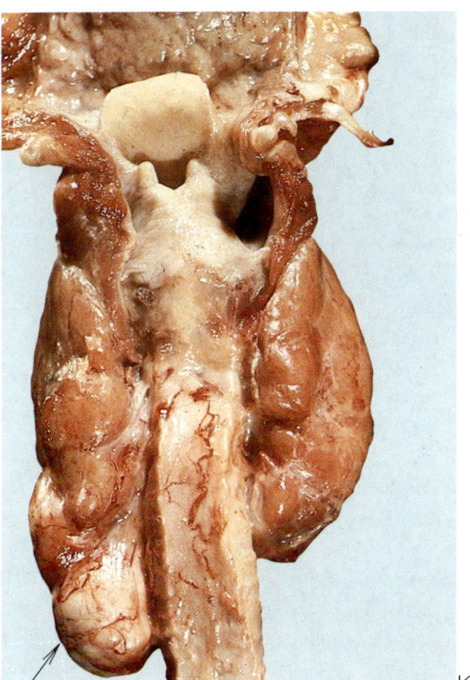

K42

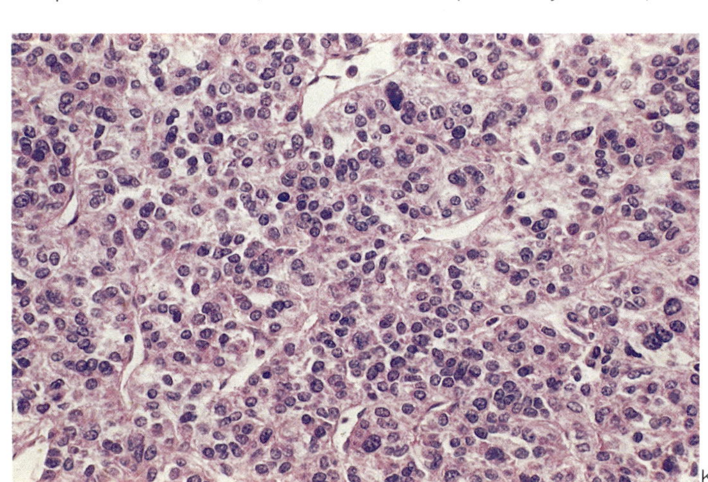

K43

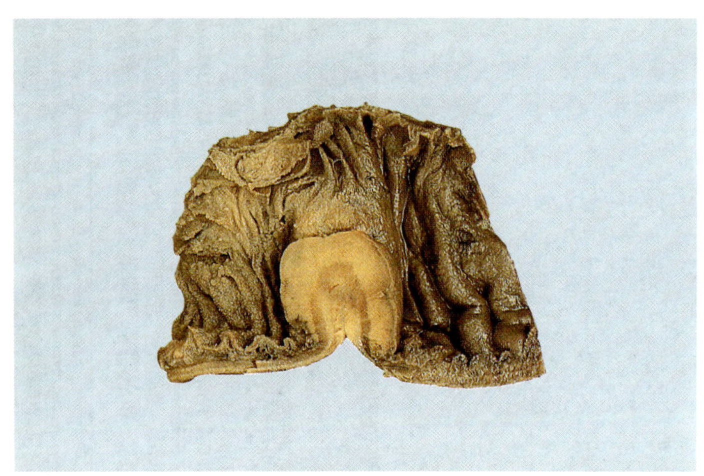

Fig. K44.   Carcinoid tumor of the ileum. A nonencapsulated but well-defined tan submucosal mass is seen in this segment of ileum. The tumor can be seen above and below the distinct muscularis propria, and infiltrates the fat. Although the tumor had spread to regional lymph nodes, the liver was not involved and there was no carcinoid syndrome.

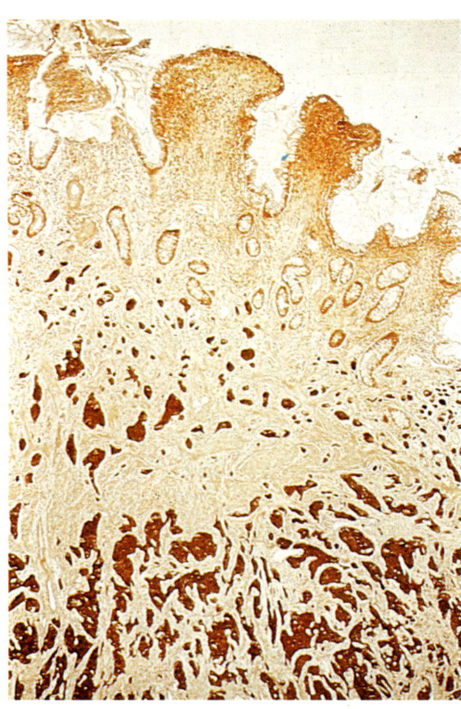

Fig. K45.   Carcinoid tumor of the ileum. Tumor cells infiltrate the submucosa and mucosa and are seen as silver-positive nests, ribbons, and sheets of cells within the intestinal wall connective tissue. The silver impregnation methods demonstrate the serotonin-containing endocrine granules.   (Masson-Hamperl)

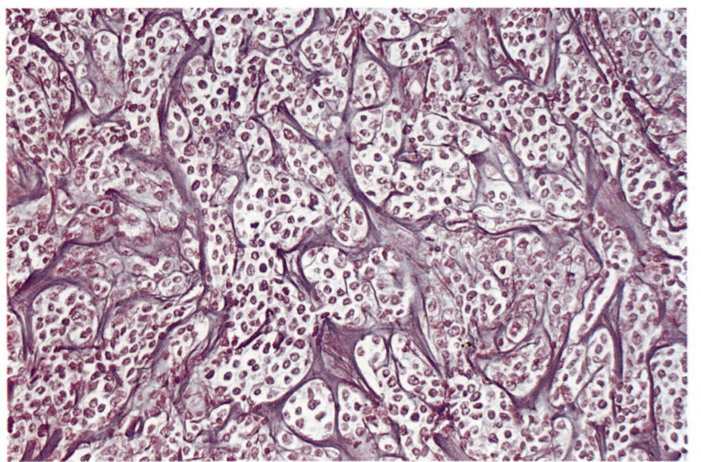

Fig. K46.   Carotid body tumor (paraganglioma; chemodectoma). This endocrine tumor has a thin capsule and consists of nests of large polyhedral cells grouped in an organoid pattern ("zellballen"), separated by loose connective tissue with a richly vascular stroma. The tumors are usually chemically inactive, but may mimic pheochromocytoma when they are functional. Histologically identical tumors can be found in the aortic bodies, the glomus jugulare (Otani tumor), and the ganglion nodosum of the vagus nerve. (elastica-Gomori)

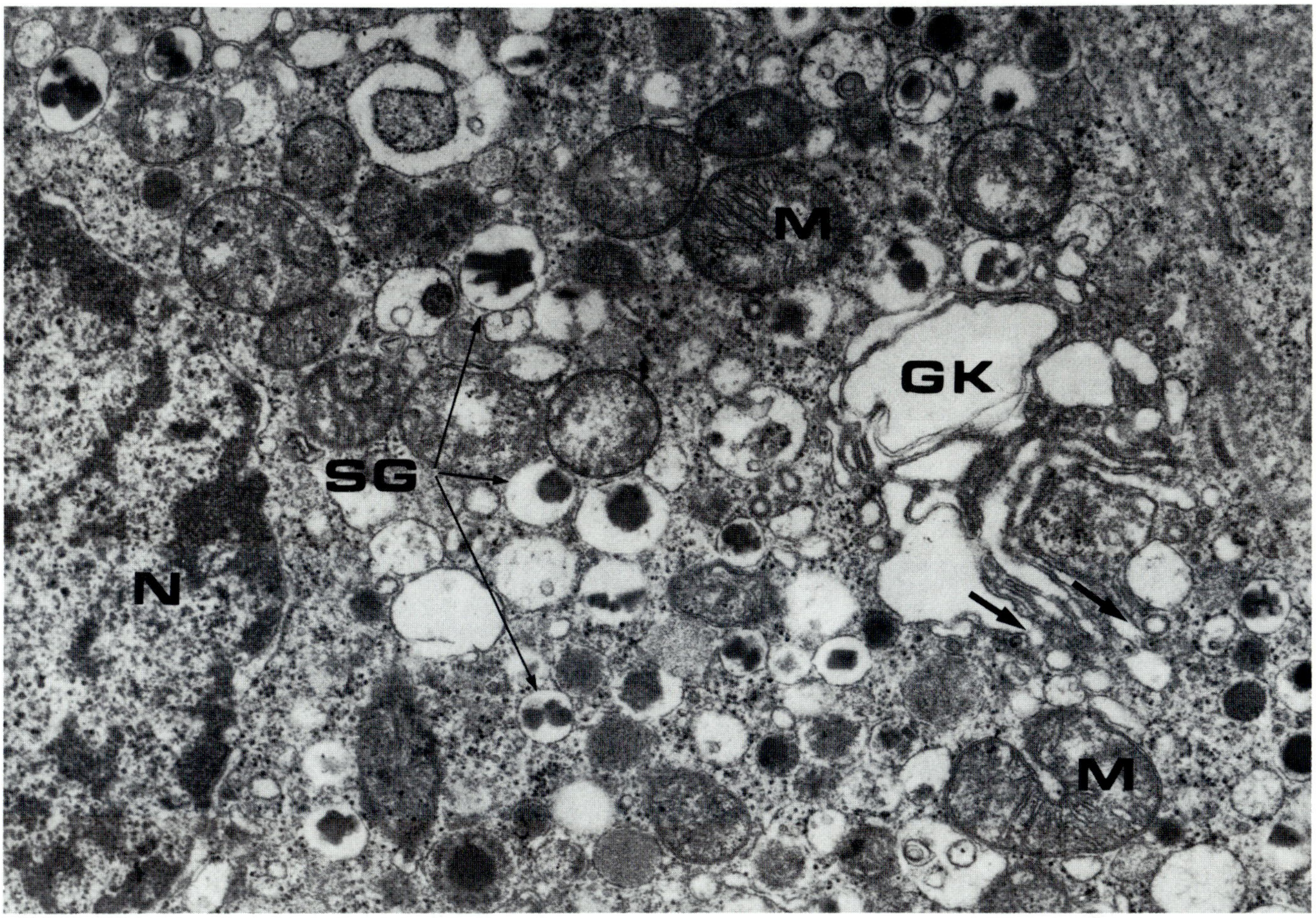

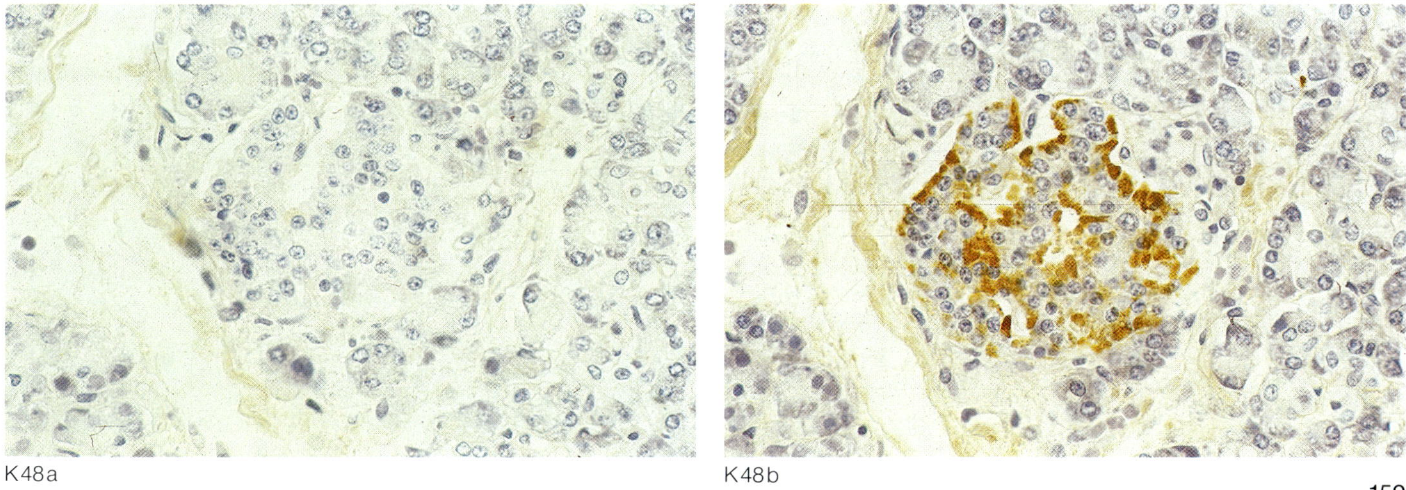

Fig. K47.   Ultrastructure of a B-cell of the human pancreas. The cytoplasm contains many secretory granules (SG) within which there are crystalline aggregates of insulin. There are scattered mitochondria (M) and partly dilated Golgi apparatus (GK) in which the early stages of secretory granule formation can be identified *(arrow).* The cell nucleus (N) is to the left.   (magnification 21 450×)

Fig. K48.   Pancreas from type I (insulin dependent) diabetes mellitus of short duration. Insulin cannot be demonstrated in the islet of Langerhans by immunocytochemistry studies (a), whereas glucagon containing cells are present in the same islet (b).

K48a

K48b

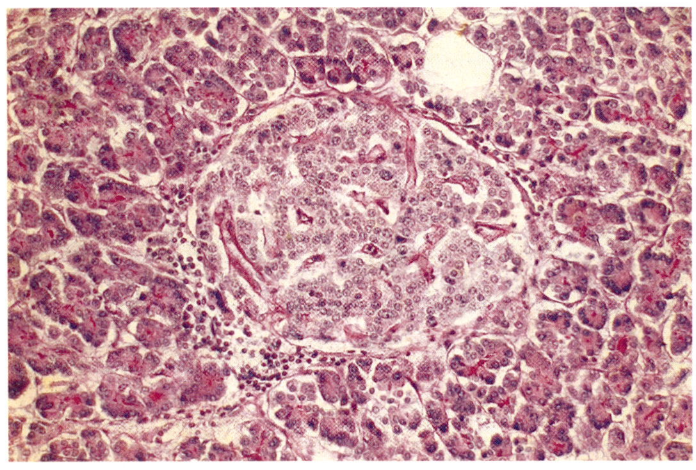

Fig. K49. Pancreas from a patient with type I diabetes mellitus of short duration. The cells of the islet of Langerhans are intact. There is a surrounding lymphocytic infiltrate. This inconsistent finding is thought to represent an autoimmune process, and is found most often in juvenile-onset diabetes mellitus.   (hematoxylin-eosin)

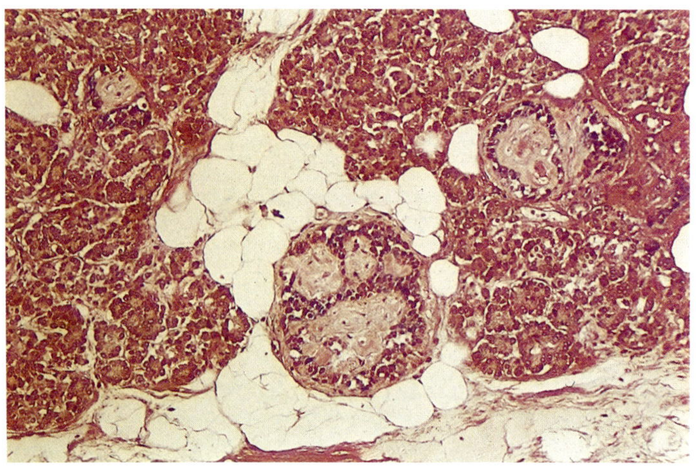

Fig. K50. Pancreas from type II (noninsulin dependent) diabetes mellitus. Three islets can be identified in this photomicrograph surrounded by acini, fat, and connective tissue. Eosinophilic amorphous amyloid surrounds the capillaries of the islets, compressing and displacing the islet cells. This change has been found in non-diabetics as well as diabetics, and is not necessarily associated with systemic amyloidosis. B-cell stain blue in this aldehyde-fuchsin preparation.

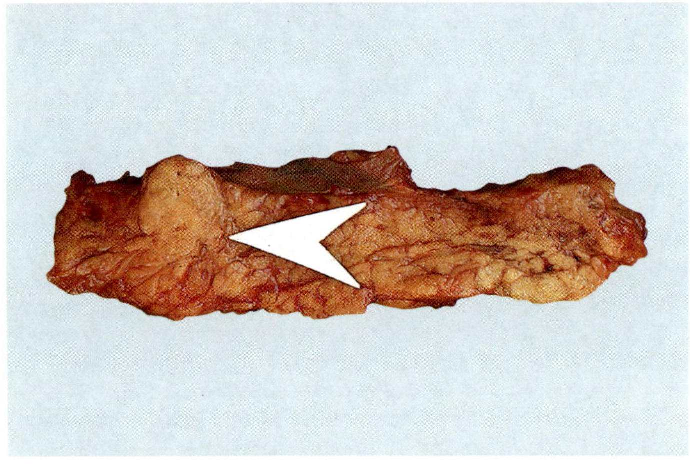

Endocrine Tumors of the Pancreas   (K51–K53)
G. Klöppel

Fig. K51. Insulinoma *(arrow)*. This patient had a hypoglycemia syndrome. Functionally and immunocytochemically this proved to be an insulin-secreting tumor of the pancreas. The tumor was in the mid-body. There were no metastases evident at the time of surgery.

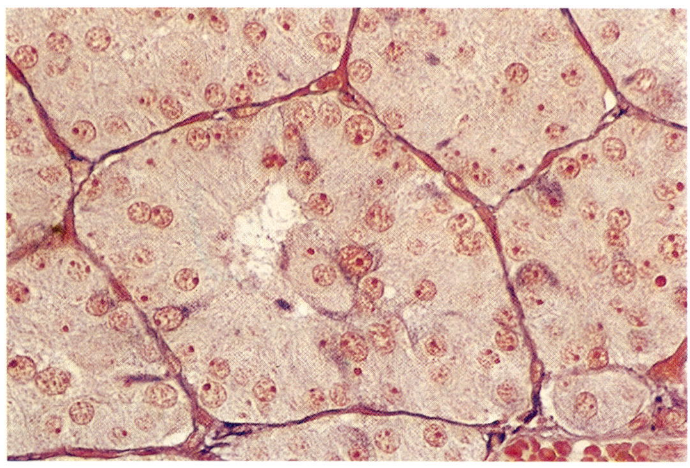

Fig. K52. Insulinoma. Occasional tumor cells stained blue with the aldehyde-fuchsin reaction, consistent with insulin activity.

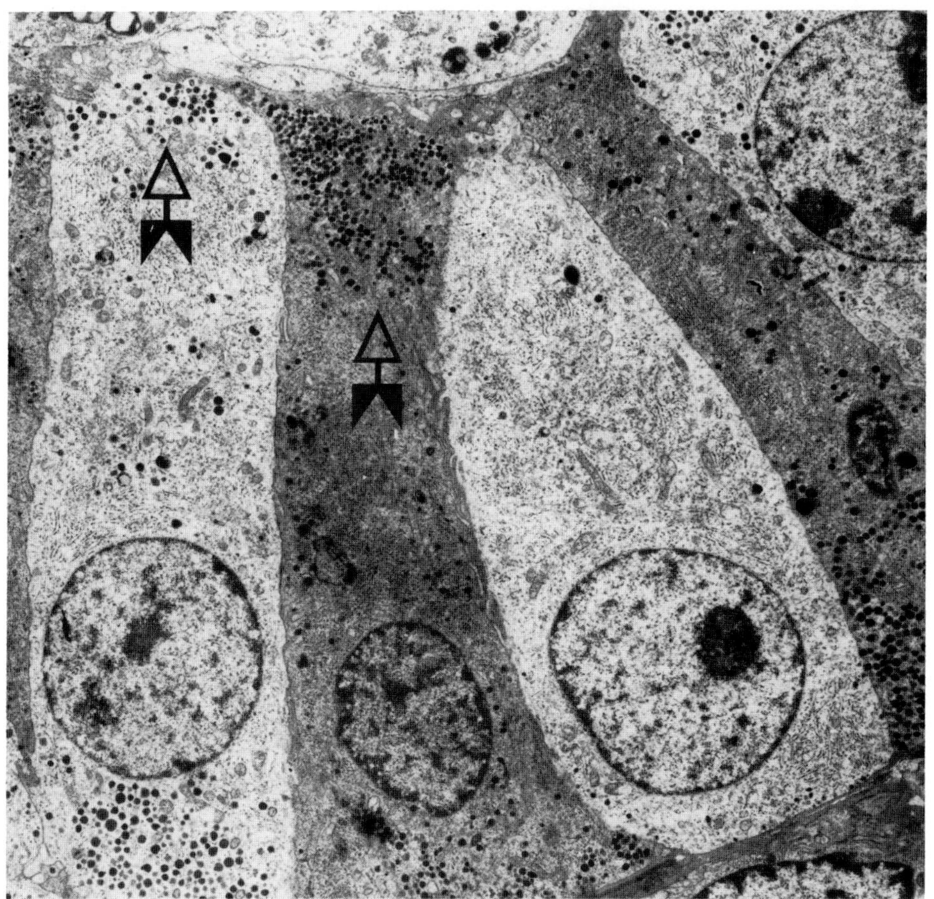

Fig. K53. Ultrastructure of an endocrine tumor of the pancreas. The tumor cells are arranged in parallel fashion with a concentration of secretary granules at the apical poles *(arrows)* where the release of the hormonal material takes place. These tumors can produce various hormonally-active polypeptides and can cause a variety of hormone-induced signs and symptoms.

L. Nervous System

H. Noetzel, F. Gullotta

The structure of the brain and spinal cord is particularly complex; because of this, malformations can cause a wide variety of morphologic and clinical alterations. Severe malformations are not compatible with life, whereas slight malformations can cause developmental disorders of varying degree. This is also true of perinatal brain damage. Since the brain is not completely developed just prior to birth, significant sequelae may result from a variety of injuries, including hypoxia, perinatal infections, and birth trauma. In contrast, disorders of the vascular system generally occur in later years. They are due mostly to the arteriosclerotic disorders and may be complicated by thromboses or subsequent hemorrhages. Small hemorrhages can occur without major sequelae, depending on the site of injury. Large hemorrhages often produce functional disorders which may be incompatible with life. Brain infarctions may follow arterial thrombi and emboli, but may also result when there are thromboses of the cerebral veins and the sinuses of the dura mater. Clinical manifestations of these events depend on the site of injury. Inflammatory disorders of the nervous system also produce variable affects depending on the site of their occurrence. Generally, infections involve the brain after hematogenous spread. Locally spread infections follow trauma, occasionally are due to otitis media, and rarely may be due to cranial osteomyelitis. Although the morphologic features of some of the infectious disorders, such as tuberculosis, syphilis, and the viral encephalitides are well recognized, the clinical manifestations may be entirely nonspecific and confusing.

A number of forms of encephalitis have become increasingly important in recent years. These include herpes encephalitis, toxoplasma encephalitis, and cytomegalovirus encephalitis. Slow viruses may also affect the central nervous system. The encephalitides in these cases have characteristic degenerative changes, generally without significant inflammatory reaction. In some of these disorders there may be demyelinization. The principal disorder caused by demyelinization is, of course, multiple sclerosis. The specific etiology and pathogenesis of this disorder are still not understood.

Hypoxic disorders are particularly injurious to the central nervous system, since nerve cells have a specially high demand for oxygen. The brain and spinal cord may also be affected by a variety of metabolic disorders, including those associated with chronic alcoholism, hypovitaminosis, and many disorders involving lipid, carbohydrate, and protein metabolism. The neurolipidoses are particularly important.

Traumatic injuries to the brain may cause severe damage, depending on the localizations and intensity of the injury. Injuries to the head, even if the cranium remains intact, may be associated with hemorrhages and concomitant brain edema.

Intracranial tumors may arise from the meninges, the nerve tissue itself, and the supporting connective tissue of the brain, and may be metastatic. Tumors which are biologically benign can cause significant impairment or death because of their location or their increasing size in an enclosed space. The prognosis of brain tumors varies considerably, depending on site and rate of growth. Prognosis can often be predicted by evaluating the histopathologic features of the tumor.

Finally, the brain is particularly susceptible to the effects of aging. Generalized atrophy of the brain may occur in the absence of severe vascular insufficiency. In some patients the atrophy may be a morphologic observation only, whereas in others there may be progressive development of dementia.

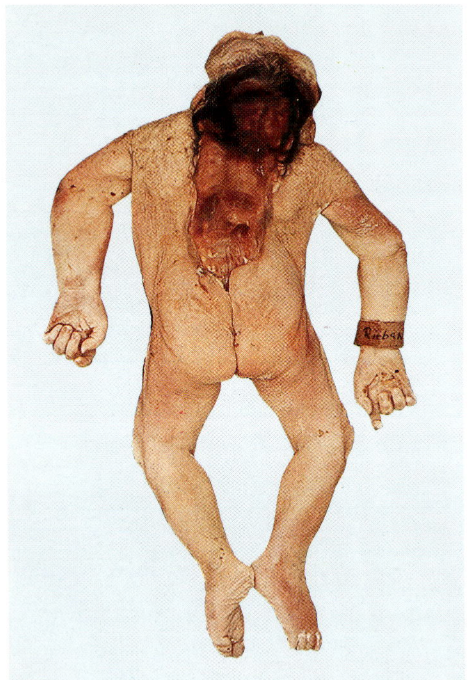
L1

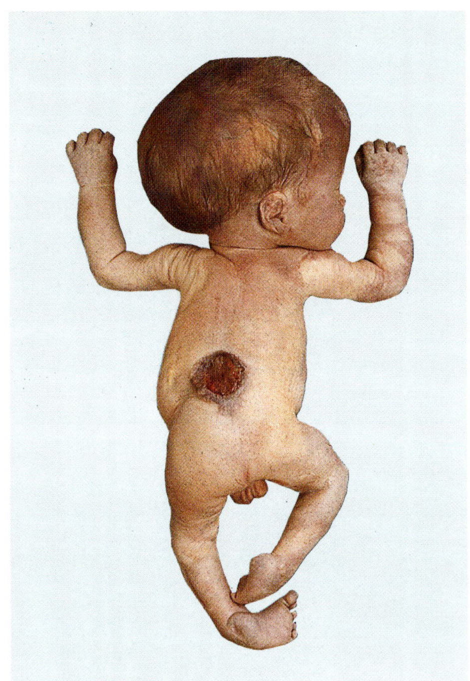
L2

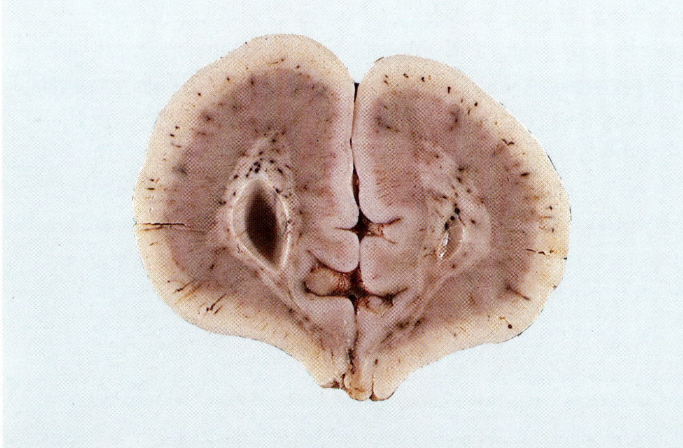
L3

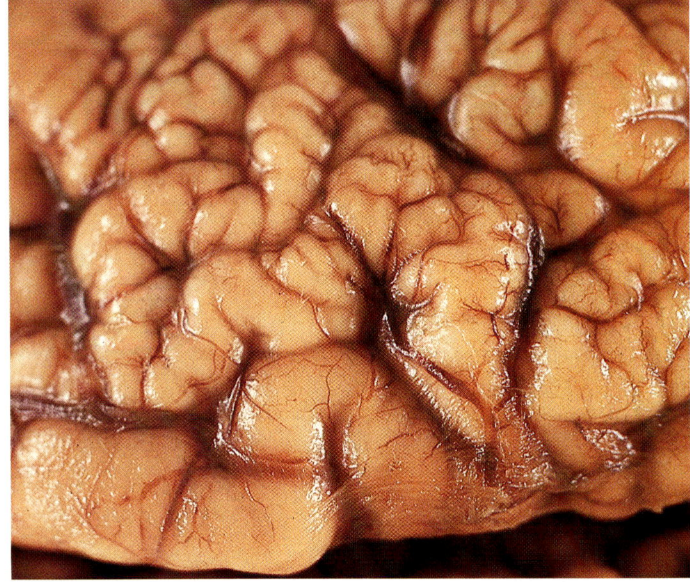
L4

Malformations *(L1–L5)*

Fig. L1. Anencephaly. This is the most severe form of craniorachischisis in which the cranium and the upper portion of the spine are completely absent. The brain consists of malformed embryonic nerve tissue irregularly mixed with portions of the choroid plexus and the vascularized leptomeninges. In this type of malformation the facial structures may be relatively well formed, although the orbit and eyes frequently protrude, causing the typical "frog's facies".

Fig. L2. Small lumbar meningo-myelocele with internal hydrocephalus. This malformation is relatively common and may not always be associated with hydrocele. In this case the defect is easy to see since it is associated with a relatively large spina bifida. In some cases the defect may be quite small, without an obvious meningocele, and the site of the defect may have a prominent covering tuft of hair with only a tiny fistula present. Meningitis may be a complication even in these small defects. This patient also had the Arnold-Chiari malformation, in which there was caudal displacement of the medulla and vermis of the cerebellum below the level of the foramen magnum, contributing to the hydrocephalus.

Fig. L3. Lissencephaly (agyria). There is complete absence of gyrus formation. The only suggestion of gyrus formation is in the midline.

Fig. L4. Microgyria. Rarely there may be an exaggeration of gyrus formation in which the overall architecture of the brain developed. Many of the gyri show additional subdivisions. This is thought to be due to an injury to the development of the cortex which occurs during the last trimester of pregnancy. These malformations tend to occur in areas supplied by the major cranial arteries and could reflect some disturbance in oxygenation.

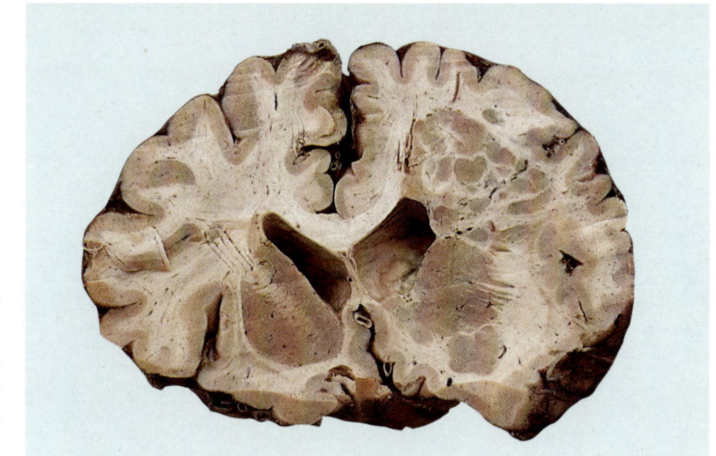

Fig. L5. Heterotopic brain tissue in the right cerebral hemisphere. The right medullary area is markedly deformed by several islands of grey matter which are obviously displaced from the cortical surface. These well-formed masses of nerve cells probably were displaced during the migration of neuroblasts from the subependymal layer to the cortex. It has also been suggested that this injury may be due to a transient defect in oxygenation.

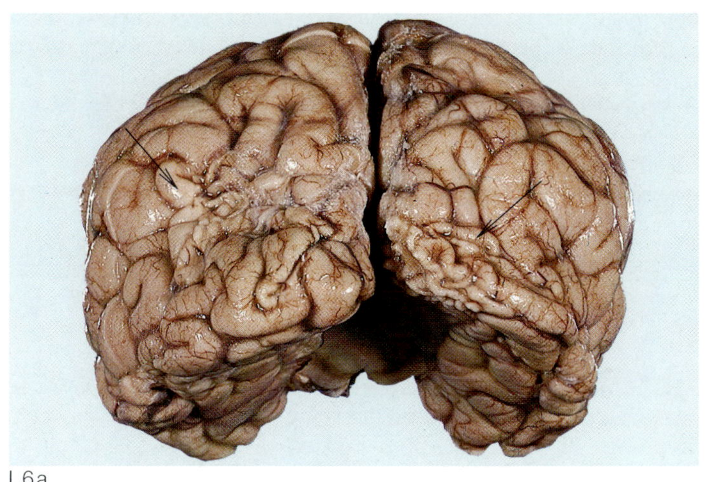

L6a

Perinatal Brain Injuries (L6–L10)

Fig. L6. Ulegyria. This is a form of brain scar that develops when brain development is almost complete. It is thought to follow a local vascular disturbance with secondary ischemia. *a)* The left occipital lobe has an area of deformity *(arrow)* in which the brain tissue appears contracted. *b)* In this cross-section the ulegyria is seen as a markedly retracted, atrophic segment of brain at the upper half of the photograph, and does not impinge on the ventricle.

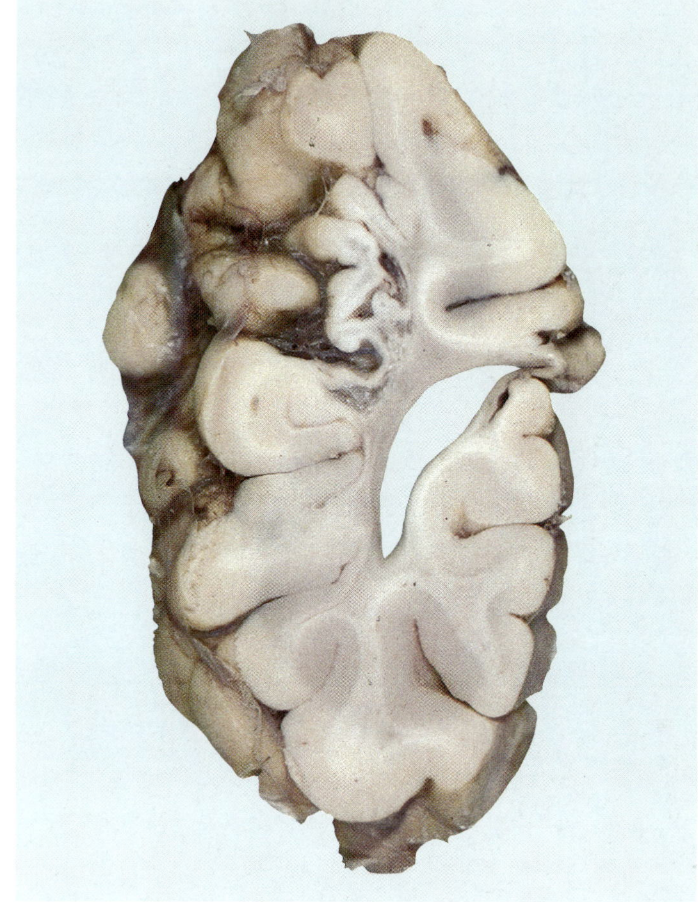

L6b

Fig. L7. Porencephaly. The brain shows multiple cystic spaces involving both cerebral hemispheres. These changes can follow necrosis of brain tissue, whether of hypoxic, viral, or unknown causes. The contour of the cerebral cortex is generally well-preserved, but it is irregularly sclerotic with absence of the oxygen-sensitive ganglion cells. Porencephalic cysts can communicate to the ventricles as well as to the external surface of the brain so that cerebrospinal fluid can flow in more than one direction. This photograph is of the classic form of porencephaly, although the term has now come to be used for almost any cysts occurring in an infant brain.

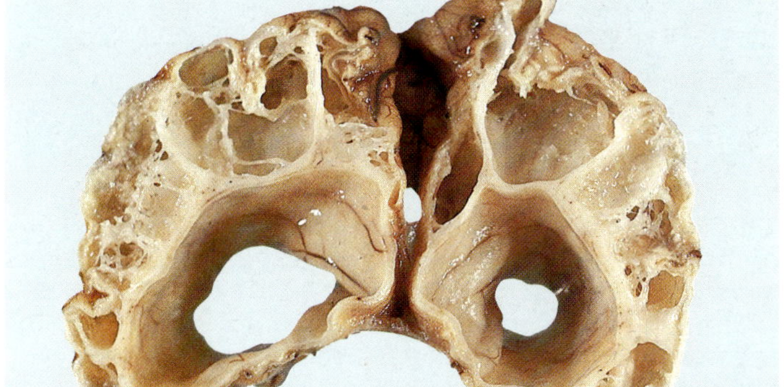

L7

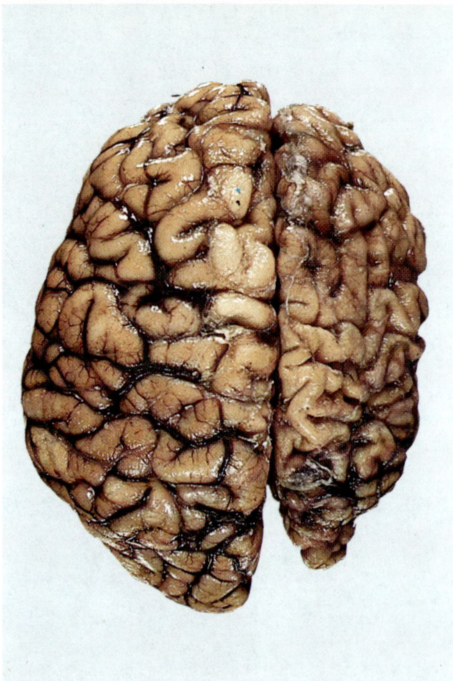

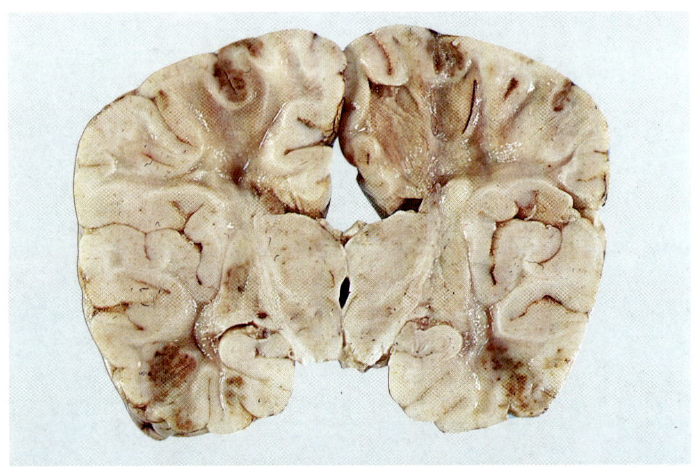

Fig. L8. Cerebral hemiatrophy. The right half of the cerebrum is both markedly diminished in size and also sclerotic, while the left cerebrum is normally developed. The pathogenesis of hemiatrophy is not clear. Among the potential causes are vascular insufficiency on one side of the brain, external pressure from a subdural hematoma, or pressure from a subdural "hygroma" (accumulation of serous fluid resembling cerebrospinal fluid in the subdural space). The atrophic brain generally manifests immediately in the perinatal period and should be regarded as a secondary injury rather than a primary malformation.

Fig. L9. Cerebral edema and necrosis due to ischemic injury. The well-defined hemorrhagic infarcts are easily seen. The edema of the brain can be appreciated by the almost complete loss of sulcal indentations. The medullary portion is irregularly necrotic as a consequence of this ischemic injury. If there is a period of survival following the injury, these changes can lead to the development of cerebral cysts (porencephaly) *(see Fig. L 7).*

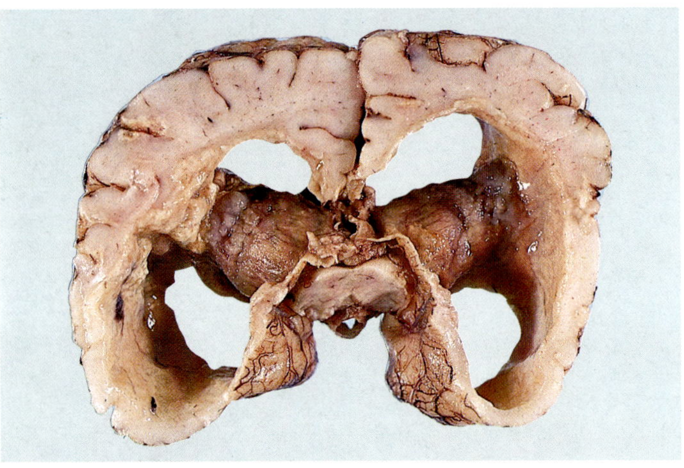

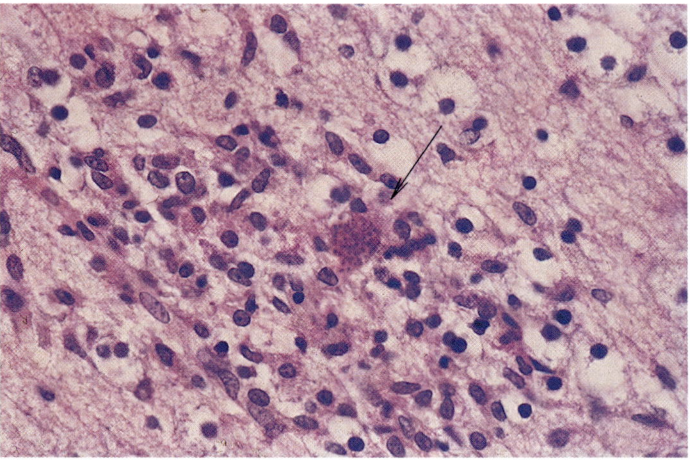

Fig. L10a. Congenital toxoplasmosis. Severe internal hydrocephalus is obvious. The greatly enlarged ventricles, and consequent necrosis and thinning of the surrounding brain, follow inflammatory injury and stenosis of the aqueduct of Sylvius. The ependymal lining and most of the subependymal medulla is completely destroyed.

Fig. L10b. Toxoplasma cysts *(arrow)* were found on histologic study of this brain. When acquired transplacentally, toxoplasmosis can lead to chronic destructive meningo-encephalitis with development of hydrocephalus, as seen here, cerebral microcalcifications which may not be clinically manifest, and choroidoretinitis which can lead to blindness.

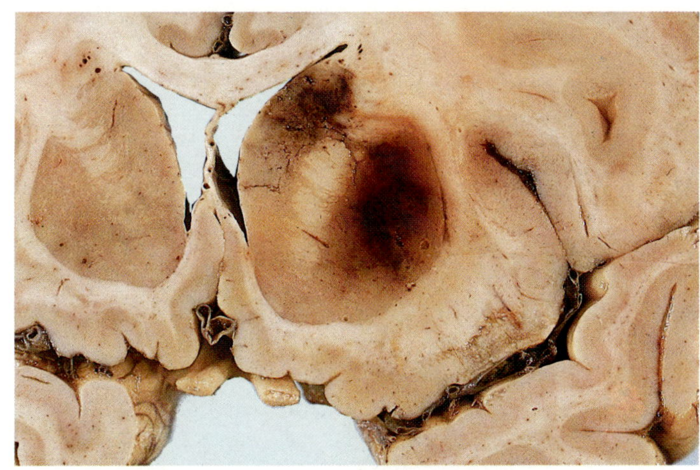

Fig. L 11.   Fresh hemorrhagic infarct in the area supplied by the lenticulostriate artery following embolism to the middle cerebral artery. The left ventricular space is somewhat compromised because of the edema of the underlying brain. The hemorrhagic necrosis also involves the internal capsule, although the changes are not as obvious as those of the caudate nucleus and putamen. Cerebral swelling, following infarction generally reaches a maximum during the first 3–5 days and disappears after approximately two weeks.

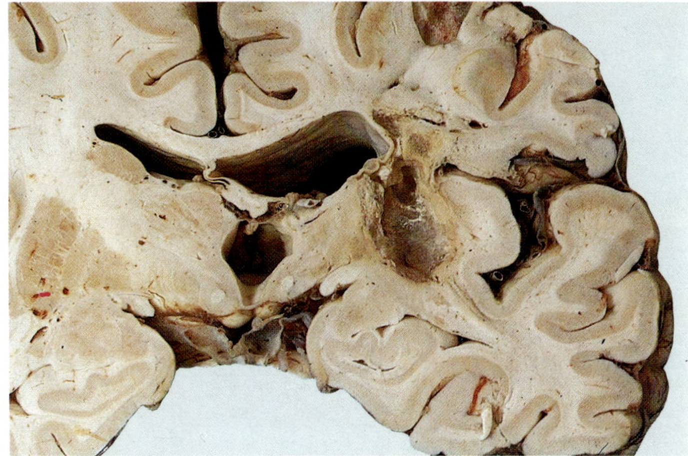

Fig. L 12.   Old cystic infarct in the region of the right basal ganglia. Completely healed brain infarctions, unlike those in other organs, are converted into fluid-filled cavities which characteristically have sharply circumscribed edges. The brownish discoloration is due to hemosiderin. The right internal capsule is degenerated and the thalamus is shrunken, with secondary dilatation of the right cerebral ventricle and the third ventricle.

Fig. L 13.   *a)* Severe atherosclerosis involving the vertebral and basilar arteries with aneurysmal dilatation obvious at the distal part of the right vertebral and the first portion of the basilar. *b)* The vessels of the circle of Willis and the cerebellum have been removed to expose the broad irregular grey areas of repressed brain. This is the surface appearance of cystic infarcts. Atherosclerotic plaques can be seen in the cut edges of the posterior cerebral arteries at the junction of the cerebral peduncles and the hippocampus.

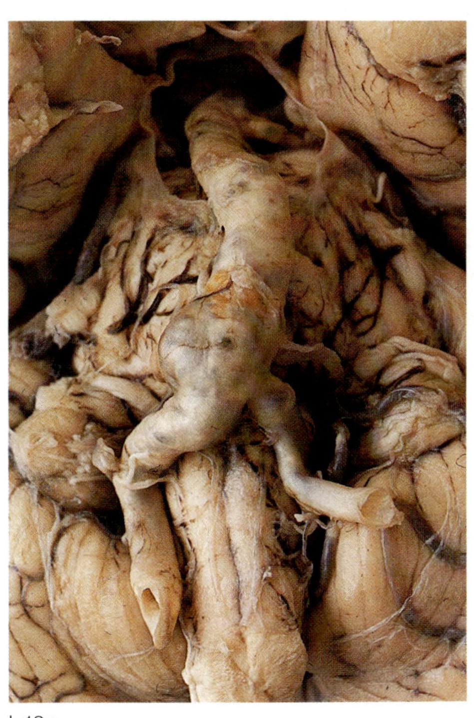

L 13a

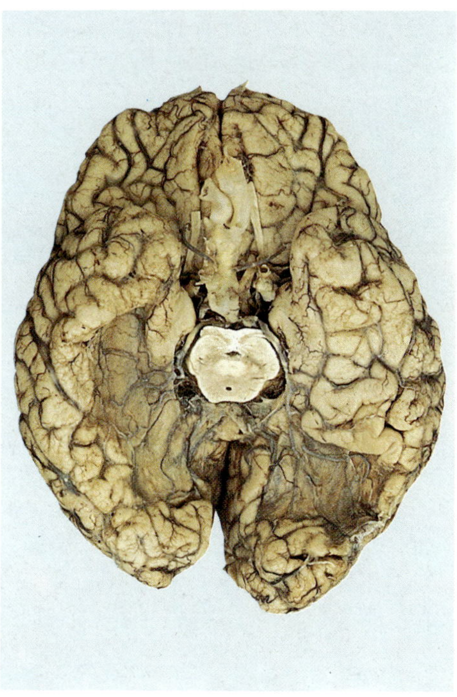

L 13b

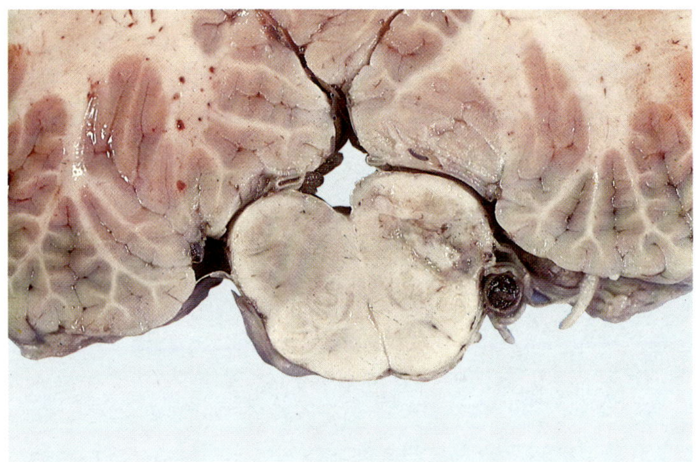

Fig. L 14. Wallenberg's syndrome. This is a clinical syndrome reflecting the involvement of the lateral medullary structures located dorsal to the inferior olivary nucleus. In this patient thrombotic occlusion of the right vertebral artery led to infarction of the medulla oblongata. Patients may be ataxic and may have disturbed pharyngeal function and altered phonation, as well as abnormalities of sensation.

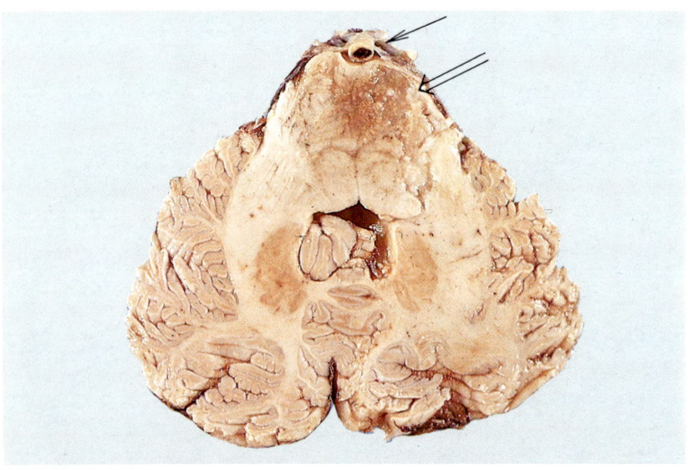

Fig. L 15. The basilar artery *(single arrow)* is atherosclerotic and thrombosed and there is partial necrosis *(double arrow)* of the pons.

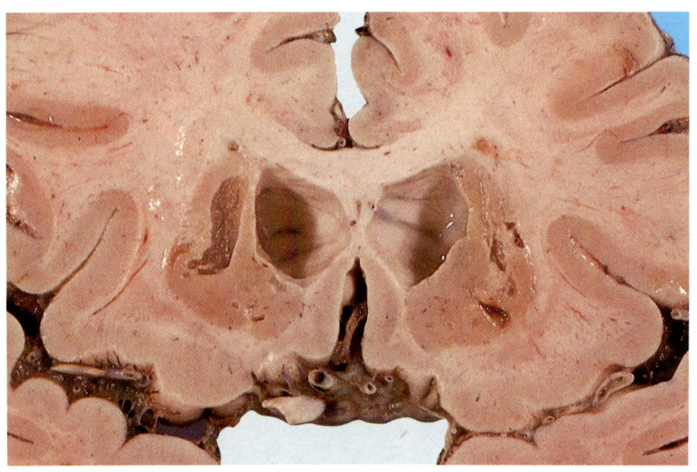

Fig. L 16. Lacunes in a patient with essential hypertension. These destructive brain lesions are secondary to ischemic infarction and almost always are seen in the basal ganglia, in the thalamus, internal capsule, pons, and convolutional white matter. Lacunes are generally from 0.2 to 15 cmm and are often overlooked at the time of autopsy because they are so small. With complete healing, lacunes become visible as cavities with sharply circumscribed edges. These small infarctions are almost always due to atherosclerosis affecting the middle cerebral artery and basilar arteries, and their branches, and are similar in etiology to cerebral cysts *(Fig. L 12)*.

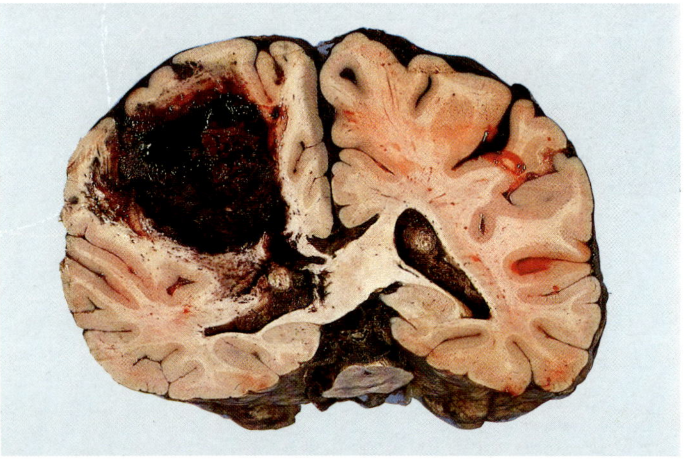

Fig. L 17. Recent, extensive cerebral hemorrhage in a patient with hypertension. There is massive destruction of the left cerebral hemisphere with formation of an intracerebral hematoma. Immediately surrounding the hemorrhagic area the brain is marked by numerous tiny ("flea-bite") hemorrhages. Cerebral hemorhage of this magnitude is virtually always fatal. Smaller hemorrhages, which may not lead to death, can lead to the formation of cysts *(Fig. L 12)* or, when very small, lacunes *(Fig. L 16)*.

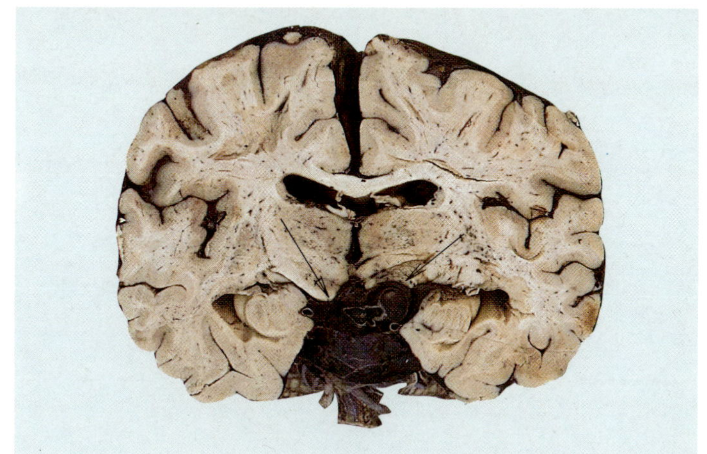

Fig. L 18.   Ruptured cerebral aneurysm *(between both arrows)* at the base of the brain, with fresh subarachnoid hemorrhage. Aneurysmal hemorrhage is almost always found at the base of the brain, in contrast to the hemorrhage following hypertension which involves the cerebral parenchyma. Aneurysmal hemorrhage involves the brain tissue only secondarily.

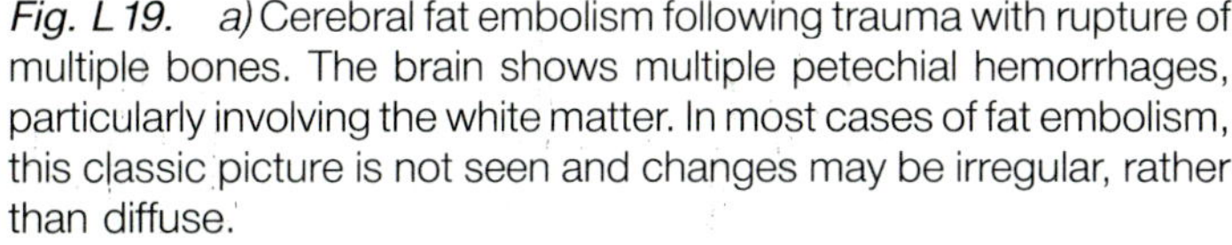

Fig. L 19.   *a)* Cerebral fat embolism following trauma with rupture of multiple bones. The brain shows multiple petechial hemorrhages, particularly involving the white matter. In most cases of fat embolism, this classic picture is not seen and changes may be irregular, rather than diffuse.
b) Histopathology of fat embolism. The capillary in this photomicrograph is distended by neutral fat, which has been stained with Sudan red. This photomicrograph is the counterpart to the gross appearance and shows the characteristic ring hemorrhage due to acute ischemia in the white matter immediately surrounding this small vessel.

L 19a

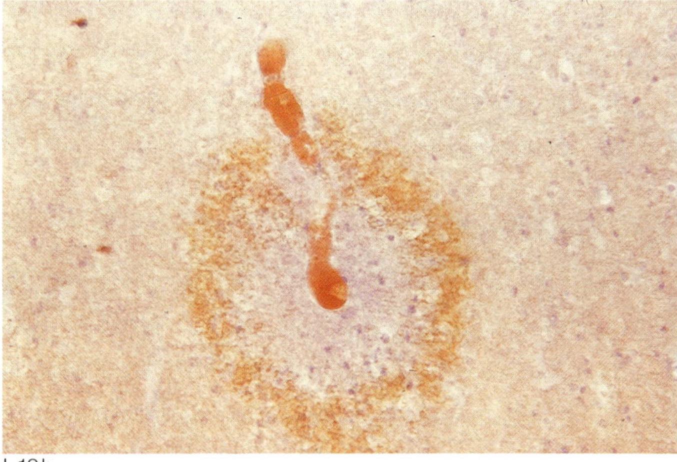

L 19b

Fig. L20.   Sinus thrombosis:
a) There is extensive hemorrhagic infarction of the left frontal region due to thrombosis of the anterior third of the superior sagittal sinus. A distended thrombosed vein, which drains into the sinus, is obvious on the cerebral convexity immediately caudal to the area of hemorrhage. The parietal, occipital, and frontal lobes are not affected.
b) Recent hemorrhagic infarct involving the right and left thalamus as a result of thrombus of the great vein of Galen. This is only rarely seen in adults, but is not infrequent in premature infants. When this type of injury is small and the patient survives, cystic lesions *(Fig. L 12)* may develop.

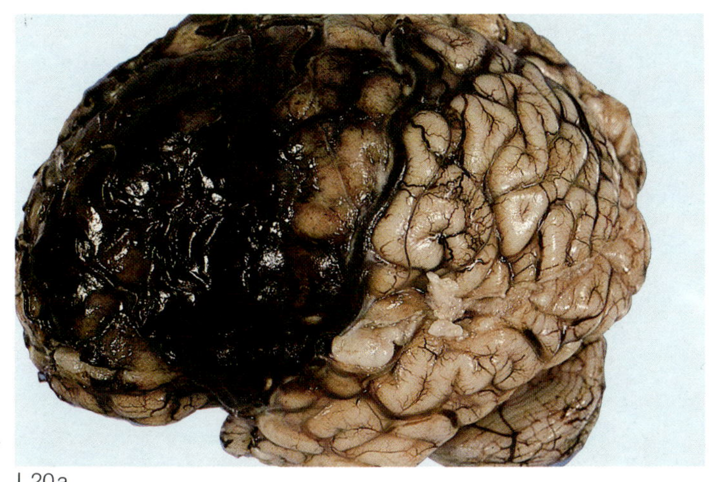

L20a

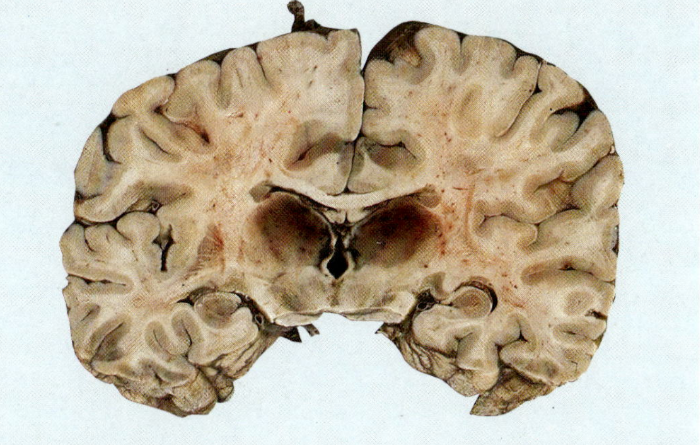

L20b

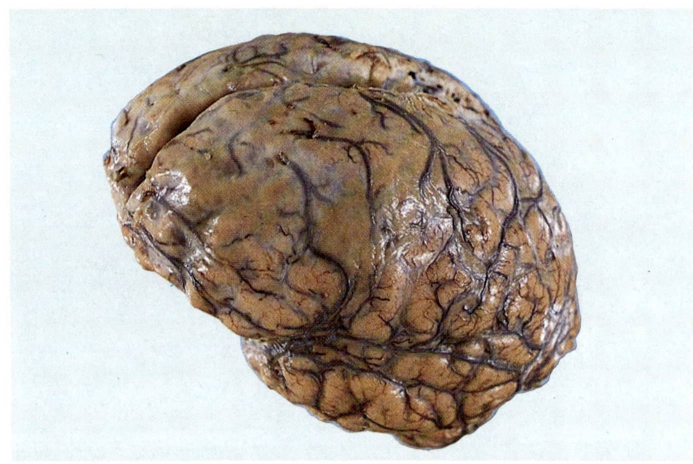

Fig. L21. Acute, purulent leptomeningitis. The leptomeninges are irregularly thick and opaque because of a covering exudate, and the veins of the convexity are accentuated. Pyogenic meningitis most often follows infection with meningococci and pneumococci, and may extend to the base and the cerebellum, as well as the spinal cord.

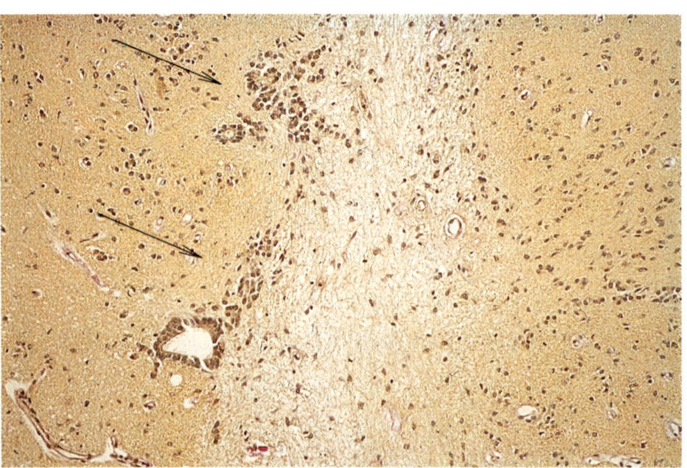

Fig. L22a. Post-inflammatory aqueduct stenosis. The aqueduct can no longer be recognized because of compression by gliotic scar tissue (pale area at the middle of the picture). The remnant of the aqueduct persists as a small ependymal lined channel (lower left) and multiple small nests of ependymal cells *(arrows)*. Inflammatory cells are no longer seen.

Fig. L22b. Hemosiderin deposits are seen in the glial scar tissue. This is evidence that the aqueductal stenosis is not the result of congenital injury, but rather a sequel of ischemic, previously hemorrhagic, necrosis. (Prussian blue reaction)

Fig. L23. Horizontal section of child's brain showing severe internal hydrocephalus due to aqueduct stenosis after meningitis. The ventricles are enormously dilated with secondary cerebral atrophy. In this photograph, the lateral ventricles, the Foramen of Monro, and the third ventricle are all greatly dilated.

Fig. L24. Tuberculous meningitis. Tuberculous leptomeningitis results from the hematogenous spread of tubercle bacilli to foci in the central nervous system and subsequent infection of circulating cerebrospinal fluid. Although the entire brain can be involved, the base of the brain is most characteristically affected. There may be considerable ischemic change because of meningeal vessel involvement directly by infectious inflammatory exudate, indirectly by secondary obliterative endarteritis, or by both processes. The ventricular cavities, especially the aqueduct, may show inflammatory changes, and there may be secondary aqueduct stenosis and hydrocephalus *(Fig. L23)*. The ischemic changes may be most prominent in the cranial nerves, brain stem ganglia, and hypothalamus.

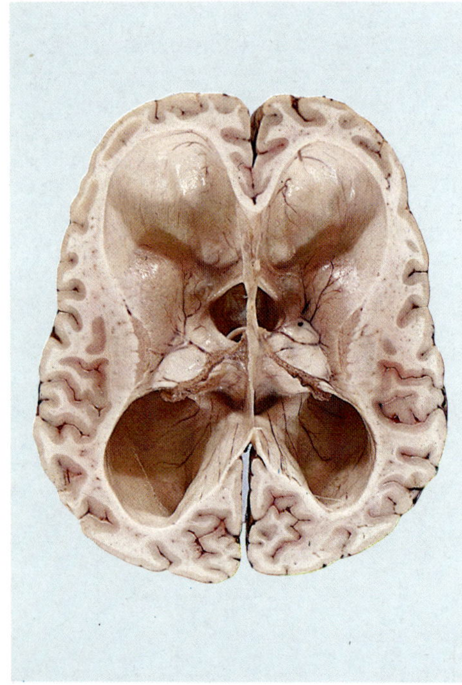

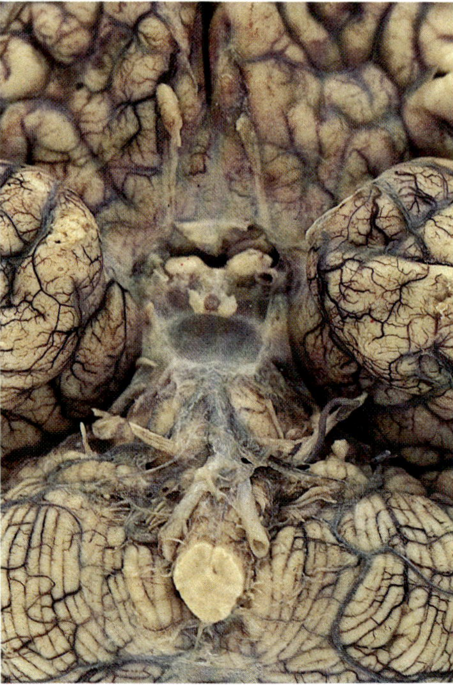

L23

L24

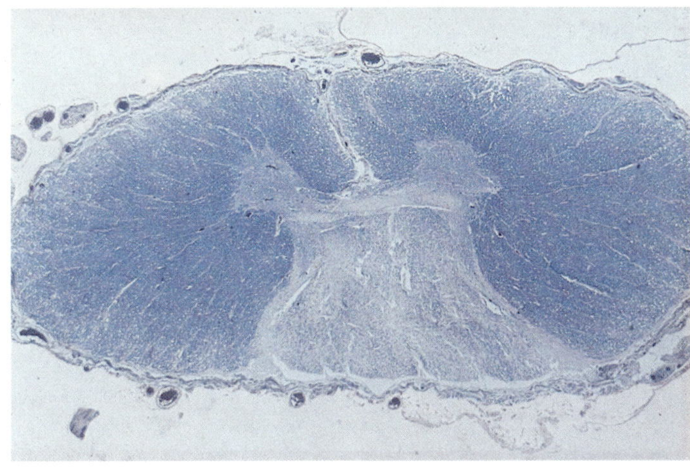

Fig. L25. Left temporo-occipital brain abscess following otitis media. Brain abscess can result from direct extension of an infectious process, in this case from the ear, or from hematogenous spread by septic emboli.

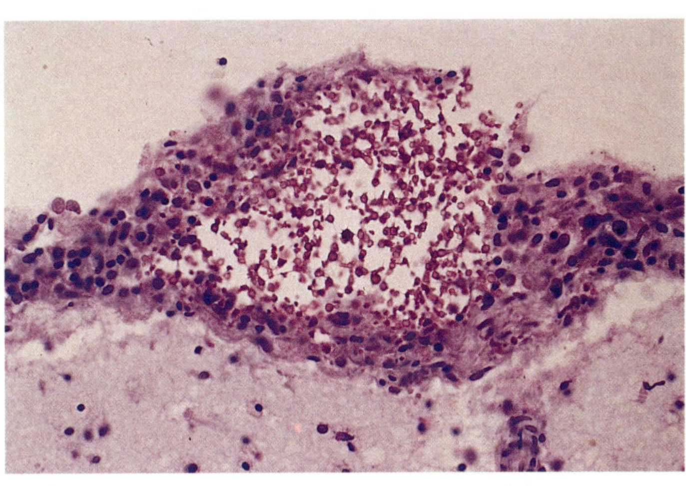

Fig. L26. Tabes dorsalis is a tertiary form of neurosyphilis in which there is atrophy and demyelination of the posterior spinal columns, seen in this photomicrograph as pale blue, and the dorsal roots. The dorsal spinal column involvement is a secondary degeneration due to ascending injury from the damaged dorsal root. Ataxia is common due to loss of position sense and is most marked in the lower extremities.   (Heidenhain)

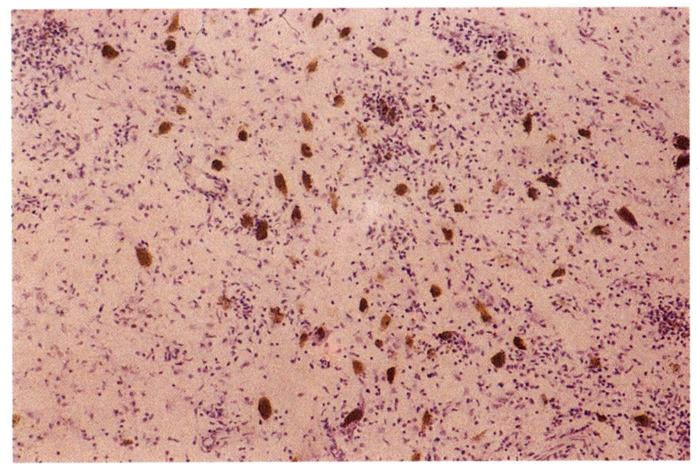

Fig. L27. Cryptococcal meningitis. This high magnification photomicrograph shows the leptomeningeal surface with an acute inflammatory exudate in which there are distinct bright red (Periodic-acid Schiff reaction) spores of *Cryptococcus neoformans.* Cryptococcosis is the most commonly recognized cerebral mycosis, but other fungal disorders (e.g. aspergillosis, candidiasis, nocardiosis) can also affect the brain particularly in immunodepressed individuals.

Fig. L28. Encephalitis lethargica (von Economo's disease), acute stage. The area of the substantia nigra has an extensive cell infiltrate consisting of lymphocytes and plasma cells. There is degeneration of melanin-containing cells with subsequent phagocytosis (neuronophagia) seen as brown pigmented cells. Cerebral Purkinje cells and ocular motor neurons can also be lost. A frequent sequel, occurring after a symptom-free interval of weeks to months, and sometimes years, is postencephalitic parkinsonism, often accompanied by mental deterioration and oculogyric crises *(Fig. L29).*

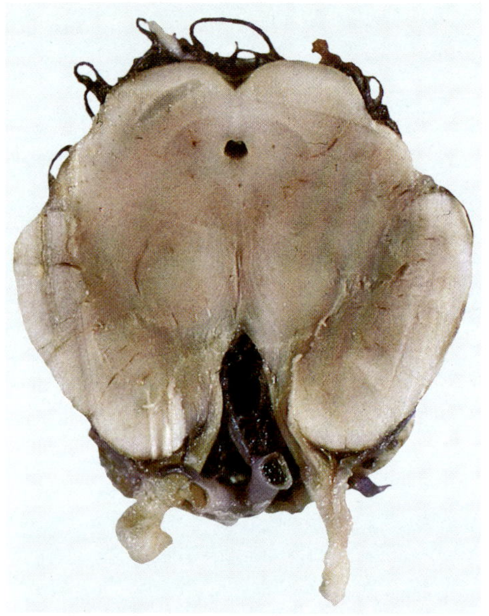

L29

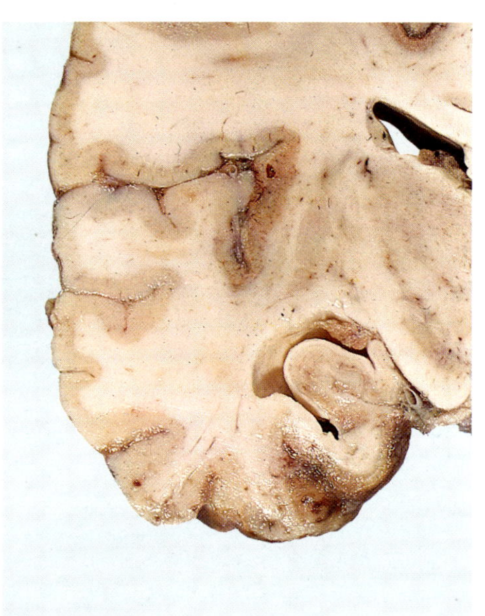

L30

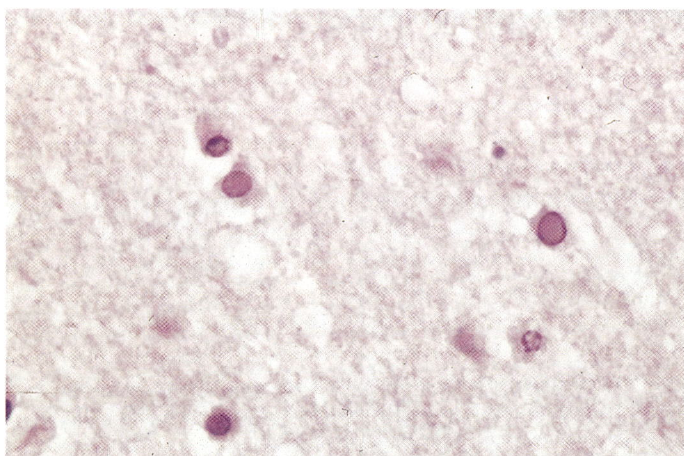

L31a

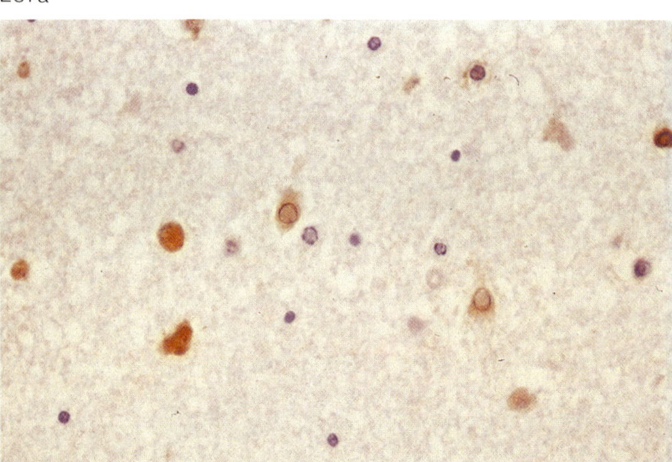

L31b

Fig. L29. Postencephalitic parkinsonism. The substantia nigra is almost completely depigmented. Extensive depigmentation is more characteristic of postencephalitic Parkinsonism than of idiopathic Parkinson's disease. In the latter condition there is patchy loss of pigmented neurons in the substantia nigra, particularly the zone of compacta and the locusceruleus. In addition, characteristic neuronal intracytoplasmic eosinophilic (Lewy) bodies are seen in idiopathic Parkinson's disease.

Fig. L30. Acute necrotizing Herpes encephalitis of the basal portion of the temporal lobe. This is the characteristic location of adult Herpes simplex encephalitis in adults who have previously been exposed to HSV-I. It is thought that the virus reaches this area after reactivation of infection in the trigemminal ganglia since the virions may be intracellular and escape immune attack. Clinically, these patients present with fever, headache, and flu-like illness. In some patients a previous dermal herpetic lesion may reappear. There may be subsequent disorientation, behavioral changes, hallucinations, and other evidence of severe encephalitis, and patients may occasionally seem to have a psychiatric illness.

Fig. L31a. Herpes encephalitis. The nuclei of glial cells are enlarged and filled with eosinophilic inclusion material which is the light microscopic representation of extensive nuclear infection by viruses.

Fig. L31b. Herpes encephalitis. This is the same case as shown above. In this photomicrograph, however, the viruses have been stained with a peroxidase-labelled monoclonal antibody to Herpes virus. The brown staining deposits can be seen in many nuclei as well as focally in the cytoplasm.

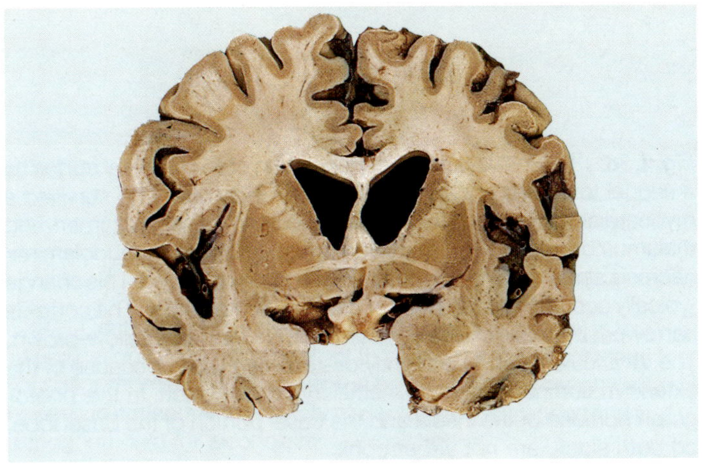

L32

Fig. L32. Creutzfeldt-Jakob syndrome. There is slight atrophy of the cerebral cortex and of the caudate nucleus, with secondary mild enlargement of the ventricles. In general, the gross appearance of the brain is not dramatic.

Fig. L33. a) Creutzfeldt-Jakob disease. The brain shows spongiform degeneration (status spongiosis) due to marked neuronal loss and replacement gliosis. The cerebral cortex of the frontal and temporal lobes is most severely affected, but the change may also be seen in the corpus striatum, thalamus, upper brain stem tegmentum, and superficial cerebellar cortex layers. These spongiform changes can be mimicked by anoxic damage and can also occur in association with a variety of inflammatory, toxic, and metabolic conditions.
b) This photomicrograph of the cerebellar cortex shows a Periodic-acid Schiff-positive storiform inclusion *(double arrow)* adjacent to a Purkinje cell *(single arrow)*. This type of inclusion, which resembles a "spiked ball", is characteristically seen in kuru and is not pathognomonic of Creutzfeldt-Jakob syndrome, but suggests that there are pathogenetic similarities between the two diseases.

Demyelinating Disorders (L34–L41)

Fig. L34. Multiple sclerosis. Sharply defined, grey-brown areas are seen irregularly in the medulla *(arrows).* These represent zones of demyelinization. These are not necrotic areas, and, at least early in the disease, there is no loss of neurons and clinical manifestations may wax and wane.

Fig. L35. Uremic polyneuropathy with segmental, discontinuous loss of myelin. In this photomicrograph, stained with the Kluver-Barrera reaction, myelin stains blue and it is clear that segments of the nerve completely lack a myelin covering.

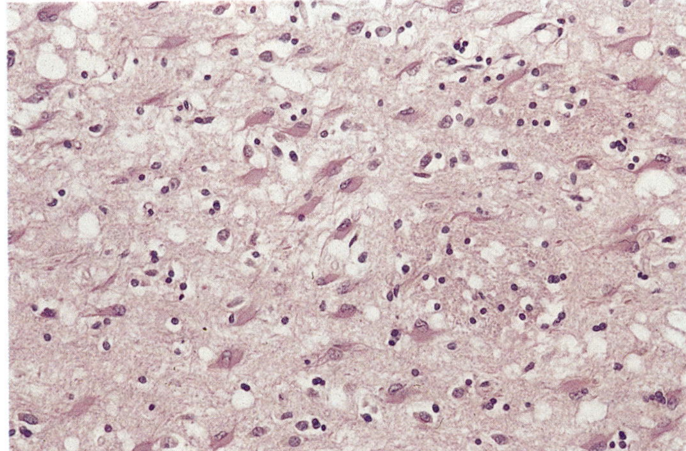

L33a

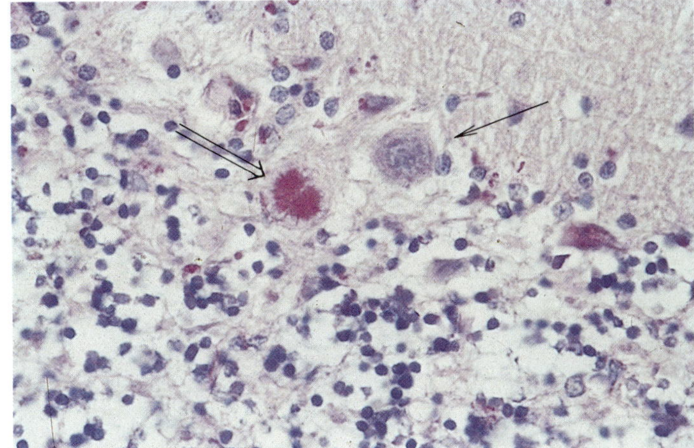

L33b

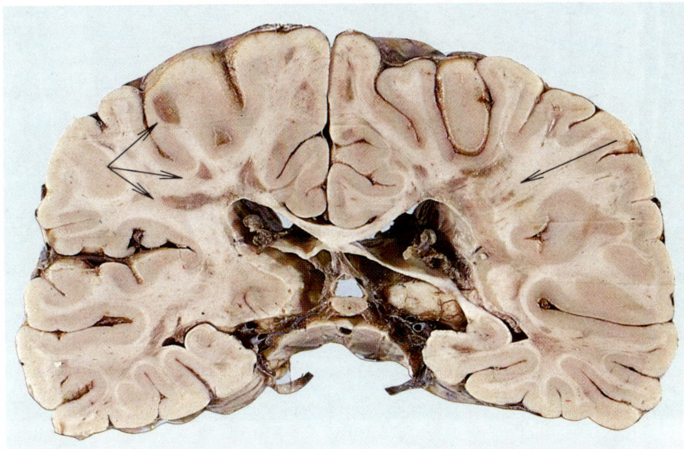

L34

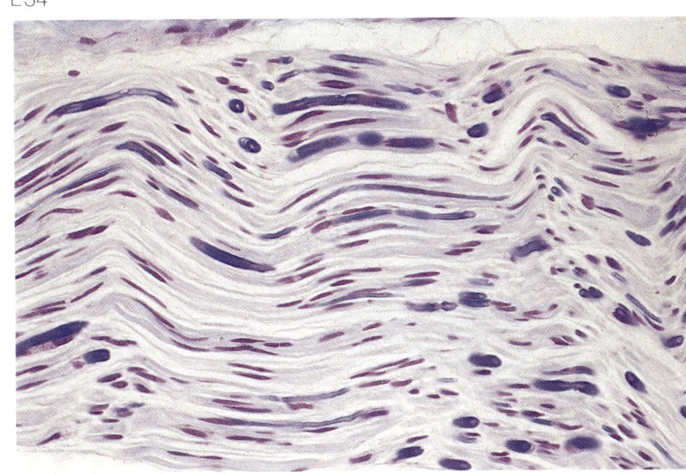

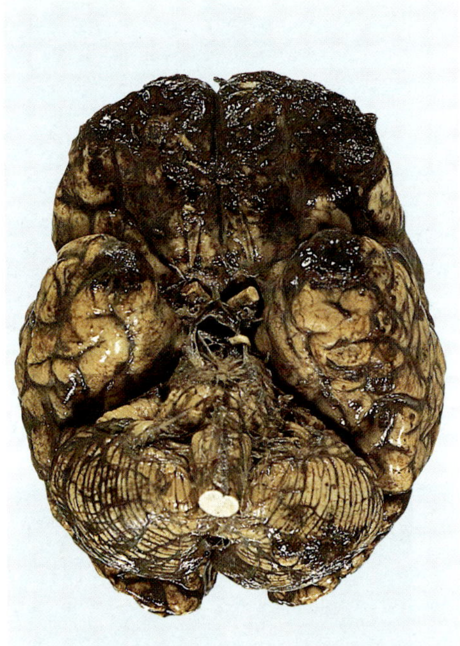

L42

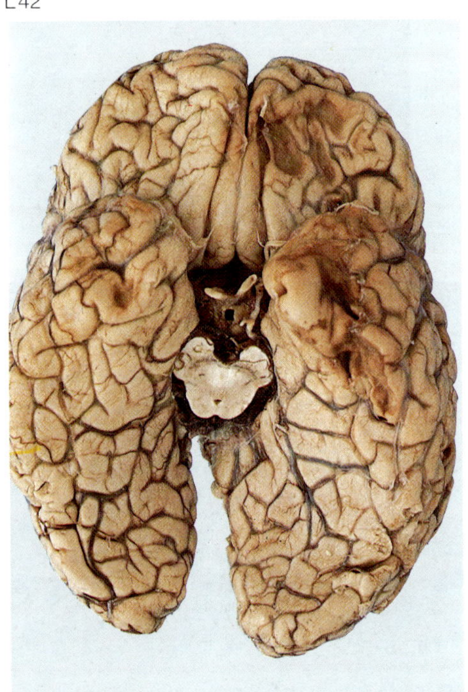

L43

Fig. L42. There is recent, extensive brain damage following a motorcycle accident. Hemorrhage covers the frontal lobes and cerebellar lobes in this photograph of a typical cerebral contusion. There is also severe cerebral edema. Contusions form at the site of cranial impact called "coup contusions", while those opposite the cranial impact are known as "countrecoup contusions".

Fig. L43. This brain shows evidence of prior contusions, most marked in the left frontal and temporal lobes (right side of the photograph), but there is a similar lesion in the right temporal lobe. The lesions are brown because of the extensive deposition of hemosiderin as a sequel to previous hemorrhage. Cerebral lacerations in these locations are often found in countrecoup injuries after contusions on the cerebral convexity. These lacerations often appear as irregular branching cleft-like defects along the gyral surface.

Fig. L44. Recent, post-traumatic subdural hematoma. This low magnification photomicrograph through both frontal lobes shows a large left-sided hematoma with marked compression of the underlying brain. A fresh contusion can also be seen at the base of the left frontal region in the gyrus rectus.

Fig. L45. Cerebellar herniation due to acute increase of intracranial pressure. The cerebellar tonsils are bilaterally constricted, corresponding to their herniation through the foramen magnum. The medulla oblongata is secondarily compressed. Herniation of the cerebellum also contributes to vascular compression, with anoxia, and characteristically there is cardiorespiratory failure.

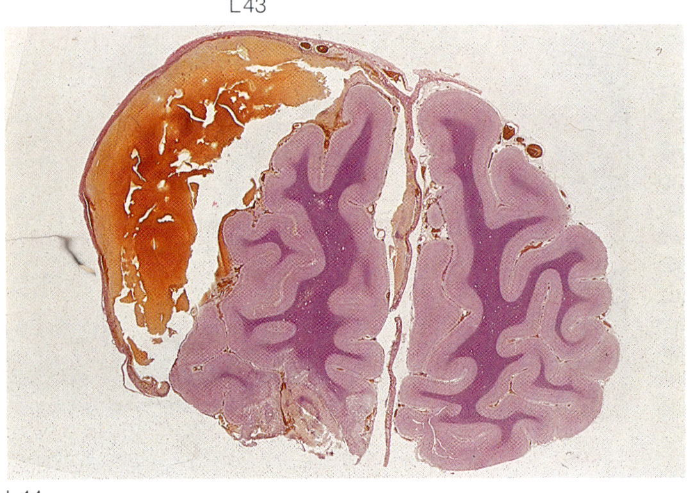

L44

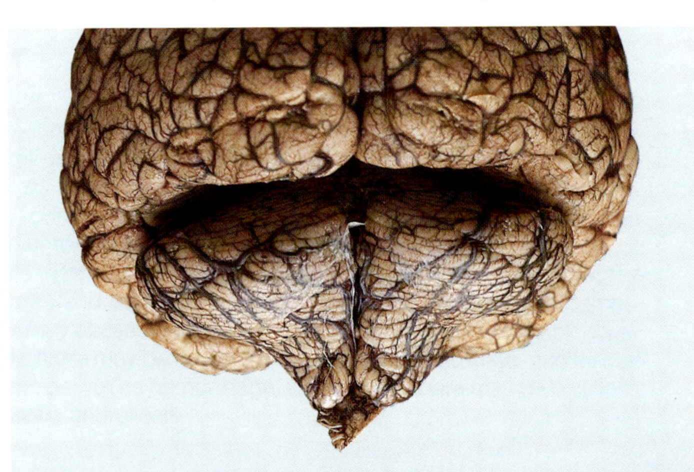

L45

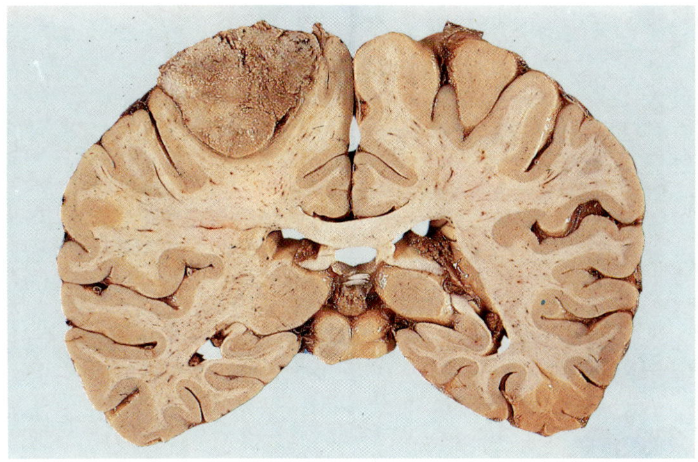

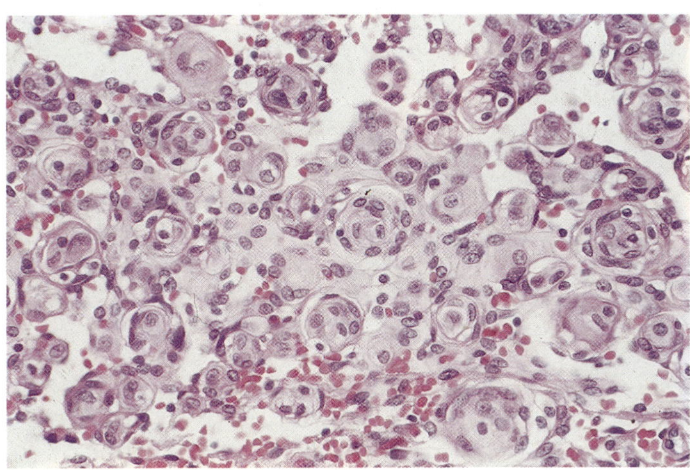

Fig. L46a.   Large meningioma in the area of the left cerebral convexity. Meningiomas are the most common of all meningeal tumors. Although they arise on the dura mater, they may compress the brain, as in this case, as they grow increasingly larger. The underlying cerebral cortex is atrophied. Despite large size, these tumors may not manifest clinically and may sometimes be found at autopsy.

Fig. L46b.   Photomicrograph of transitional meningioma showing characteristic whorls of tumor cells. These whorls may subsequently become calcified, forming psammoma bodies. (hematoxylin-eosin)

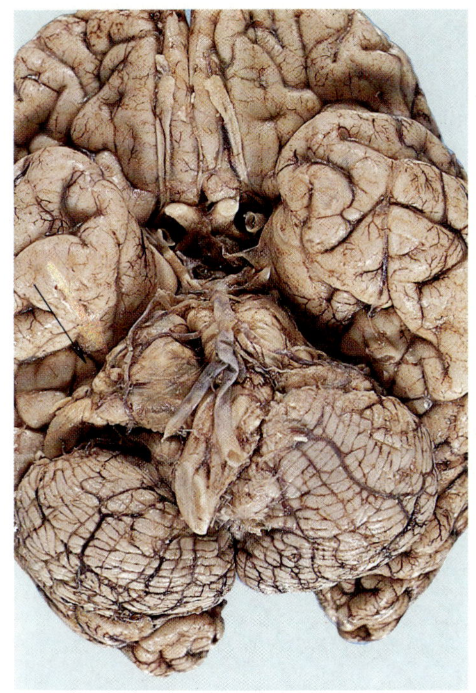

Fig. L47a.   Acoustic neurinoma at the right cerebello-pontine angle *(arrow)*. These tumors are neurolemmomas (Schwannomas) and arise from the cells of the nerve sheath. As these benign tumors fill the cerebello-pontine angle they distort the brain stem and the trigeminal and other cranial nerves, which may become stretched over its surface. They may cause internal hydrocephalus and brain stem compression, with subsequent cardio-respiratory arrest. Because the tumors arise from the nerve sheath, nerve function itself may be affected and symptoms involving the nerve from which they arise may be encountered.

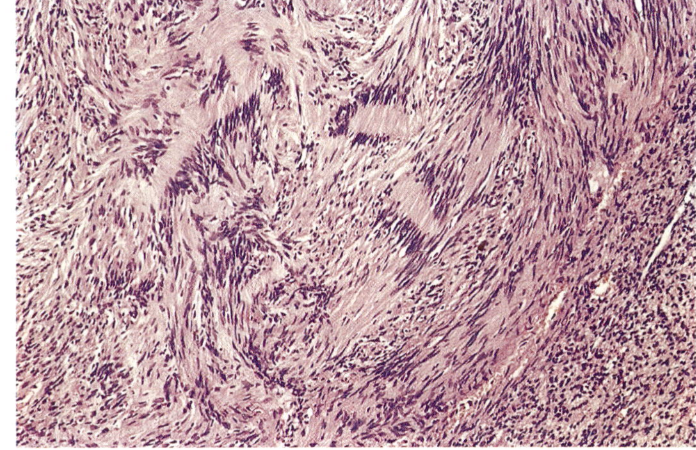

Fig. L47b.   Photomicrograph of an acoustic neurinoma (neuro-lemmoma). These tumors are usually solid and fibrous and histologically consist of interlacing bands of spindle-shaped cells which characteristically tend to have nuclei of adjacent cells aligned in parallel columns ("palisading"). This arrangement is seldom absent and is useful for diagnosis.   (hematoxylin-eosin)

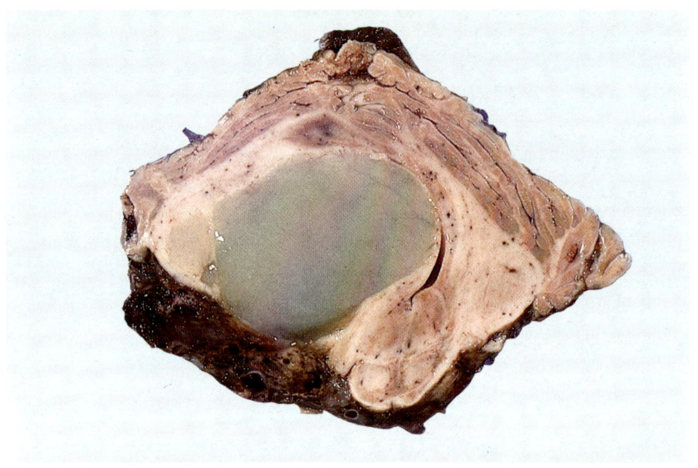

Fig. L48a. Cerebellum in von Hippel-Lindau syndrome. A large cyst filled with gelatinous material replaces most of the right cerebellar hemisphere and compresses the left side with almost complete obliteration of the fourth ventricle. At the lower edge of the cyst there is a compressed capillary hemangioma.

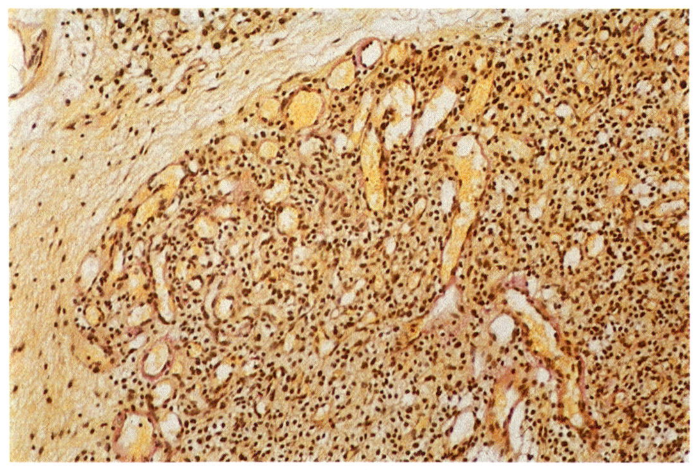

Fig. L48b. Photomicrograph of a capillary hemangioma. There is extensive proliferation of small, endothelium-lined vascular spaces, sharply delineated from the surrounding cerebellar tissue. Hemangioblastomas may also occur in von Hippel-Lindau syndrome, and the cerebral vascular tumors may be associated with cystic disease of the pancreas and kidneys, syringomyelia, and cutaneous angiomas. (van Gieson)

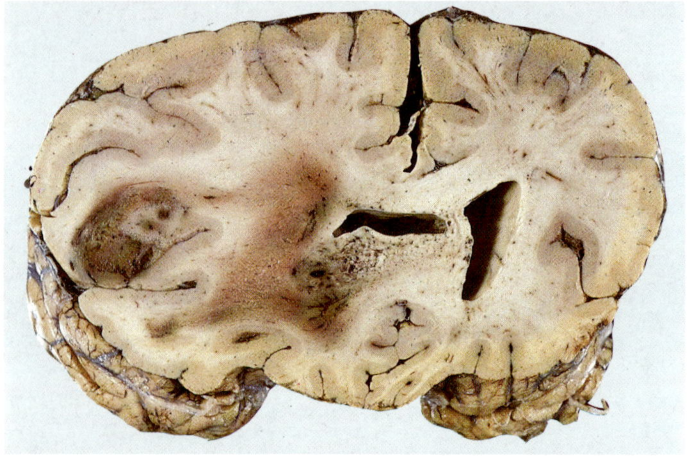

Fig. L49a. Gliobastoma multiforme of the right fronto-parietal region. The cerebral hemisphere is infiltrated by a poorly defined hemorrhagic and necrotic tumor which has greatly enlarged the hemisphere, and caused marked displacement of the anterior horn of the right ventricle. The tumor is not circumscribed and the interface between brain tumor and normal tissue is not easily recognized.

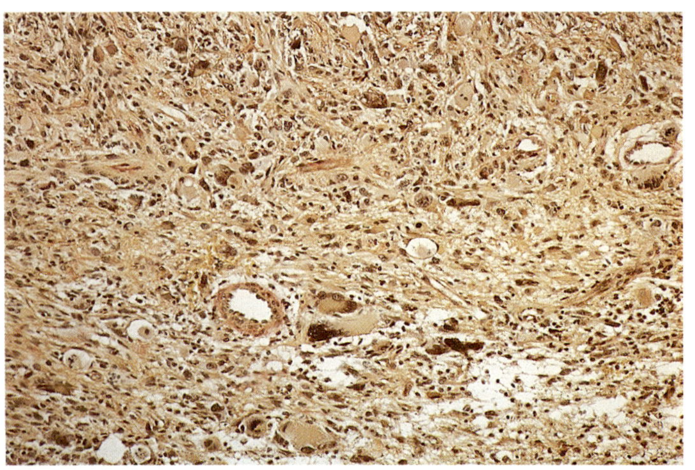

Fig. L49b. Photomicrograph of a glioblastoma multiforme. The tumor is highly cellular with marked pleomorphism and many mitoses. The tumor is highly vascular with proliferation of small blood vessels. The capillary endothelial cells are characteristically swollen. A few multinucleated giant tumor cells are present. Other features of glioblastoma multiforme, not seen in this photomicrograph, are necrosis and hemorrhage, and palisading of tumor cell nuclei around blood vessels and at the periphery of necrotic areas. The name glioblastoma multiforme derives from the macroscopic appearance of the tumor *(Fig. L49a)* which is varied because of the irregular distribution of viable tumor, necrotic tumor, and hemorrhage. (van Gieson)

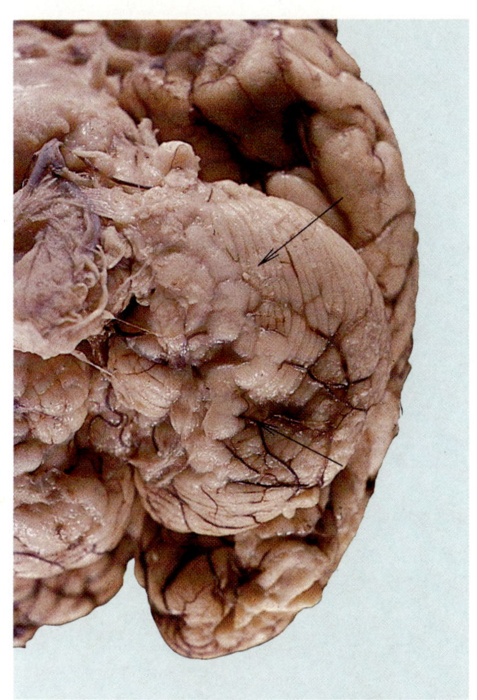

Fig. L50a. Cerebellar medulloblastoma. This tumor is visualized from the inferior aspect of the cerebellum. The cerebral hemispheres can be seen, slightly out of focus, above the cerebellum. The tumor is soft, grey-white, and poorly defined *(arrows)*. The tumor arises from the cerebellum and extensively infiltrates the surrounding leptomeningeal tissues. This tumor arises almost exclusively in the cerebellum and is most common under the age of ten years, occurring more often in males than in females. Most of the tumors are midline, but a few arise in the lateral cerebellar hemisphere or in the cerebello-pontine angle. The tumor tends to protrude into the left ventricle, sometimes occluding it, and may spread widely within the subarachnoid space.

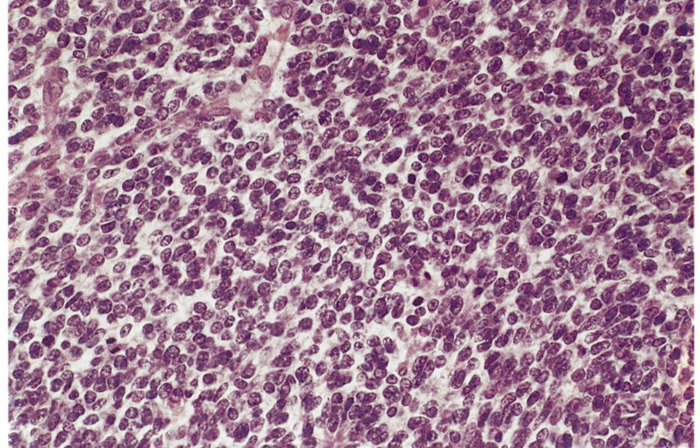

Fig. L50b. Photomicrograph of a medulloblastoma. This highly cellular tumor consists of undifferentiated small cells with hypochromatic round or slightly elongated nuclei. Primitive neurons can sometimes be recognized, and there may be rosette formation. These tumors resemble the adrenal neuroblastoma. Mitoses may be abundant.   (hematoxylin-eosin)

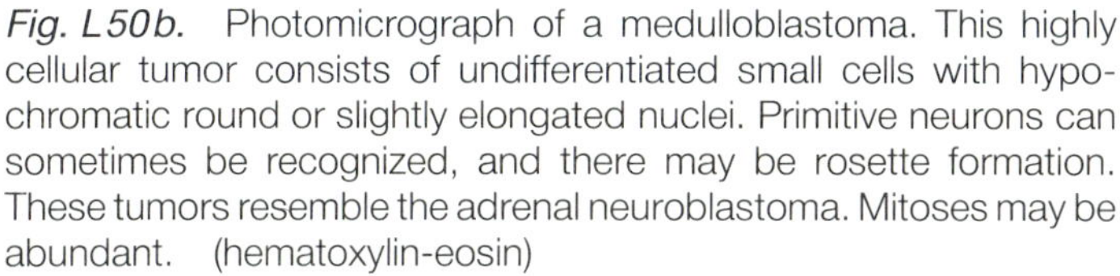

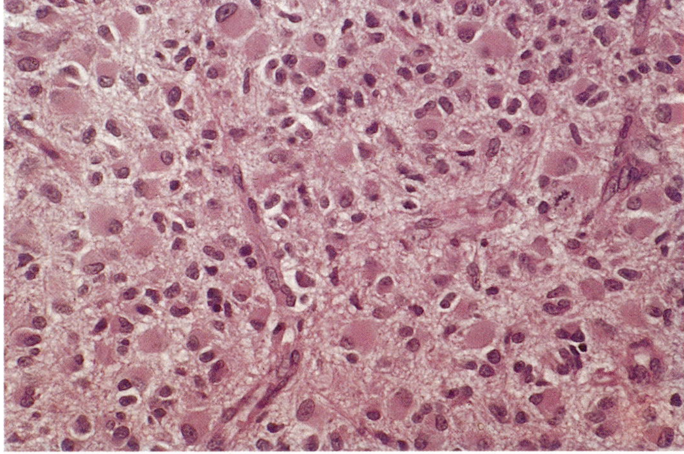

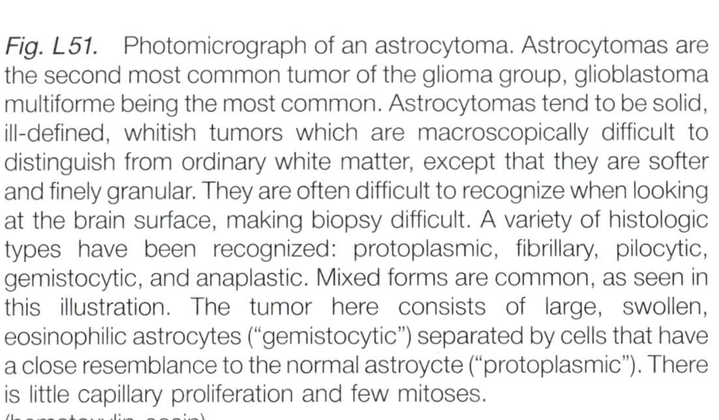

Fig. L51. Photomicrograph of an astrocytoma. Astrocytomas are the second most common tumor of the glioma group, glioblastoma multiforme being the most common. Astrocytomas tend to be solid, ill-defined, whitish tumors which are macroscopically difficult to distinguish from ordinary white matter, except that they are softer and finely granular. They are often difficult to recognize when looking at the brain surface, making biopsy difficult. A variety of histologic types have been recognized: protoplasmic, fibrillary, pilocytic, gemistocytic, and anaplastic. Mixed forms are common, as seen in this illustration. The tumor here consists of large, swollen, eosinophilic astrocytes ("gemistocytic") separated by cells that have a close resemblance to the normal astroycte ("protoplasmic"). There is little capillary proliferation and few mitoses.
(hematoxylin-eosin)

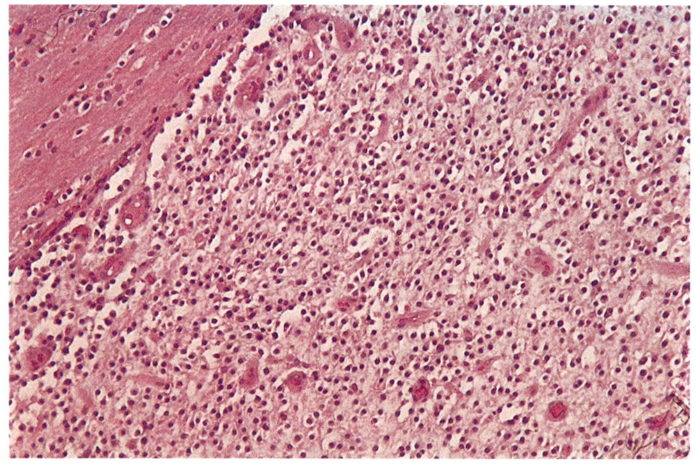

Fig. L52. Oligodendroglioma. Despite the fact that oligodendrocytes greatly outnumber the other cells of the brain, this tumor is relatively uncommon. It generally arises in the cerebral white matter, particularly the frontal lobes, and usually becomes manifest in adult life. Symptoms suggest that growth has occured over a relatively long period, often for years. Tumor oligodendrocytes may differ little from normal oligodendrocytes. The nucleus of each is surrounded by a halo of clear cytoplasm imparting a "fried egg" appearance as seen here. The proliferation of cells which closely abut each other contributes to an overall honeycomb appearance. Nuclear size and shape may vary, particularly in the central parts of the tumor. The tumor is moderately vascularized with fine capillaries. In this case there is a relatively sharp delineation from the adjacent non-tumorous brain tissue. This is not seen in every case and the margin of the tumor may be difficult to identify.   (hematoxylin-eosin)

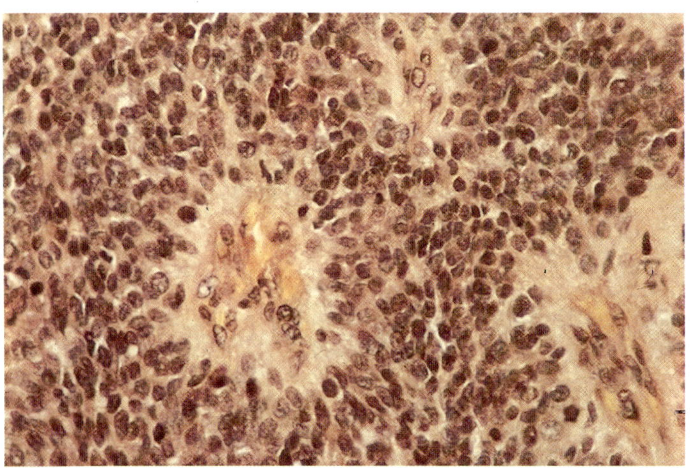

Fig. L53. Photomicrograph of an ependymoma. Ependymomas develop from the lining of the ventricular system and, consequently, commonly grow in the ventricles. Ependymoma is slow growing, occurring mostly in young people. The cells are typically epithelial in appearance and tend to be grouped around small spaces so that they resemble glandular acini. In other areas, as in this photomicrograph, they are arranged in a rosette-like pattern around blood vessels. When the tumor has this characteristic appearance, it is relatively easy to diagnose. In some cases, however, the tumor may be quite anaplastic and may resemble glioblastoma multiforme. (van Gieson)

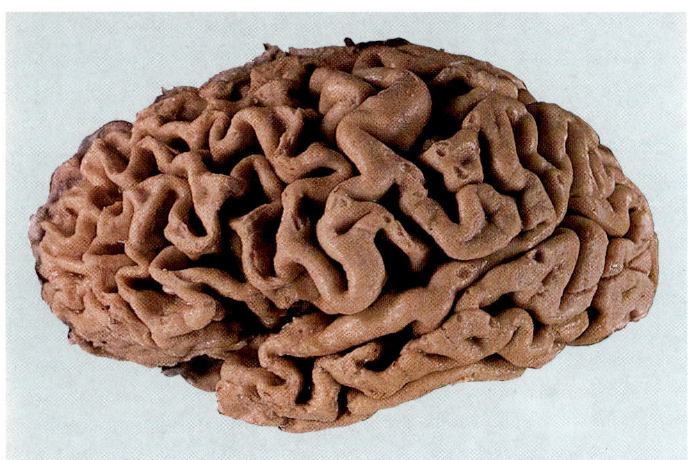

Atrophy *(L54)*

Fig. L54. Pick's disease. Pick's disease is a peculiar form of localized atrophy of the brain. This rare condition occurs mainly in the later years of life, and women are more often affected than men. Symptoms depend on the parts of the brain affected. In this case there is severe atrophy of the gyri of the frontal, parietal, and temporal lobes, with almost complete sparing of the occipital lobe. The sulci are secondarily greatly widened.

M. The Eye

M. Vogel

The eye is affected by a variety of diseases. Clinically, conjunctival and corneal lesions are particularly important. For the pathologist, disorders of the posterior portions of the eye are often of greatest interest. As example, choroidal melanoma may be seen. This tumor grows from the choroid into the interior of the ocular bulb, often producing retinal detachment. The retina may also be affected by diabetes mellitus. In diabetes mellitus there is a special form of micro-angiopathy in which there are micro-aneurysms, hyalinizations, exudate formation, and vascular occlusions. Retinal detachment may occur spontaneously because of degeneration, or as a reflection of inflammation or tumors. The retina may also demonstrate a highly malignant tumor of children, the retinoblastoma. This tumor can be sporadic but may also occur as an autosomal dominant inherited disorder. Glaucoma is one of the most frequent of eye diseases and is found in approximately 2% of the population above the age of 40. Characteristic changes occur in the iridocorneal angle; there may be secondary degeneration of the optic disc and optic nerve if treatment is not effected.

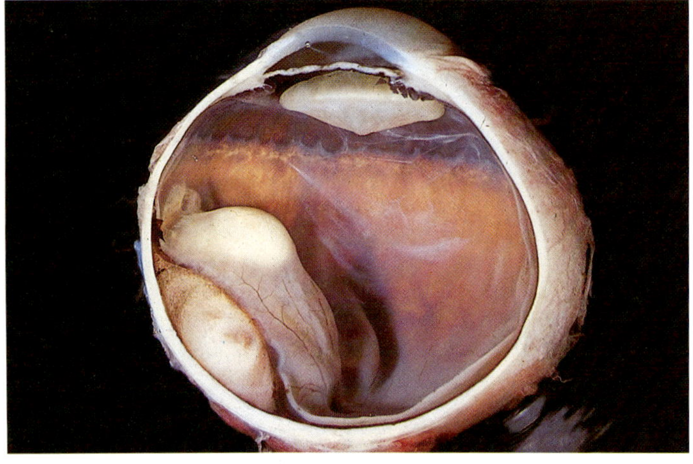

Ocular Melanoma *(M1–M3)*

Fig. M1. Malignant melanoma arising from the choroid. This large exophytic tumor has broken through Bruch's membrane and is in the sub-retinal space. The retina is markedly distorted and degenerated as it overlies the tumor. The lens is secondarily displaced. These tumors may be highly malignant in behavior, often metastasizing to the liver. In contrast, melanomas arising at the iris rarely metastasize.

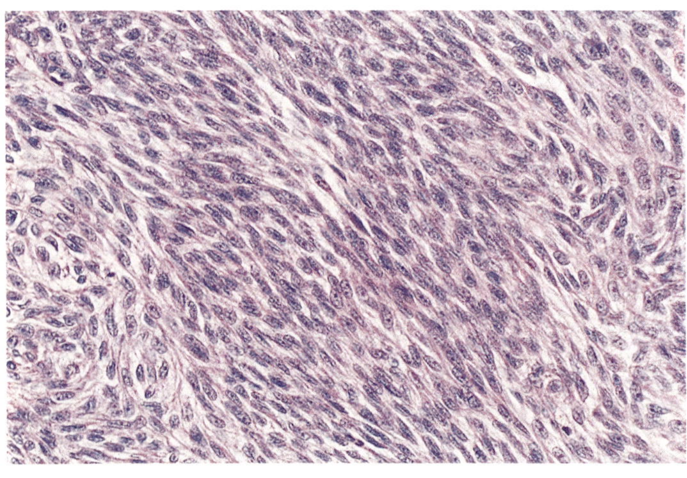

Fig. M2. Spindle cell melanoma of the choroid. This tumor consists predominantly of slender, spindle-shaped cells with elongated nuclei and small nucleoli (spindle A). There is almost no recognizable melanin pigment. In other areas, larger cells with prominent nucleoli (spindle B), can be seen.   (hematoxylin-eosin)

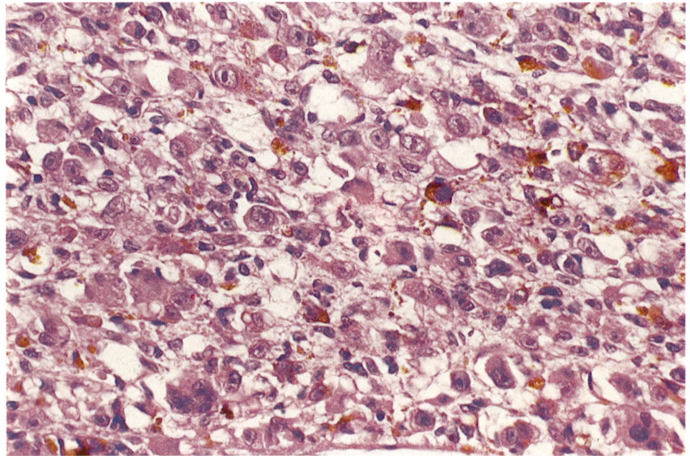

Fig. M3. Epithelioid cell melanoma of the choroid. The cells are large, irregular, with abundant cytoplasm and round nuclei with prominent nucleoli. Many of the cells contain melanin pigment; there are occasional multinucleated forms. The cells tend to be loosely arranged and appear as noncohesive small groups.   (hematoxylin-eosin)

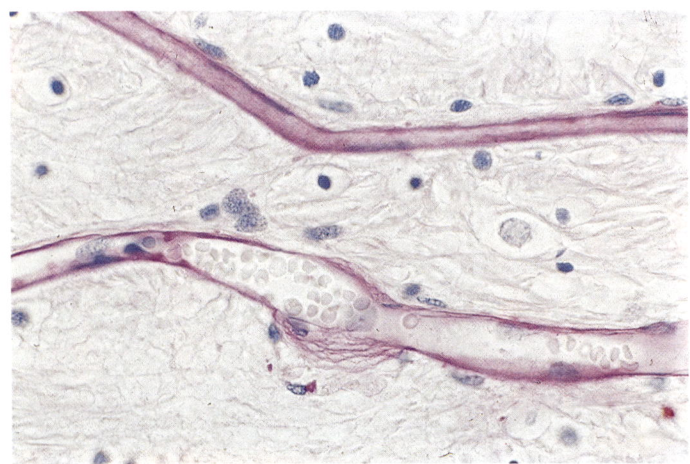

Retinal Disorders *(M4–M9)*

Fig. M4. Diabetes mellitus. Occular diabetes mellitus is one of the leading causes of blindness in industrialized countries. In this photomicrograph the retinal capillaries have varying caliber due to degeneration of intralumenal pericytes and loss of endothelial cells. In the middle of the lower capillary, a micro-aneurysm is seen. The lumen of the capillary above is obliterated and there are no red blood cells within.   (PAS)

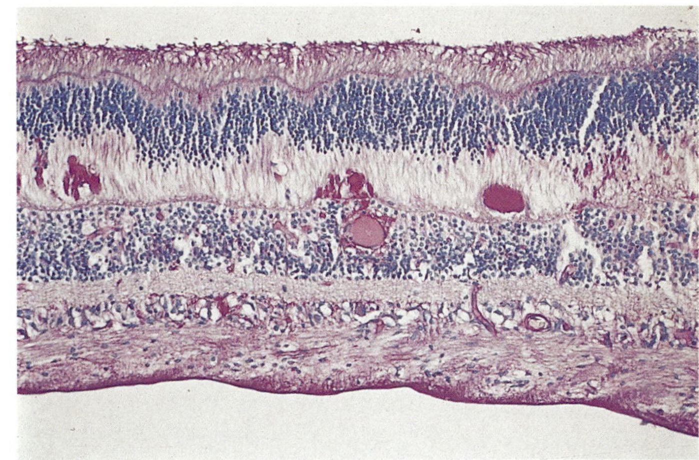

Fig. M5. Diabetic retinopathy. Multiple scattered exudates are in the outer plexiform layer of the retina. In addition there is considerable edema. A micro-aneurysm is at the center. (PAS)

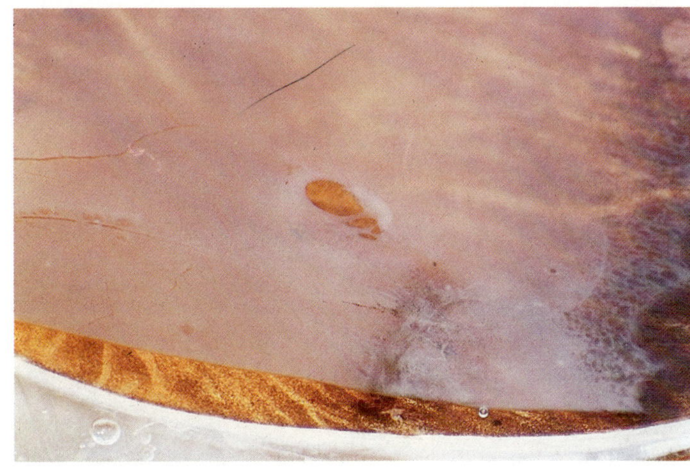

Fig. M6. Retinal tear. A sharply outlined clear area, formed from four small defects, is seen in the center in the equatorial region of retinal degeneration.

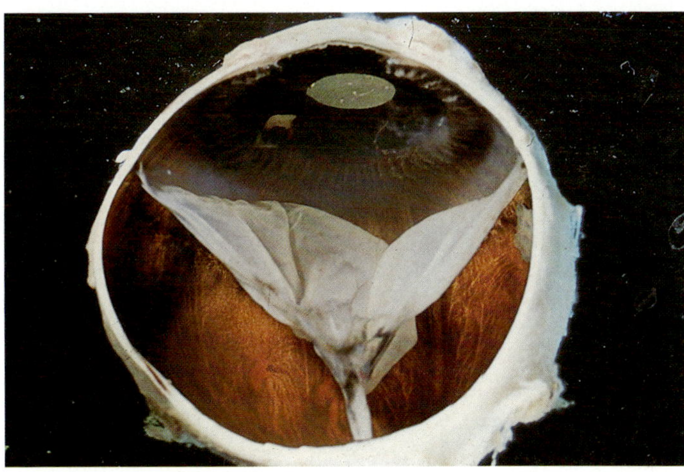

Fig. M7. Total retinal detachment with contraction of the vitreous body. The retina forms a freely moving membrane.

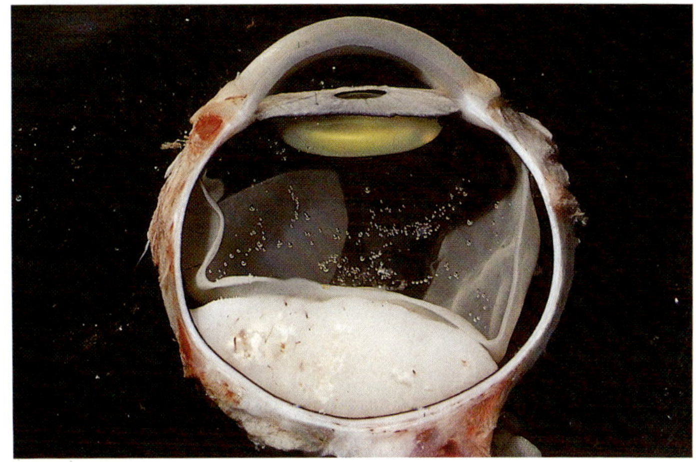

Fig. M8. Retinoblastoma. A large tumor is at the posterior eye, beneath the retinal membrane. The tumor has areas of necrosis and calcification.

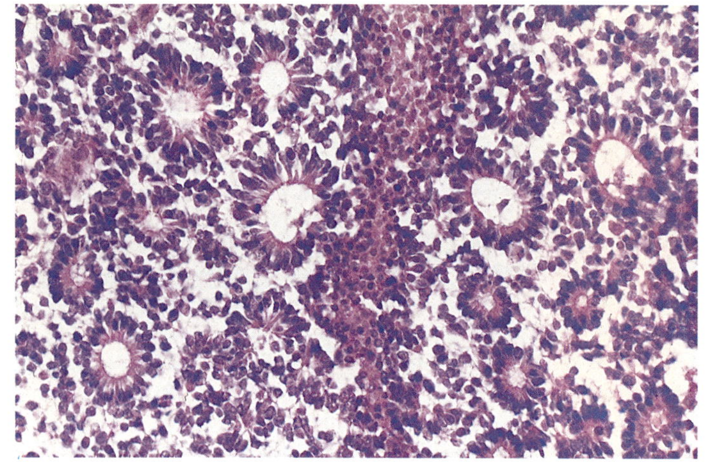

Fig. M9. Retinoblastoma. The tumor cells form typical rosettes. There is considerable nuclear pleomorphism and the nuclei have abundant chromatin. Retinoblastoma, in contrast to melanoma, occurs almost exclusively in children. Prognosis depends on the extent of the tumor and is quite poor if the optic nerve has been infiltrated.   (hematoxylin-eosin)

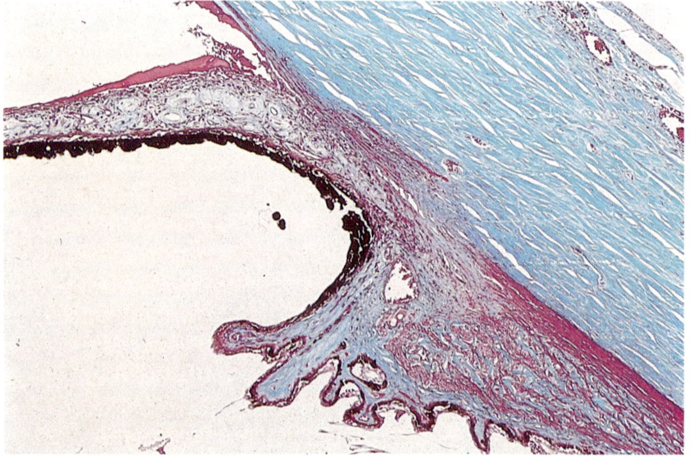

Glaucoma   *(M 10 – M 11)*

Fig. M 10. Iridocorneal angle from a patient with glaucoma. This section shows a region of the corneal limbus. The cornea is blue, the iris is to the left, and the ciliary body is at the lower portion of the photomicrograph. The trabecular network is at the area of juncture of iris, ciliary body, and cornea. Obstruction to flow of aqueous humor, in this case, is due to adhesions of the iris to the cornea (anterior synechiae).   (Masson trichrome)

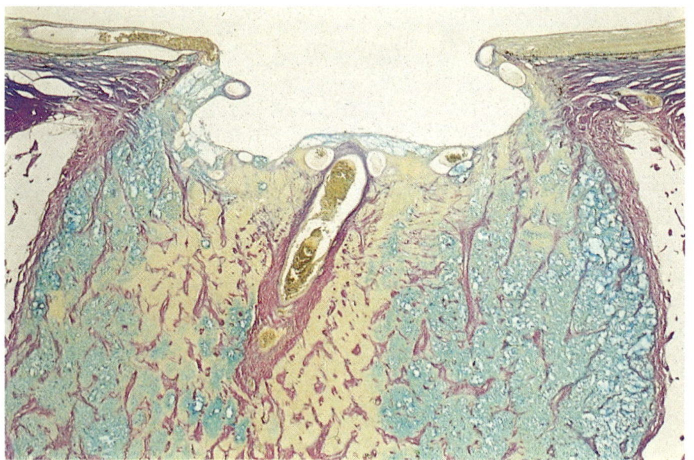

Fig. M 11. Late stage of chronic glaucoma showing "cupping" (deep excavation) of the optic disc and degeneration of optic nerve. Microcystic change, at the periphery of the optic nerve, is part of the degeneratory process.

N. Skeletal Muscles

F. Gullotta

Muscle biopsy is widely employed as an easily performed diagnostic tool to provide important information about the various diseases of skeletal muscles. In this way the various forms of neurogenic atrophies can be differentiated. These are diseases of the skeletal muscles due to degenerative disorders of the motor neurons. The most frequent hereditary muscle disease is progressive muscular dystrophy which occurs in various clinical forms. The myotonic disorders are a group of chronic, generally autosomal, dominantly inherited, muscle disorders, which clinically manifest as myotonic reactions, with prolonged muscle contractions elicited by voluntary movements or exogenous stimuli. In recent years a variety of forms of congenital myopathies have been recognized. The glycogen storage diseases, particularly Pompe's type, may manifest with involvement of skeletal muscle. Inflammations, relatively rare, may be bacterial, fungal, or, on occasion, parasitic. An example of parasitic myositis is trichinosis. Polymyositis is a relatively uncommon muscle disorder associated with autoimmune type inflammation.

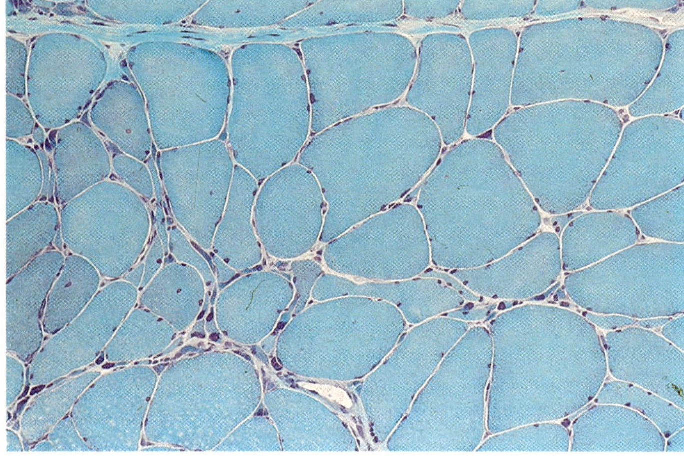

Fig. N1. Neurogenic (denervation) atrophy. In this cross-section, the typical pattern of neurogenic atrophy is seen. There are scattered, small fibers with concave cellular margins, appearing compressed by adjacent intact fibers, some of which may be secondarily hypertrophied. The atrophic fibers have relatively prominent nuclei due to persistence of sarcolemmal membrane. There is no fibrosis or interstitial inflammation.
(Cryostat section; trichrome; magnification 50×)

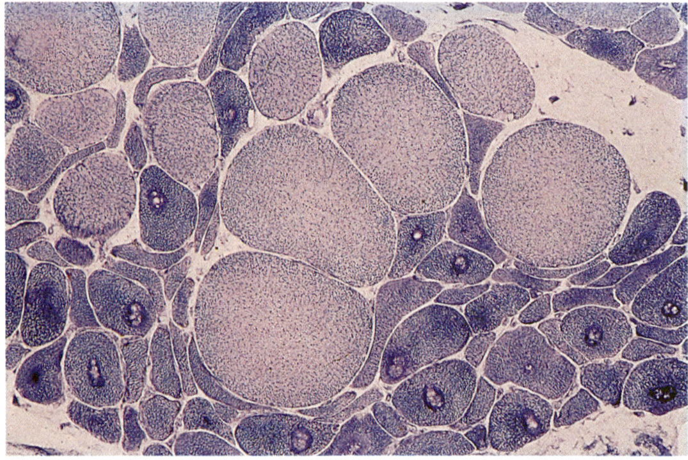

Fig. N2. Neurogenic atrophy. Many of the atrophic fibers show "target" formation. This diagnostic pattern is usually restricted to type I fibers and is best seen, as in this case, in sections studied with histochemical techniques. The fibers have a central zone lacking enzyme activity, surrounded by a zone of increased activity, and then a zone of normal activity.
(Cryostat section; NADH-tetrazolium-reductase; magnification 64×)

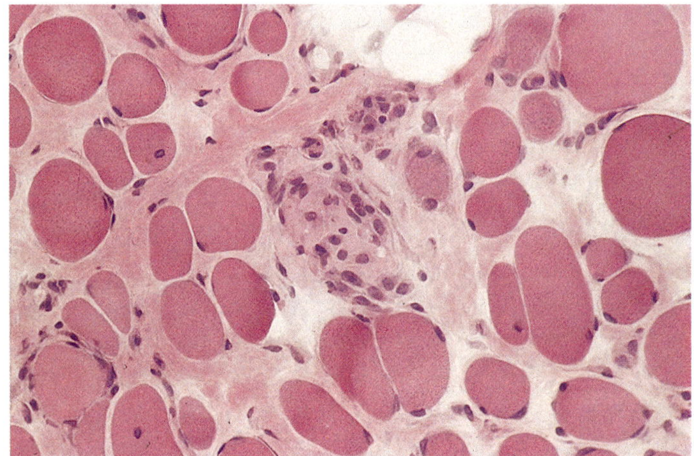

Muscular Dystrophies and Myopathies   *(N3–N9)*

Fig. N3. Progressive muscular dystrophy, early stage. The muscle fibers are surrounded and separated by fibrous connective tissue. Some fibers show internal nuclei, evidence of regeneration. A necrotic fiber at the center is undergoing phagocytosis. Fat cells are seen at the upper portion of the photomicrograph.
(Cryostat section; hematoxylin-eosin; magnification 64×)

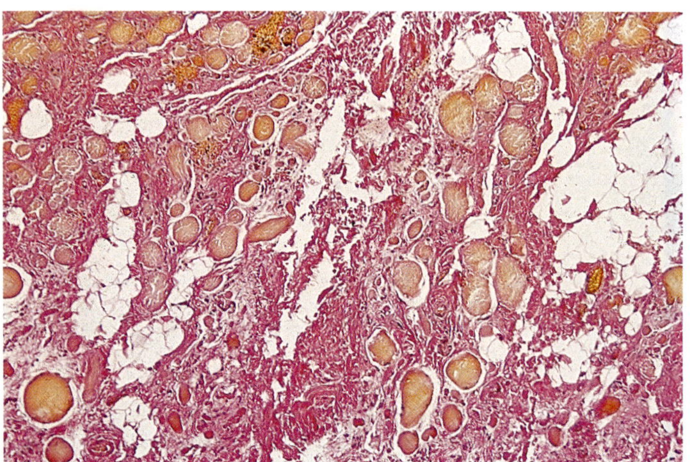

Fig. N4. Progressive muscular dystrophy, late stage. There is almost complete loss of muscle fibers (yellow) and replacement by fat and fibrous tissue. This fat and fibrosis imparts the pseudohypertrophic appearance of the affected muscles. In young men with severe sex-linked (Duchenne type) muscular dystrophy, the gastrocnemius muscles are most affected.
(van Gieson; magnification 40×)

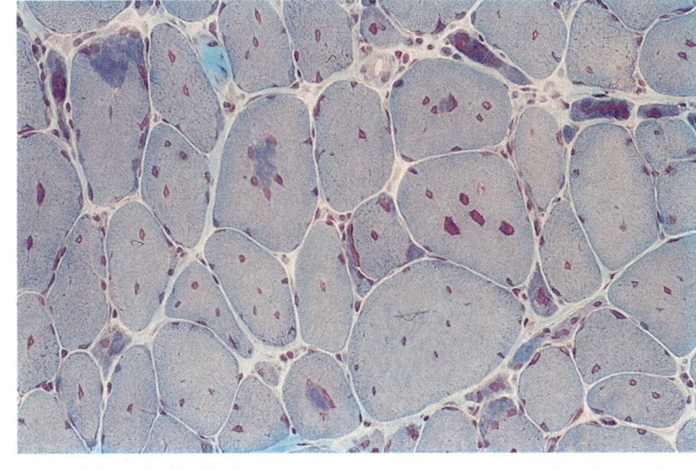

Fig. N5. Myotonic dystrophy. This autosomal-dominant disorder may have extraskeletal manifestations, including cardiac involvement, cataracts, gonadal atrophy, and mental deficiency. The caliber of the muscle fibers is increased, and there are many internal nuclei. In one area, characteristic dark sarcoplasmic masses are prominent. Ring fibers are present, best seen at the lower mid-portion of the photomicrograph. There is relatively little necrosis or phagocytosis in this form of muscular dystrophy, and fatty and fibrous infiltration are not prominent.
(Cryostat section; trichrome; magnification 64×)

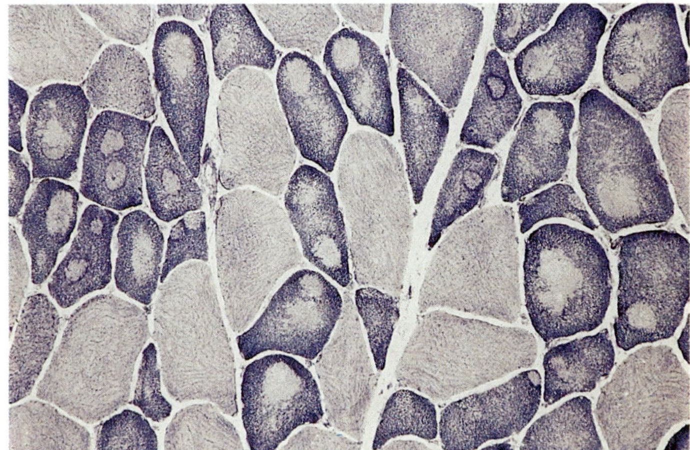

Fig. N6. Central core disease. The type I fibers (dark) have one or more round, enzyme-free areas ("cores") imparting a resemblance to target fibers *(Fig. N2).* The cores are surrounded by fibrils with increased enzymatic activity. This group of congenital myopathies occurs sporadically and is seldom familial. Diagnosis is established by histochemical enzymatic studies.
(Cryostat section; NADH-tetrazolium-reductase; magnification 64×)

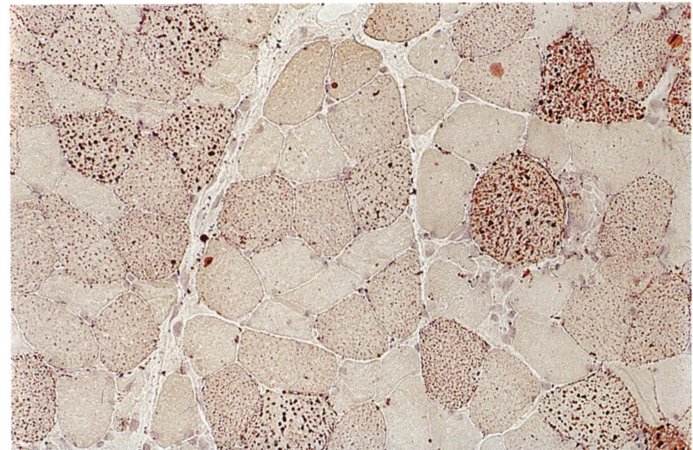

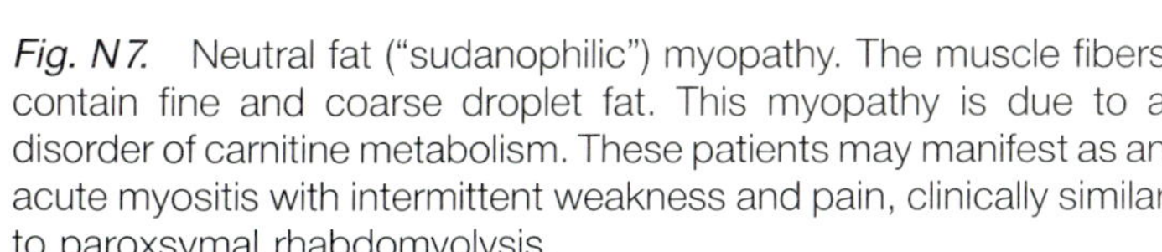

Fig. N7. Neutral fat ("sudanophilic") myopathy. The muscle fibers contain fine and coarse droplet fat. This myopathy is due to a disorder of carnitine metabolism. These patients may manifest as an acute myositis with intermittent weakness and pain, clinically similar to paroxsymal rhabdomyolysis.
(Cryostat section; Oil red 0; magnification 50×)

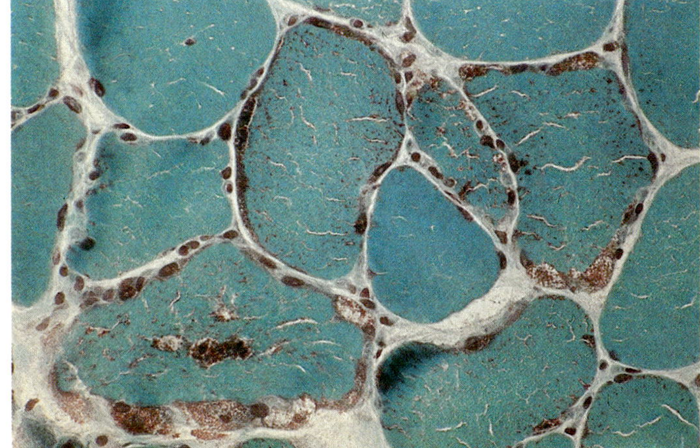

Fig. N8. Mitochondrial ("ragged red fiber") myopathy. There are prominent collections of mitochondria seen beneath the sarcolemmal membrane as red, finely granular bodies. The fibers are secondarily hypertrophied. The changes are nonspecific and may follow a variety of muscle disorders. The mitochondria are themselves abnormal *(Fig. N9).*
(Cryostat section; trichrome; magnification 100×)

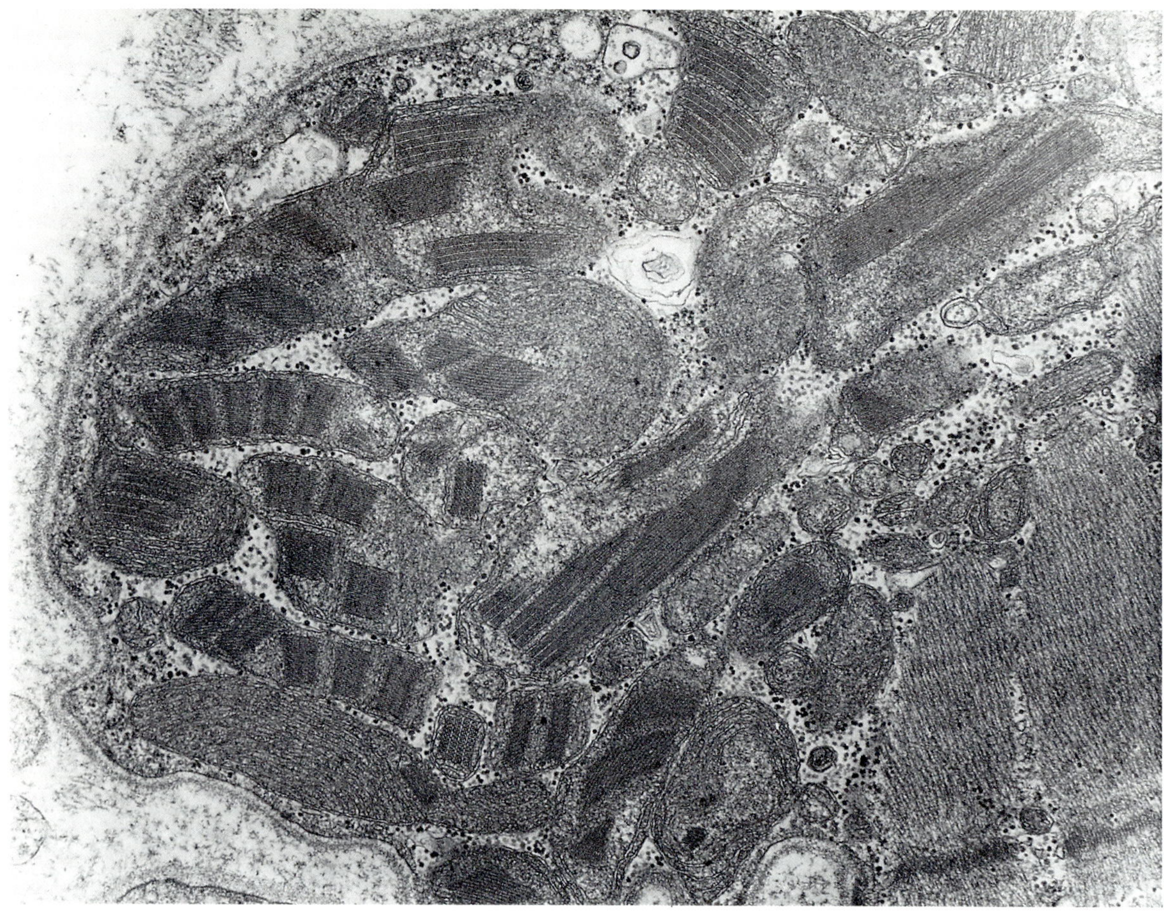

Fig. N9. Electron micrograph of a muscle fiber from a mitochondrial myopathy *(Fig. N8)*. Most of the mitochondria are markedly distorted and contain crystalline structures. These changes follow hyperplasia of the mitochondrial cristae and inner membranes, and are associated with mitochondrial dysfunction. (magnification 15,000×)

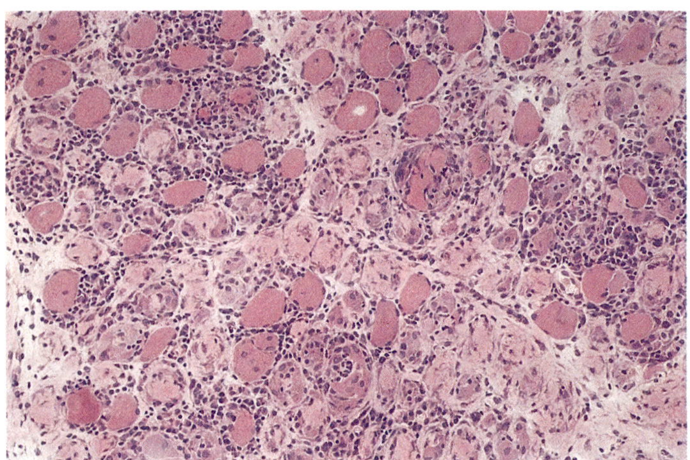

Inflammatory Myositis   *(N10)*

Fig. N10. Severe chronic polymyositis. There is an intense chronic inflammatory cell infiltration with many necrotic muscle fibers and marked phagocytic activity. This inflammation is followed by interstitial fibrosis and muscle atrophy and can be difficult to distinguish from progressive muscular dystrophy.
(Cryostat section; hematoxylin-eosin; magnification 40×)

O. Skeletal System

W. Remagen

The skeletal system is affected by both local diseases and systemic disease.

A variety of metabolic disorders may affect the bones with their manifestations dependent on a number of features, including local stress. Among the metabolic disorders are osteoporosis, osteomalacia, rickets, Paget's disease, and other forms of osteosclerosis. Although these conditions are systemic in nature, they may express at only a single or a few sites. The bones may also, of course, be affected by genetic and hormonal disorders.

Abnormalities of circulation that affect the bones are relatively uncommon. Circulatory disorders are generally exogenous in nature, due to either trauma or, in many instances, therapeutic intervention. Aseptic necrosis of the bone, for example, may follow steroid therapy. It may also develop spontaneously. Osteomyelitis, infection of the bone, may develop because of hematogenous spread from a remote site or, not infrequently, after traumatic fracture in which the integrity of the skin is interrupted.

In recent years bone tumors and tumor-like lesions have been carefully studied as therapeutic approaches have become more specific. Tumors may originate from virtually all cells of the skeletal system, and there is a full range of benign, low-grade malignant, and highly malignant tumors.

The joints and associated structures are affected by degenerative, immune, metabolic, and traumatic disorders, as well as proliferative conditions whose precise nature is not well understood.

The joints and juxta-articular tissues are subject to disorders that often reflect the constant stress these structures undergo. The degenerative disorders of the articular structures are generally grouped as arthroses. The major forms of arthritis, rheumatoid arthritis and osteoarthritis, differ in their clinical expression and in their pathogenesis. Osteoarthritis is most likely a degenerative disorder as a concomitant of aging. Rheumatoid arthritis, in contrast, can be grouped as one of the autoimmune disorders, although the precise pathogenesis has not been completely elucidated. The tendons and other connective tissue structures are also subject to inflammatory disorders, often in conjunction with those of the articular structures.

Fascial disorders occur particularly in the extremities. They are generally biologically benign but may be difficult to treat and eradicate. One of the most common tumors affecting the tendon sheath is the so-called giant cell tumor which is biologically innocuous. Another tumor that arises in the periarticular structures is the synovial sarcoma. This tumor can be highly malignant.

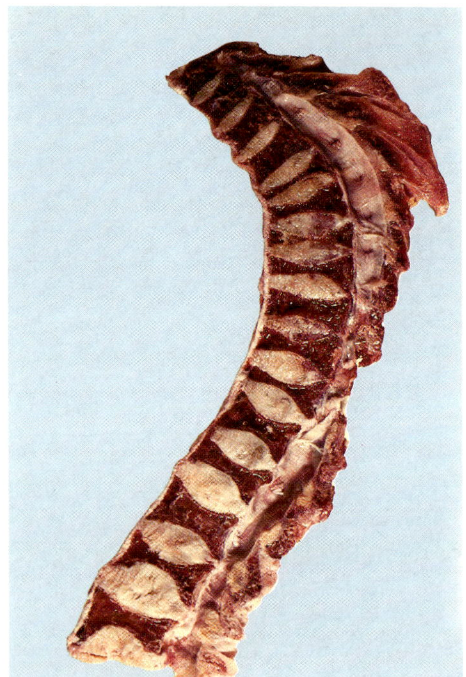

Fig. O1.   Sagittal section of the thoracic and lumbar spine in a patient with severe osteoporosis. Many of the vertebral bodies are collapsed, and there is irregular widening of the intervertebral discs. There is marked kyphosis.

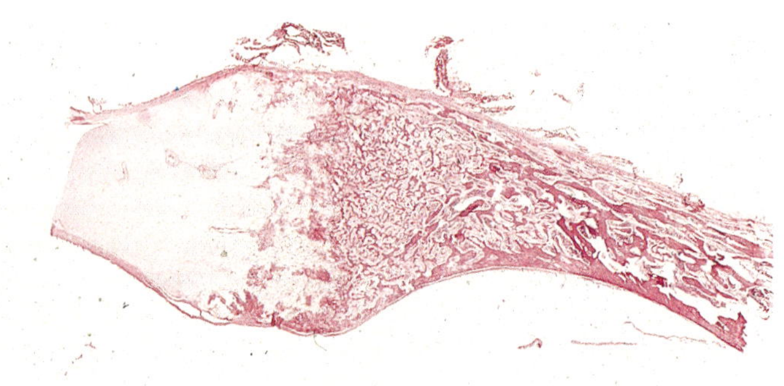

Fig. O2.   Rickets. The growth plate is widened and irregular with disordered architecture. The usual regular columnar arrangement of chondrocytes is lost, and the zone of provisional calcification disappears. Cartilagenous islands extend into the metaphysis where there is osteoid formation but impaired mineralization. The bone is osteomalacic and weakened. Because of this, the legs may be bowed.   (hematoxylin-eosin)

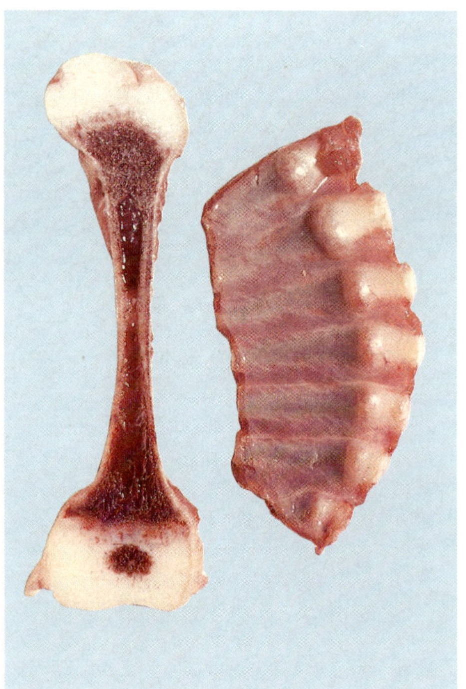

Fig. O3.   Section of the femur and portion of the rib cage, including costochondral junctions, from an infant with rickets. The growth plates seen in the femur are quite irregular, and the area of the poorly-formed epiphyseal line is widened. The ribs show the widening of the costochondral junctions which may be palpable ("rachitic rosary").

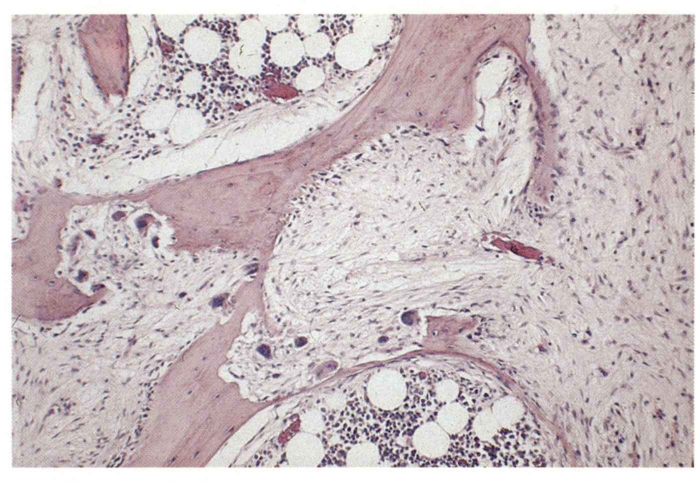

Fig. O4. Renal osteomalacia. The bony trabeculae are irregular with clusters of osteoclasts seen in scalloped areas, with marked peritrabecular fibrosis. The osteoclasts are large, dark cells, most of which are multinucleate. Uninvolved marrow is seen above and below. The extent of the defect in mineralization cannot be appreciated in this decalcified hematoxylin-eosin section.

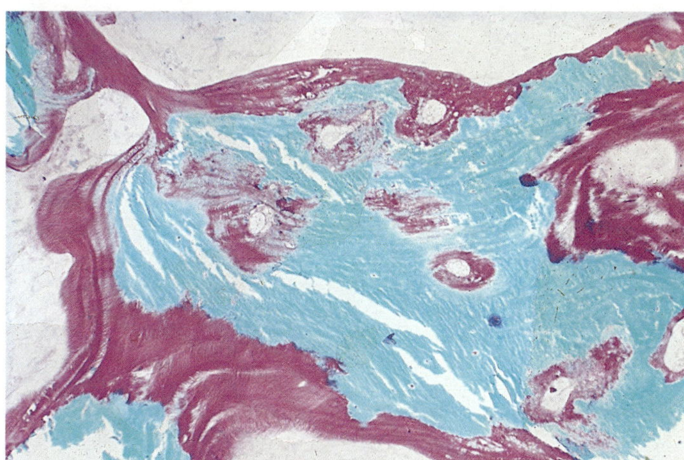

Fig. O5. Osteosclerotic form of renal osteodystrophy. This is a nondecalcified bone section stained with the Goldner method. Mineralized bone is seen as green material, and the nonmineralized bone (osteoid) is red. The osteoid is at the periphery of the broad area of bone formation. The relatively thin zone of nondemineralized bone is laminated. Normally the osteoid zones are not so wide.

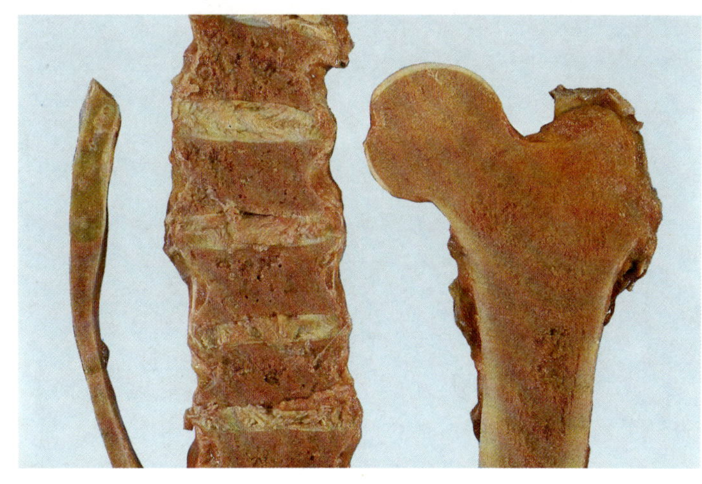

Fig. O6. Osteosclerosis. Sections of rib, vertebral bodies, and proximal femur. The marrow spaces are stony hard, and neither soft marrow nor the trabecular pattern of bone *(see Fig. O9)* can be discerned.

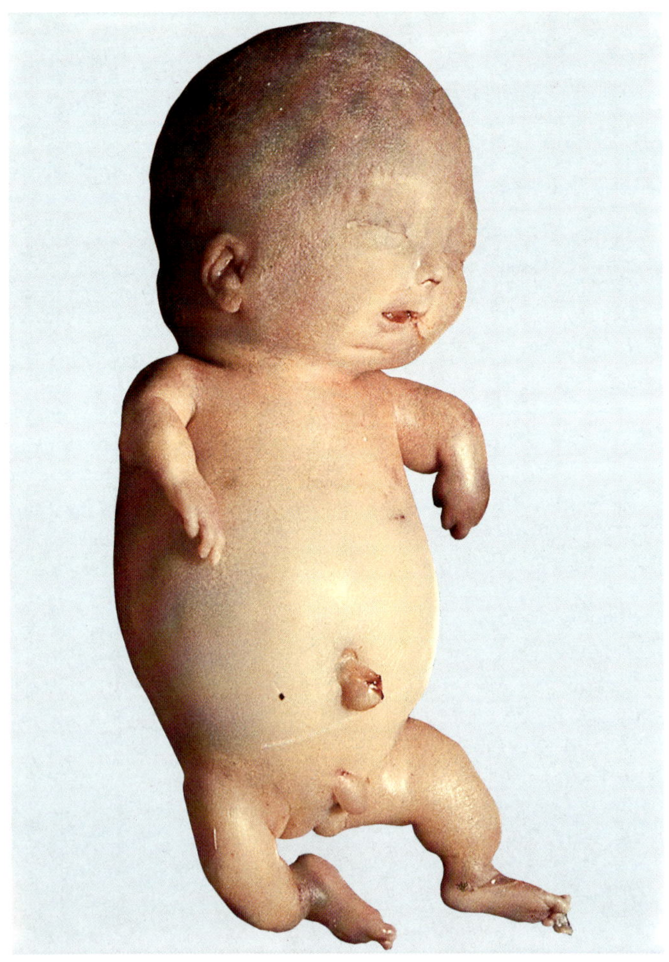

Fig. O7. Osteogenesis imperfecta. This hereditary connective tissue disorder usually becomes manifest during life by a predisposition to multiple fractures. In this case there were multiple intrauterine fractures with resultant deformities of the extremities. This fetus died from severe hydrops.

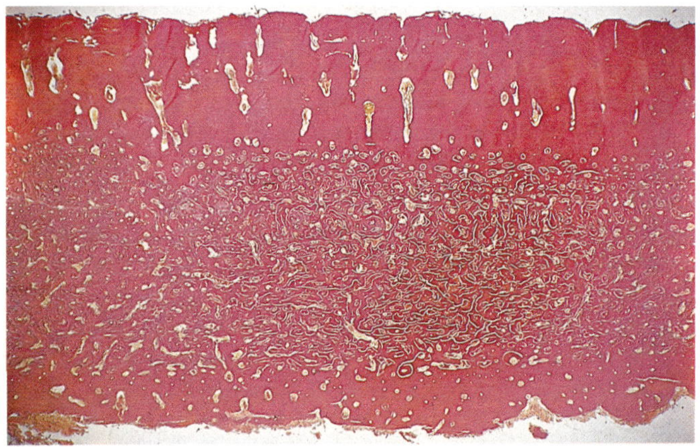

Fig. O8. Osteopetrosis. This condition is characterized by the overgrowth of bone, with sclerosis, causing marked thickening of the bony cortex and narrowing of the marrow cavity. Despite the excess bone production, the skeleton is quite brittle and fractures easily occur. Cortical bone, above and below, is markedly thinned, and the marrow space is almost obliterated.   (van Gieson)

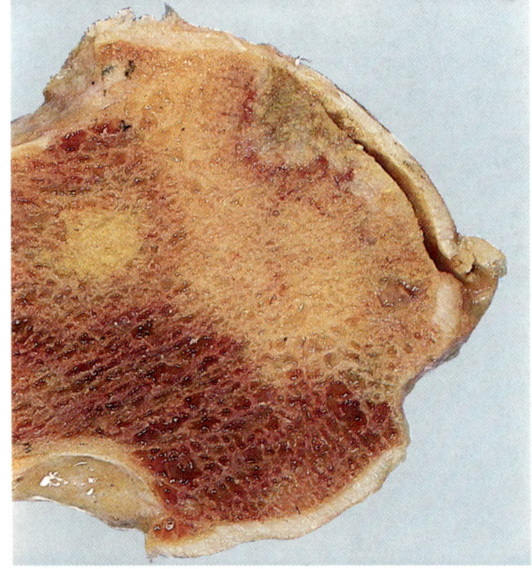

Vascular and Inflammatory Disorders   (O9–O14)

Fig. O9. Aseptic necrosis of the head of the femur. This is the typical picture showing the subchondral fissure, visible on x-ray, which follows the loss of trabeculae. Also seen is a wedge-shaped zone of acute necrosis rimmed by a red line indicating an acute inflammatory response. The overlying articular surface is irregularly indented.

Fig. O10. Chronic osteomyelitis of the proximal tibia. An irregular cavity formed of necrotic tissue contains a yellow-gray mass of devitalized bone ("sequestrum"). The necrotic inflammatory exudate has fallen out after sectioning. The cavity extends to the periosteal surface (right). The bone immediately surrounding the cavity is markedly sclerotic, as evidence of the reparative activity.

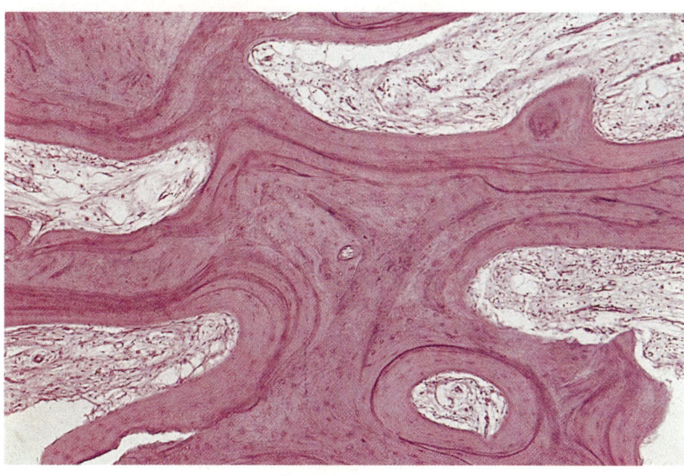

Fig. O11. Chronic osteomyelitis. In this photomicrograph the reparative responses to osteomyelitis are easily seen. The bone trabeculae show evidence of marked new bone formation, seen as approximately parallel "cement lines" imparting a laminated appearance. This is the sclerotic zone. The marrow space is slightly fibrotic and there are scattered chronic inflammatory cells. (hematoxylin-eosin)

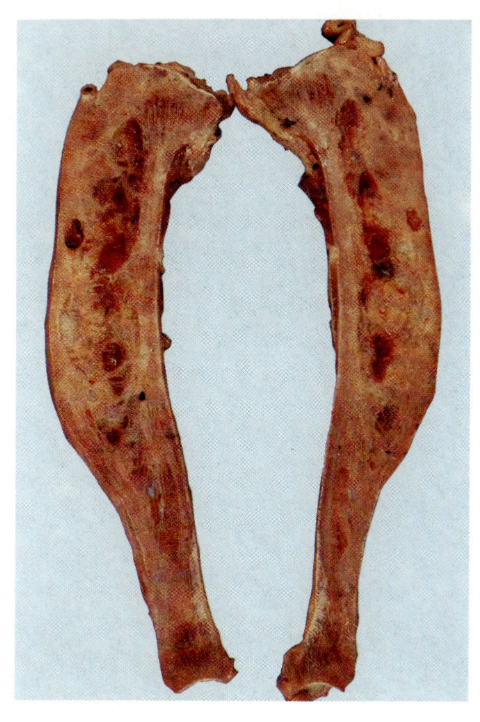

Fig. O12. Paget's disease of bone. Sagittal section of the tibia showing the typical advanced form. The bone is markedly deformed ("osteitis deformans"). The bony proliferation obliterates the cortex and extends irregularly into the marrow space. Although the overall size of bone is increased due to both cortical and trabecular thickening, the bone is soft and can be porous.

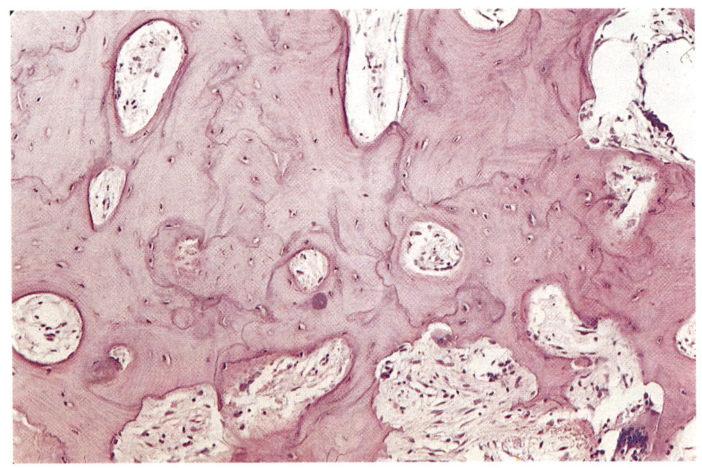

Fig. O13. Paget's disease of bone. The pathognomonic feature of Paget's disease is shown here. The bone has tile-like or mosaic pattern of mineralization. This is the stage of mixed osteolysis and osteogenesis, and a group of osteoclasts can be seen at the lower margins of bone. Compare the irregular, almost jigsaw puzzle pattern of mineralization in this photomicrograph with the parallel organization of normal reparative response *(Fig. O11).* (hematoxylin-eosin)

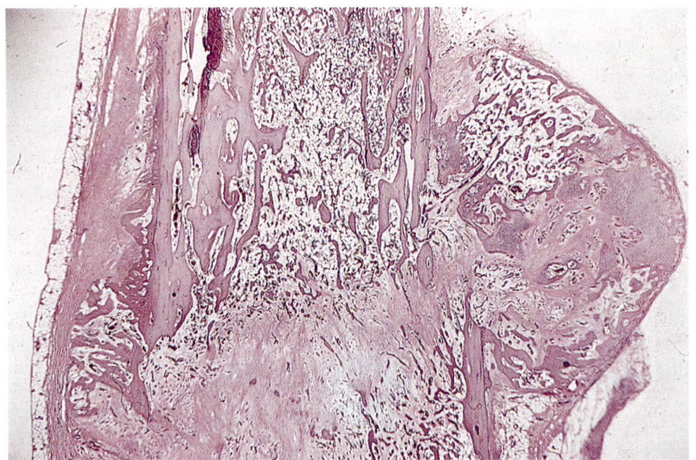

Fig. O14. Healing fracture. Fracture healing is a dynamic continuous process with three stages. The hematoma at the fracture site is organized to form a soft "pro-callus". This pro-callus is converted to fibrocartilaginous callus which firmly binds fragments of bone. Finally the fibrocartilaginous callus is replaced by osseous callus, which is remodeled with usage to approximate or equal the pre-fracture form. In this photomicrograph nodular masses of callus are seen outside the cortex and periosteum. The fibrocartilage is undergoing enchondrial ossification.   (hematoxylin-eosin)

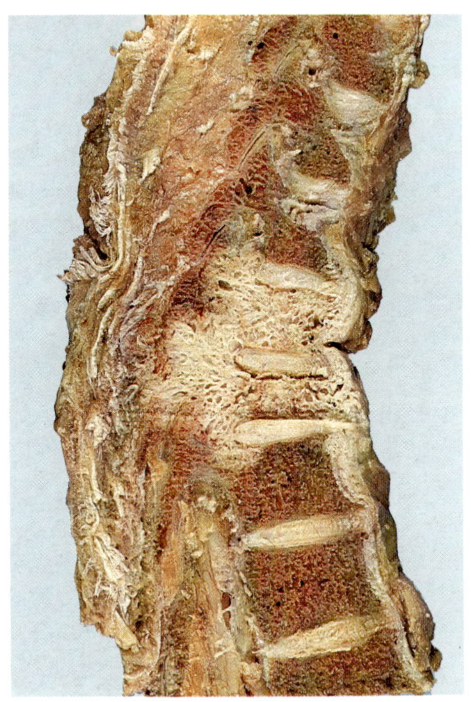

Tumors and Tumor-Like Conditions   *(O15–O24)*

Fig. O15. Sagittal section of lower thoracic vertebrae (T5–T12) showing metastatic carcinoma, from a primary site in the lung, almost completely destroying T8 and T9. The tumor extends posteriorly and compresses the spinal cord. Bone metastases are common in metastatic carcinoma, particularly those arising in lungs, breast, and prostate.

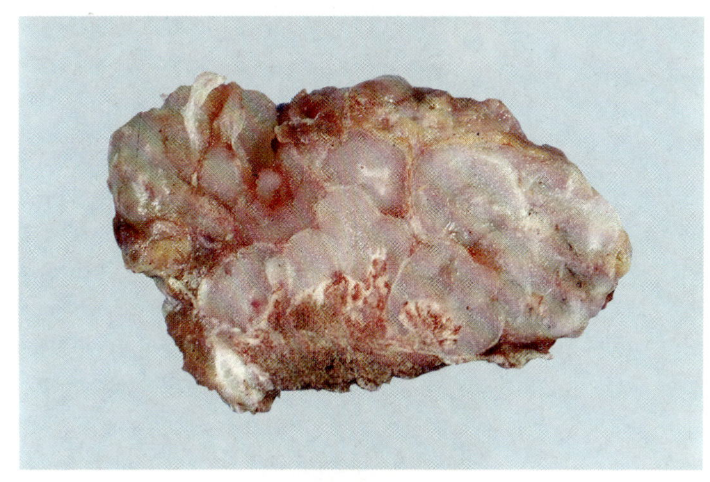

Fig. O16.   Large osteochondroma (exostosis) arising from a pelvic bone. The typical blue-white opalescent appearance of the irregular cartilaginous cap is well seen. These lesions result from abnormal epiphyseal bone growth, resulting in a cartilage-capped bony mass projecting from enchondral bones. These may be solitary or, in hereditary syndromes, multiple. Malignancy (chondrosarcoma usually) develops in approximately 5% of the patients with the hereditary form of the disease.

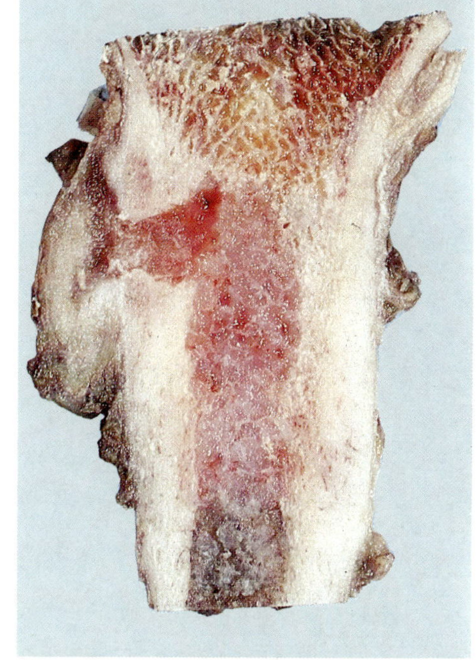

Fig. O17.   Resection of the proximal femur with a chondrosarcoma. The proximal resection line (above) is through the lower portion of the greater trochanter. Most of the lower portion of the marrow space contains irregular blue-white semitransparent tumor masses of chondrosarcoma. The previous biopsy site is seen as a cortical defect at the upper left. A portion of the fibula was used to replace this resected segment. There was good response for seven years, at which time recurrence was noted in the surrounding soft tissue.

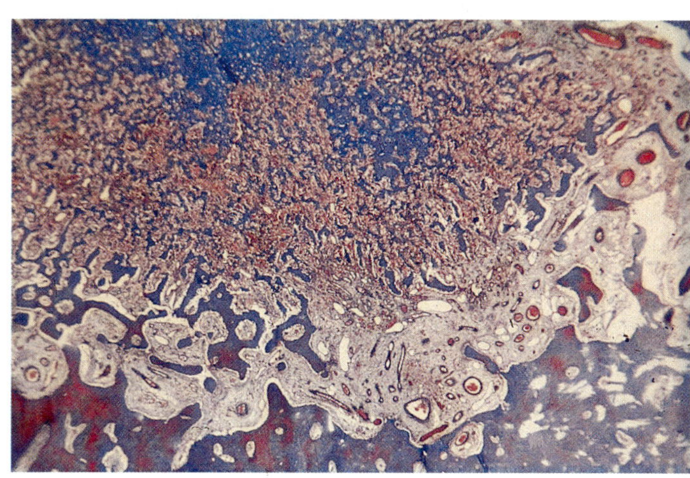

Fig. O18.   Osteoid osteoma. This small benign neoplasm has no malignant potential. Typically this is a painful lesion which responds to aspirin. There is a central "nidus" composed of irregularly branching, partially mineralized osteoid (above) surrounded by densely sclerotic bone. The radiograph is characteristic showing a small radiolucent area, the nidus, surrounded by densely radio-opaque sclerotic bone.   (Masson trichrome)

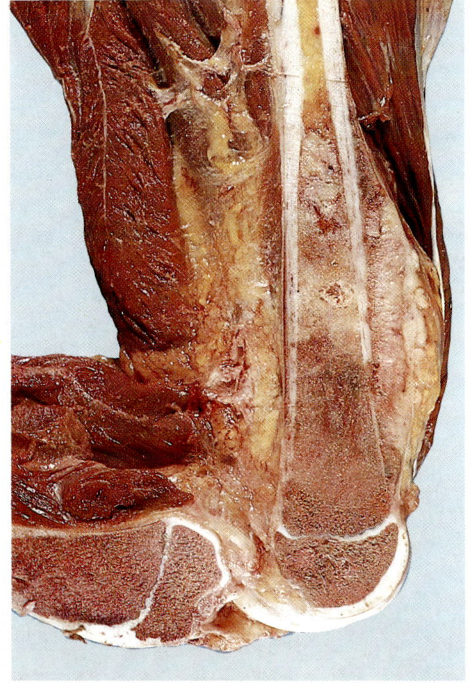

Fig. O19.   Sagittal section of the distal femur and proximal tibia from a 17-year-old man with osteogenic sarcoma. The epiphyseal plates have not yet fused. The tumor is seen as a fleshy gray-white noncircumscribed mass, lifting and filling the periosteal space (right), and also extending into and up the marrow cavity. The proximal marrow (above the tumor) is fatty, whereas the rest of the marrow appears hematopoietically active.

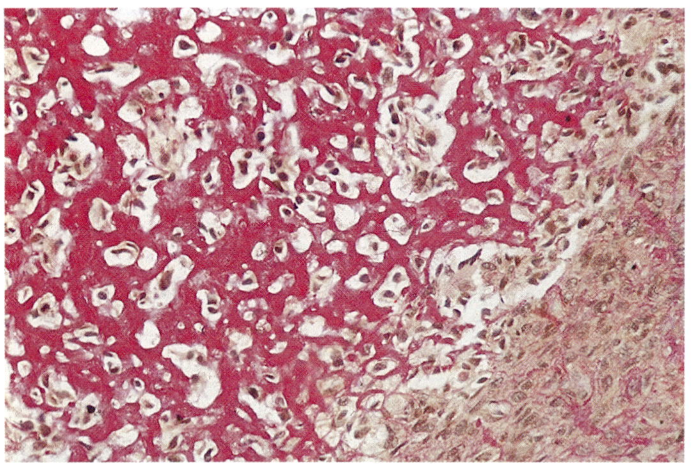

Fig. O20.   Osteogenic sarcoma. This aggressive malignancy of mesenchymal cells characteristically forms osteoid and/or bone directly from tumor cells. There are irregular osteoid bands (red) in this photomicrograph, between which there are many bizarre, often multinucleated, tumor cells. These tumors vary greatly in cellular components and there may be differing amounts of osteoid, cartilage, connective tissue, and vascular elements.   (van Gieson)

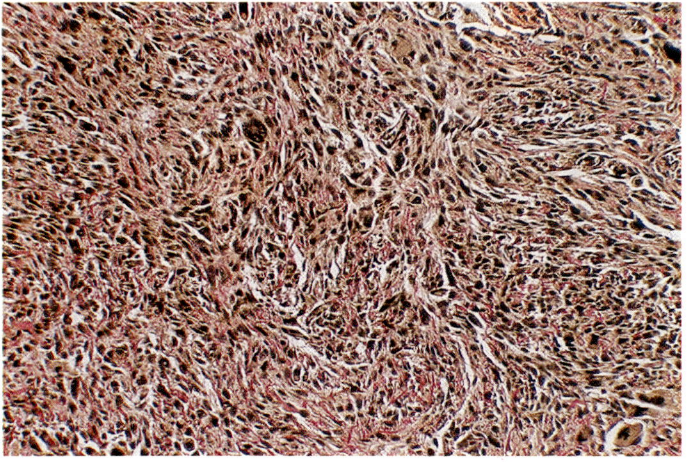

Fig. O21.   Malignant fibrous histiocytoma. This tumor arises in soft tissues or bone. Histologically these tumors may consist of densely-packed spindle cells with large hyperchromatic, often multinucleate tumor cells. A bizarre giant cell, with approximately ten nuclear lobes, is seen near the middle of the photomicrograph. Characteristically, as in this case, the tumor cells are arranged as interlacing bundles with areas of storiform pattern. A small amount of collagen (red) is seen between tumor cells.   (van Gieson)

Fig. O22. Ewing's sarcoma. The cell of origin of this highly malignant primary bone tumor is uncertain. These tumors arise within the marrow cavity and consist of sheets of undifferentiated small round or oval cells with prominent nuclei and scanty cytoplasm. The tumor cells are glycogen-rich, as shown in these photomicrographs by the PAS positivity (left) which is not present after diastase digestion (right).

Fig. O23. Fibrous dysplasia is a benign disorder characterized by slowly proliferating uniformly cellular fibrous tissue within which there are irregularly formed trabeculae of woven bone. In this photomicrograph the bone is red. The irregularity of the trabeculae has been likened to Chinese characters. The background of mature connective tissue is moderately cellular. There are sinusoidal vascular spaces in this case and scattered clusters of chronic inflammatory cells.   (van Gieson)

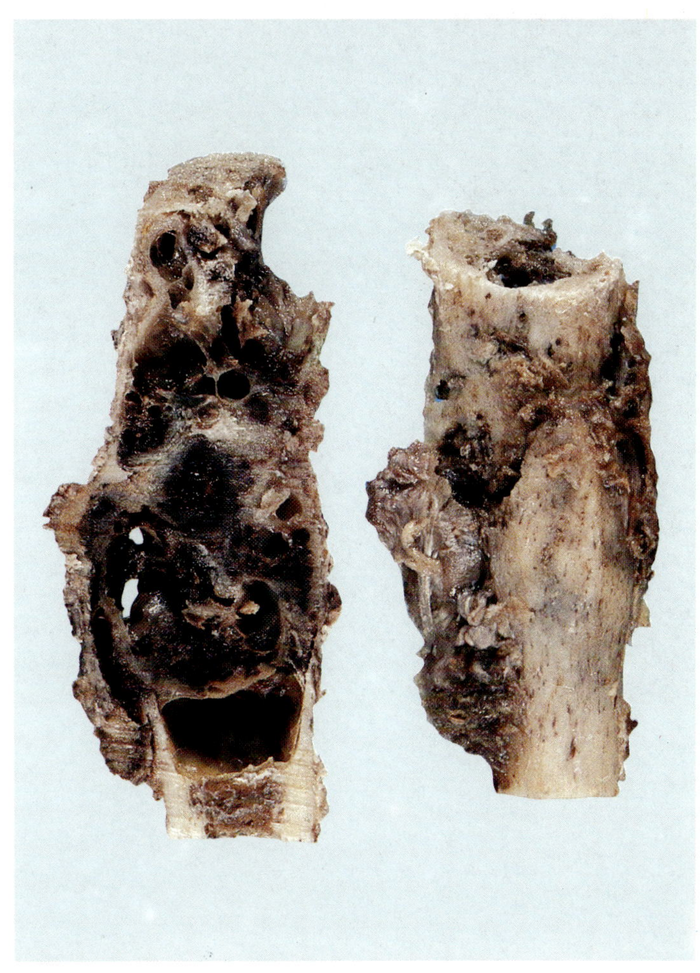

Fig. O24. Aneurysmal bone cyst. This is an expansile mass of blood-filled spaces of varying size, which usually presents as pain and swelling. In this case the multicystic hemorrhagic mass replaces almost the entire bone, with only a small portion of the metaphysis at the lower edge of the mass. A thin shell of reactive bone is seen at the upper left. The cystic spaces are filled with dark red granulation tissue, and there was considerable blood, which is no longer present after the spaces were opened.

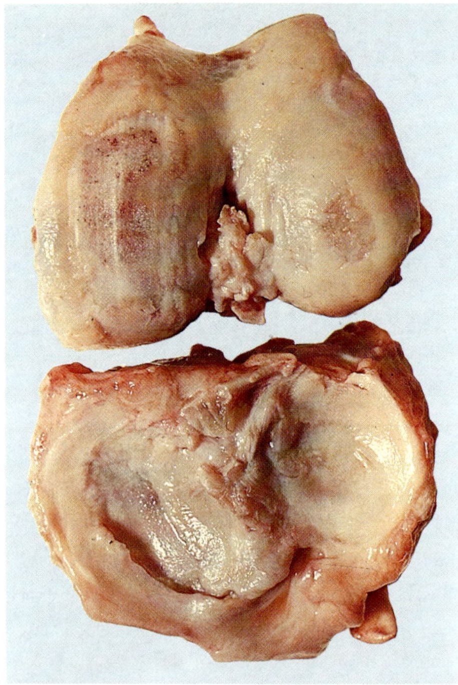

Fig. O25.   This photograph of an opened left knee joint shows a severe osteoarthritis (degenerative joint disease). The knee joint is the largest and most complex joint in the body and is subject to the stresses of its hinge action requirements as well as weight bearing. The lower end of the femur is at the upper portion of the picture, and its corresponding joint space with menisci and ligaments is below. The medial articular surface is to the left. In this case there is marked destruction of the cartilage exposing subchondral bone which, in some areas, becomes highly polished (eburnation). The medial meniscus (medial semi-lunar cartilage; left) is frayed, and the lateral meniscus (lateral semi-lunar cartilage; right) is almost completely effaced.

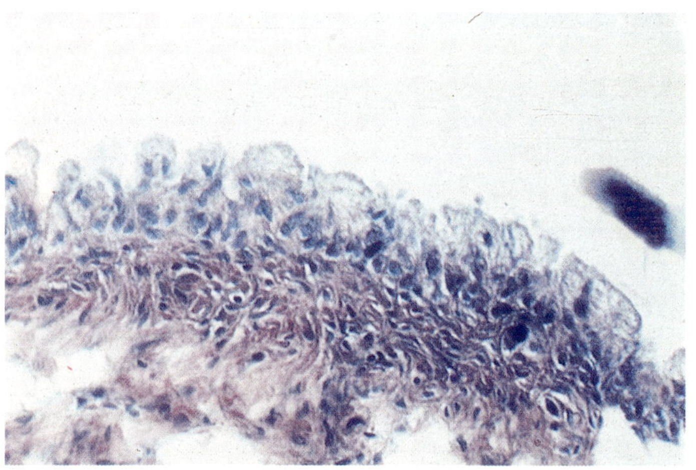

Fig. O26.   Proliferative synovitis of rheumatoid arthritis. This photomicrograph is of a synovial biopsy from a patient with chronic rheumatoid arthritis. In this Giemsa-stained preparation there is marked proliferation of the synovial lining (above). The cells are hypertrophied and multilayered and there is increased vascularity and hyperplasia of the subsynovial connective tissue. There is a sparse lymphocytic infiltrate.   (Giemsa)

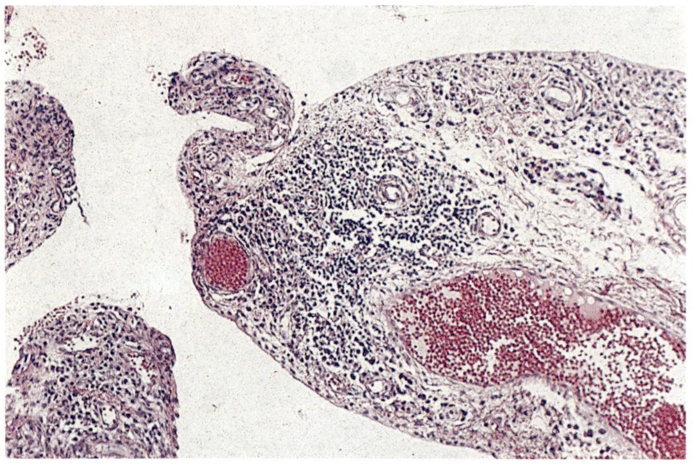

Fig. O27.   Excised synovium from a patient with rheumatoid arthritis. Three villus-like synovial fragments are seen in this low magnification photomicrograph. Dilated and congested blood vessels are easily seen, and there is intense stromal infiltration by lymphocytes and plasma cells with formation of a lymphoid nodule. This polypoid villus mass ("pannus"), which may have varying degrees of inflammation and necrosis, eventually erodes into the underlying articular cartilage contributing to significant joint dysfunction.   (hematoxylin-eosin)

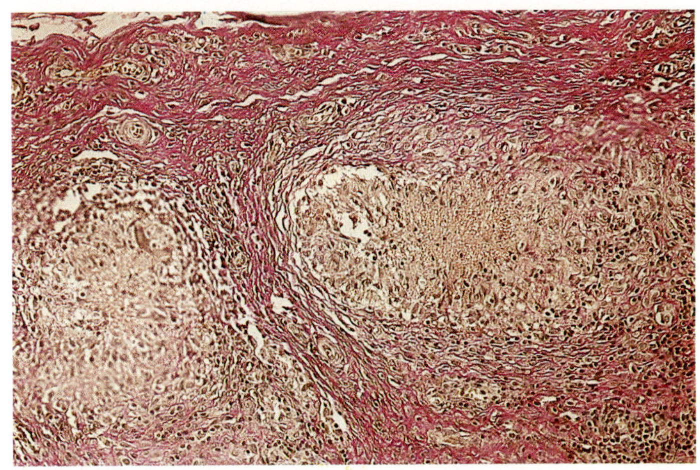

Fig. O28. Rheumatoid nodules in the periarticular connective tissue, from a patient with rheumatoid arthritis. These distinctive granulomas may occur in the joint structures, skin, lung, pleura, pericardium, heart and spleen, and are indistinguishable from the nodules sometimes seen in patients with rheumatic fever. They are characterized by a central focus of fibrinoid-type necrosis, surrounded by proliferating, generally radially oriented chronic inflammatory cells, including histiocytes, lymphocytes and plasma cells, and fibroblasts. This radial orientation creates the distinctive appearance of a granuloma with peripheral palisading. (van Gieson)

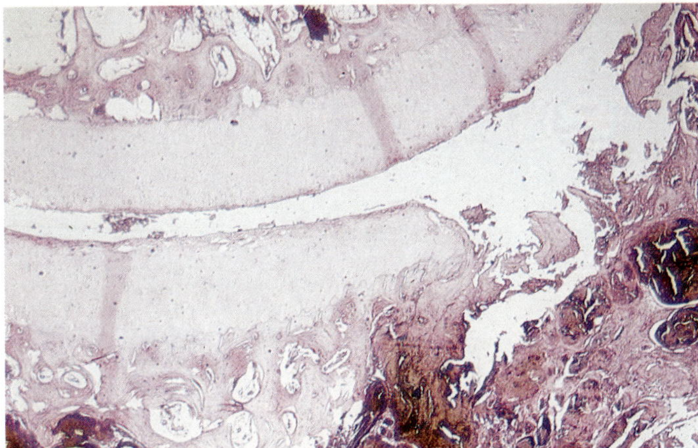

O29a

Fig. O29. Gout. Joint tissues and gouty arthritis shown in low magnification photomicrographs with both usual light microscopy *(a)* and with polarized light microscopy *(b)*.

In *(a)*, there are two cartilagenous structures with associated lamellar bone. The lower cartilage is partially destroyed by a chronic inflammatory process (middle right and lower left) composed of proliferating fibroblasts, lymphocytes, histiocytes, and foreign body type giant cells. The giant cells are at the lower right edge of the photomicrograph, but are not easily seen with this degree of magnification.   (hematoxylin-eosin).

In *(b)* the brightly birefringent material, consisting of amorphous or crystalline aggregates of urates, is easily seen corresponding to the areas of destruction present in *(a)*. The background bone and cartilage is weakly birefringent

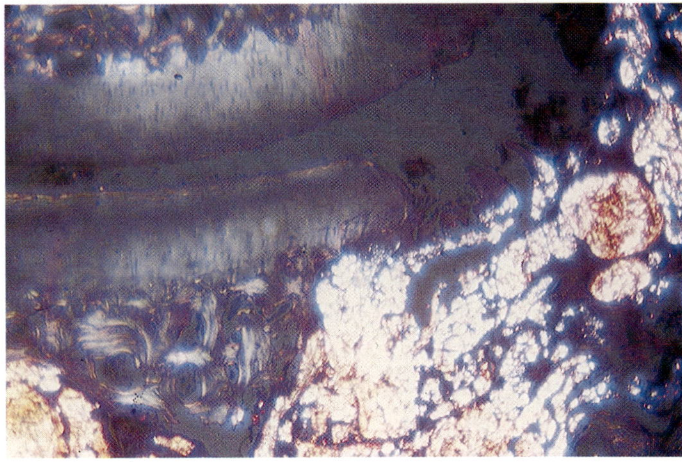

O29b

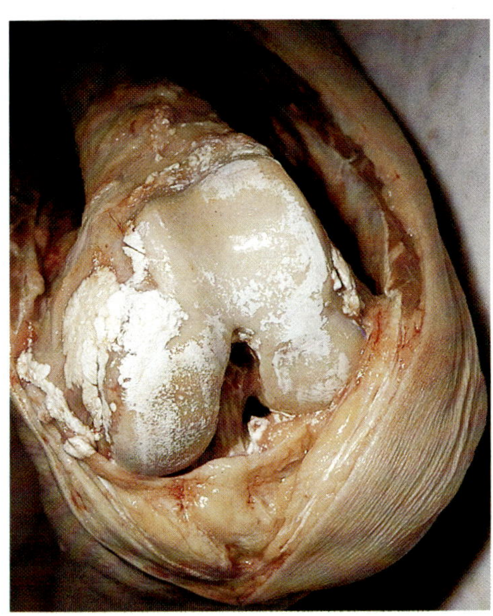

Fig. O30. Gouty arthritis. This photograph shows the opened left knee joint with extensive white deposition of urates on articular surfaces of the femoral condyles, and in periarticular connective tissues. The stage of urate encrustation of articular surfaces, as seen here, is associated with synovial proliferation and pannus formation and, eventually, bone destruction.

199

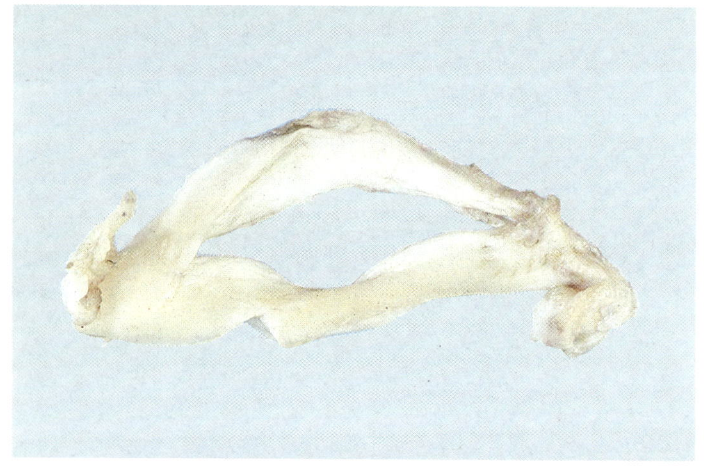

Fig. O31. Resected right medial meniscus with a longitudinal tear. The medial meniscus is more often involved than the lateral one, probably because it is more securely attached to supporting structures than the lateral meniscus, and less capable of adaptation to sudden positional changes. The torn fragment can become displaced and cause "locking" of the joint, as well as contribute to damage of synovial and joint capsule tissues. The fibrocartilage of a damaged meniscus has little or no reparative capacity. In recent years this type of surgical specimen has become extremely unusual since most meniscal resections are performed through an arthroscope, and the cartilage is removed as multiple small fragments.

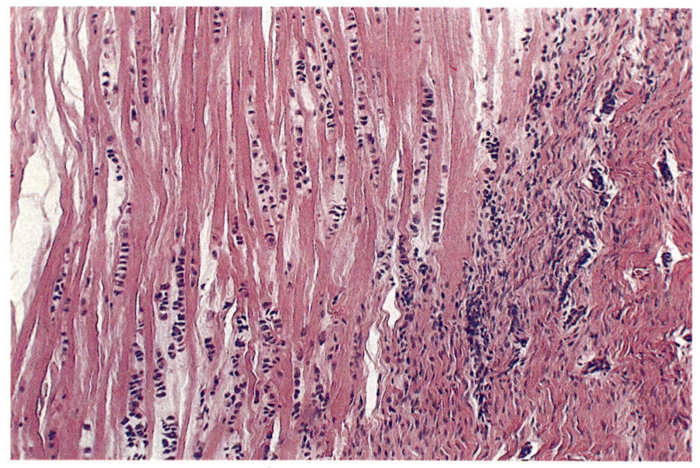

Fig. O32. Stenosing tenosynovitis occurring at the radiostyloid process (de Quervain's disease). The inner portion of the tendon sheath (left) is stretched, and there is increased interstitial collagen. The outer portion is fairly unchanged and consists of capillary-rich connective tissue. The thickening of the tendon sheath causes pain by compressing the extensor pollicis brevis and abductor pollicis longis tendons. The etiology is unknown. This is a relatively uncommon problem for the pathologist.   (hematoxylin-eosin)

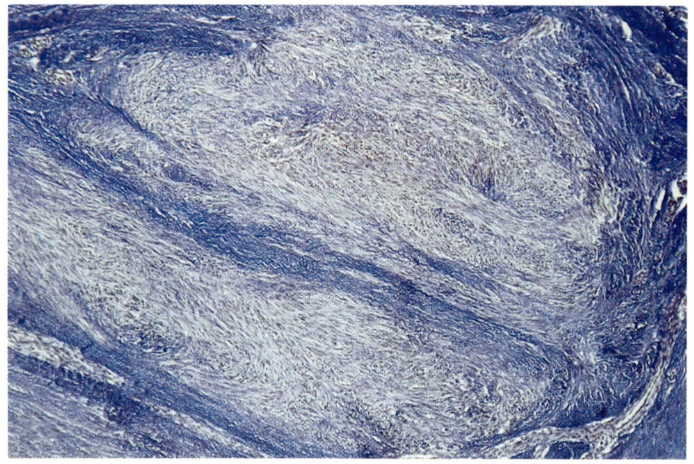

Fig. O33. Dupuytren's contracture. Fibromatoses are a group of fibroblastic proliferations that may aggressively infiltrate adjacent tissue, but are not thought to be neoplastic. They may occur at varying sites, including the neck (fibromatosis colli), the feet (plantar fibromatosis), the penis (Peyronie's disease) and, as in this case, the fascia of the palm. The palmar fascia becomes extensively replaced by proliferation of collagen-rich fibroblastic tissue which entraps tendons and leads to flexion contractions of the hands and fingers. In this photomicrograph we see abundant blue collagen surrounding and infiltrating the palmar aponeurosis.   (Ladewig)

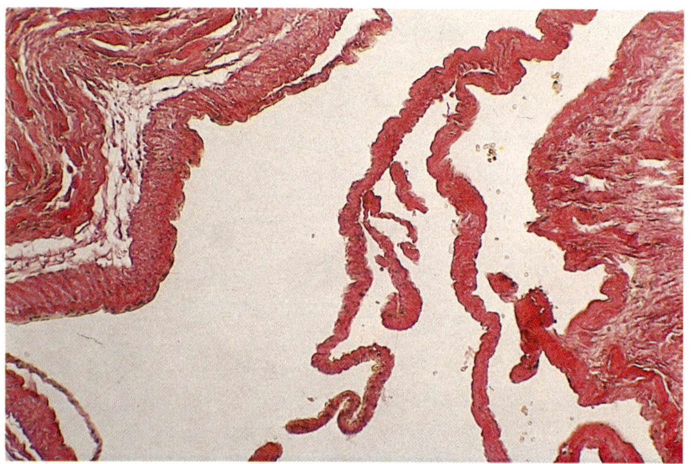

Fig. O34. Ganglion (cyst). These lesions occur on the dorsum of the wrist and hands, and are not true cysts. Instead they result from mucoid degeneration of the fibrous tissue of tendon sheaths, ligaments, and aponeuroses. In this photomicrograph there is the characteristic picture of cyst-like spaces, almost always without a lining, and varying amounts of collagenous connective tissue (red). The ganglion is commonly located near the small joints of the wrist. At one time the ganglion was known as the "Bible" tumor because of the 19th century practice of treating them by slamming a heavy book, such as a Bible, on them to collapse the lesion. Today, local excision is relatively easy and much preferred.   (van Gieson)

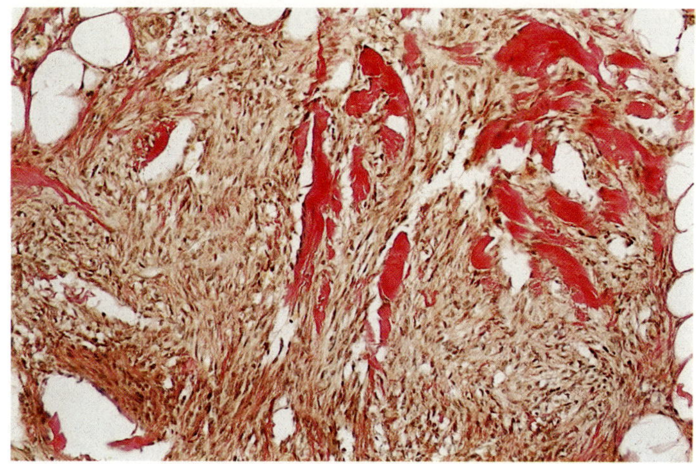

Fig. O35. Nodular fasciitis. This nonneoplastic lesion is another, more aggressive form of fibromatosis which may clinically and histologically be mistaken for a sarcoma, and is sometimes called pseudosarcomatous fasciitis. The histologic pattern is that of an exuberant, nonencapsulated and noncircumscribed growth of somewhat atypical fibroblasts which may be cytologically difficult to distinguish from true sarcoma cells. In this photomicrograph bundles of fibroblasts interconnect irregularly, contain newly-formed capillaries, and surround the stretched and distorted collagenous connective tissue of the fascia.   (van Gieson)

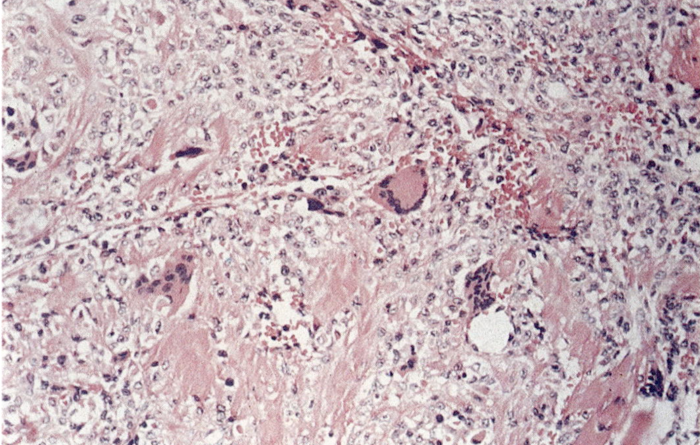

Fig. O36. Benign giant cell tumor of tendon sheath. These nodular lesions of tendon sheaths consist, as in this photomicrograph, of haphazardly arranged histiocytes, which contain varying amounts of lipid, as well as lymphocytes, fibroblasts, and giant cells, of both the foreign body and osteoclast type. These lesions are relatively common, and it is not entirely agreed that they are truly tumors. Instead they may be a localized form of tenosynovitis.
(hematoxylin-eosin)

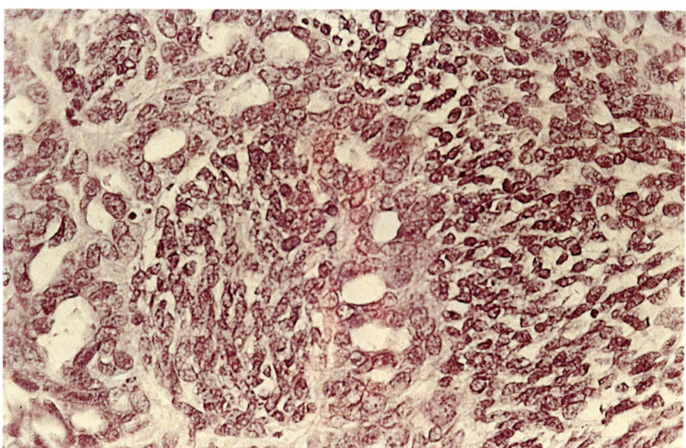

Fig. O37. Synovial sarcoma is an uncommon malignant tumor that arises most often from the deep juxta-articular soft tissues of the extremities. The characteristic, and definitive, histologic feature of the tumor is the finding of spaces lined by plump synovial cells. These gland-like structures may be difficult to identify since the bulk of these tumors consists of undifferentiated malignant spindle cells. The spaces are not true glands and lack a basement membrane, as well as cytochemical features of epithelial cells. Despite their resemblance to gland epithelium, these cuboidal and columnar cells are the neoplastic counterpart of synovial cells.
(hematoxylin-eosin)

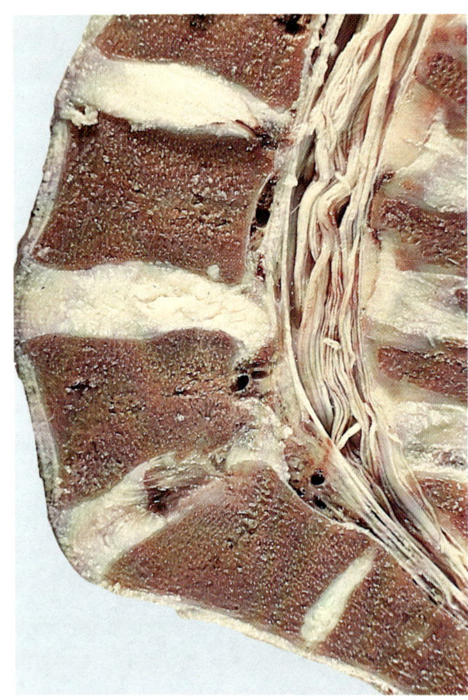

Fig. O38.   Intervertebral disc prolapse. This is a photograph of a sagittally sectioned lower vertebral column showing vertebral bodies L3–S2, and the spinal canal containing the cauda equina. The intervertebral discs between L4/L5 and L5/S1 are dorsally prolapsed into the spinal canal. In this location, since the cauda equina is relatively unfixed in position and there is room for compression, there may not be signs or symptoms secondary to this phenomenon. When evidence of cord compression is seen, the prolapse must be reduced to prevent permanent damage.

P. Skin

F. Vakilzadeh, E. Macher, K. Wolff

Skin is susceptible to a great variety of disorders. Skin disease may be the result of exogenous factors, may reflect disorders of the epidermis, dermis, and subdermal connective tissue, and may also be a manifestation of systemic disorders. Many of the hereditary conditions may manifest as diseases of the skin. Infectious disorders often affect the skin. This is particularly true with viral diseases in which the skin may be affected primarily, as in molluscum contagiosum, or may show changes as a part of a widespread viral infection. Bacteria have been well known as causes of skin infections. The common pyogenic bacteria may lead to pyogenic infections of the skin. Nonpyogenic bacteria, including tuberculosis, may also infect the skin. Tuberculosis might be separated from other granulomatous diseases of the skin and subcutaneous tissue, including foreign body reactions and sarcoid. A variety of autoimmune disorders also affect the skin. Many of them lead to cutaneous manifestations involving the epidermis or the epidermal-dermal interface. Systemic lupus erythematosus, of course, is well recognized as a disease which may have cutaneous manifestations. Discoid lupus erythematosus is also well recognized and the deposition of immune complexes in the skin can be shown in both of these conditions. One of the most frequent skin diseases is psoriasis. The etiology of this disorder is unclear. Another common skin condition is lichen planus which clinically is generally recognized as a papillary disorder.

Skin tumors are similarly varied in etiology, histogenesis, and manifestations. There are well recognized premalignant conditions, skin tumors which have relatively low capacity for metastases, and destructive skin tumors. The pigment-forming tumors, both benign and malignant, are among the most common particularly in temperate and tropical zones. Benign nevi are frequently seen and must be clinically and morphologically distinguished from the highly malignant melanomas. The skin may also be involved by malignant lymphoproliferative disorders. One of the most important of these is mycosis fungoides, a malignancy of T-cells.

Only a small segment of cutaneous pathology is covered in this chapter. An understanding of dermatopathology requires knowledge of clinical and pathologic features, and is best achieved by observing the lesion in the clinical setting and studying it after biopsy.

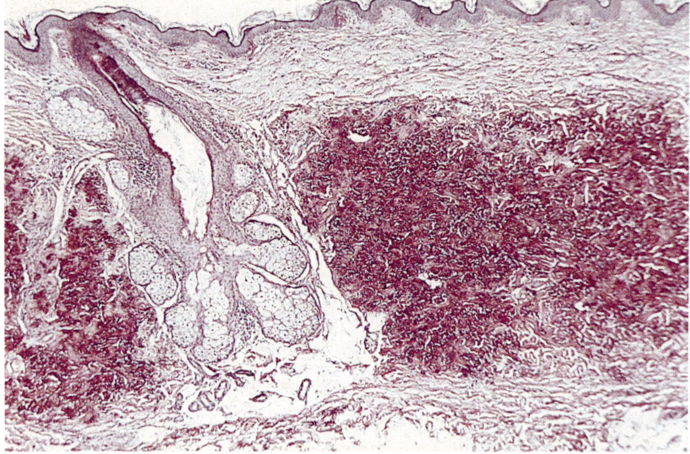

Fig. P1.   Pseudoxanthoma elasticum. This is a hereditary disease in which yellowish plaques and papules are distributed symmetrically in abnormally loose skin of the neck, axilla, groin, and cubital and popliteal spaces, with less frequent involvement of other parts of the body. The elastic fibers are usually easily seen, even in routine preparations stained with hematoxylin eosin, as masses of curved, small, partially calcified curled bodies which tend to concentrate in the mid-dermis.   (hematoxylin eosin-elastica)

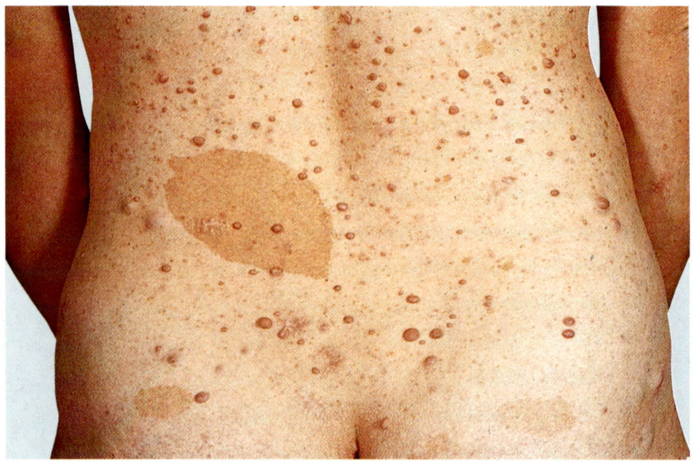

Fig. P2.   Neurofibromatosis (von Recklinghausen's disease). Multiple cutaneous and subcutaneous neurofibromas are obvious. In addition, there are three separate irregular flat pigmented (café au lait) areas. This is the typical external appearance of this autosomal dominant disease. In some patients these skin tumors may be so numerous as to cover almost the entire body.

Viral Diseases   (P3–P4)

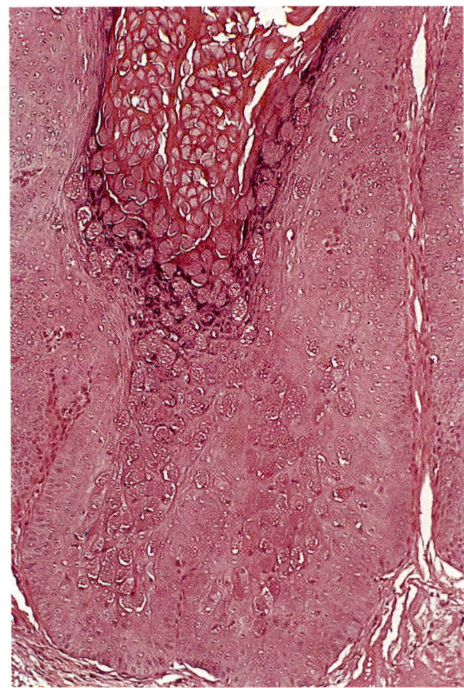

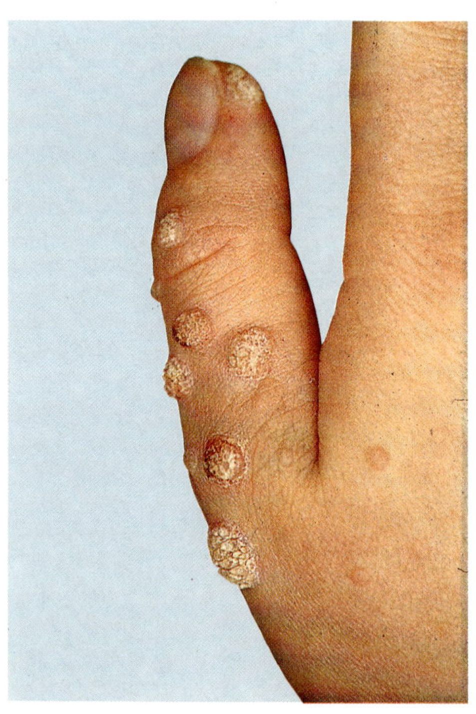

Fig. P3.   Molluscum contagiosum. This mildly contagious auto-inoccuable disease is characterized by large, homogeneously smooth, brightly eosinophilic inclusions ("molluscum bodies").
(hematoxylin-eosin)

Fig. P4.   Verucca vulgaris. This is the common wart, due to papilloma virus infection.

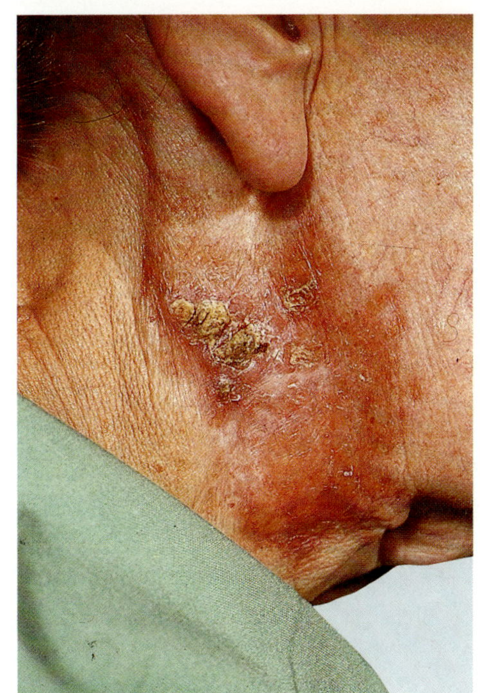

Fig. P5.   Cutaneous tuberculosis ("lupus vulgarus"). This is the most common form of cutaneous tuberculosis and is relatively rarely seen. Flat, soft, brownish skin lesions resembling tumors lead to superficial ulceration and, ultimately, drainage from sinus tracts.

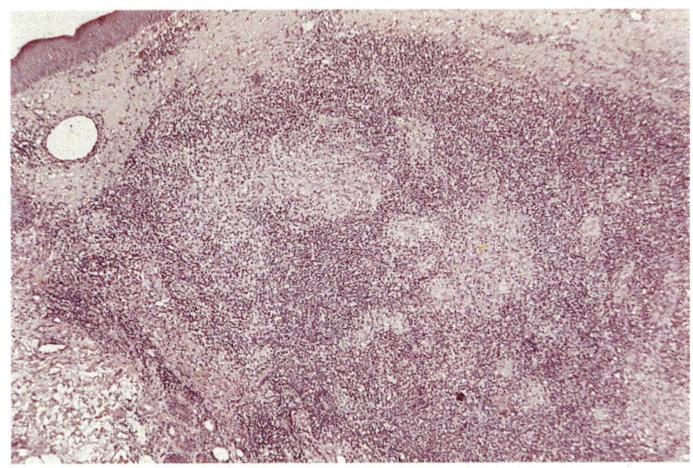

Fig. P6.   Photomicrograph of cutaneous tuberculosis showing typical epithelioid granulomata with Langhans giant cells. The intact epidermis is to the left. The granulomata are surrounded by sheets of lymphocytes.   (hematoxylin-eosin)

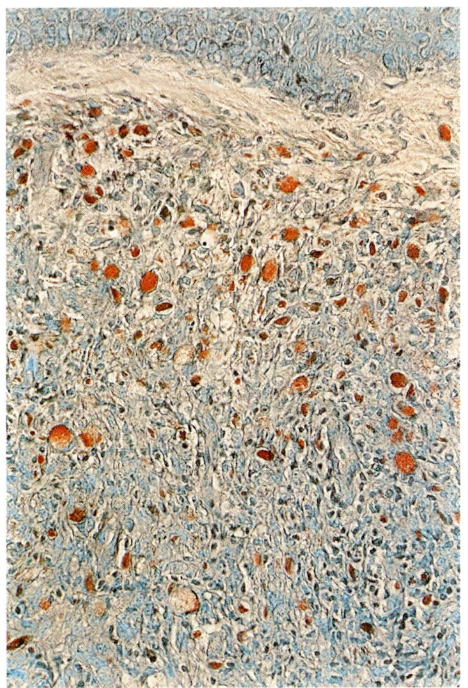

Fig. P7.   Lepromatous leprosy. There is a relatively uniform infiltrate of large histiocytic (Virchow) cells which contain innumerable lepra bacilli. The characteristic infiltrate is typically separated from the epidermis by a narrow rim of compressed connective tissue.   (Giemsa)

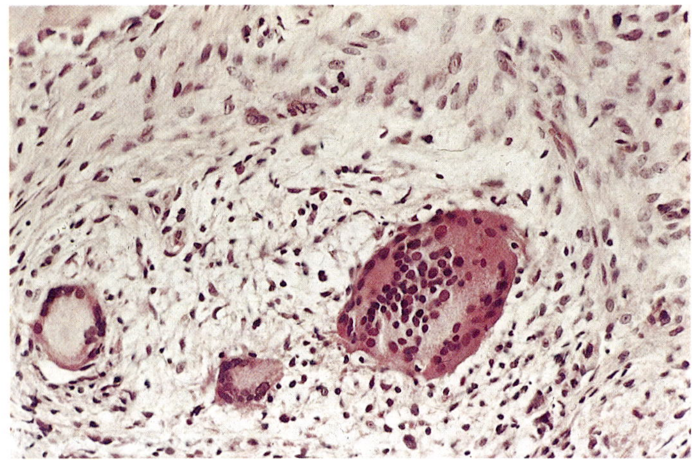

Fig. P8.   Foreign body granuloma of the skin. Large foreign body giant cells, with multiple nuclei, are seen surrounded by histiocytes and lymphocytes. These giant cells, which occasionally contain as many as 100 nuclei, are formed by the fusion of histiocytes. (hematoxylin-eosin)

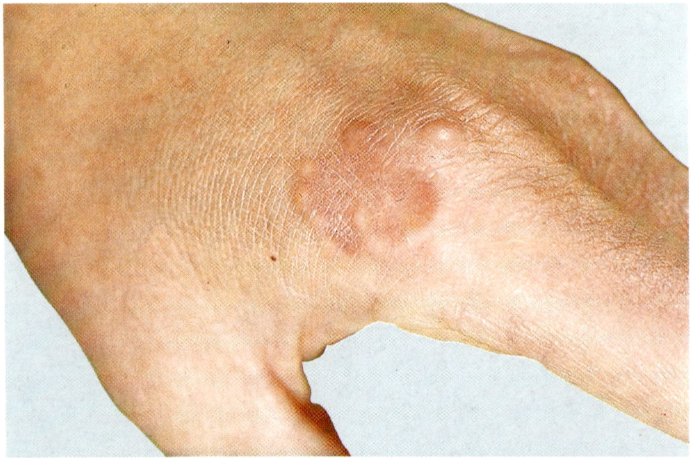

Fig. P9a.   Granuloma anulare. This is a chronic eruption, generally asymptomatic, in which there is a ringlike arrangement of papules or nodules. This is a typical location, on the dorsum of the fingers and hand, but the lesion may also occur on the elbows, neck, feet, and buttocks. The etiology is unknown. The lesions tend to regress spontaneously.

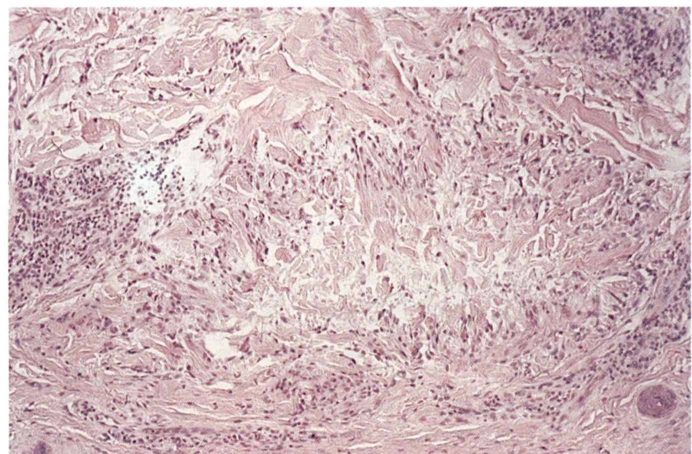

Fig. P9b.   Photomicrograph of granuloma anulare. This lesion resembles a rheumatoid nodule and consists of an oval, granulomatous lesion with a central necrotic area and peripheral radially arranged (palisading) histiocytes with sparsely distributed lymphocytes.   (hematoxylin-eosin)

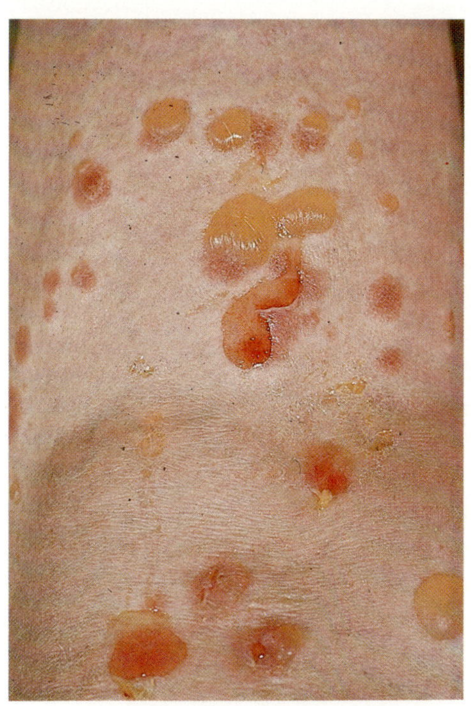

Fig. P10.   Pemphigus vulgaris. Multiple soft bullous lesions, which bleed secondarily, are seen on the skin. Pemphigus refers to a group of bullous disorders of unknown etiology, most of which were fatal before corticosteroids were available. Both sexes are equally affected, and the diseases affect mainly those between 40 and 70 years of age. Pemphigus often begins in the mucous membranes of the mouth, and skin may not be involved for a number of months. The several varieties of pemphigus include pemphigus vulgaris, pemphigus foliaceus, and pemphigus vegitans, which are differentiated primarily on the basis of the acuteness of the disease or the type of lesions accompanying the vesicles.

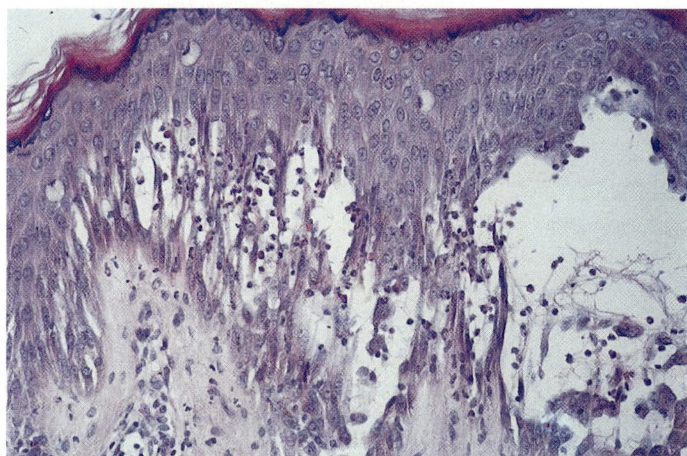

Fig. P11a.   Pemphigus vulgaris with bullous formation. There is superbasilar dissolution with accumulation of serous fluid in the formed space. The basal layer of cells is preserved. The superficial layers form the covering of the bulla. Isolated clusters of epithelial cells are present, along with a few inflammatory cells, in the bulla. These isolated acantholytic cells are known as Tzanck cells. (hematoxylin-eosin)

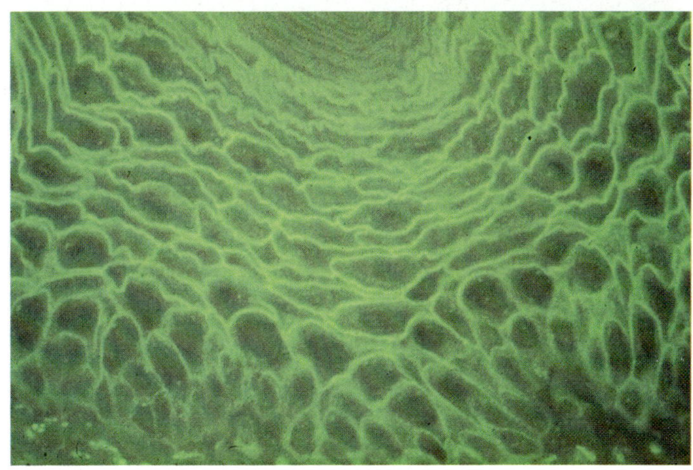

Fig. P11b.   Immunofluorescent microscopy of pemphigus showing fixation of antibodies in the intercellular space of the epidermis.

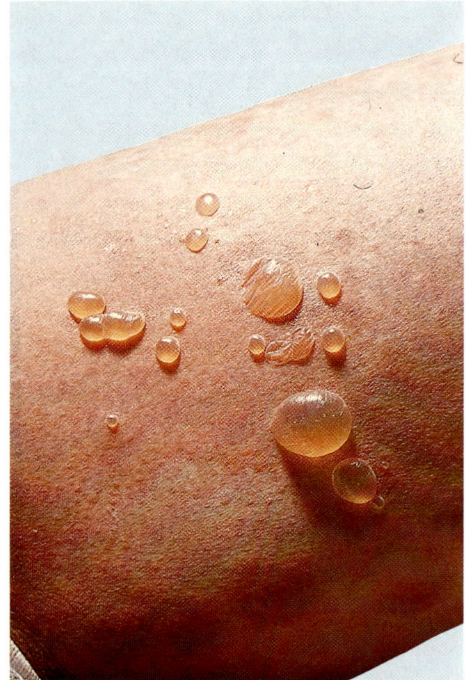

Fig. P 12. Pemphigoid. Pemphigoid is thought to be a variant of erythema multiforme bullosum, as is the Stevens-Johnson syndrome. Pemphigoid, on occasion, may be associated with visceral cancer. The bullous lesions in this photograph have faint circular erythematous zones.

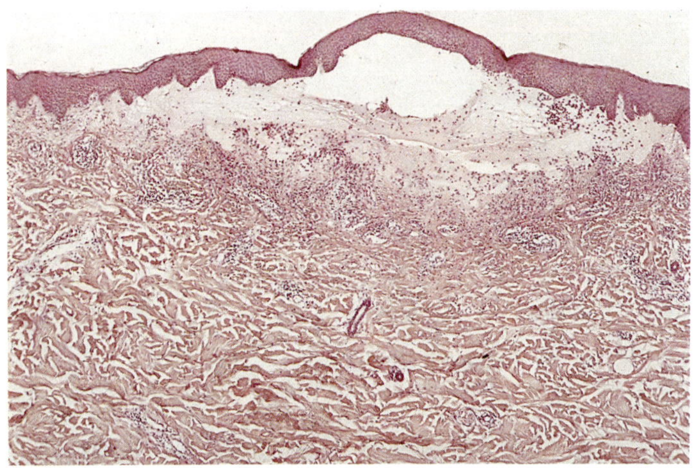

Fig. P 13a. Photomicrograph of bullous pemphigoid. The bulla forms between the epidermis and dermis. There is a relatively sparse dermal reaction, and Tzanck cells are absent. (hematoxylin-eosin)

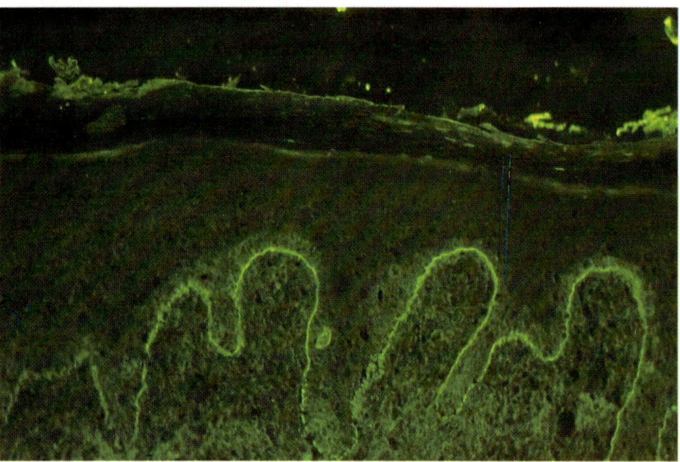

Fig. P 13b. Immunofluorescent study of bullous pemphigoid shows deposition of antibasement membrane antibodies.

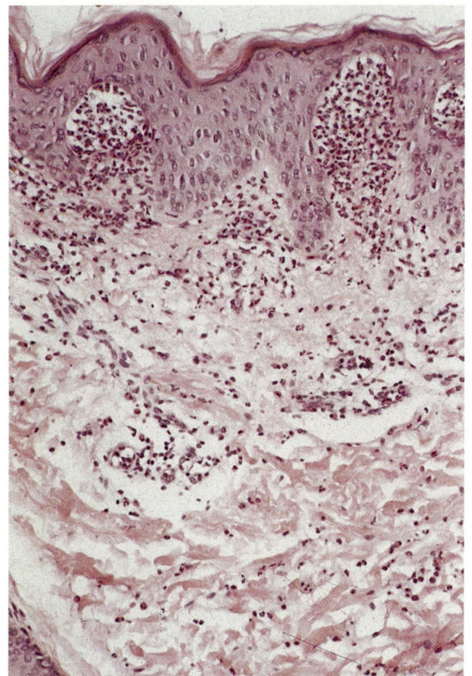

Fig. P14. Dermatitis herpetiformis (Duhring's disease). This condition is symmetrically distributed as groups of lesions in the scapular region, on the buttocks, or on the extremities. Most often there are vesicles which may be tiny or relatively large, but some of the lesions may be erythematous macules or papules. The etiology is unknown. Some patients with dermatitis herpetiformis also have celiac sprue *(Fig. G32)*. In this typical photomicrograph there is a collection of serum, fibrin, neutrophilic, and eosinophilic leukocytes in an area of cleavage of the epidermis from the underlying dermis at the tip of the dermal papilla. (hematoxylin-eosin)

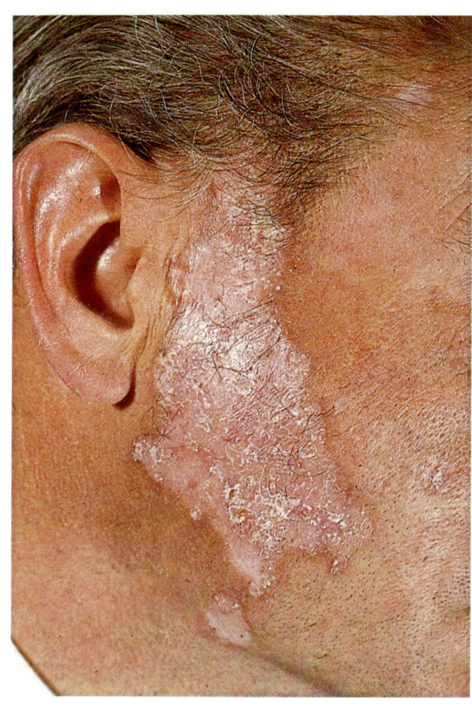

P 15a

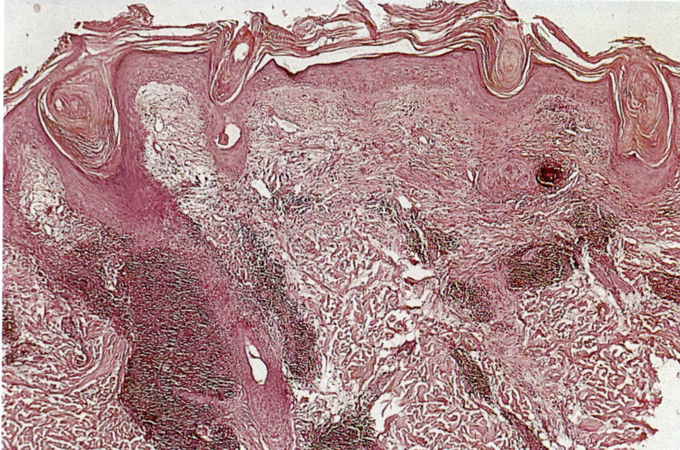

P 15b

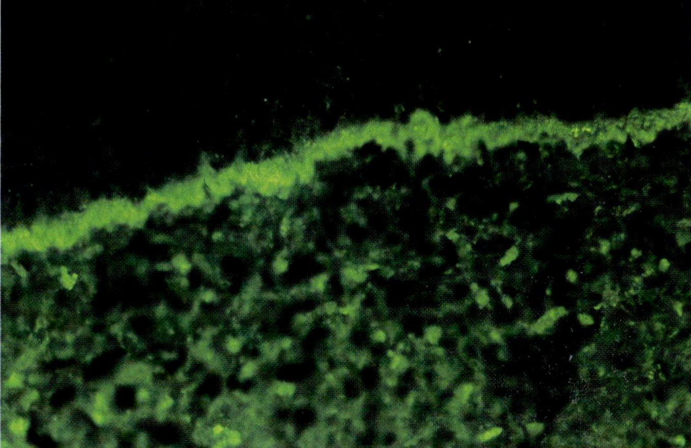

P 15c

Fig. P15. Discoid lupus erythematosus.
a) A large, well defined ("discoid") irregular plaque-like area of skin is covered with lichenoid scales, and there is an erythematous border.
b) Photomicrograph showing epidermal atrophy, hyperkeratosis particularly over hair follicles, and focal perivascular lymphocytic infiltrates.
c) Immunofluorescence showing band-like deposition of immune complexes in the basement membrane. (hematoxylin-eosin)

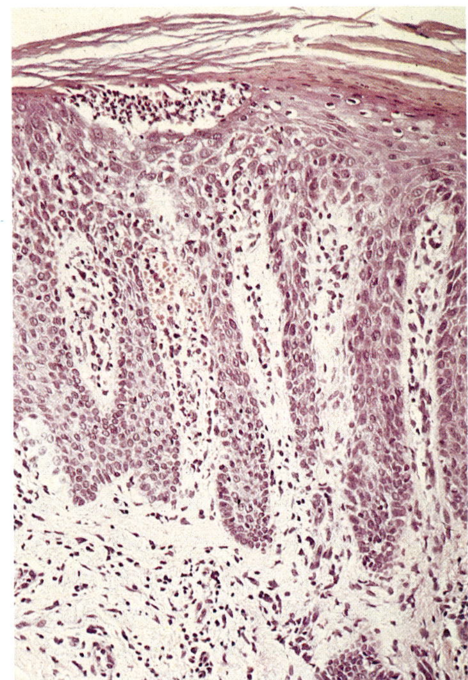

Fig. P 16.   Psoriasis. Psoriasis is characterized by reddish-brown papules covered with silvery-white scales. The condition tends to be symmetrical and most prominent on the knees and elbows. This chronic condition may be resistant to therapy. In this photomicrograph there is characteristic parakeratosis, elongation, clubbing, and fusion of rete pegs, thinning of the epidermis above dermal papillae, and accumulation of acute inflammatory cells in the Malpighian layer (micro-abscesses of Munro).   (hematoxylin-eosin)

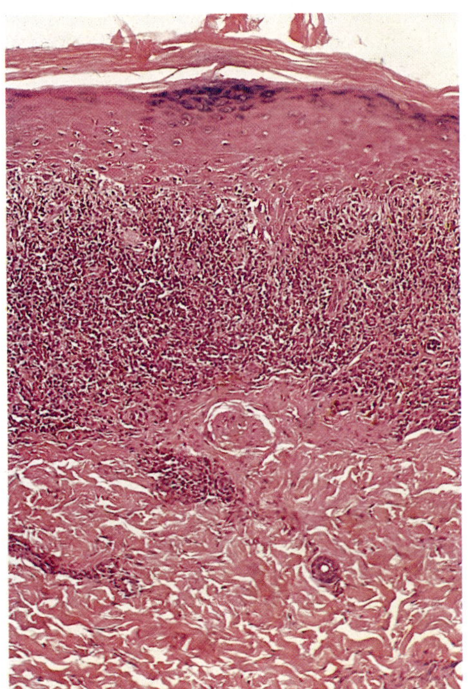

Fig. P 17.   Lichen planus. This condition is generally easily recognized as irregular, violaceous, flat, shiny, pruritic papules which are distributed symmetrically along the flexor aspects of the wrists, forearms, and legs. This condition generally resolves spontaneously. This photomicrograph shows characteristic hyperkeratosis and acanthosis with prominence of the stratum granulosum. There is slight degeneration of the basal layer and a dense band-like mononuclear infiltrate consisting of lymphocytes and histiocytes, sharply limited to the papillary and subpapillary portions of the dermis.   (hematoxylin-eosin)

Tumors   (P 18 – P 28)

Fig. P 18.   Bowen's disease.
a) Irregular, erythematous, scaling patches on the skin superficially resembling psoriasis.
b) In this photomicrograph the usual epidermal architecture is replaced, and there is loss of squamous maturation, proliferation of large cells without the usual nuclear orientation, multinucleated epithelial cells, many atypical mitoses, and dyskeratosis. (hematoxylin-eosin)

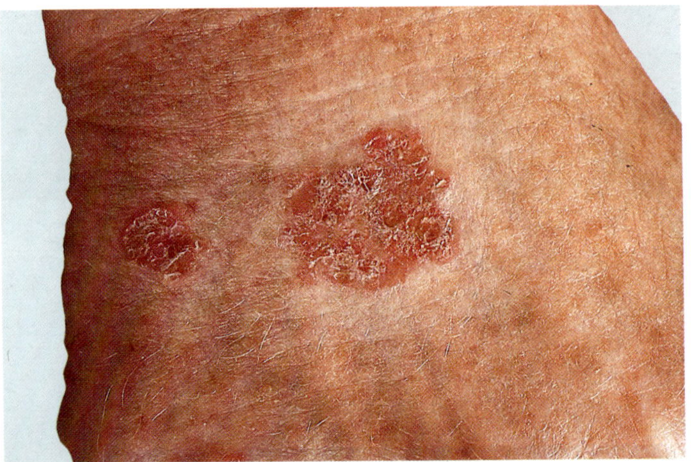

P 18a

P 18b

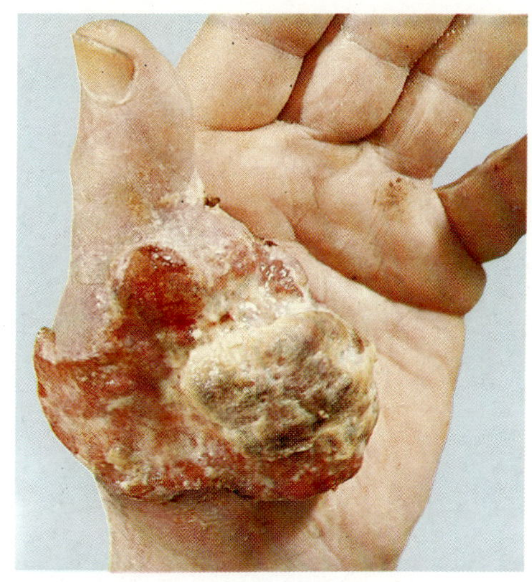

Fig. P19. Large squamous cell carcinoma of the hand. Histologically, this is keratinizing squamous cell carcinoma with extensive necrosis. Squamous cell carcinoma may occur in any part of the body, but there is a predilection for exposed areas such as the face and, as in this case, hands. Chronic irritation predisposes to squamous cell carcinoma, and a number of factors including heat, various carcinogens, and arsenic have been incriminated. However, the most important pathogenetic factor is ultraviolet light from sun exposure.

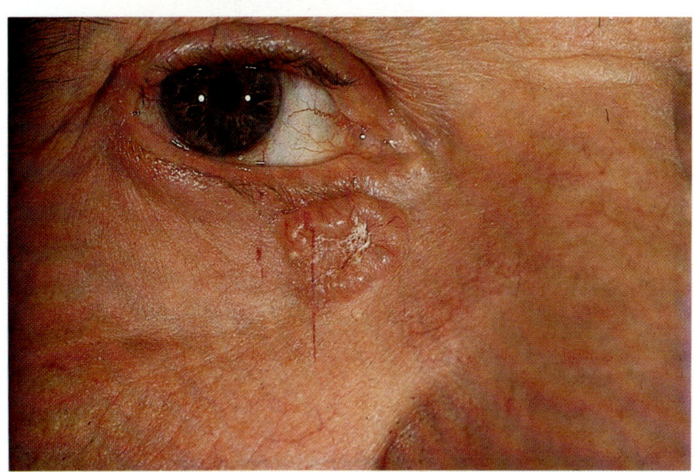

Fig. P20a. Basal cell carcinoma of the lower eyelid. Although metastases are infrequent with basal cell carcinomas, these neoplasms do progress, erode, and infiltrate neighboring bone and cartilage. They occur predominantly in blonde, fair-skinned people in the region of the face bounded by the hair line, ears, and upper lip, but may occur in any part of the body. The edges of this irregular tumor are raised and nodular and there is an irregular flat central zone of ulceration.

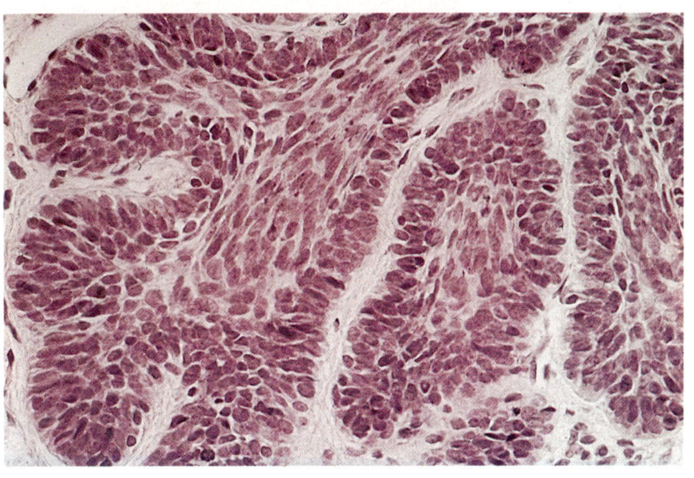

Fig. P20b. Photomicrograph of basal cell carcinoma. Nests of closely packed, relatively uniform, oval cells with dark nuclei are separated by central zones of more polyhedral cells without intracellular bridges. The nests are often rimmed, as in this case, by a layer of similar cells arranged in a fairly uniform radial pattern reminiscent of the vertically arranged basal cells of the normal epidermis.   (hematoxylin-eosin)

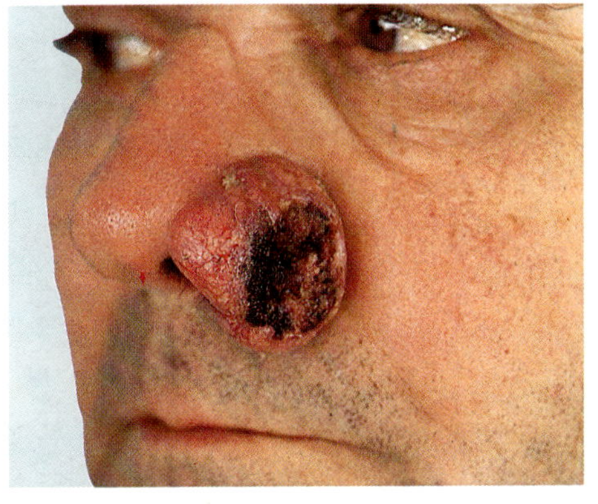

Fig. P21. Keratoacanthoma. This raised, coarsely granular hyperkeratotic squamous tumor, with a central necrotic crater, is often difficult to distinguish from a squamous cell carcinoma. These lesions are essentially keratinous masses with prominent pseudoepitheliomatous hyperplasia at their bases and periphery.

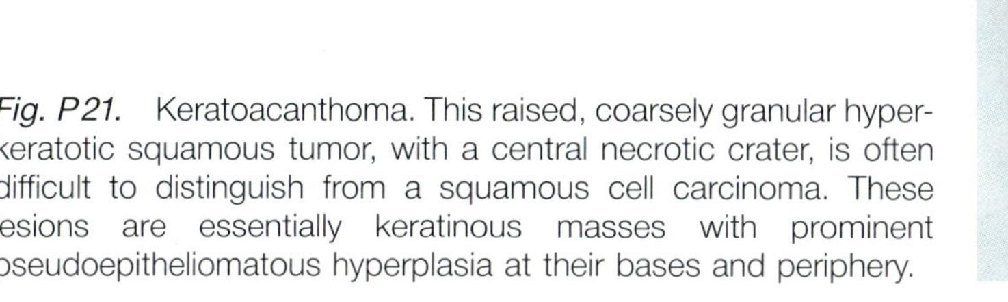

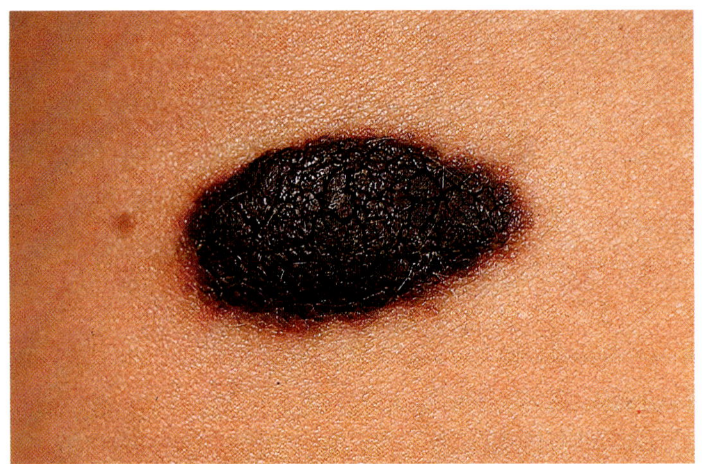

Fig. P22a.   Darkly pigmented nevus. Benign nevi may occur within the dermis, in which case they are biologically innocuous, and at the dermal epidermal junction, where they are a direct forerunner of malignant melanoma. Fortunately, malignant transformation of junctional nevi occurs relatively infrequently. Compound nevi, including both the intradermal and junctional components may occur. Blue nevi consist of interlacing bundles of spindle cells with relatively long cytoplasmic processes and varying degress of pigmentation, which appear blue through the intact skin.

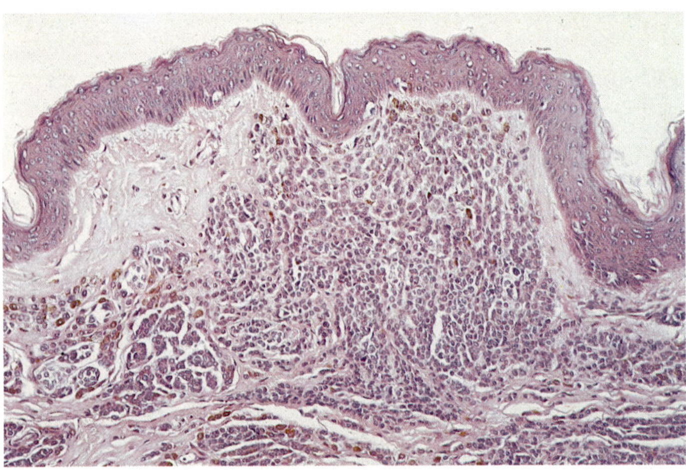

Fig. P22b.   Intradermal nevus. The characteristic nevus cells have relatively pale cytoplasm in small uniform nuclei. The cells tend to occur in spherical nests. This lesion is not associated with malignant change.   (hematoxylin-eosin)

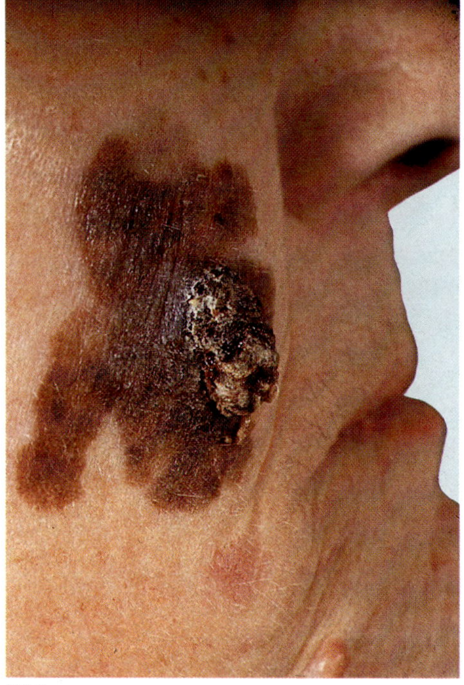

P23a

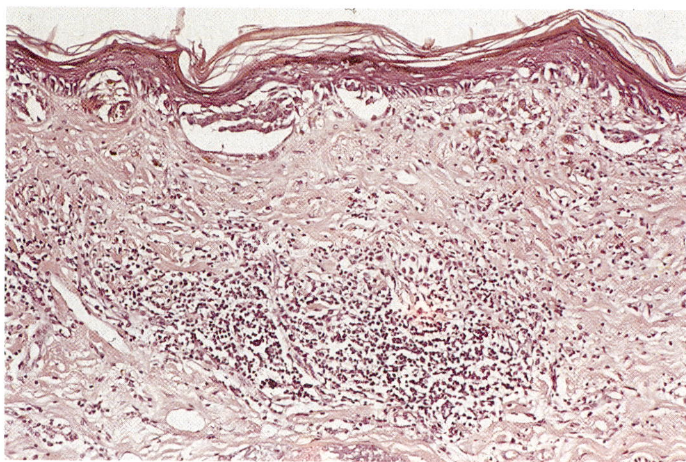

P23b

Fig. P23.   Malignant melanoma, lentigo maligna variant. *a)* The tumor spreads out horizontally as an irregularly pigmented lesion with focal nodularity. *b)* Histologically, there are many atypical, spindle-shaped melanocytes in flat and spherical clusters immediately beneath the epidermis, with single, barely perceptible in this lower power photomicrograph, tumor cells migrating upward into the epidermis.   (hematoxylin-eosin)

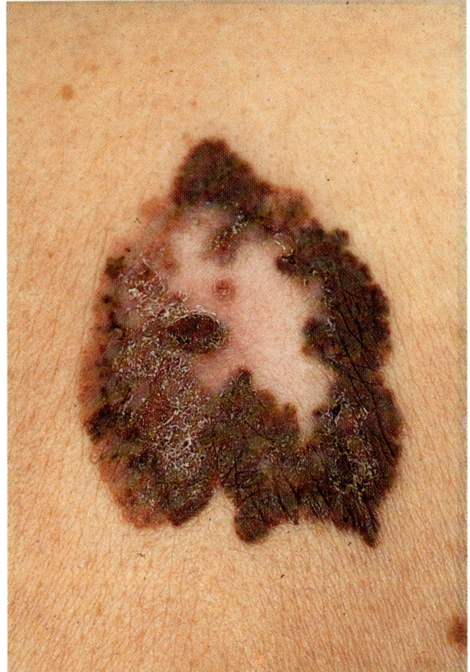

P24a

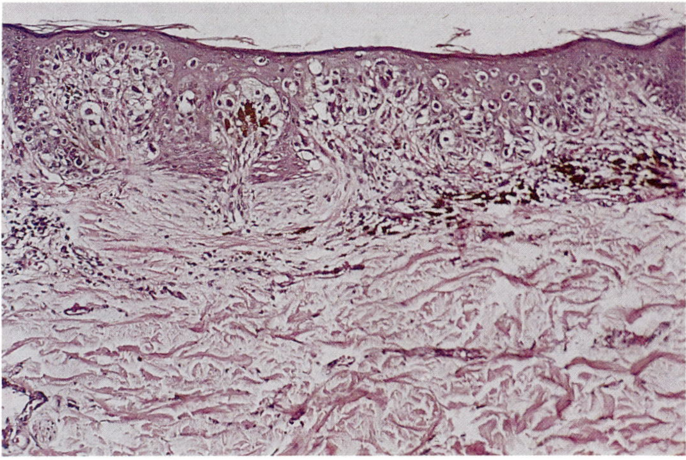

P24b

Fig. P24. *a)* Malignant melanoma, superficial spreading variant. The tumor edges are irregular and, in places, poorly defined. There are scattered hyperkeratotic scales and a central pale zone of spontaneous regression. *b)* Histologically nests of melanoma cells are spreading throughout the lower epidermis, with invasion both downward into the dermis and, as single cells, up into the epidermis. (Stains a, b: hematoxylin-eosin)

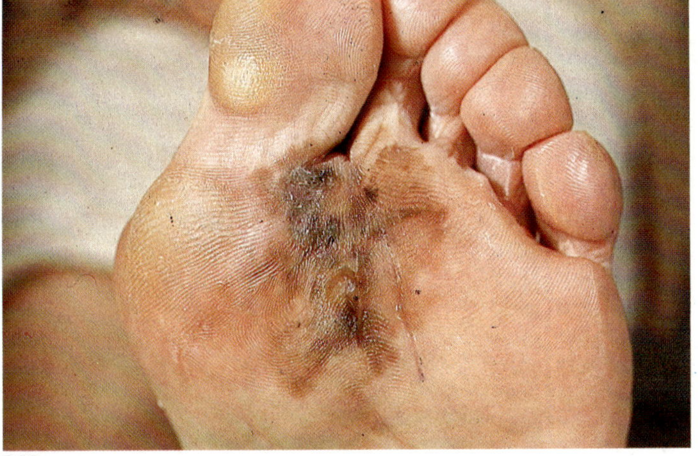

P25a

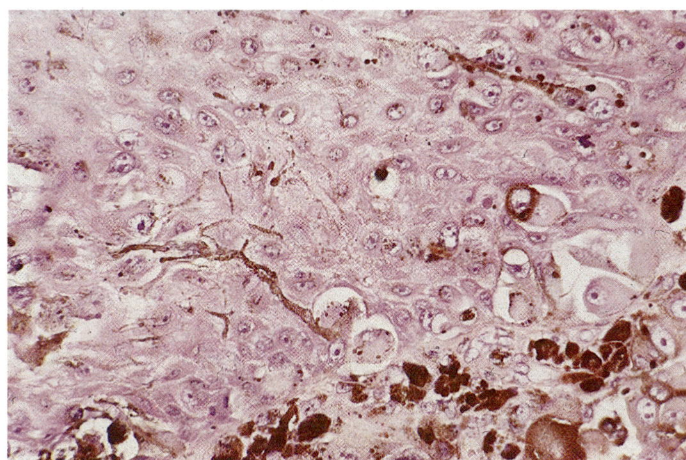

P25b

Fig. P25. Malignant melanoma, acral lentiginous variant.
a) The tumor is poorly defined, irregularly pigmented, and hyper-keratotic.
b) Highly atypical, darkly pigmented tumor cells are at the lower portion of the picture. Some of the intradermal tumor cells have long branching dendrites. (hematoxylin-eosin)

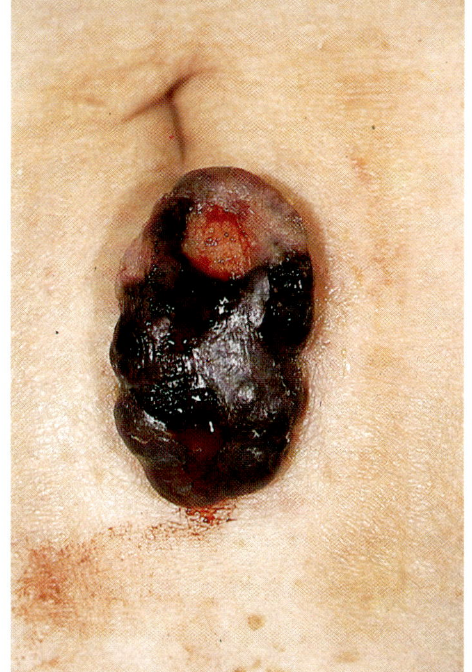

Fig. P26. Malignant melanoma, nodular variant. A large, irregular, brown-black tumor mass protrudes on the skin. There are areas of hemorrhage and necrotic ulceration.

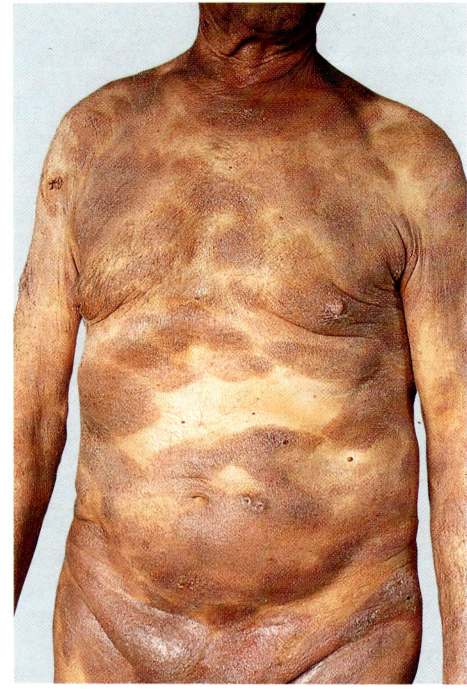

Fig. P27. Mycosis fungoides, infiltrative stage. There is diffuse involvement of the skin by a flat, expansive, irregularly nodular, erythematous and focally hyperkeratotic process. This malignant proliferation of T-cells involves the epidermis, dermis, and subdermal tissue, and, in as many as 70 percent of cases, there may also be visceral involvement at the time of death.

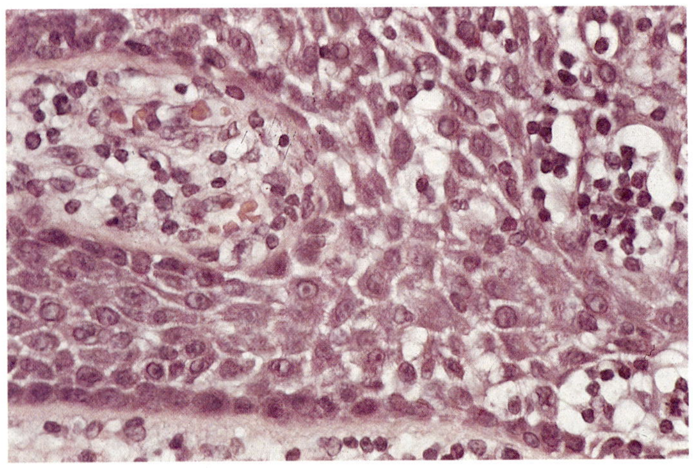

Fig. P28. Photomicrograph of mycosis fungoides showing small intraepidermal "micro-abscesses" of Darier-Pautrier. These "micro-abscesses" are microscopic foci of malignant T-cells that have extended into the epidermis.   (hematoxylin-eosin)

Q. Urinary Tract

W. Rotter

The kidneys serve major metabolic functions. The formation and excretion of urine serves to delicately balance both fluid equilibrium and mineral metabolism. In addition to these activities, the kidneys are most likely responsible for normal red blood cell production as the principal source of erythropoietin. Although some of the functional activities of the kidneys are not completely understood, in general there are morphologically identifiable structures which correspond to the various activities of the kidneys. In addition to epithelial and mesenchymal components, the kidneys are highly vascular organs. The glomeruli participate in the blood filtration process and production of urine. In addition the interstitium is highly vascular. Diseases of the vessels may lead to major functional as well as morphologic sequela.

Although renal malformations are present at birth, they may not manifest until a relatively advanced age. Atherosclerosis may affect the kidneys directly, by involvement of renal arteries and arterioles, or indirectly because of cardiac or aortic disease. Renal hypertension has characteristic morphologic features in the kidneys and, of course, affects other parts of the cardiovascular system.

A group of diseases which involve the kidneys may be dissimilar in pathogenesis and many clinical features, but have the common clinical finding of massive proteinuria, hypoproteinemia, peripheral edema, and hyperlipemia. This constellation of findings is known as the nephrotic syndrome and may be due to immune complex disorders, circulatory diseases, or metabolic disorders, and may also occur in pregnancy and may be hereditary.

The noninflammatory glomerulopathies are morphologically characteristic and may reflect a variety of pathogenetic mechanisms. Glomeruli may be injured by metabolic, vascular, and toxic mechanisms, in addition to inflammatory phenomena. In many cases of noninflammatory glomerulopathy, the nephrotic syndrome is a manifestation, but this is not always the case.

The inflammatory glomerulonephritides are generally a reflection of immunologic injury. A variety of morphologic patterns may be identified. These patterns reflect differing pathogenetic mechanisms and are often associated with varying clinical manifestations. The glomerulonephritides may be acute or chronic and may cause hypertension, as well as disordered urinary excretion. Chronic glomerulonephritis, no matter the pathogenesis, leads to shrunken ("end-stage") kidneys.

The interstitial nephritides are also important. The term interstitial nephritis refers to a variety of acute and chronic inflammatory processes that predominantly involve the renal interstitial tissue. To a great degree, interstitial inflammation may be secondary to glomerular, vascular, and renal tubular disorders. Longstanding interstitial nephritis may also lead to an end-stage kidney.

Calcium metabolism is particularly important in the kidney since calcium salts may precipitate in the tubules. This may be due to local tubular injury ("dystrophic calcification") or may reflect systemic hypercalcemia ("metastatic calcification"). The cellular deposition of calcium salts leads to tubular dysfunction. In general these forms of nephrocalcinosis are not thought to be a part of the pathogenesis of renal stone formation. Renal stone formation is thought to be due to both excessive concentration of the various constituents of renal stones as well as local physico-chemical alterations which predispose the mineral precipitation. Renal stones may lead to tubular injury and renal obstruction with subsequent development of pyelonephritis.

The most important malignant tumor of the kidney is the renal cell carcinoma ("hypernephroma") which is thought to arise from epithelial cells of proximal convoluted tubules. The macro- and microscopic features are characteristic. Renal cell carcinoma has a great propensity for metastasis and may spread to virtually any part of the body.

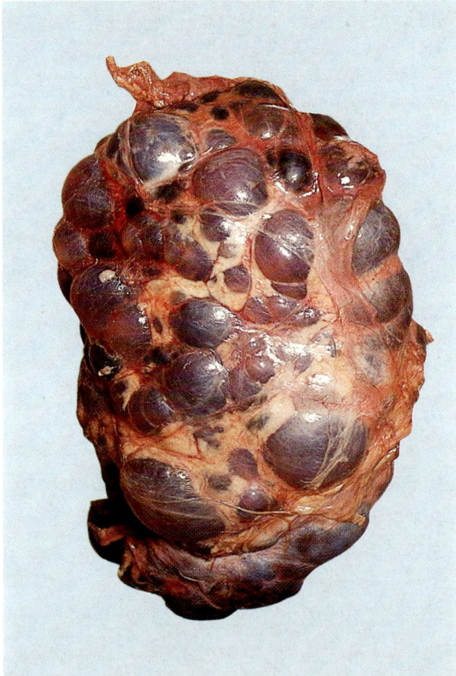

Renal Malformations *(Q1–Q2)*

Fig. Q1.   Adult polycystic disease of the kidney (Potter type III). This kidney is approximately 25 cm long and 6 cm wide. The surface is coarsely nodular because of the varying size of the cysts. The parenchyma is almost completely destroyed and replaced by the cysts which are lined by renal tubular epithelial cells and contain an ultrafiltrate of urine.

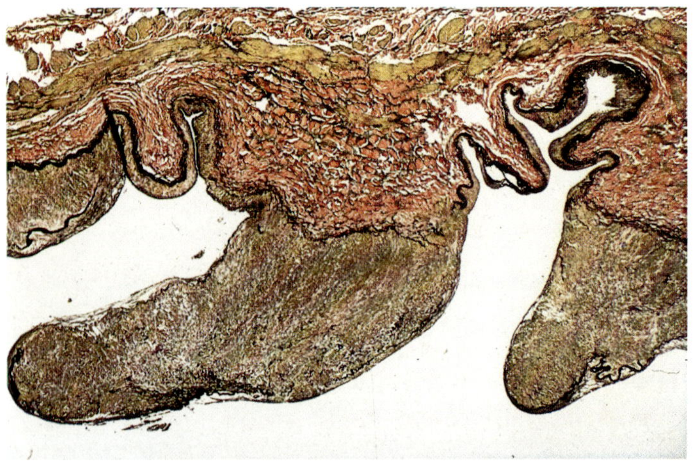

Fig. Q2.   Fibromuscular hyperplasia of the renal artery. This is a form of intimal and muscular hyperplasia which is relatively rare and causes hypertension, particularly affecting young women. In this photomicrograph the greatly proliferated intima can be seen protruding, in multiple areas, into the lumen. The underlying internal elastic membrane is frayed, and the muscle and its elastic fibers are thickened.   (van Gieson-elastica)

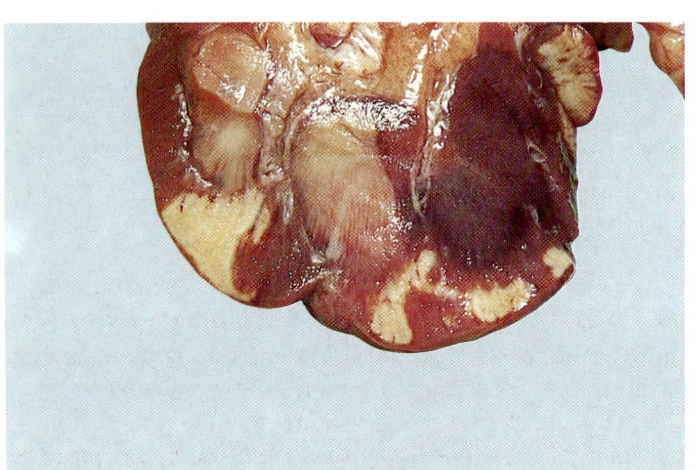

Circulatory Disturbances *(Q3–Q7)*

Fig. Q3.   Multiple renal infarcts. The infarct on the left shows the characteristic wedge shape, with the base at the periphery and the apex pointing towards the renal hilum. The yellow represents completely necrotic renal tissue. The infarct is bordered by a thin erythematous rim, representing vascular dilatation and congestion as a part of the inflammatory response. A similar thin erythematous line lies between the infarcts and the capsule; this is the area supplied by capsule arteries.

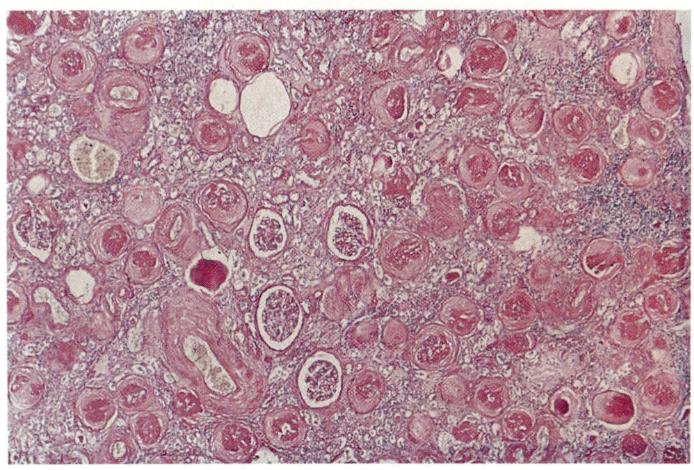

Fig. Q4. Focal atrophy of the kidney. In this photomicrograph the cortex shows extensive tubular atrophy and glomerular sclerosis. Because of the tubular atrophy the glomeruli are relatively close together and appear to be increased in number. There is a moderate amount of nonspecific, secondary interstitial inflammation. This type of change follows longstanding, severe vascular insufficiency. (hematoxylin-eosin)

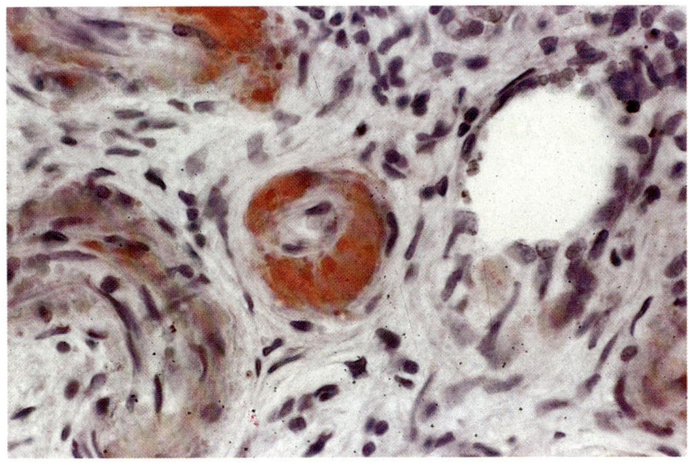

Fig. Q5. Nephrosclerosis. These kidneys are smaller than normal. They weighed approximately 100 gm each rather than the usual 150 gm. The surfaces are marked by coarse nodularity which are reflections of atrophic areas *(Fig. Q4)* separated by bulging zones of intact and hyperplastic tubules. The coarseness of the nodularity indicates that the disease is primarily arterial, rather than arteriolar.

Fig. Q6. Arteriolar nephrosclerosis. The arteriole in the center of the photomicrograph is almost completely occluded by the accumulation of mural sudanophilic (lipid) material which has completely replaced the media. This kidney would also be reduced in size, but the surface would be finely granular since the primary disease is in arterioles.

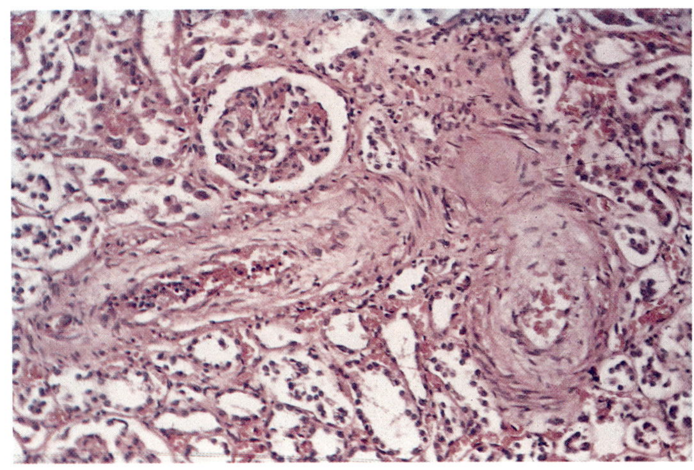

Fig. Q7. Malignant nephrosclerosis. A small artery, in the renal cortex, shows marked intimal proliferation and fibrosis with narrowing of the lumen. This patient clinically manifested with hypertension refractory to treatment.   (hematoxylin-eosin)

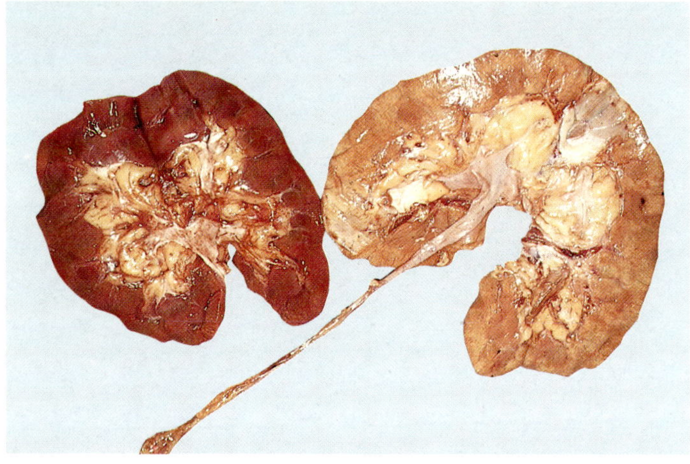

Nephroses   *(Q8–Q9)*

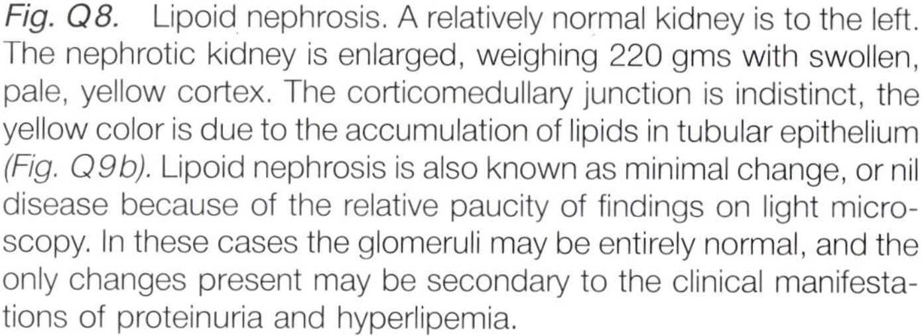

Fig. Q8.   Lipoid nephrosis. A relatively normal kidney is to the left. The nephrotic kidney is enlarged, weighing 220 gms with swollen, pale, yellow cortex. The corticomedullary junction is indistinct, the yellow color is due to the accumulation of lipids in tubular epithelium *(Fig. Q9b)*. Lipoid nephrosis is also known as minimal change, or nil disease because of the relative paucity of findings on light microscopy. In these cases the glomeruli may be entirely normal, and the only changes present may be secondary to the clinical manifestations of proteinuria and hyperlipemia.

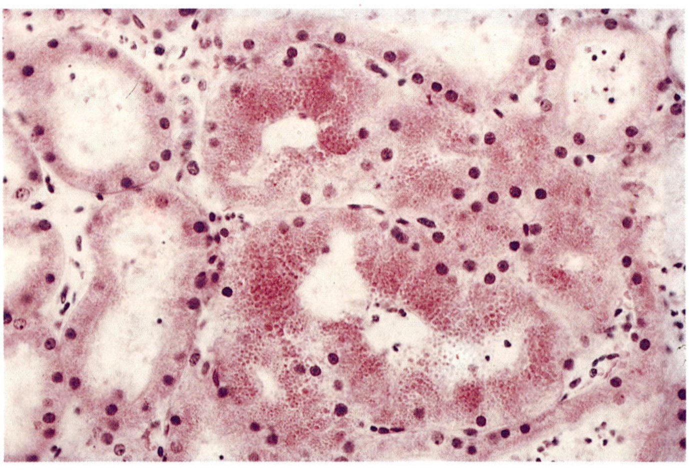

Fig. Q9a.   Photomicrograph of renal tubules showing hyalin droplets due to reabsorption in a patient with nephrotic syndrome. This morphologic manifestation is due to proteinuria. Protein is seen as homogeneous, eosinophilic droplets in epithelial cells. (hematoxylin-eosin)

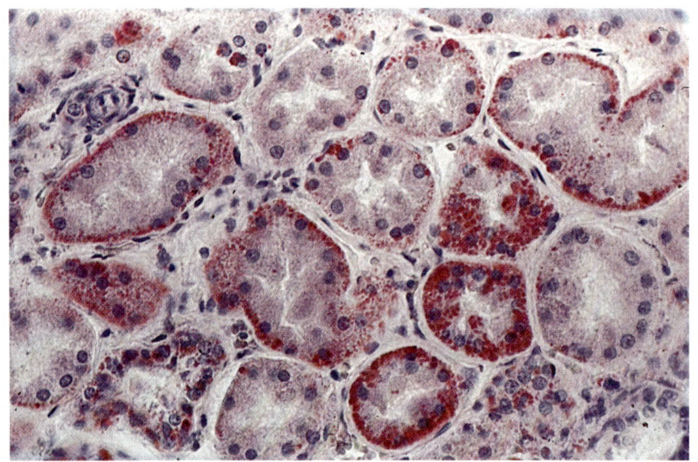

Fig. Q9b.   Fatty droplets in renal epithelial cells. There is reabsorption of fat in patients with nephrotic syndrome who are hyperlipemic. The fat, stained red with Sudan, is seen as uniform fine droplets in renal tubular epithelium.

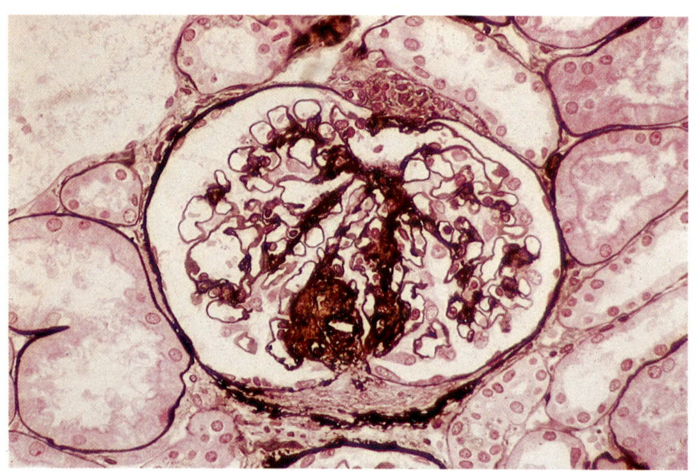

Noninflammatory Glomerulopathies   *(Q10–Q13)*

Fig. Q10.   Focal segmental glomerulosclerosis. In this condition there is focal sclerosis of glomerular lobules with thickening of basement membrane and the development of adhesions and fibrinoid nodules. An adhesion between the formed glomerular lobule and Bowman's capsule is seen at the lower portion of the photomicrograph. This condition initially manifests as nephrotic syndrome but tends to be resistant to steroid therapy and, in many cases, may progress to renal failure. In contrast to lipoid nephrosis, this condition is more common in adults.   (PAS-methenamine-fuchsin).

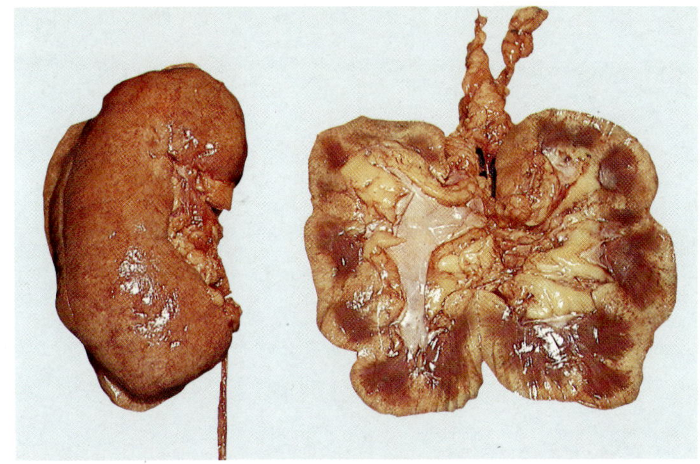

Fig. Q11. Renal amyloidosis. The kidneys are enlarged and have a smooth surface. The cortex is quite pale and is waxy to the touch. The pale cortex contrasts dramatically with the red renal medulla.

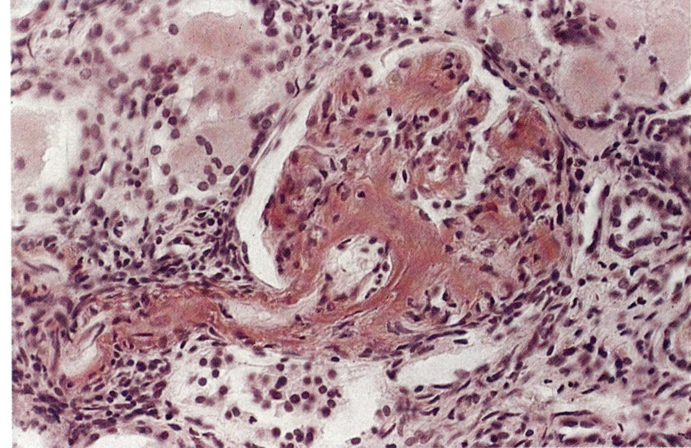

Fig. Q12. Renal amyloidosis.

Fig. Q12a. Homogeneous deposits of amyloid can be seen in this photomicrograph of a renal glomerulus after staining with Congo red. The amyloid can be seen in the wall of the afferent arteriole, in the mesangium, and glomerular loops. The tubules contain pale, hyalin protein material that stains faintly with Congo red, but it is not amyloid.

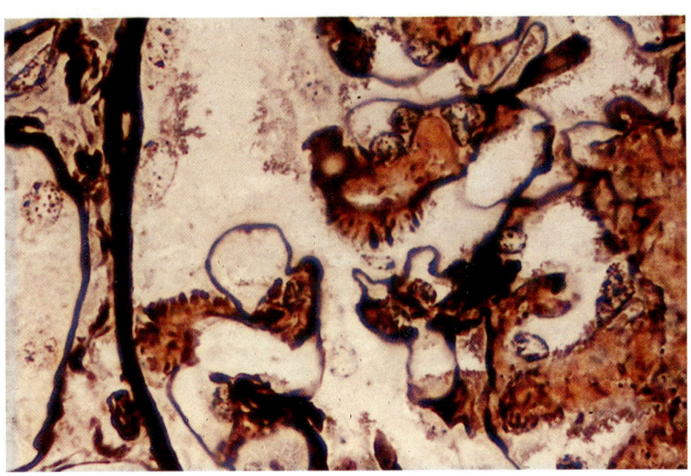

Fig. Q12b. After staining with PAS-methenamine silver, the basement membranes of the glomerular capillaries and the Bowman's capsule appear black. The amyloid, which is present both on the epithelial and endothelial sides of the glomerular basement membrane is argyrophobic and, therefore, stains brown. Spikelike argyrophilic extensions of the basement membrane can be seen between amyloid deposits. These spikes resemble those seen in membranous glomerulonephritis *(Fig. Q19).*

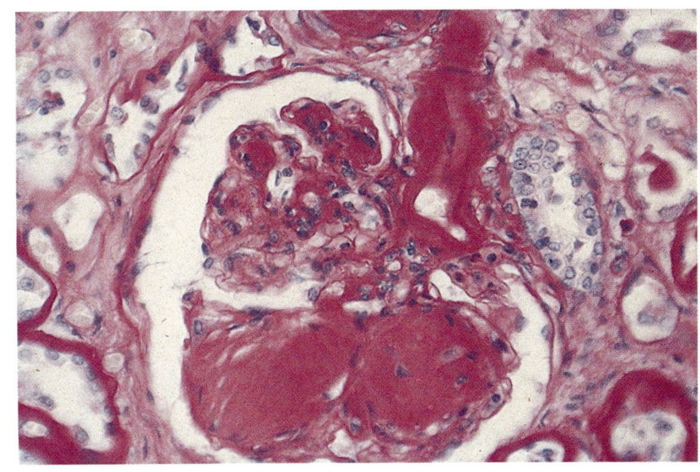

Fig. Q13. Diabetic glomerulosclerosis (Kimmelstiel-Wilson disease). The mesangium contains nodular masses of homogeneous PAS-positive material which completely obliterates the capillary channels. Similar material is seen in the wall of the afferent arteriole. The few remaining capillaries are characteristically displaced to the periphery.

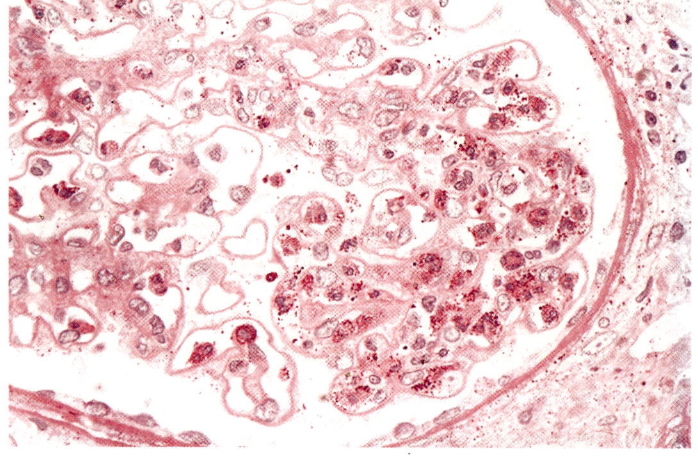

Fig. Q14.   Acute poststreptococcal glomerulonephritis. The kidney in this form of acute diffuse glomerulonephritis is moderately swollen and may be either pale or congested. The glomeruli are enlarged. There is an increase in the cellularity of the glomerular tuft because of the dilatation of capillary channels by swollen endothelial cells and acute inflammatory cells with a relative paucity of red blood cells. Electron microscopy and immunofluorescence microscopy show "humps" of immune complex deposits between basement membrane and podocytes.   (PAS)

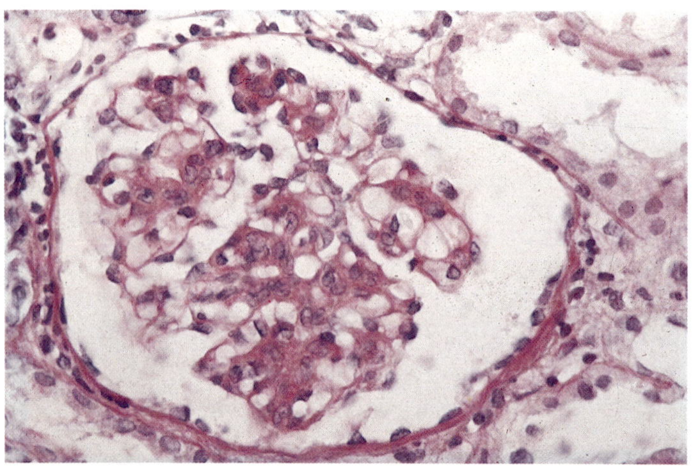

Fig. Q15.   Mesangial proliferative glomerulonephritis. The mesangium is expanded with little or no involvement of capillary lumena. The mesangium contains mononuclear cells, of mesangial origin, with clusters of four or more cells per mesangial area. There may be increased mesangial matrix and, in advanced cases, mesangial sclerosis. Capillary endothelial cells are essentially unchanged. Immunofluorescent studies demonstrate the deposition of immune complexes.   (hematoxylin-eosin)

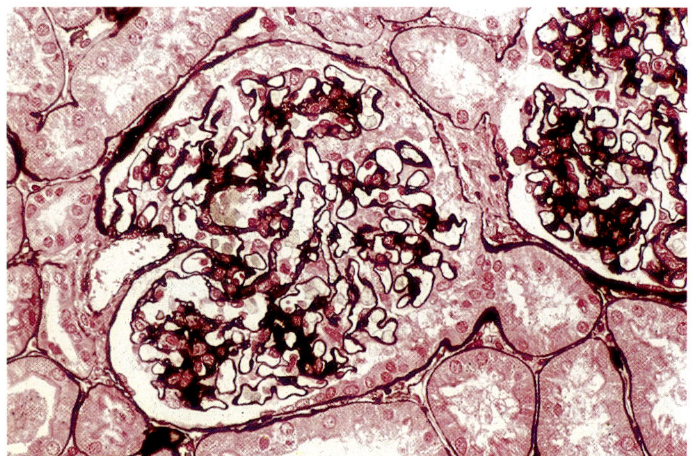

Fig. Q16.   Segmental mesangial proliferative glomerulonephritis with sclerosis. The capillary lumens are completely patent, and there is no proliferation of endothelial cells. The mesangia of some of the lobules is widened with proliferation of mesangial cells and increase of argyrophilic fibrillar material. Immunofluorescence demonstrates diffuse immune complex nephritis.   (PAS-methenamine-fuchsin)

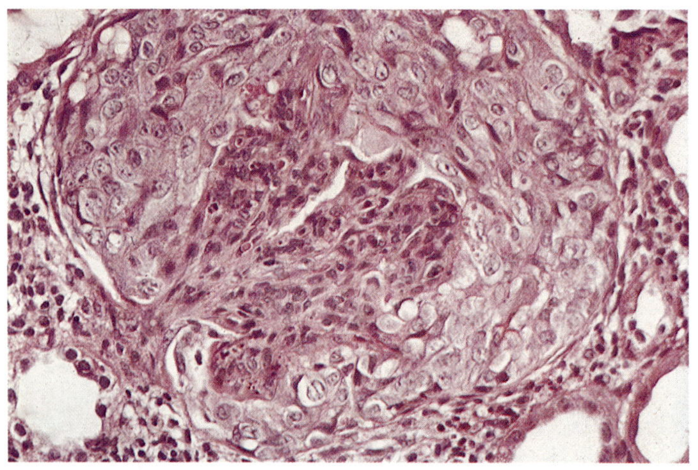

Fig. Q17.   Diffuse crescentic glomerulonephritis (extra-capillary glomerulonephritis). The glomerulus is markedly compacted and bloodless, and Bowman's space is filled with a cellular crescent. The crescents derive from the proliferating Bowman's capsule lining (parietal epithelium) with some participation of podocytes (visceral epithelium), monocytes, and polymorphonuclear leukocytes. A few polymorphonuclear leukocytes are seen in the collapsed capillaries and at the area of the glomerular hilus (lower left). Immunofluorescent studies demonstrate immune complex deposition. (hematoxylin-eosin)

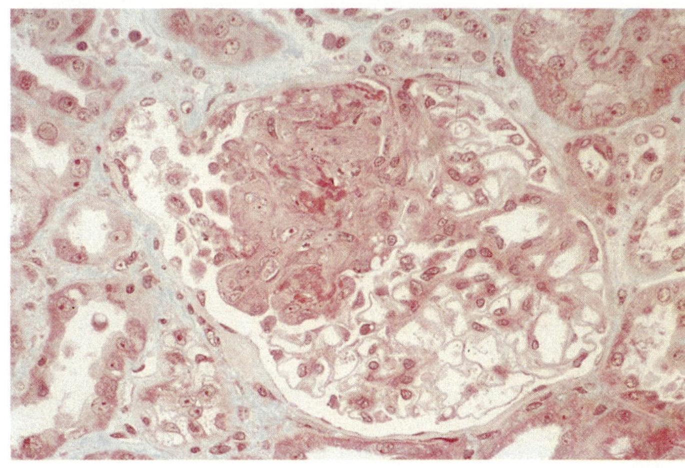

Fig. Q18.   Necrotizing anti-glomerular-basement membrane glomerulonephritis.

Fig. Q18a.   A portion of the glomerulus is completely necrotic (red, to the left) and there is focal, slight mesangial proliferation to the right of the glomerulus. The beginning of the proximal tubule system is seen at the upper left of Bowman's capsule. Immunofluorescent studies demonstrate a linear deposition of antibodies to IgG and C_3 on the basement membrane. This picture is characteristic of Goodpasture's syndrome.   (Trichrome)

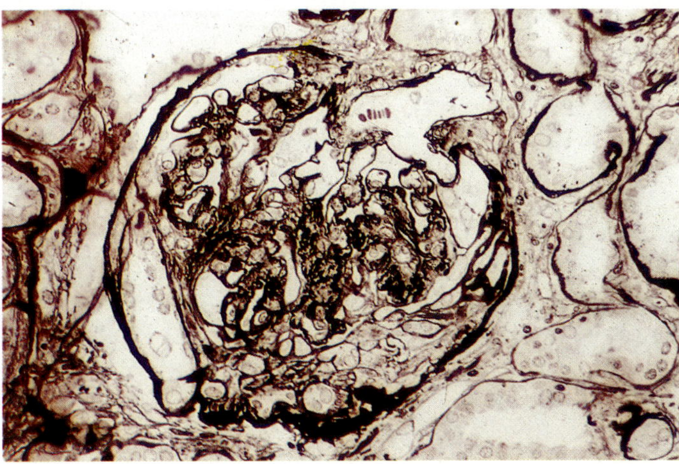

Fig. Q18b.   This is the second biopsy from the patient depicted in *Fig. Q18a,* and was obtained after a course of immunosuppressive therapy and hemodialysis. The hilus of the glomerulus is at the top right. The glomerulus itself is partially compressed by a crescent. The capillary loops adjacent to this crescent are extensively compressed and sclerotic, and the proliferation of the crescent separates lobules. A few intact capillaries are seen.   (PAS-methenamine)

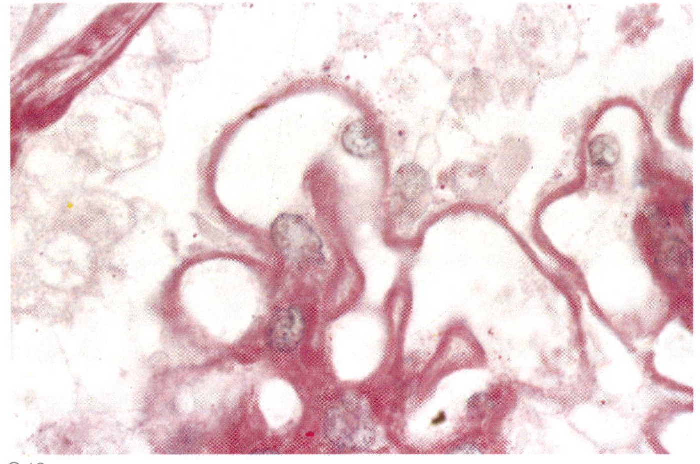

Q19a

Fig. Q19. Membranous glomerulonephritis.

Fig. Q19a. In this high magnification photomicrograph, after staining with periodic acid Schiff reagent, the capillary walls are seen to be uniformly thickened. The capillary lumens are relatively wide and there is no endothelial proliferation. In general, the mesangial areas (not shown here) are unaffected. Immunofluorescent studies demonstrate granular deposits of IgG and C_3 along the periphery of the capillary loops.

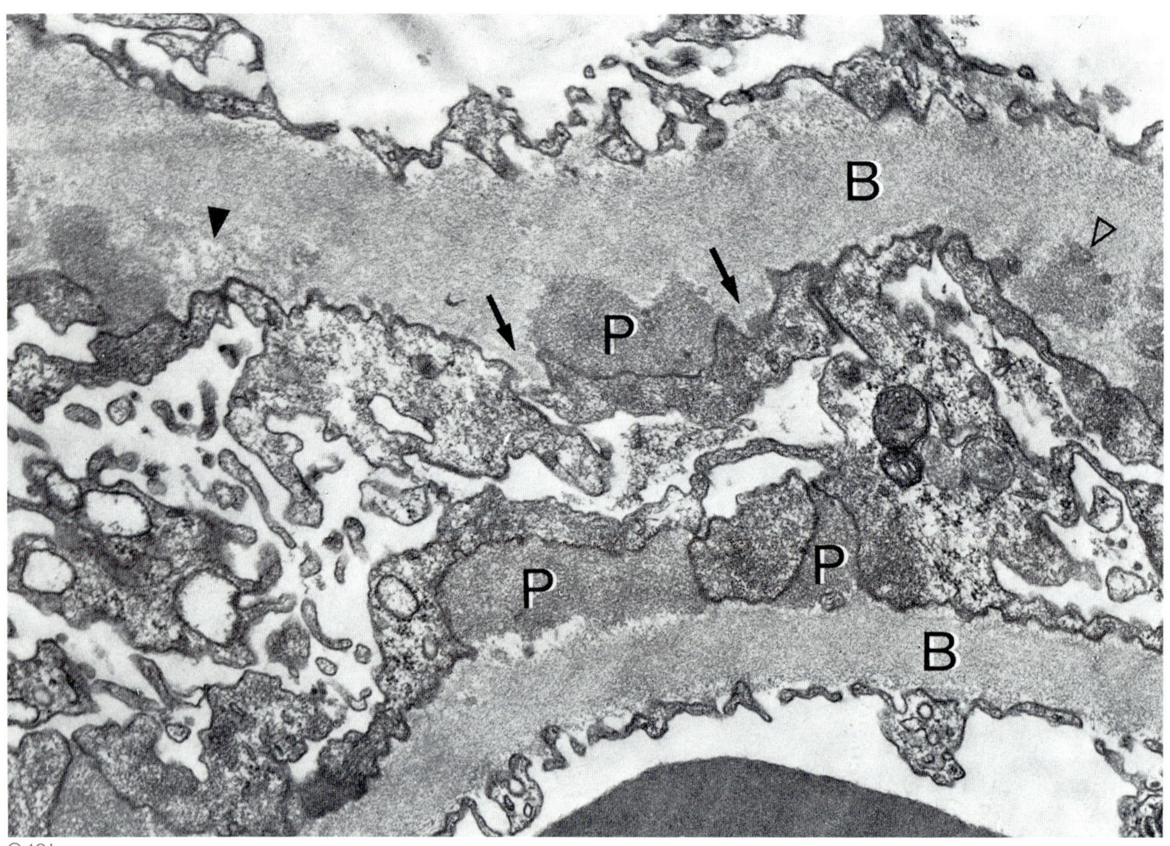

Q19b

Fig. Q19b. Electron micrograph of the basement membrane (B) showing immune deposits (P). Newly formed basement membrane material partially surrounds immune deposits forming "spikes" *(arrows)*. The open arrowhead, to the right, shows an immune deposit partially incorporated into basement membrane material. The closed arrowhead shows completely incorporated immune deposit material.

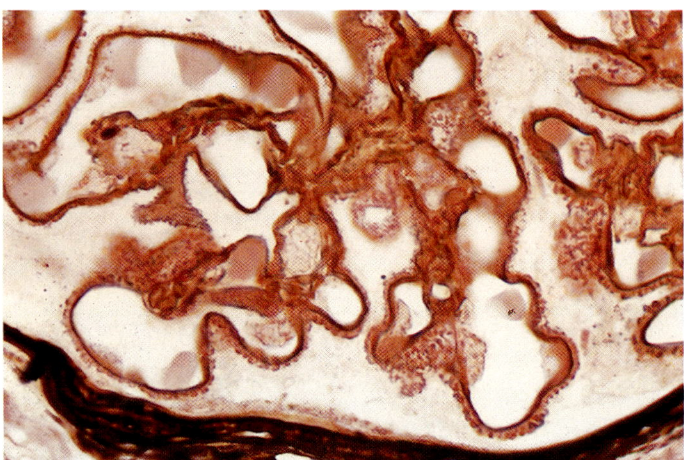

Q19c

Fig. Q19c. This PAS-methenamine-fuchsin-stained biopsy shows deposition of granular immune complexes on the basement membrane (red) separated by the argyrophilic spikes. There is no cellular proliferation, and capillary openings are completely patent.

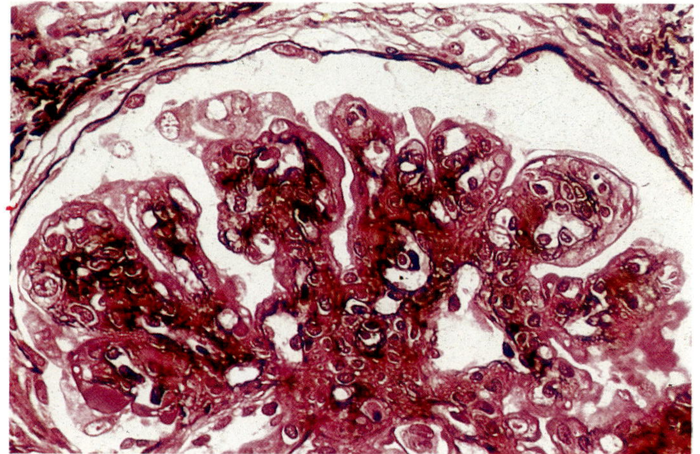

Fig. Q20. Membrano-proliferative glomerulonephritis (diffuse mesangio-capillary glomerulonephritis). The glomerulus is enlarged, and the mesangial areas are expanded by increased numbers of cells and proliferation of mesangial matrix. The lobules are accentuated. The capillary wall is thickened and, in areas, has a "double contour" appearance due to duplication of basement membrane. The glomerular capillaries are almost completely occluded and the glomerulus is relatively bloodless. Fuchsinophilic (red) subendothelial deposits, representing immune complex, are seen in the upper mid portion of the photomicrograph. Podocytes are swollen. Immunofluorescent studies confirmed the presence of IgG, IgM, and C_3. (PAS-methenamine-fuchsin)

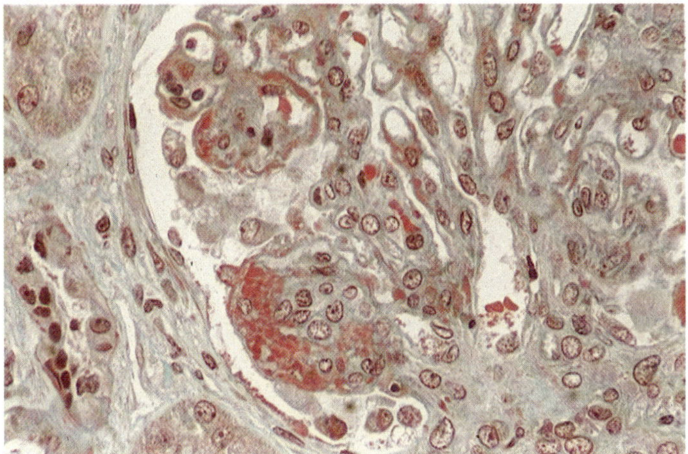

Fig. Q21. Diffuse lupus nephritis showing cellular proliferation and sclerosis. The lobule to the lower left shows mesangial proliferation with obliteration of capillaries. Mesangial cells and matrix (blue-green) are increased. At the periphery of the lobule there are abundant fuchsinophilic (red) deposits representing the deposition of immune complex and fibrinogen. At the upper left a lobule has slightly increased mesangium with only partial obliteration of capillaries. There is focal subendothelial fuchsinophilic deposit forming thickened capillary loops ("wire loops"). In the mid portion of the glomerulus the capillaries are relatively well-preserved. Immunofluorescence demonstrated granular deposition of IgG and C_3. (trichrome)

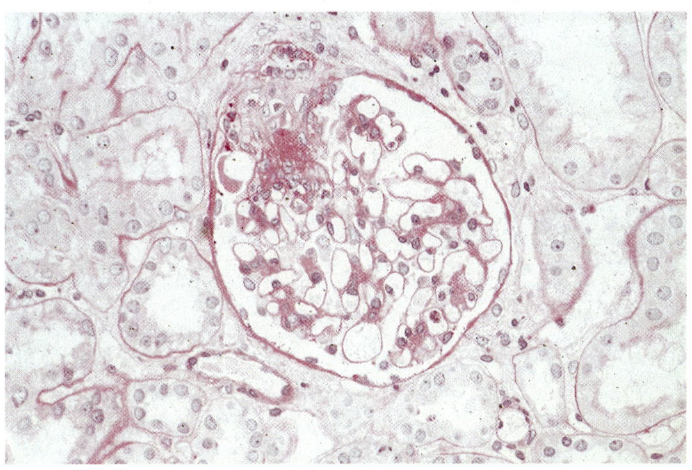

Fig. Q22. Nephritis of Henoch-Schoenlein purpura. In most patients with this condition glomerular disease is mild and self-limited. There may be diffuse mesangial proliferation and focal and segmental thrombosis, with necrosis and crescent formation. In this photomicrograph there is a characteristic triangular shaped area of sclerosis, at the upper left of the glomerulus, with adjacent, slightly thickened and sclerotic Bowman's capsule. The remainder of the glomerulus is unremarkable. (PAS)

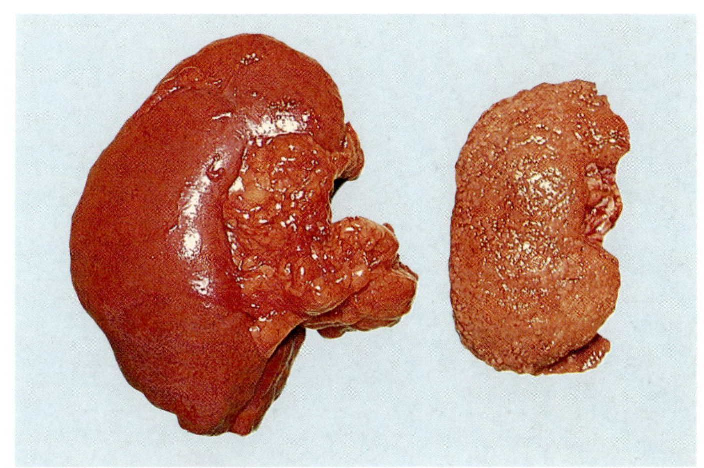

Fig. Q23. Chronic glomerulonephritis. A normal kidney is to the left. A shrunken, pale kidney, with a finely granular surface, represents the end-stage of chronic glomerulonephritis. Compare this kidney to the end-stage kidney of atherosclerosis *(Fig. Q5).*

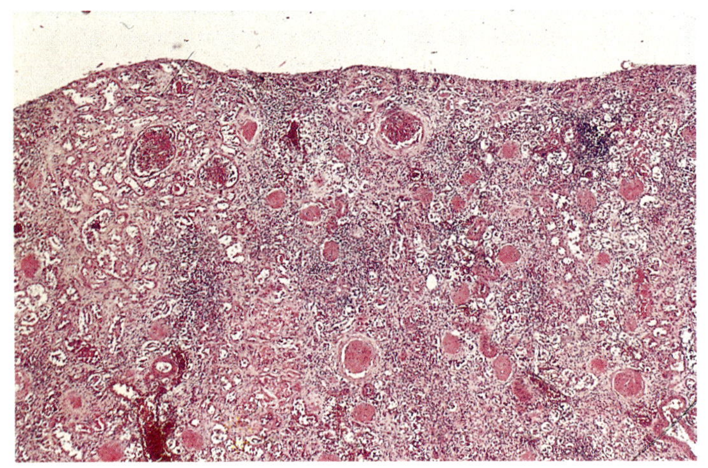

Fig. Q24. Chronic glomerulonephritis. This photomicrograph of the end-stage kidney of chronic glomerulonephritis shows almost complete atrophy of tubules and marked hyalinization of glomeruli. The number of glomeruli is reduced and, because of the tubular atrophy, they are relatively close together. The interstitium is infiltrated by many lymphocytes. A few of the tubules are dilated, and filled with darkly eosinophilic proteinaceous fluid. The kidneys in end-stage glomerulonephritis may weigh as little as 50 gms each. In many cases of end-stage kidney the pathogenetic mechanism cannot be appreciated since glomerular, vascular, and interstitial disorders can all result in the typically shrunken and diffusely scarred and sclerotic kidney.   (hematoxylin-eosin)

Pyelonephritis   *(Q25–Q28)*

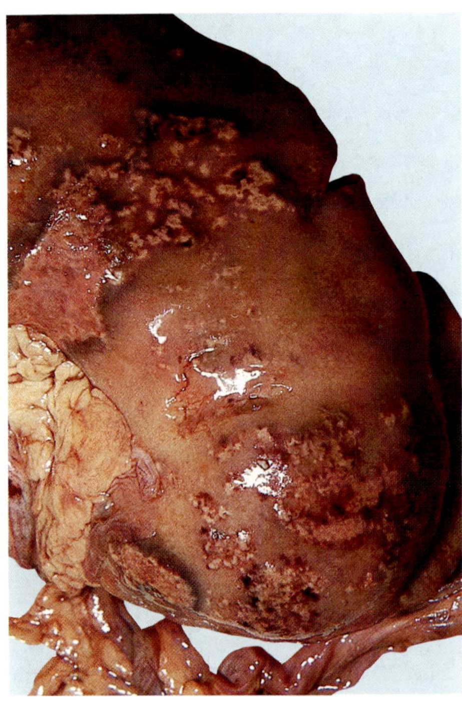

Fig. Q25. Hematogenous pyelonephritis. This kidney is marked by many pyogenic foci consisting of central, yellow, necrotic areas surrounded by erythematous inflammatory rims. In contrast to ascending pyelonephritis, where the accumulation of polymorphonuclear leukocytes is in the tubules, hematogenously spread pyelonephritis tends to involve interstitium more than tubules.

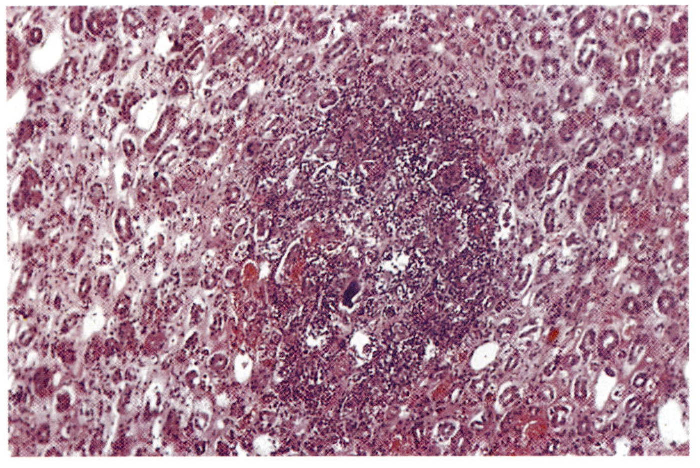

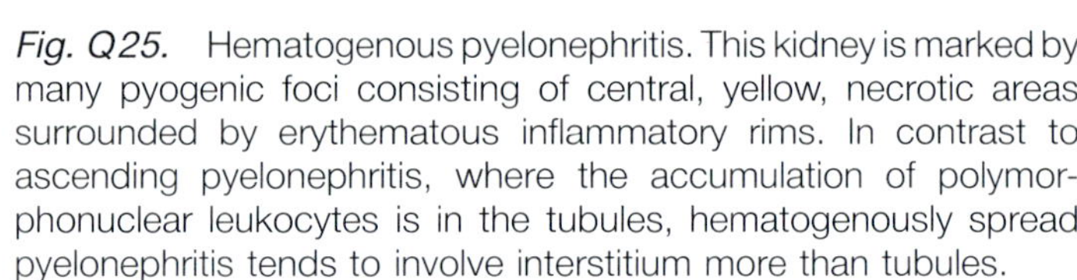

Fig. Q26. Hematogenous pyelonephritis in a patient with sepsis. The central portion of the photomicrograph shows a pyogenic focus with many polymorphonuclear leukocytes partially obliterating the usual architecture of the kidney. A number of tubules are trapped and collapsed within the acute inflammatory exudate. With time, liquifactive necrosis would predominate and an abscess would form, resembling the necrotic foci macroscopically visible in *Fig. Q25.* (hematoxylin-eosin)

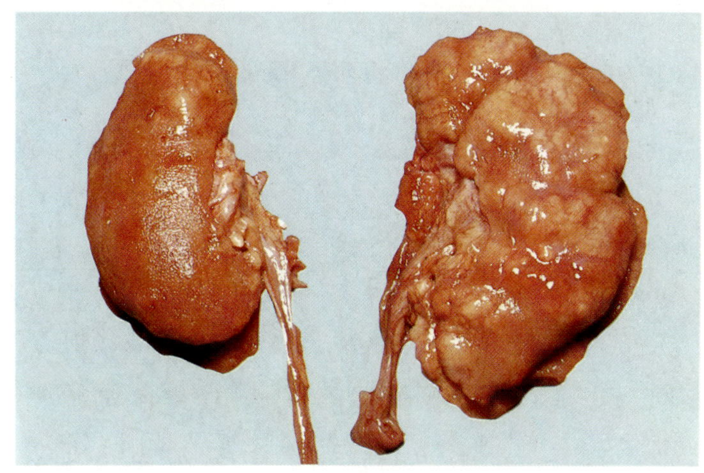

Fig. Q27. Chronic pyelonephritis. The right kidney has large irregular broadbased scars. At this stage renal function may not be completely compromised. The kidney on the left is shrunken and has a finely granular surface. This is an end-stage kidney, not dissimilar from that seen in Fig. Q23. In this instance, clinical and historical evidence led to the diagnosis of end-stage kidney due to chronic pyelonephritis.

Fig. Q28. Chronic pyelonephritis.

Fig. Q28a. This photomicrograph shows an area of renal scarring in which the surface is depressed, and the usual architecture is replaced by fibrous tissue. The scar, in this section, has a broad surface and a few dilated residual tubules are seen containing concentrated urine. The kidney to the right and left of this scar is relatively unchanged.

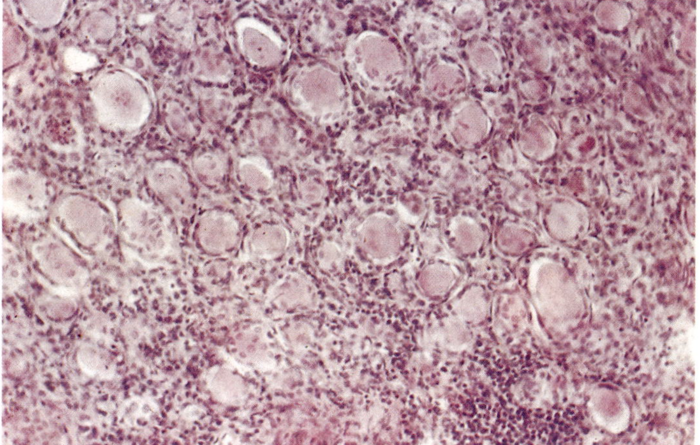

Fig. Q28b. In this photomicrograph there are many dilated tubules filled with proteinaceous fluid representing concentrated urine. The tubular epithelial cells are flattened. The clustering of tubules, with their eosinophilic contents bears a resemblance to thyroid follicles and has been called "thyroidization" of the kidney. This change is not pathognomonic and can be seen in advanced nephrosclerosis, as well as in chronic pyelonephritis. (hematoxylin-eosin)

Nephrocalcinosis and Urolithiasis   *(Q29–Q31)*

Fig. Q29. Nephrocalcinosis. Previously necrotic tubular epithelial cells become calcified (dystrophic calcification). The dark blue masses of calcium almost completely obliterate the tubular lumen. This patient died of toxic nephropathy from mercuric chloride poisoning.

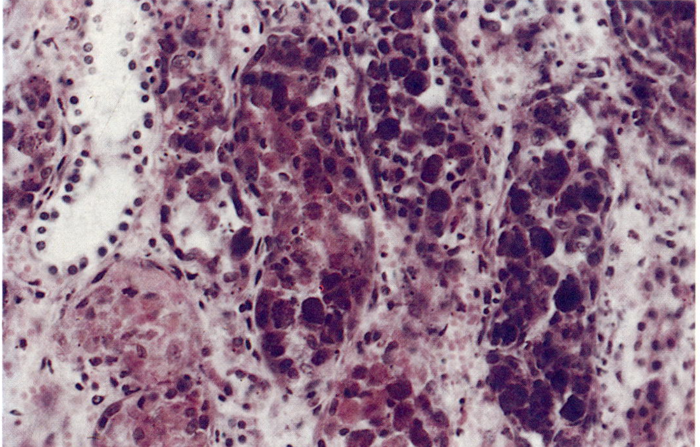

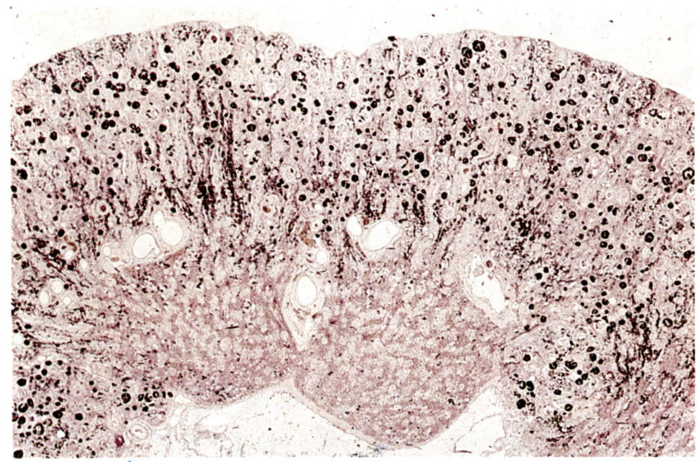

Fig. Q30. Metastatic nephrosclerosis in a patient with hypercalcemia. There is extensive deposition of calcium salts (black) in the tubular lumens and tubular epithelium, in the interstitial connective tissue, in vessel walls, and in the glomeruli.   (von Kossa)

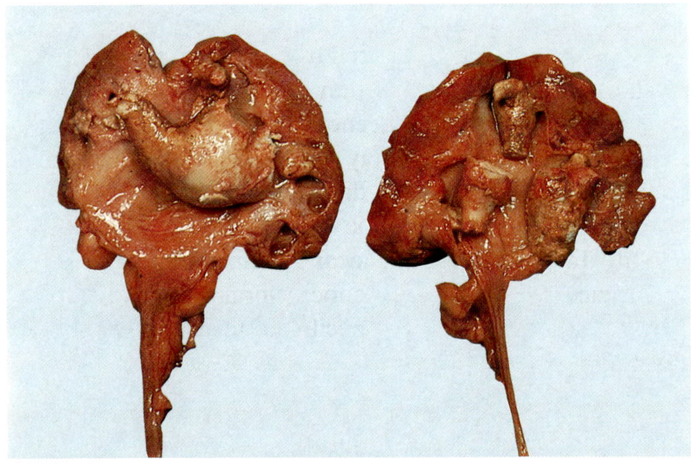

Fig. Q31. Nephrolithiasis. The kidneys show severe hydronephrosis and the pelves contain large irregular ("staghorn") calculi. These calculi were predominantly composed of uric acid and developed in a patient with chronic myelogenous leukemia.

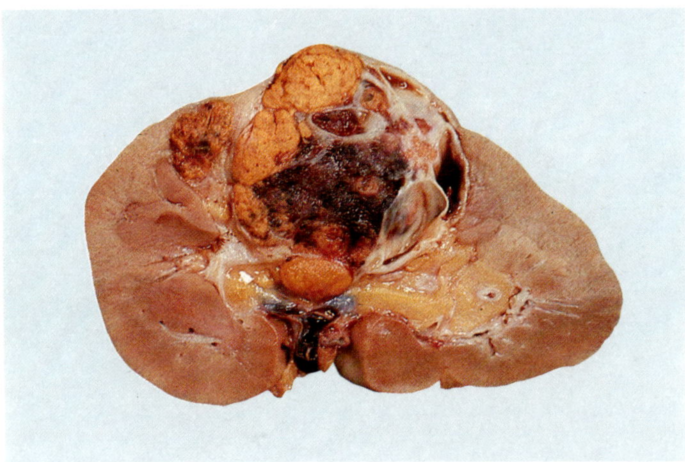

Tumors   *(Q32–Q33)*

Fig. Q32. Renal cell adenocarcinoma. A six-inch tumor fills the midportion of the kidney, elevating and infiltrating the renal capsule. This is the typical macroscopic appearance of a renal cell carcinoma ("hypernephroma"). The tumor is irregularly bright yellow, with areas of hemorrhage, necrosis, and sclerosis. A small satellite-like extension of tumor is to the left of the main mass.
(Photograph: Courtesy of H.P. Lange)

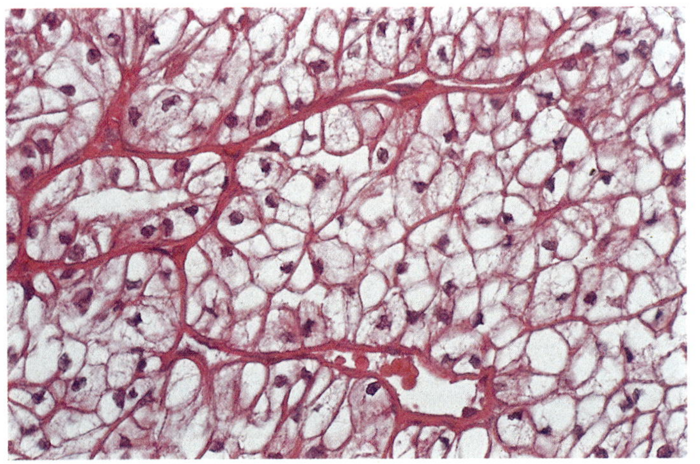

Fig. Q33. This photomicrograph shows the typical appearance of a renal cell carcinoma. This section was taken from the yellow area and shows large polygonal epithelial cells with pale, almost clear cytoplasm and relatively small, only slightly pleomorphic nuclei. The tumor is extremely vascular, permitting its easy visualization on angiographic studies. The clarity of the cytoplasm is due to the high lipid content of these cells, explaining the yellow appearance on macroscopic examination.
(hematoxylin-eosin; photograph: Courtesy of H.P. Lange)

R. Male Sexual Organs

G. Dhom, F. Städtler

Hypogonadism is a general term for functional disorders of the testes in which there is decreased spermatogenesis. This may be due to disorders of the seminiferous tubules, as well as of the hormone-secreting Leydig cells. Primary hypogonadism is not uncommon and can be a pre- or postpubertal manifestation. In Klinefelter's syndrome the testis is poorly developed. In the undescended testicle spermatogenesis may be impaired. In addition, there are a variety of acquired disorders which affect spermatogenesis and may lead to infertility. Secondary male infertility follows pituitary insufficiency. The term tertiary hypogonadism is used when the deficiency is due to a hypothalamic lesion.

The testes and epididymes may be affected by a variety of inflammatory disorders, either singly or together. Granulomatous orchitis is one form of testicular inflammation.

Testicular tumors are particularly important. Germ cell tumors are common and, with the advent of monoclonal antibodies to identify specific cell products, have become better understood.

The prostate gland is affected by benign proliferations which cause urethral obstruction. Particularly important in elderly men is prostatic adenocarcinoma. Both benign and malignant conditions may contribute to nonspecific manifestations of prostatic disease. Inflammatory diseases of the prostate may be difficult to differentiate clinically from prostatic adenocarcinoma. The histologic appearance of prostatic adenocarcinoma may be an indicator of prognosis, and specific patterns are used in classification.

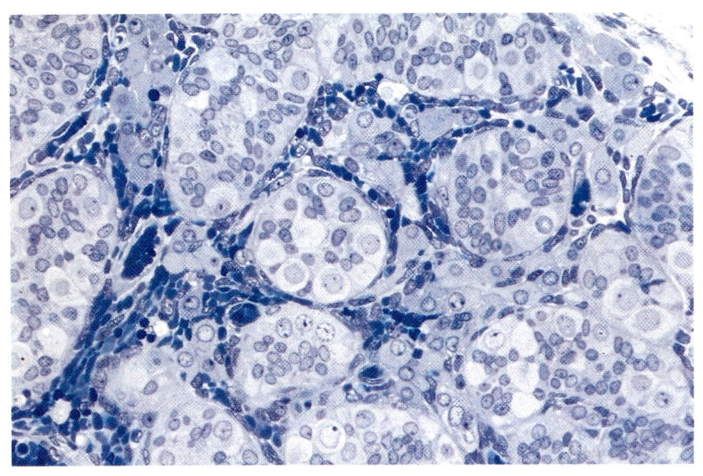

Fig. R1. This one micron section is of a normally developed, descended testicle in a 6-year-old male who had an undescended testicle on the other side. The tubules in the center of the photomicrograph are approximately 60 microns in diameter which is normal. The tubules appear solid. Immature forms of Sertoli cells and spermatagonia are seen. The spermatagonia sit on the basement membrane and have well-defined, round, pale-staining cytoplasm, and round central nuclei.   (Unna)

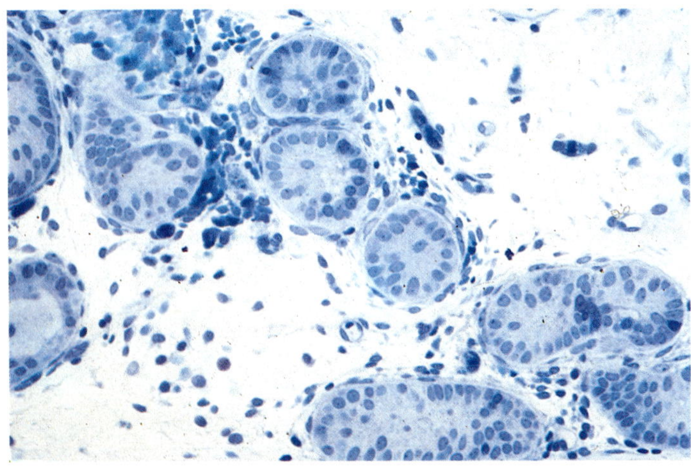

Fig. R2. Partially atrophic undescended testicle from the same patient as in *Fig. R1.* The tubules have a diameter of 44 microns and are fully formed. There is a single layer of tubular epithelium which consists mostly of immature Sertoli cells. The intervening stroma is fibrotic.   (Unna)

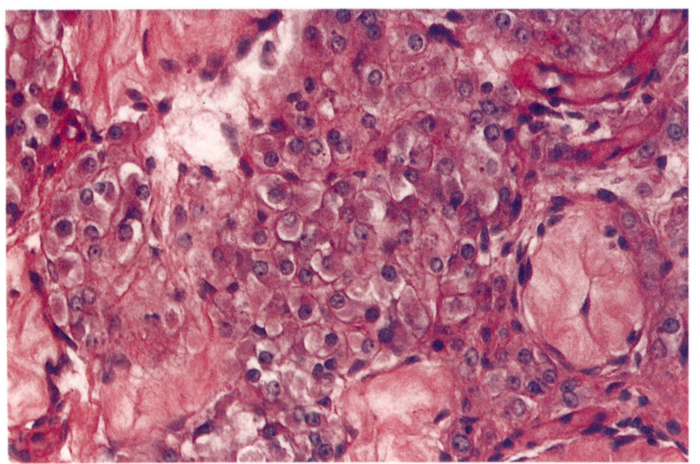

Fig. R3. Klinefelter's syndrome. This is a characteristic histopathology in which there are sheets of hyperplastic polyhedral Leydig cells in between atrophic seminiferous tubules. Spermatogenesis is completely absent.   (PAS)

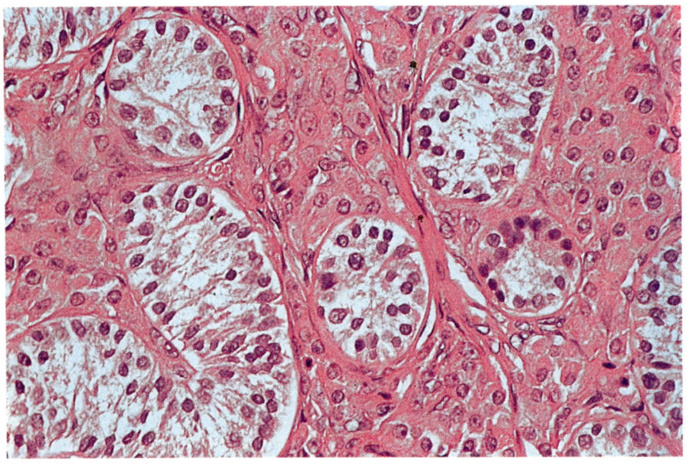

Fig. R4. Characteristic histopathology of testicular feminization syndrome. There is marked hyperplasia of Leydig cells. The seminiferous tubules are poorly developed and resemble the prepubescent testis. The seminiferous tubules contain mostly Sertoli cells, but a few primary spermatoagonia are seen.
(hematoxylin-eosin)

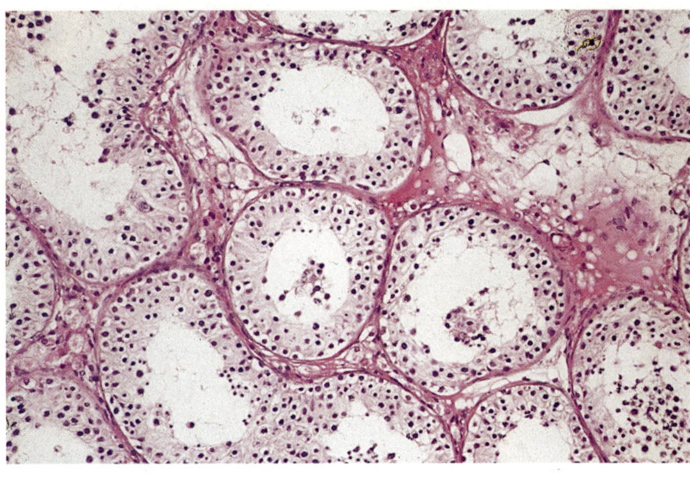

Fig. R5. Testicular biopsy in a 30-year-old man with infertility. There is primary hypogonadism with markedly reduced spermatogenesis. Spermatogonia are arrested at the spermatid stage. Mature spermatozoa are not seen. The interstitium is slightly edematous, and there are the usual small clusters of Leydig cells. (hematoxylin-eosin)

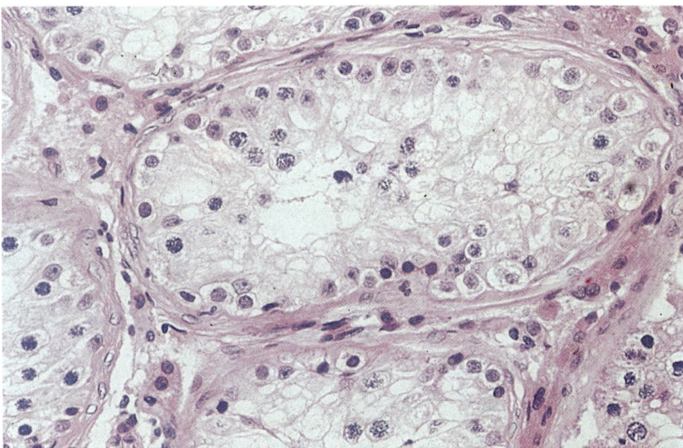

Fig. R6. Advanced, primary postpuberty hypogonadism with arrest of spermatogenesis. The tubules contain only spermatogonia and Sertoli cells. Mature spermatocytes are not seen. The etiology of impaired spermatogenesis is often difficult to determine from study of the biopsy.   (hematoxylin-eosin)

Inflammation and Tumors   *(R7–R15)*

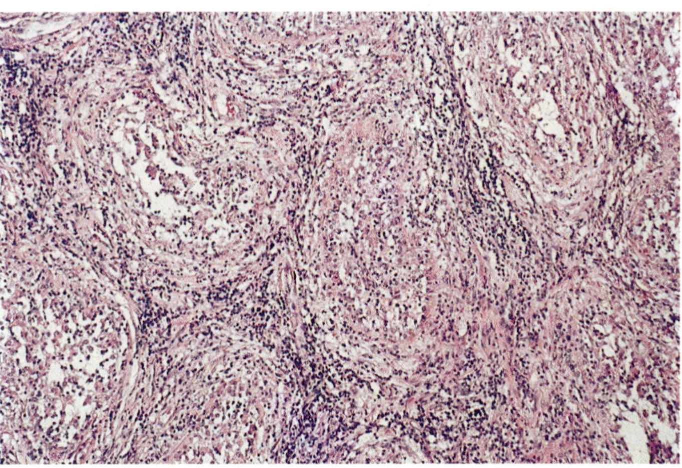

Fig. R7. Nonspecific granulomatous orchitis. The testicular tissue is extensively destroyed by the massive inflammatory infiltrate. The seminiferous tubules are almost completely obliterated and do not contain recognizable spermatozoa. Sertoli cells are similarly difficult to recognize. True granulomas are not seen and the granulomatous appearance results from the inflammatory cells incompletely obliterating the usual tubular architecture.   (hematoxylin-eosin)

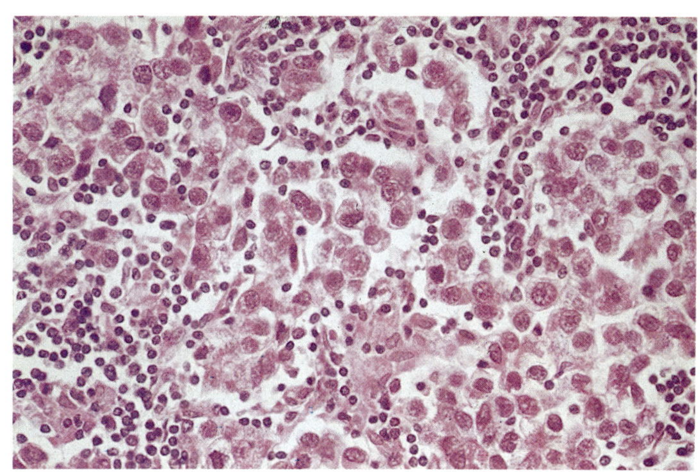

Fig. R8. Germinoma (seminoma). In this photomicrograph sheets of malignant cells are seen. They are round to slightly polyhedral, fairly uniform, with prominent large nuclei in which there are obvious nucleoli. Mitoses are rare. There is a moderate amount of surrounding lymphocytic infiltration.   (hematoxylin-eosin)

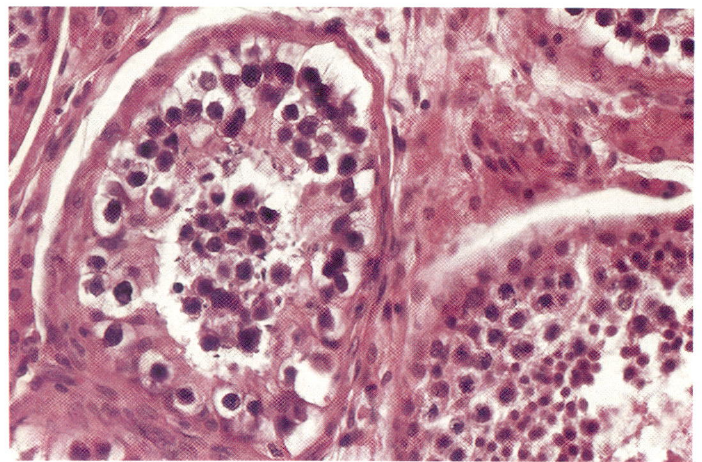

Fig. R9.   Testicular biopsy in a patient with infertility. Two seminiferous tubules are well-visualized in this photomicrograph. The one to the left shows markedly abnormal cells resembling primary spermatogonia. The tubule to the right shows usual maturation. Because of a number of markedly dysplastic seminiferous tubules similar to this the testicle was removed and, in another area, showed a typical invasive germinoma.   (hematoxylin-eosin)

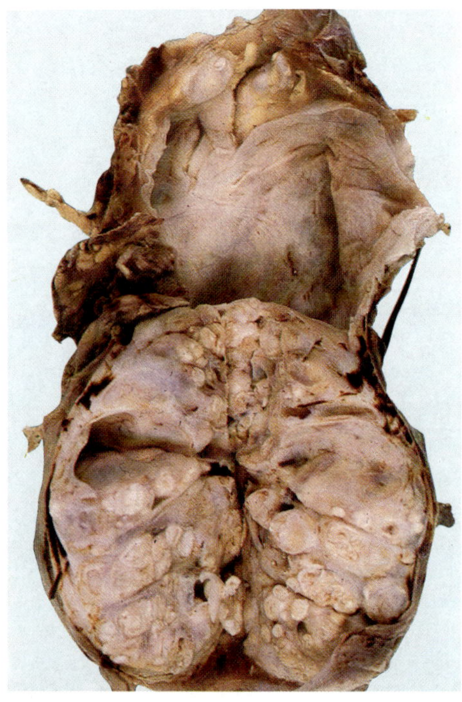

Fig. R10.   Section of a testicle with a mature teratoma. Multiple cysts contain keratin and sebaceous material as well as watery and viscid fluid. The testicle is almost completely replaced, although a thin rim of residual testicular parenchyma is immediately beneath the tunica albugina. Teratomas in the testis have a high incidence of malignancy, in contrast to those of the ovary *(Figs. S17–S19)* which are almost always benign.

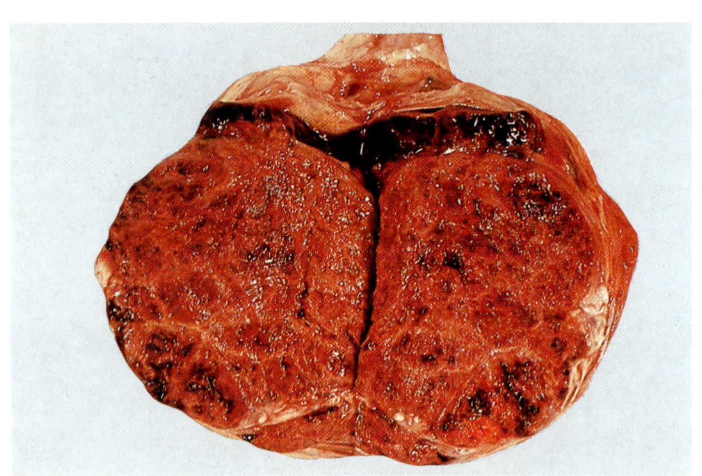

Fig. R11.   Section of a testis with a choriocarcinoma. Large portions of the tumor are hemorrhagic and necrotic. Areas of hemorrhage and necrosis in testicular tumors must be carefully sectioned for the presence of trophoblast-like cells.

Fig. R12. Photomicrograph of a mature teratoma showing an area resembling intestinal epithelium. To the lower left and the upper portion of the photomicrograph are the edges of two cysts, each of which is lined by keratinizing squamous epithelium. The small cyst at the right hand border of the photomicrograph is lined by respiratory-type epithelium. A lymphoid nodule is in the wall of the intestine-like structure.   (van Gieson)

Fig. R13. Photomicrograph of a choriocarcinoma. Pseudo-papillary structures contain syncytial trophoblasts. There is virtually no stroma. Immunohistochemical staining with a monoclonal antibody showed the presence of human chorionic gonadotrophin. (hematoxylin-eosin)

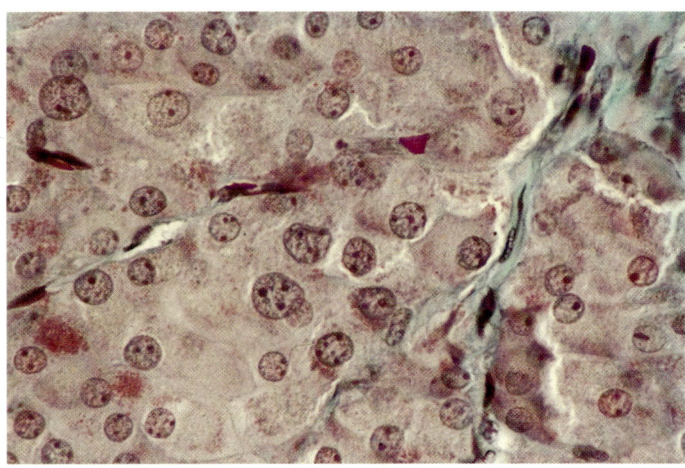

Fig. R14. Photomicrograph of an interstitial (Leydig) cell tumor. Sheets of epithelial-like polyhedral cells with abundant cytoplasm are seen. The nuclei show only slight pleomorphism, but contain one or more enlarged nucleoli. The characteristic Reinke crystalloid is not seen in this photomicrograph.   (Goldner)

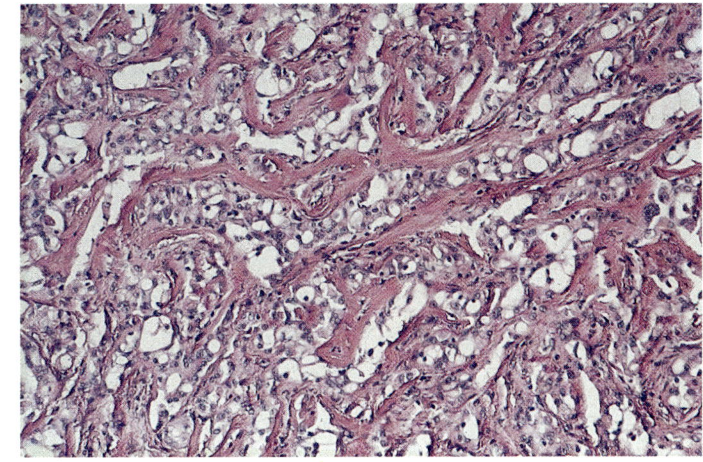

Fig. R15. Adenomatoid tumor of the epididymis. Flattened and irregular glandlike spaces are seen with lining cells resembling epithelium. The stroma is fibrous and there are strands of smooth muscle. This tumor is thought to arise from mesothelial cells and shows characteristic elaborate microvilli with the electron microscope.   (hematoxylin-eosin)

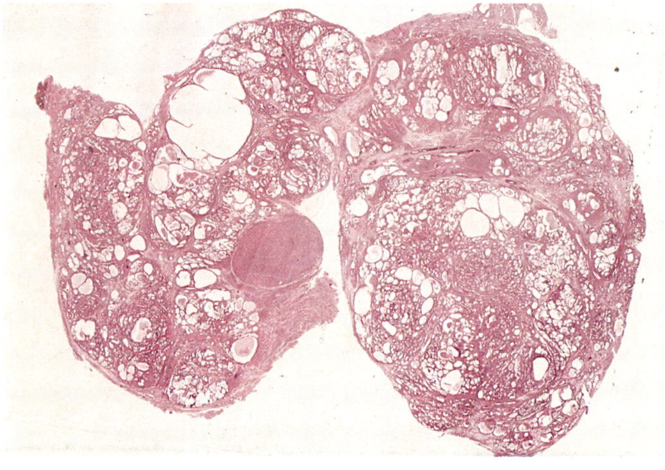

Fig. R16.   Fibroadenomatous hyperplasia of the prostate. There is proliferation of glandular spaces forming irregular nodules, separated by fibrous connective tissue. To the left of center the small, uniformly eosinophilic area is a nodule consisting entirely of stromal cells.   (hematoxylin-eosin)

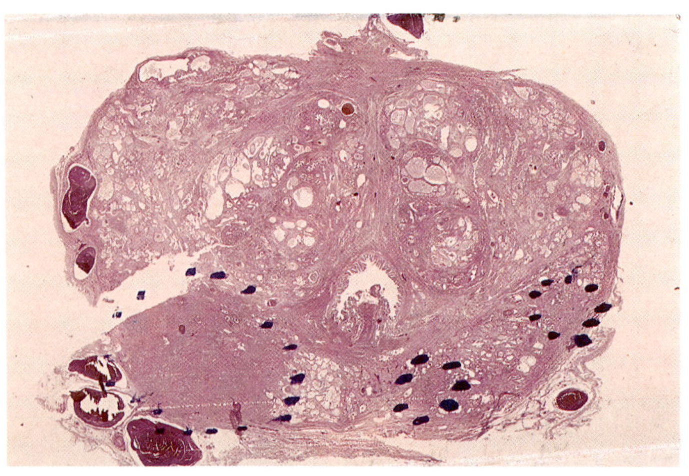

Fig. R17.   Clinically occult prostatic adenocarcinoma. Three small areas of adenocarcinoma, encircled by ink dots, were found at autopsy in the prostate of this elderly man who had no clinical manifestations of prostatic adenocarcinoma during life. The incidence of prostatic adenocarcinoma increases with age.

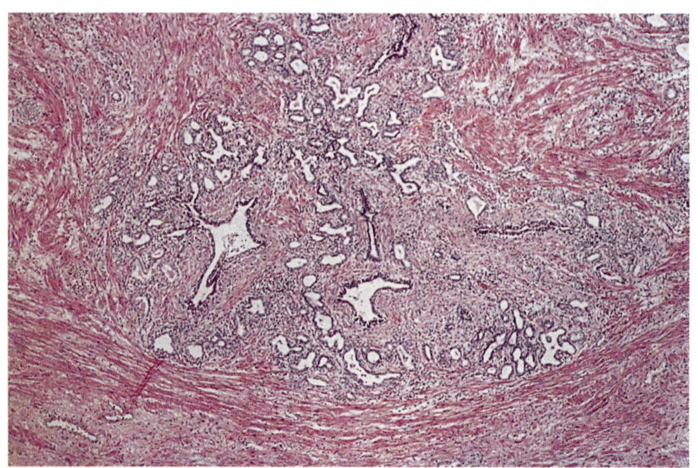

Fig. R18.   Focal prostatic hyperplasia. In this patient a few excretory ducts are surrounded by prominent glandular spaces with a moderate amount of fibrous connective tissue. The remainder of the prostate, in this patient, was atrophic.

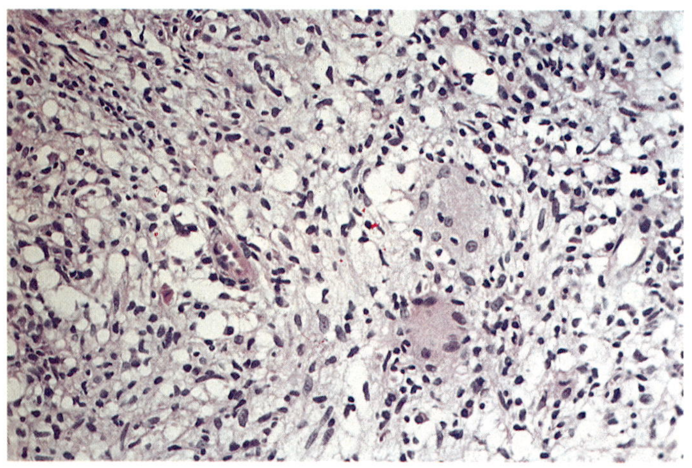

Fig. R19.   Granulomatous prostatitis. In this high-magnification photomicrograph, there are two large multinucleated giant cells, a few epithelioid histiocytes, many lymphocytes, and a few eosinophils. Granulomatous prostatitis may, on occasion, show areas of necrosis and may resemble tuberculosis. In most cases, however, acid fast bacilli cannot be identified.   (hematoxylin-eosin)

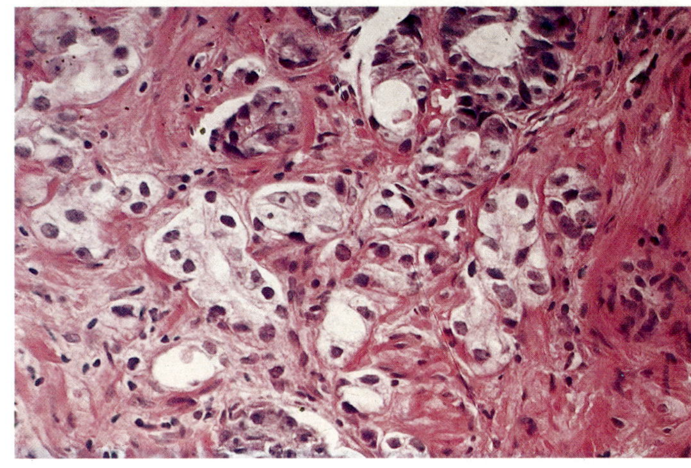

Fig. R20. Well-differentiated prostatic adenocarcinoma. In the normal prostate two cell layers can be seen lining the glands. In adenocarcinoma there is only a single layer of tumor cells which characteristically show slight pleomorphism and prominent small nucleoli.

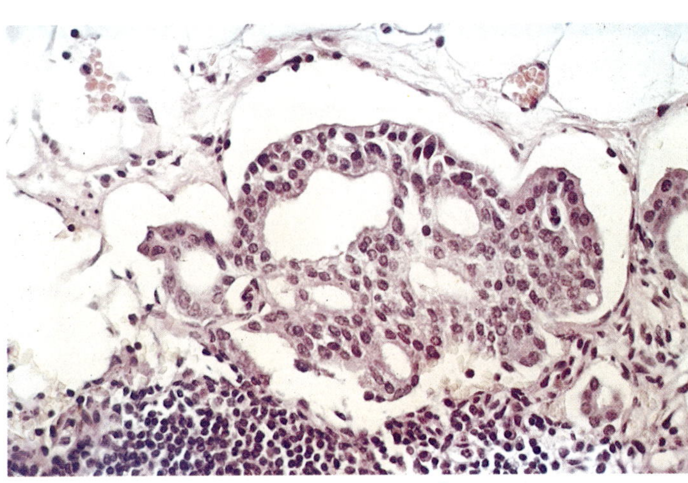

Fig. R21. Moderately well-differentiated prostatic adenocarcinoma. A group of irregular closely-apposed glands containing obviously pleomorphic nuclei and large nucleoli are seen. (hematoxylin-eosin)

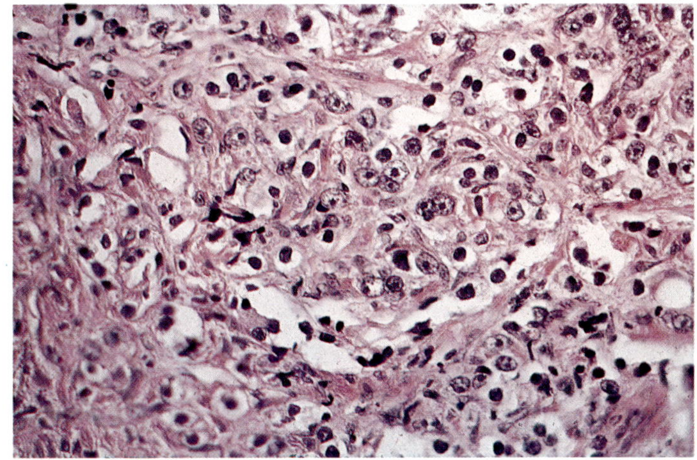

Fig. R22. Cribriform adenocarcinoma of the prostate, metastatic to a lymph node. Tumor cells are present in the peripheral sinus. The lymph node parenchyma is to the lower portion of the photomicrograph. (hematoxylin-eosin)

Fig. R23. Poorly differentiated prostatic adenocarcinoma. Tumor cells are arranged in sheets. The nuclei are markedly pleomorphic, and the nucleoli are characteristically prominent. (hematoxylin-eosin)

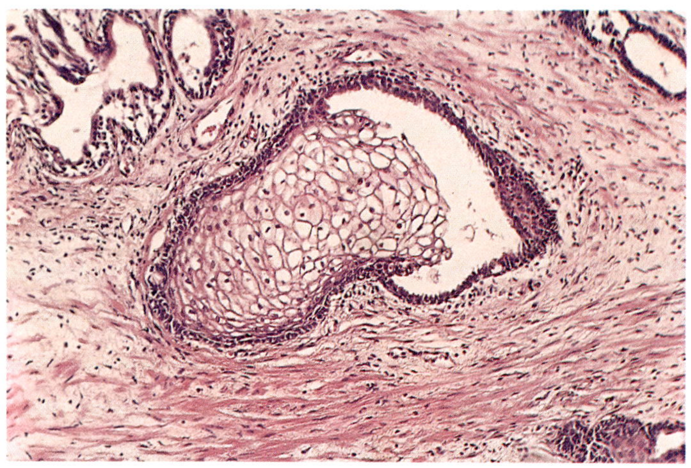

Fig. R24.   Squamous metaplasia in an excretory duct of the prostate. This change is characteristically found in men who receive estrogen therapy for prostatic adenocarcinoma and is, in itself, entirely benign.

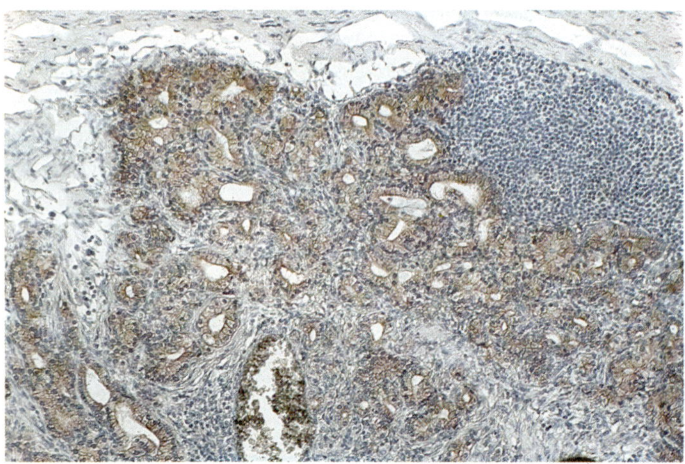

Fig. R25.   Prostatic adenocarcinoma metastatic to a lymph node. The etiology of the tumor was demonstrated by the immunoperoxidase method in which monoclonal antibody to prostate-specific antigen was utilized.

S. Female Reproductive System

J. H. Holzner

The ovary is affected by a number of disorders in which there is diminished activity. These contribute to characteristic clinical pictures. There may also be syndromes due to hypersecretion, some of them contributing to uterine and breast neoplasia. Benign ovarian cysts are quite frequent. They may be quite large as well as serous or mucinous. Benign cysts are often clinically silent until they become large enough to palpate or until they contribute to acute abdominal distress because of torsion. Para-ovarian cysts are also frequent. The ovary may be affected by a variety of tumors, both benign and malignant, which are morphologically and functionally quite diverse. In contrast to the testis, teratomas of the ovary are almost always benign. Malignant tumors, of course, arise in the ovary. Tumors of the surface epithelium are the most common group of ovarian neoplasms and include the majority of ovarian carcinomas. Other malignant tumors arise from germ cells or gonadal stroma. The latter group, which constitutes approximately five percent of ovarian tumors, may be hormonally active. Ovarian tumors occur at all ages, but at different degrees of frequency. Dysgerminomas, yolk sac tumors, and embryonal carcinomas, as well as teratomas are tumors of predominantly younger patients. In contrast, carcinomas mostly affect older individuals. The tumors of the ovary are generally homologous to those of the testis. The ovaries may also be the site of metastatic carcinoma and as many as six percent of ovarian malignancies are secondary. The eponym "Krukenberg tumor" is reserved for metastatic carcinoma which is mucin-secreting with signet ring cells, desmoplastic, and usually arising from a primary in the stomach or pancreas.

The fallopian tubes are often affected by inflammatory conditions, which may lead to pyo- or, eventually, hydrosalpinx. Carcinoma of the fallopian tube is rare.

Female hormonal activity is reflected in the morphologic variations of the endometrium. Direct correlations can be made between histopathologic features of endometrium and hormonal state. Hyperestrogenism contributes to endometrial hyperplasia and carcinoma, whereas hypoestrogenism is the basis for endometrial hypoplasia and atrophy.

Uterine neoplasms can arise in the endometrium, the myometrium, and even from serosal mesothelium. Epithelial tumors arise from endometrium as well as from the squamous epithelium of the cervix. The most common tumors of the uterus are benign leiomyomas. These manifest as tumor masses which can contribute to urinary frequency when anterior, constipation when posterior, and uterine bleeding when submucosal. The uterus may also be enlarged because of adenomyosis and stromal hyperplasia.

The most common malignant tumors of the female reproductive system arise in the endometrium of the uterine corpus and in the cervix, particularly at the region of the squamo-columnar junction. With the widespread utilization of Pap smears, cervical carcinoma has markedly decreased in incidence. Carcinoma of the cervix affects women at the end of the reproductive period, but can also occur in younger women. In most cases cervical squamous cell carcinoma is preceded for as long as a decade, by various stages of squamous dysplasia. It is in these early stages that the cytologic studies are particularly useful in preventing the development of the full-blown malignancy. Carcinoma of the cervix tends to occur in women who are multi-parous. In contrast, endometrial carcinoma is more often found in nulliparous women, many of whom can be shown to have idiopathic or therapeutically induced hyperestrogenism. Uterine sarcomas are relatively rare.

Pregnancy may be complicated by a variety of disease processes. Postpartum endometritis is relatively uncommon, as are the trophoblastic neoplasms. Extrauterine pregnancies primarily affect the fallopian tubes and, when there is tubal rupture and hemorrhage, can be life-threatening. Study of the histopathology of the endometrium, showing characteristic changes of pregnancy without fetal or placental tissue, can assist in establishing the diagnosis of ectopic pregnancy.

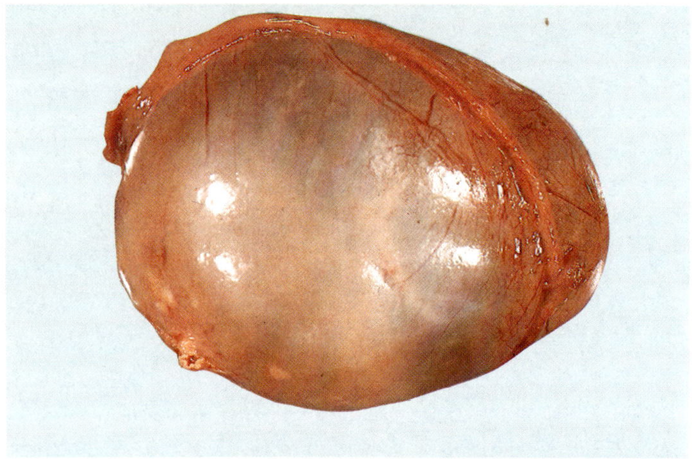

Fig. S1.   Para-ovarian cyst. Para-ovarian cysts originate from remnants of wolffian ducts. They are located mostly in the mesosalpinx and, consequently, are covered by mesothelial cells. The fallopian tube is often stretched over the cyst, as in this case where it appears as a curved thickening at the upper and right-hand portions of the cyst. A small ovary is seen at the lower left portion of the cyst. The ovary is atrophic.

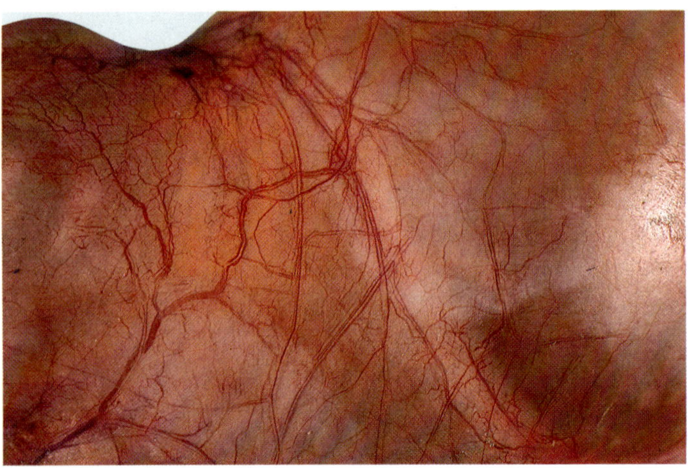

Fig. S2.   Para-ovarian cyst. Two vascular networks can be seen, one deep to the other. These represent the vessels of the cyst wall and those of the peritoneal layer covering the cyst. This feature, of two vascular networks, is useful in differentiating para-ovarian from ovarian cysts.

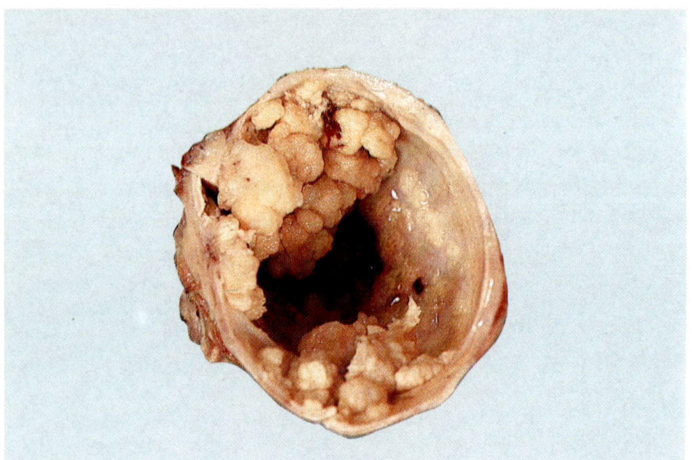

Fig. S3.   Papillary cystadenocarcinoma of the ovary is the most common malignant tumor of the ovary. Papillary ovarian malignancies may be serous, mucinous, or mixed. Ovarian carcinoma may be bilateral. Mucinous carcinoma, which is less common than serous, has a higher incidence of bilaterality. The cyst in this case is almost completely covered by nodular accumulations of papillary projections.

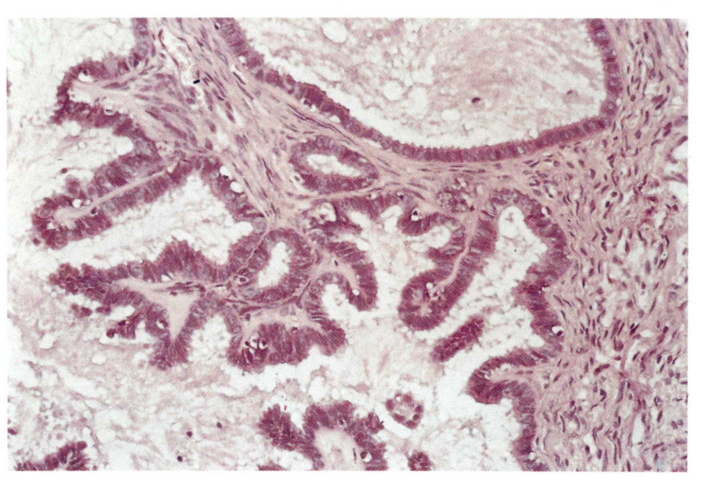

Fig. S4.   Serous papillary cystadenoma of the ovary. The photomicrograph shows papillary excrescences on the inner aspect of the ovary consisting of a single layer of fairly uniform epithelial cells which resemble fallopian tube epithelium. Many of the cells are ciliated, although that cannot be appreciated in this medium magnification. The benign nature of this tumor is suggested by the lack of proliferation and maintenance of a single cell layer, the lack of infiltration of the underlying stroma, and the lack of mitoses. (hematoxylin-eosin)

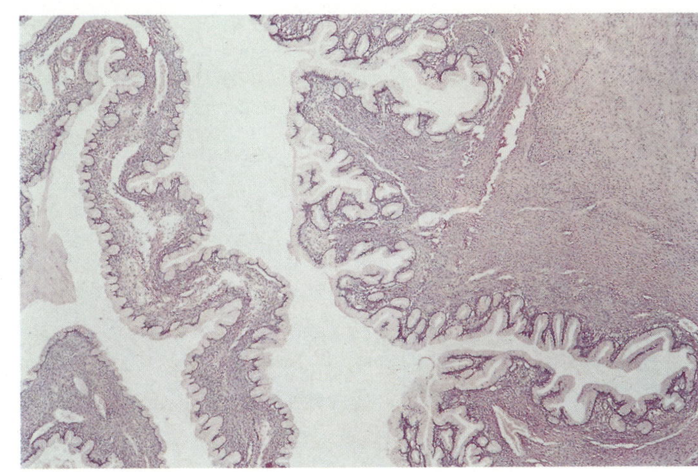

a

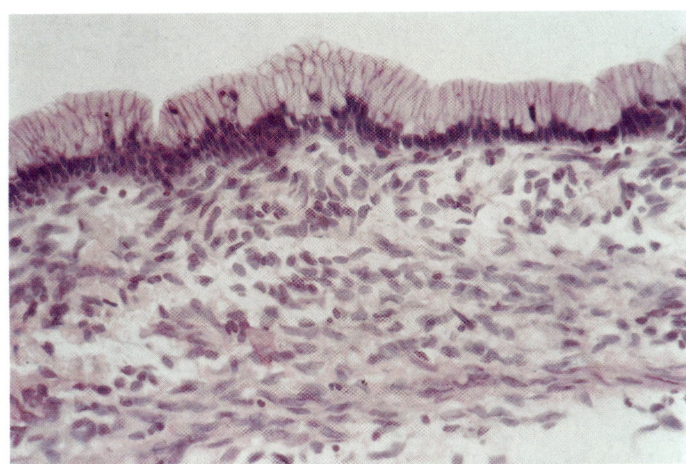

b

Fig. S5a–b. Mucinous cystadenoma of the ovary. Mucinous cystadenoma is often multi-loculated. The inner surface may be smooth and sticky, as a reflection of mucous production, or may be irregularly covered by papillary projections. In the low magnification photomicrograph, *(a)* portions of two adjacent cyst spaces are seen lined by tall, uniform, mucous-secreting epithelium with small, round basally situated nuclei; *(b)* mitoses are not seen. (hematoxylin-eosin)

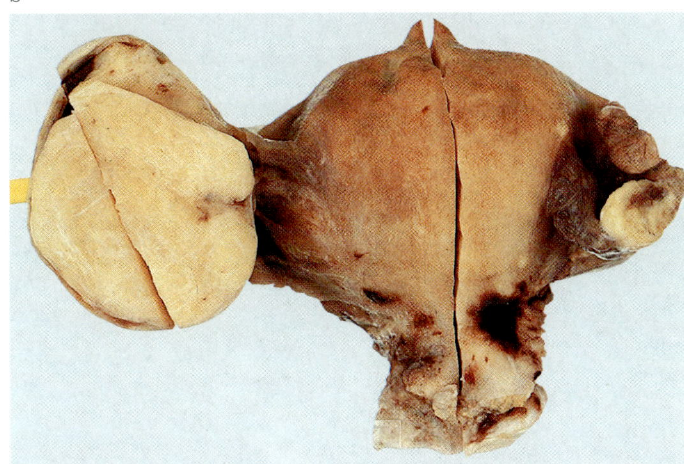
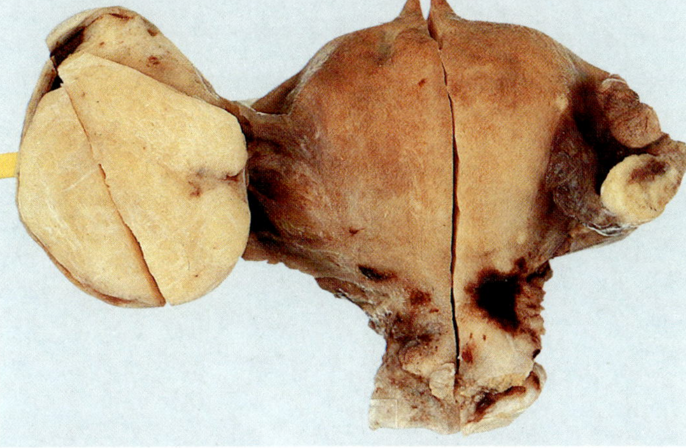

Fig. S6. Clear cell carcinoma of the ovary. The yellow color of the tumor reflects the lipid content of the malignant epithelial cells which make up this neoplasm. This tumor tends to be soft because of the almost complete lack of fibrous stroma. In general lipid cell tumors are biologically benign.

Fig. S7. Clear cell carcinoma of the ovary, mesonephric type. In this photomicrograph glandular spaces are lined by tall irregular vacuolated cells which vary considerably in size. Many of the cells are quite tall, projecting far above their neighbors, imparting a "hob nail" appearance. Some of the cells have eosinophilic cytoplasm. There is no convincing evidence to support the concept of mesonephric origin, although the term persists.   (hematoxylin-eosin)

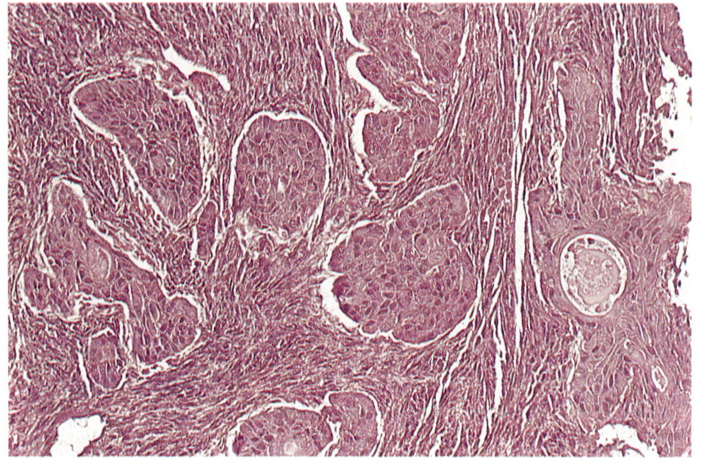

Fig. S8. Brenner tumor of the ovary. Brenner tumors are solid grey or pale yellow masses of fibrous tissue which may contain tiny cysts. Histologically the pattern of scattered, irregular epithelial masses in a background of fibrous tissue is distinctive. The epithelial component consists of ovoid cells with clear cytoplasm, vesicular nuclei, and a characteristic nuclear groove. The tiny cysts that are occasionally grossly visible are almost always lined by benign mucinous epithelium. In some cases, Brenner tumors may be found as a minor component of a mucinous cystadenoma. Malignant Brenner tumors are distinctly unusual. (hematoxylin-eosin)

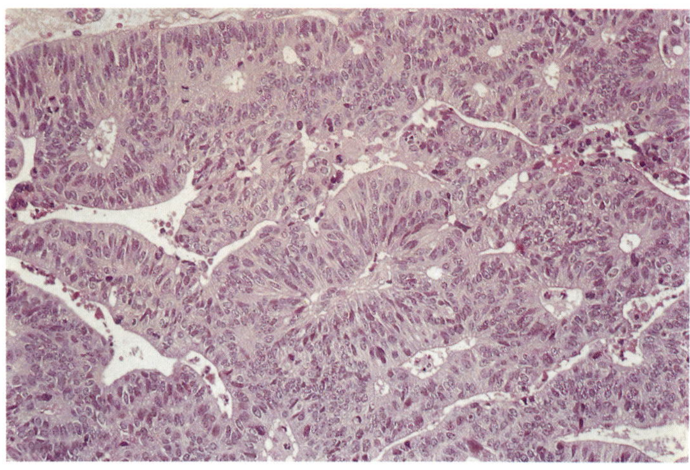

Fig. S9. Poorly differentiated ovarian carcinoma. In this photomicrograph there are solid nests and cord-like accumulations of undifferentiated tumor cells, with scattered gland forms. The tumor cells are highly pleomorphic, with large nuclei and numerous mitoses. A specific cell of origin cannot be determined from this histology. (hematoxylin-eosin)

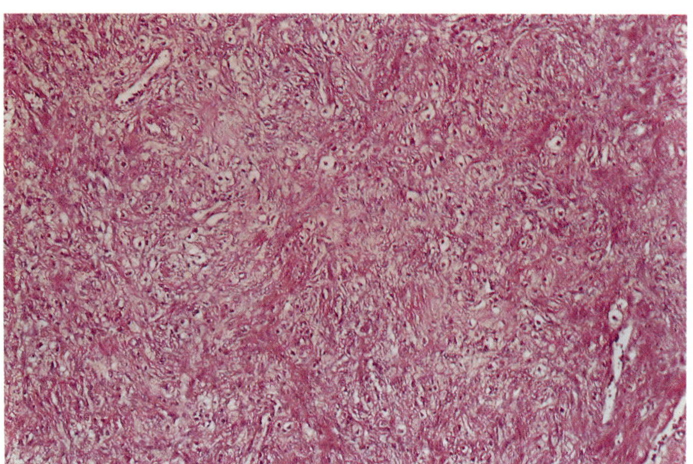

Fig. S10. Thecoma. Thecoma is one of sex cord stromal tumors which tends to be a large, firm, fibrous, well-delineated mass and can be hormonally active contributing to hyperestrogenism. Histologically plump spindle and round cells are scattered in a collagenous background. Some of the cells are vacuolated and contain lipid, which contributes to the characteristic yellow appearance seen macroscopically. (hematoxylin-eosin)

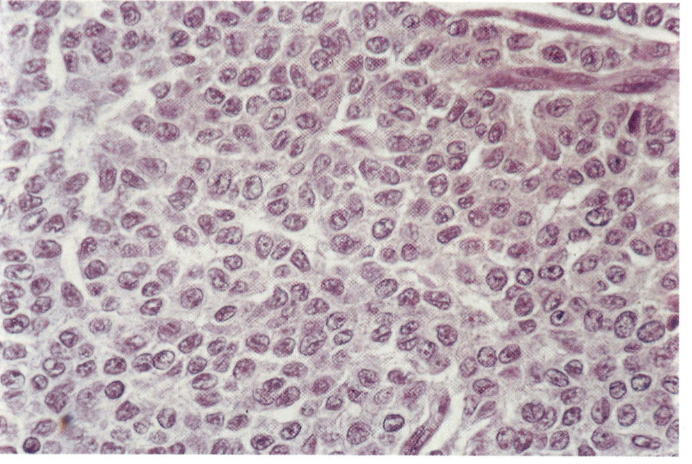

Fig. S11. Granulosa cell tumor. Granulosa cell tumors also derive from ovarian stroma. They can form a variety of histologic patterns. They may be microfollicular and macrofollicular, resembling graafian follicles, but may also be trabecular, solid, and insular. These patterns do not seem to have clinical correlation. Macroscopically, granulosa cells tumors are large yellow-brown, soft masses with areas of hemorrhage and cystic change. In general, granulosa cell tumors are hormonally inactive or may contribute to hyperestrogenism, although cystic macrofollicular tumors may produce androgenic effects. Thecomatous areas may be seen. (hematoxylin-eosin)

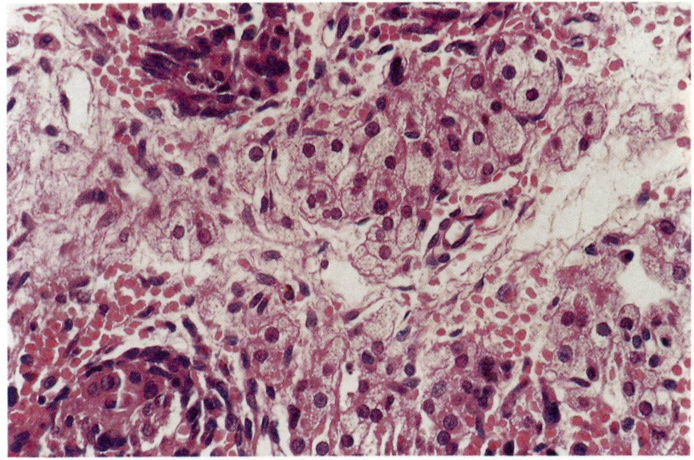

Fig. S12.   Sertoli-Leydig cell tumor (androblastoma). Sertoli-Ley-dig cell tumors arise from the same female sex cord stromal tumors as granulosa-theca cell tumors and contain female sex chromatin. Many of them are hormonally inert, although some produce andro-gens and masculinize the patient. In this low magnification photo-micrograph the tumor appears to be primarily sarcomatous in pattern with only a few tubular or epithelial elements evident. In between the sarcomatous cells, however, are interstitial-type cells, resembling Leydig cells, which contribute to the androgenic activity. (hematoxylin-eosin)

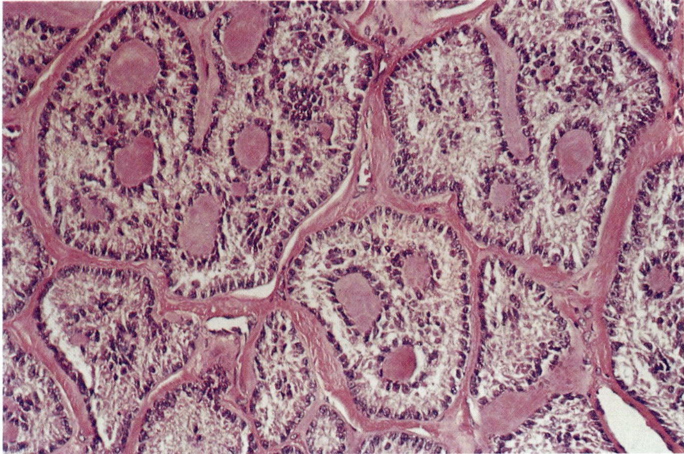

Fig. S13.   Sertoli-Leydig cell tumor. This is the same case as *Fig. S12.* In this high magnification photomicrograph, lipid-contain-ing cells are seen in a cluster to the right of the photomicrograph, with undifferentiated cells to the upper and lower left. (hematoxylin-eosin)

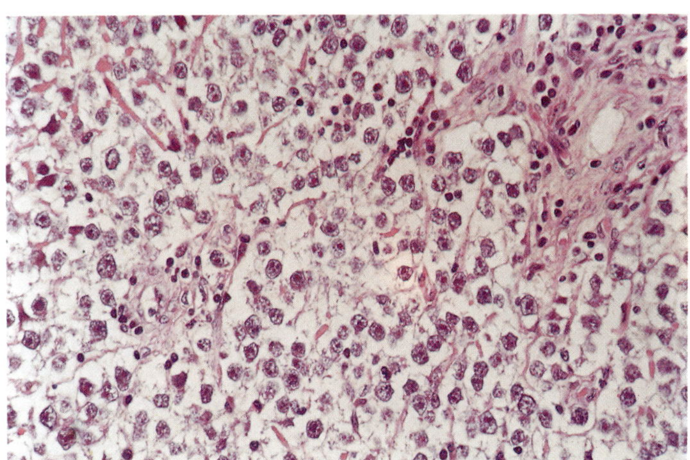

Fig. S14.   Germ cell tumor with annular tubules. This rare germ cell tumor consists of ring-like arrangements of pale, relatively large cells with abundant cytoplasm and small uniform nuclei, arranged around a hyaline-like eosinophilic center. Basement membrane material can be identified at the outside of the ring.   (hematoxylin-eosin)

Fig. S15.   Dysgerminoma. These tumors, which are homologous to the germinoma (seminoma) of the testis, are large, solid, generally encapsulated masses of soft grey-white tissue with varying degrees of hemorrhage and necrosis. Irregular clusters and sheets of poorly defined, glycogen-rich, uniform tumor cells are separated by thin connective tissue septa in which there are collapsed capillaries. There are a small number of lymphocytic cells. Approximately 10 percent of dysgerminomas are bilateral. Dysgerminoma is extremely radiosensitive and generally curable, even in the face of metas-tasis.   (hematoxylin-eosin)

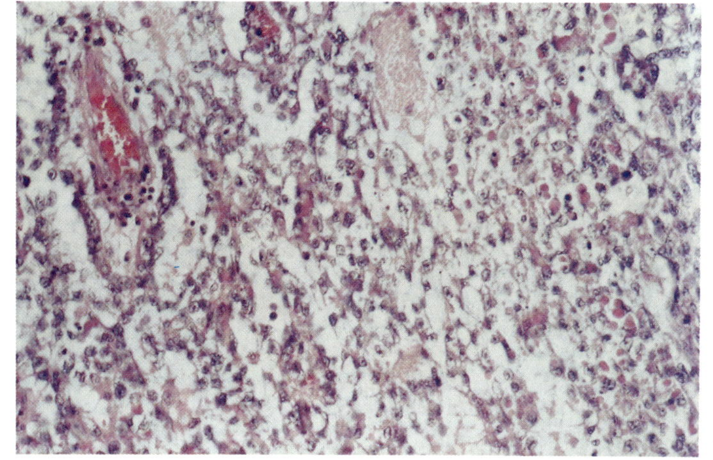

Fig. S16. Endodermal sinus (yolk sac) tumor of the ovary. Endodermal sinus tumor is a morphologically distinct entity whose characteristic histopathologic feature is the presence of isolated papillary structures surrounding a central blood vessel and lined by malignant embryonic epithelial cells. These are known as Schiller-Duval bodies, and lack basement membrane. Another distinctive feature within the tumor cells is the presence of periodic acid Schiff-positive, diastase-resistant hyaline globules which can be shown, using immunohistochemical methods, to contain alpha-fetoprotein. These tumors tend to occur in children or young women and have particularly poor prognosis.   (hematoxylin-eosin)

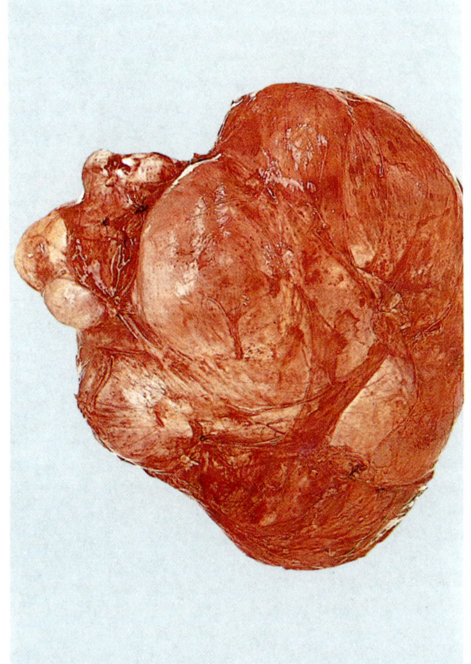

S17

S18

Fig. S17–S18. Ovarian teratoma. Benign cystic teratomas (dermoid cysts), are the most common tumors of the ovary. They tend to consist of a single dominant cyst space which can be lined by a variety of epithelial cells, but most often consist of stratified squamous epithelium of cutaneous type with sebum-elaborating glands, hair follicles, and keratin production. The accumulation of this material, which degenerates, often contributes to a strong odor when the cysts are opened. This malodorous material often appears pasty, as in the case illustrated. Teeth may be seen, as well as bone formation. The upper photograph shows the external aspect of the cyst, as it might be seen by the surgeon. In the lower photograph this cyst has been bisected, showing the accumulations of brown degenerating material and the varied appearances of the lining epithelium.

 Mature ovarian teratoma. Stratified squamous epithelium is obvious to the left. In this area there is no keratinization, and dermal appendage-type glands are not seen. The right portion of the photomicrograph consists of large irregular thyroid follicles, filled with colloid. Rarely, this entity of benign ovarian teratoma with thyroid tissue ("struma ovarii") can cause clinical manifestations of hyperthyroidism.   (hematoxylin-eosin)

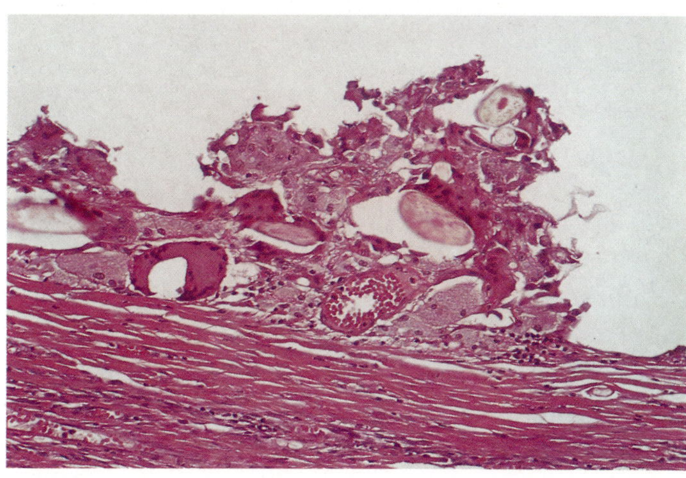

Fig. S20. **High magnification photomicrograph of a cystic teratoma** showing multinucleated giant cells and lipid-laden histiocytes, with a few hair fibers. A cross-section of a hair shaft is most easily seen at the upper right hand portion of the picture. This chronic, inflammatory, foreign body-type reaction is due to the release of lipid substance from cyst epithelial structures.   (hematoxylin-eosin)

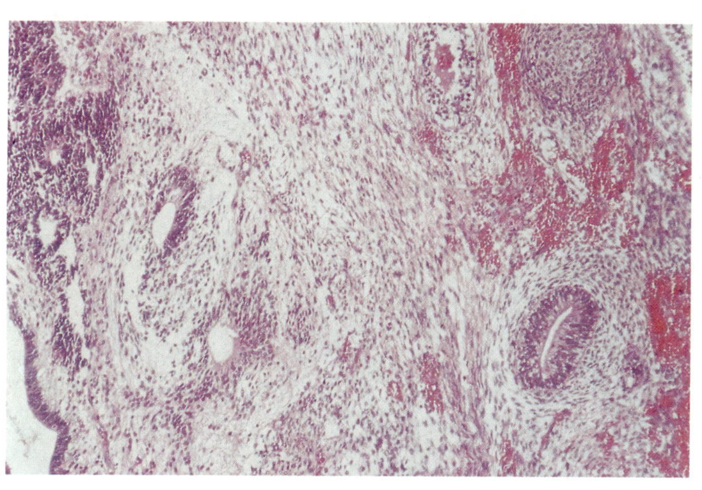

Fig. S21. **Malignant ovarian teratoma.** Immature, malignant teratomas are almost always solid. Their cellular constituents, both epithelial and mesenchymal, may be poorly differentiated. In this photomicrograph the epithelial components form undifferentiated tubular structures. The background mesenchyma is primitive in appearance.   (hematoxylin-eosin)

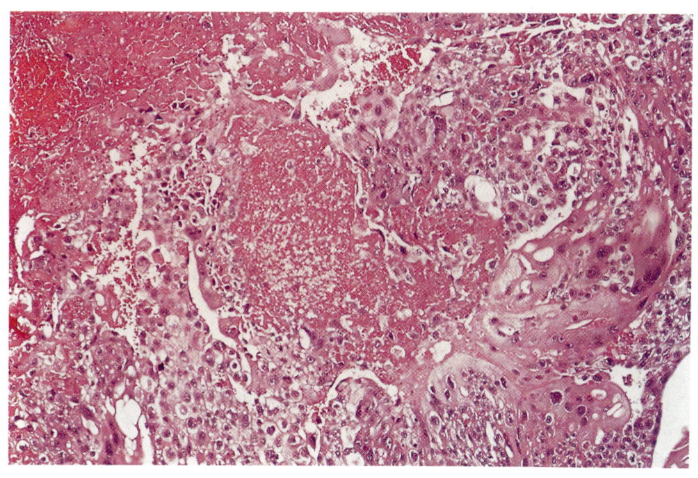

Fig. S22. **Choriocarcinoma of the ovary.** This highly malignant germ-cell tumor rarely arises in the ovary, but is histologically and macroscopically similar to that of the testis *(Fig. R11, R13).* The tumor mimics a trophoblast and consists of two cell types: basophilic, cytotrophoblastic cells with single nuclei, and large, multinucleated syncytiotrophoblastic cells. Hemorrhage and necrosis is characteristic and trophoblastic cells can be shown, using immunohistochemical methods, to contain chorionic gonadotrophin.   (hematoxylin-eosin)

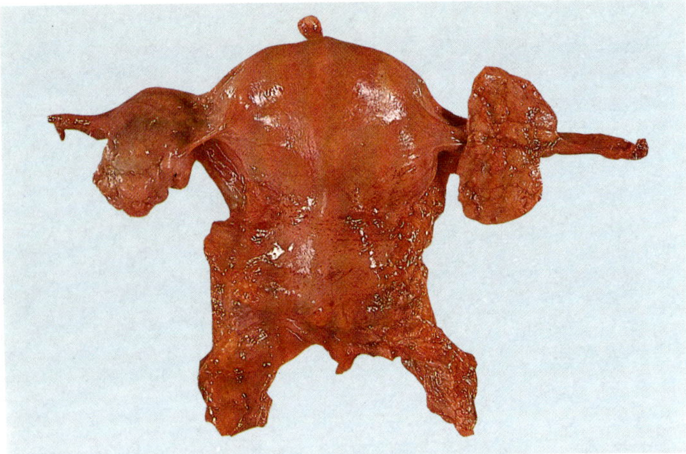

S23

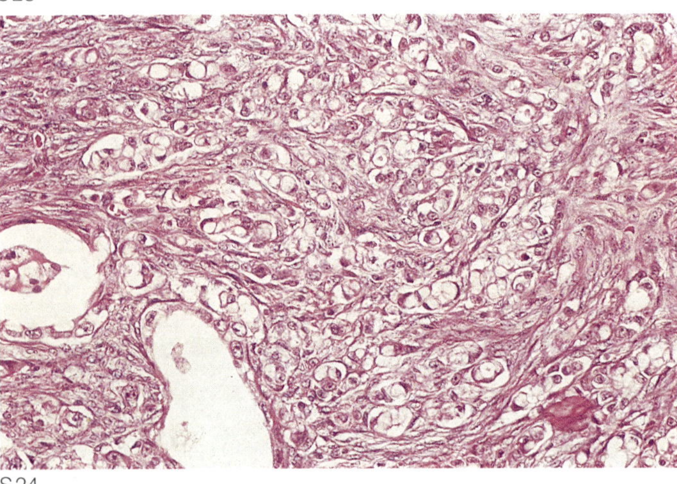

S24

Fig. S23–S24. Bilateral Krukenberg tumors. The ovaries are bilaterally enlarged. The ovary to the right of the photograph has been bisected showing almost complete replacement of the ovarian parenchyma by nodular masses of tumor.

Histologically *(S24)* abundant mucous-producing tumor cells, most of which have a signet-ring appearance, are present surrounded by abundant fibrous tissue. Because of the desmoplastic reaction these tumors are quite hard to palpation. Krukenberg tumors tend to arise from the stomach or pancreas, although metastatic carcinoma from any site may potentially affect the ovaries. (hematoxylin-eosin)

Fallopian Tubes and Endometrium *(S25–S30)*

Fig. S25. Fallopian tube adenocarcinoma. Carcinoma of the fallopian tube is quite rare. In this case the fallopian tube has been longitudinally opened and nodular masses of tumor tissue fill the lumen, which is greatly enlarged, and infiltrate through the wall. There is hemorrhage and necrosis. Histologically these tumors may be indistinguishable from the serous papillary adenocarcinoma of the ovary. The structure to the left of the fallopian tube is the vermiform appendix which was adherent to the external surface of the enlarged tube.

Fig. S26. Proliferative endometrium. This is a photomicrograph of a midstage proliferative endometrium. The glands are increasing in length and show beginning tortuosity. Mitoses are characteristically found, although they cannot be seen in this low magnification photomicrograph. The stroma also participates in the proliferative process and, at this stage, is similarly becoming increasingly cellular. (hematoxylin-eosin)

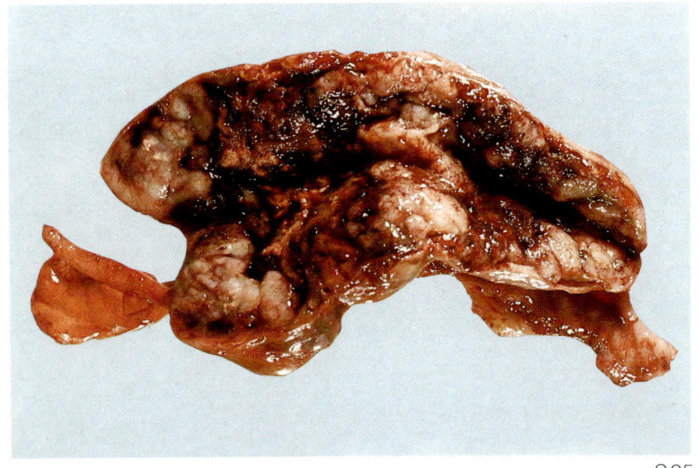

S25

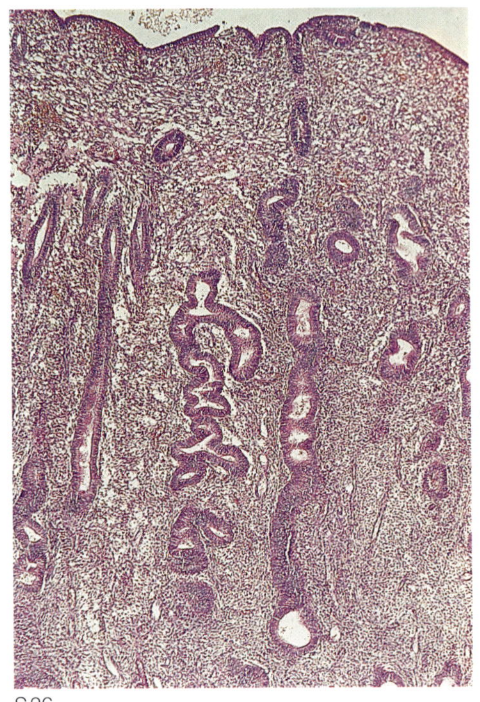

S26

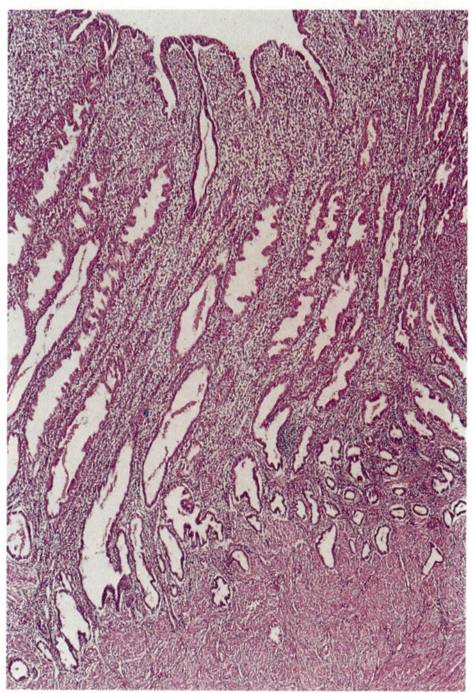

S27

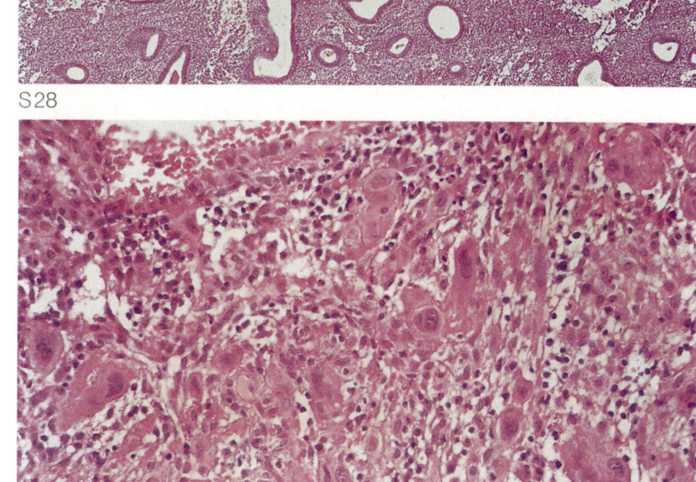

S28

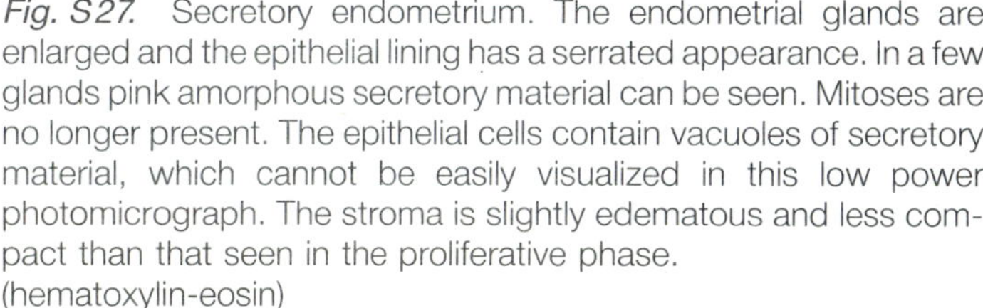

S29

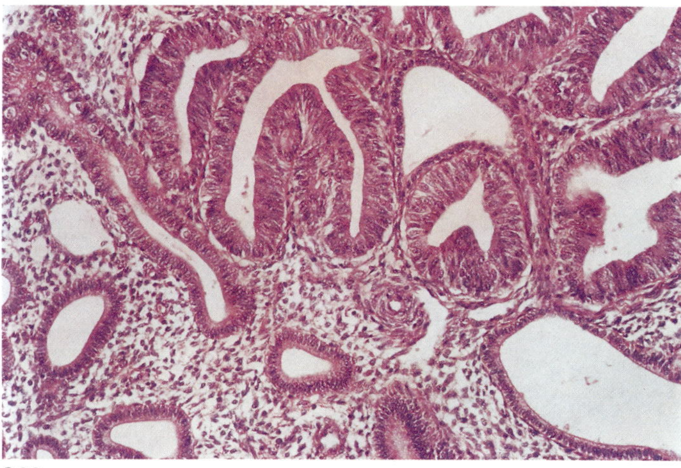

S30

Fig. S27. Secretory endometrium. The endometrial glands are enlarged and the epithelial lining has a serrated appearance. In a few glands pink amorphous secretory material can be seen. Mitoses are no longer present. The epithelial cells contain vacuoles of secretory material, which cannot be easily visualized in this low power photomicrograph. The stroma is slightly edematous and less compact than that seen in the proliferative phase. (hematoxylin-eosin)

Fig. S28. Cystic hyperplasia of the endometrium. This pattern is evidence of continuous endometrial stimulation by unopposed estrogen. The endometrial glands no longer have their usual tubular shape. The lining cells are tall and uniform with scattered mitoses, resembling the proliferative type epithelium. There is abundant stroma separating the glands, in contrast to the picture seen in adenomatous hyperplasia *(Fig. S30).* (hematoxylin-eosin)

Fig. S29. Postpartum endometritis. In this photomicrograph retained decidual tissue is irregularly infiltrated by polymorphonuclear leukocytes, lymphocytes, and plasma cells. This form of endometritis may be sterile, and may only be a reflection of the retention of placental material preventing the normal regeneration of endometrial epithelium. In other cases, particularly after contaminated deliveries, the endometritis may be severe and patients may be quite ill and can even die. (hematoxylin-eosin)

Fig. S30. Adenomatous hyperplasia of the endometrium. Endometrial glands are markedly proliferated. There are cystic glands, but most of the glands are irregular in shape. The glands are lined by highly atypical columnar epithelial cells, which are not single layered but tend to be multi-layered. Characteristically the stroma varies in amount and the proliferating glands are closely apposed (back-to-back). There is considerable cellular and nuclear atypia and many mitoses. This form of atypical adenomatous hyperplasia of the endometrium may be difficult to distinguish from well differentiated adenocarcinoma, which it often precedes. (hematoxylin-eosin)

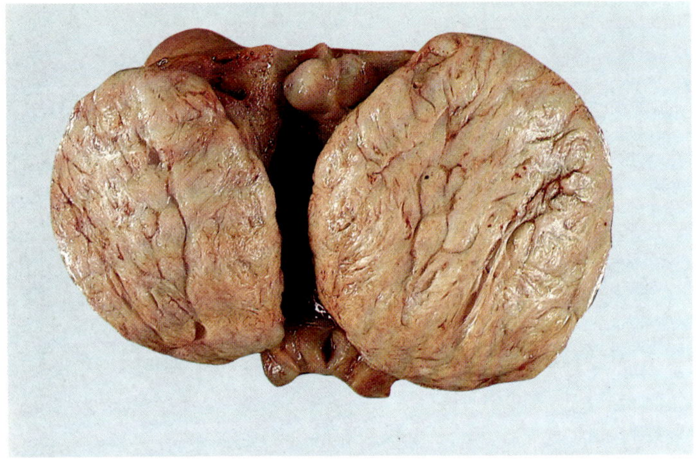

Fig. S31.   Uterine leiomyoma. A large, dominant, well circumscribed, gray tumor mass which has been bisected, occupies the entire anterior portion of this uterus. The cervical os is seen below and a small leiomyoma is seen protruding into the incised space above. The large tumor has a coarsely fascicular ("whorled") appearance on section.

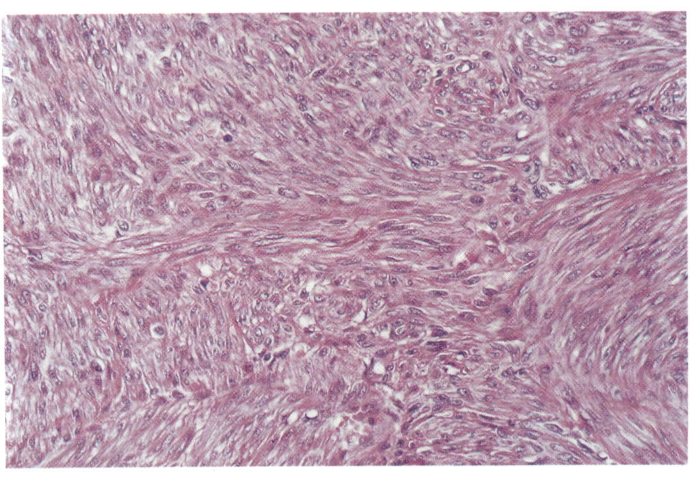

Fig. S32.   Uterine leiomyoma. Histologically, interlacing bands of elongated smooth muscle cells, with variable amounts of interstitial collagenous tissue, are characteristically seen. Mitoses are rare, although benign leiomyomas may, on occasion, show considerable necrosis.   (hematoxylin-eosin)

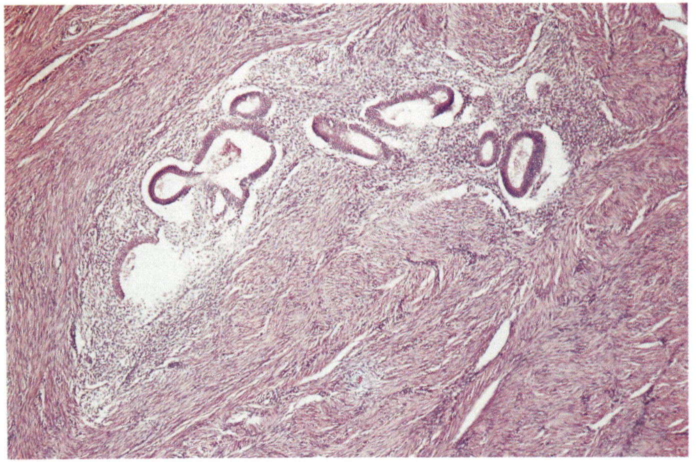

Fig. S33.   Adenomyosis of the uterus. Typically the uterus is enlarged and the myometrial wall is thickened, but well-defined tumor nodules cannot be grossly appreciated. Histologically displaced endometrial glands with accompanying stroma are found within the myometrium. Often blood-filled cysts, indicative of hormonal responsiveness, are seen. These are occasionally visible macroscopically. The finding of endometrial glands within the uterine wall does not establish the diagnosis. Uterine stroma must be confirmed before adenomyosis is diagnosed.
(hematoxylin-eosin)

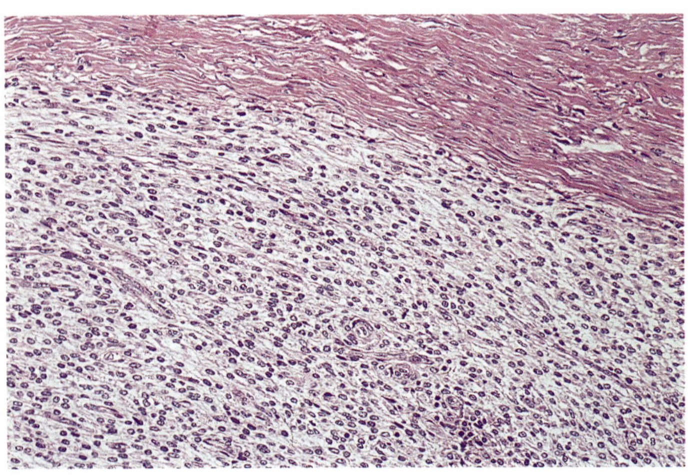

Fig. S34.   Stromal hyperplasia of the uterus. Broad sheets of uniform spindle cells, resembling endometrial stroma, are seen deep in the myometrium. The histogenesis of this phenomenon is unclear. This rare condition is almost biologically benign although, on occasion, stromal nodules, which appear histologically innocuous, may penetrate into blood vessels and may spread to distant organs such as the lung. Very rarely malignant forms of stromal proliferation can be seen.   (hematoxylin-eosin)

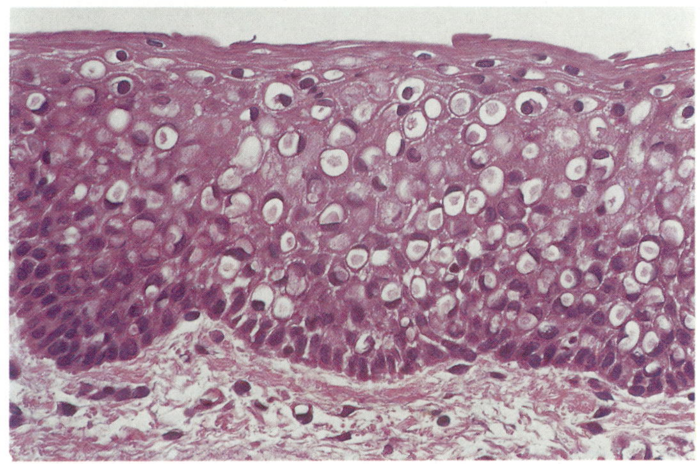

Fig. S35.   Koilocytotic atypia in a cervical condyloma. Infection of the squamous mucosa by human papilloma virus (HPV) contributes to characteristic cellular changes. A single hyperchromatic nucleus seems to float in a cellular vacuole. In some cells the nucleus is deflected to the side and the vacuole contains finely granular eosinophilic material.   (hematoxylin-eosin)

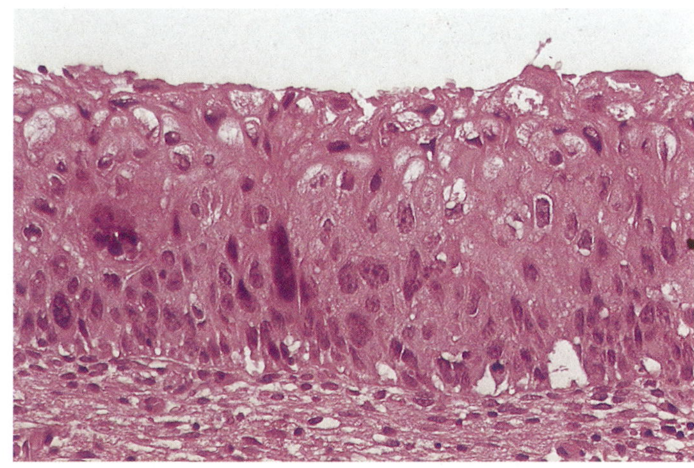

Fig. S36.   Moderate dysplasia of the cervix (CIN-2). The squamous maturation is highly abnormal, although the most superficial layers show some evidence of maturation. In the normal cervix the cytoplasmic component of cells increases as the cells come closer to the surface. Nuclei remain uniform and the nuclear axis changes from perpendicular to the basement membrane to parallel. In this photomicrograph there are many bizarre cells, some of which are multinucleated, and there is no orderly maturation except at the surface where a few cells are parallel to the basement membrane.   (hematoxylin-eosin)

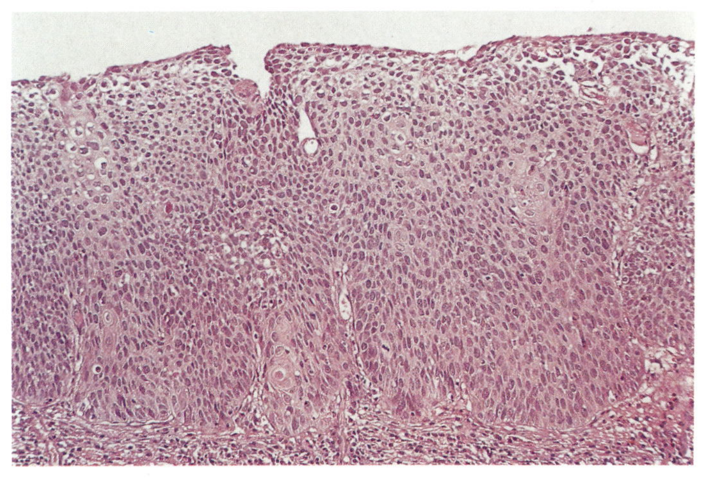

Fig. S37.   Carcinoma in-situ of the uterine cervix (CIN-3). The squamous mucosa is markedly thickened. There is complete loss of the usual pattern of maturation and atypical cells, with markedly pleomorphic nuclei, can be found at all layers. In addition dyskeratotic cells, in which keratin production is seen other than at the epithelial surface, can be identified; one is present near the lower aspect of the epithelium, at the middle of the picture. Numerous mitoses and atypical giant cells can also be seen. (hematoxylin-eosin)

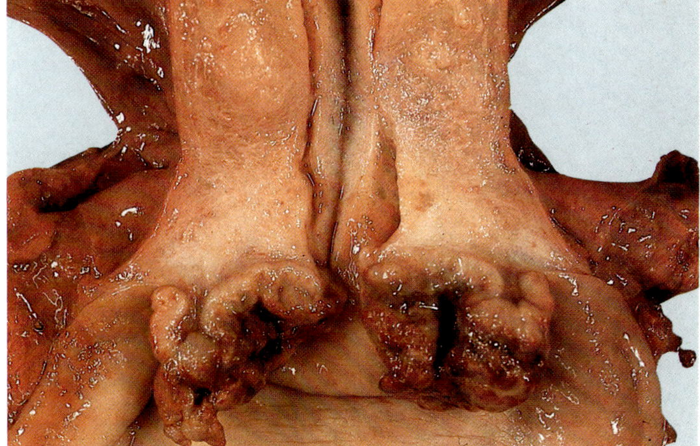

Fig. S38.   Fungating and ulcerated squamous cell carcinoma of the cervix. The external os is completely deformed by a large, exophytic, ulcerated mass of tumor. The tumor infiltrates deeply into the underlying cervical wall. In the background are other pelvic structures removed at the time of this radical hysterectomy.

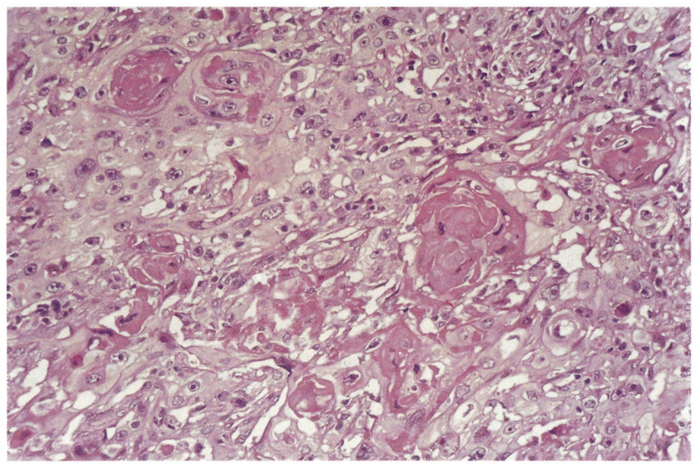

Fig. S39. Keratinizing squamous cell carcinoma of the cervix. This tumor is histologically indistinguishable from squamous cell carcinomas arising elsewhere *(Fig. E32a, Fig. G9)* and consists of sheets of squamous cells of varying differentiation with irregular keratin production, including the formation of "pearls". (hematoxylin-eosin)

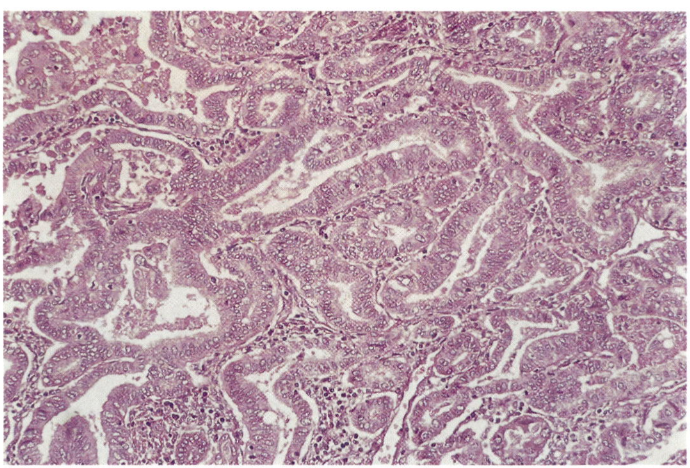

Fig. S40. Endometrial adenocarcinoma. In this moderately well differentiated adenocarcinoma of the endometrium, highly atypical proliferating glands can be seen with virtually no stroma. Many of the glands abut ("back-to-back"). Tumor cells show moderate degrees of pleomorphism, areas of stratification, and many mitoses. (hematoxylin-eosin)

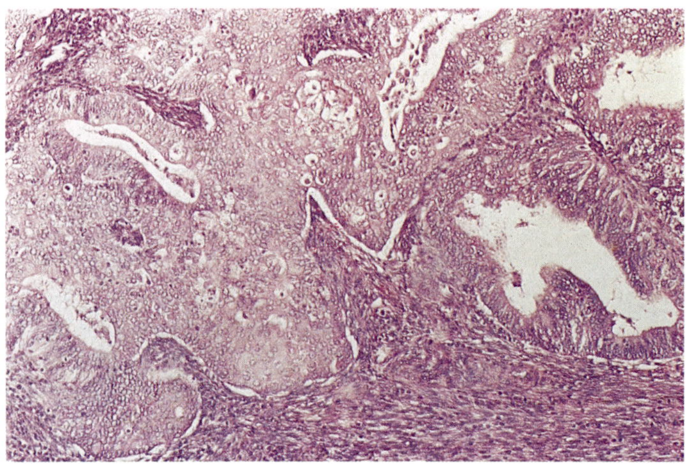

Fig. S41. Adenoacanthoma of the endometrium. This type of malignancy is rarely seen in other locations and is characterized by nests of histologically benign squamous epithelium immediately adjacent to malignant glands. In these cases the malignant potential is determined by the activity of the adenocarcinoma component. The term adenosquamous carcinoma is used to describe those tumors in which squamous and glandular elements are present and are both malignant. (hematoxylin-eosin)

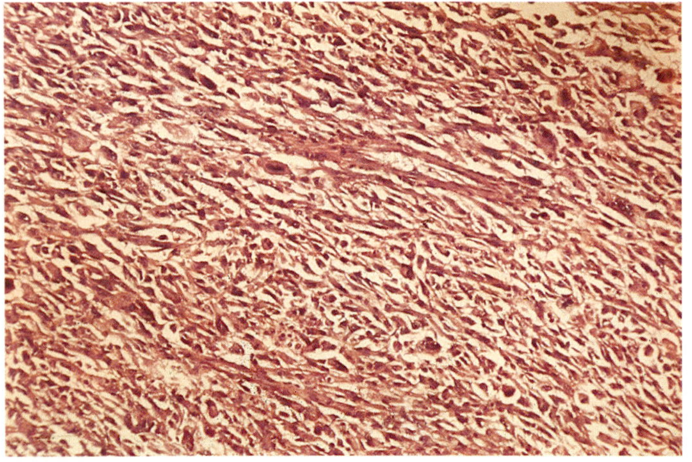

Fig. S42. Uterine leiomyosarcoma. This malignant mesenchymal tumor consists of spindle cells with obvious bizarre, often multinucleated forms in which there is considerable nuclear pleomorphism. There is some resemblance to the fascicular arrangement of the benign leiomyoma *(Fig. S32),* but the spindle cell strands are less orderly. Mitoses are scattered throughout and, in well differentiated cases, form the basis for the establishment of the diagnosis of malignancy. (van Gieson)

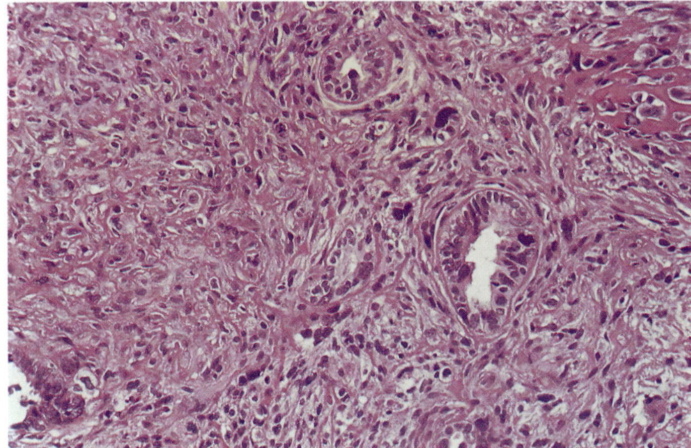

Fig. S43. Adenosarcoma of the endometrium. This is a rare mixed tumor with epithelial and mesenchymal elements in which the mesenchymal element is sarcomatous, but the endometrial glands are benign. These tumors tend to have a relatively favorable prognosis. (hematoxylin-eosin)

Fig. S44. Malignant mixed mullerian tumor (carcinosarcoma). In this tumor both the epithelial and mesenchymal elements are malignant. There may also be considerable mesenchymal differentiation, with production of smooth and striated muscle, cartilage, and bone. These patients are usually elderly and postmenopausal and the tumors often present as large polypoid endometrial masses. The prognosis is extremely poor. (hematoxylin-eosin)

Cytopathology *(S45–S49)*

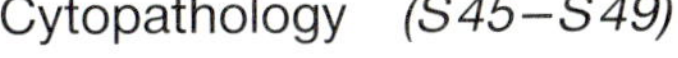

Fig. S45. This photomicrograph shows normal superficial cells obtained at the time of routine gynecological examination in women in the reproductive years. The cells are large, polygonal, with abundant eosinophilic cytoplasm and small pyknotic nuclei. This abundance of superficial cells is evidence of estrogen effect, and the smear was taken approximately two days prior to ovulation. This type of preparation is known as a Pap (Papanicolaou) smear, and is of exfoliated cells rather than a tissue section.

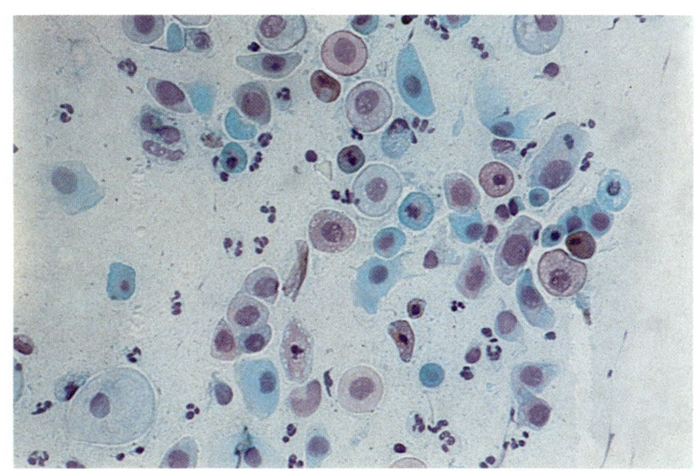

Fig. S46. Pap smear from a postmenopausal patient. Immature cells from the basal and parabasal cells predominate. They are generally round cells with a moderate amount of cytoplasm and large, somewhat pale nuclei. A few polygonal intermediate cells are found between. This pattern of epithelial atrophy may be seen in inflammatory conditions, as in this case, as evidenced by the presence of polymorphonuclear leukocytes.

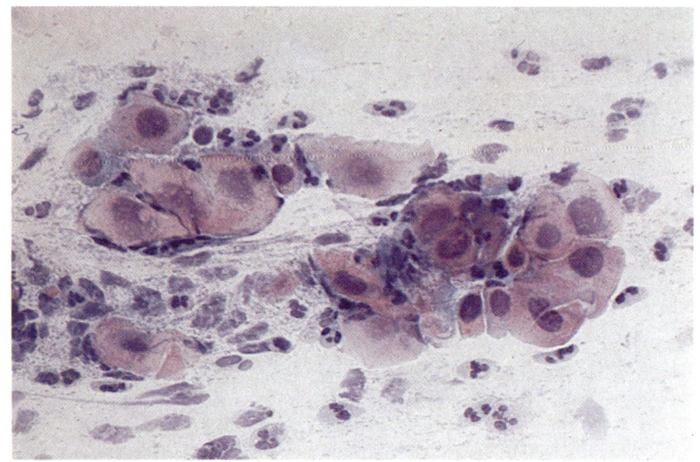

Fig. S 47. Pap smear from the uterine cervix showing moderate to severe dysplasia. The nuclei are hyperchromatic and pleomorphic, and the nuclear-cytoplasmic ratio is increased. A few of the larger cells have a tendency to be spindle in nature.

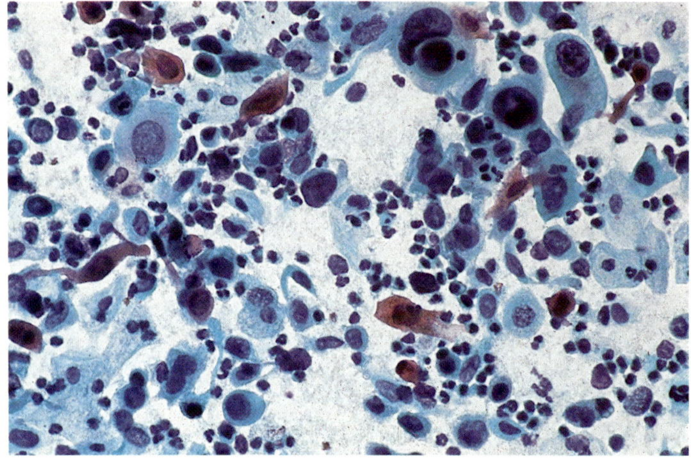

Fig. S 48. Pap smear from a patient with squamous cell carcinoma. Tumor cells show considerable variation in size and shape, with hyperchromatic pleomorphic nuclei. The cytoplasm is generally clearly defined and basophilic, although a few eosinophilic cells are seen. Many polymorphonuclear leukocytes are also seen.

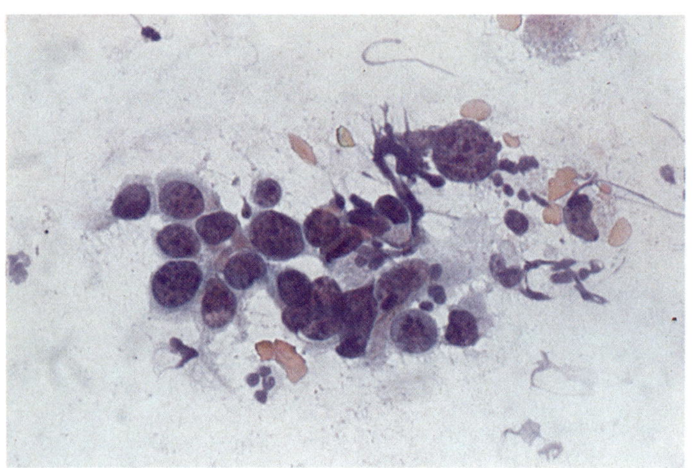

Fig. S 49. Pap smear, cytologic preparation. Pap from a patient with endometrial adenocarcinoma. Tumor cells contain scanty cytoplasm which is generally poorly defined. Nuclei are large and hyperchromatic with coarse chromatin and multiple prominent nucleoli. There is considerable variation in nuclear size and shape. Erythrocytes, evidence of bleeding, are prominent.

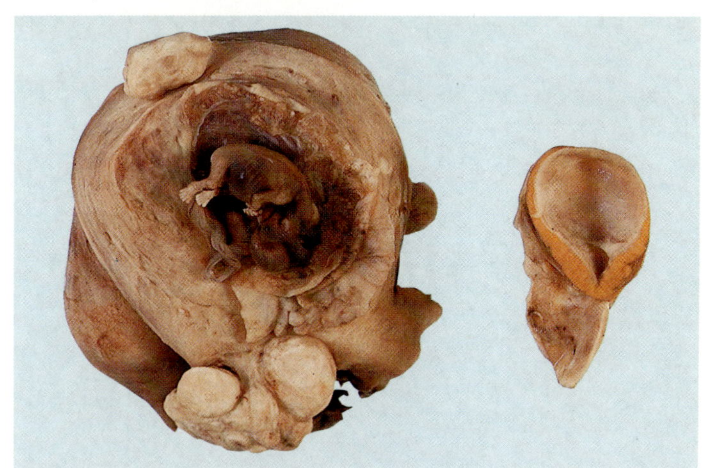

Fig. S50.   Gravid uterus removed for multiple leiomyomas. An immature fetus is seen within the opened endometrial cavity. Surrounding the cavity is reddish-yellow placental tissue. Myomas are seen at the dome of the uterus and at the lower portion of the photograph. The ovary, to the right of the photograph, is enlarged and the corpus luteum is markedly hyperplastic ("corpus luteum of pregnancy").

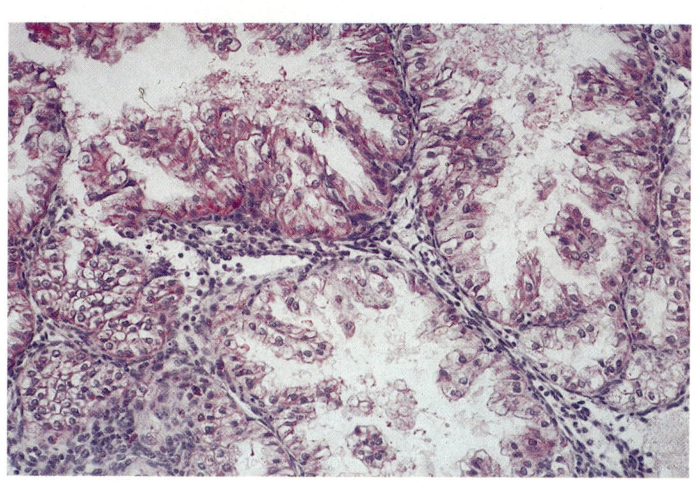

Fig. S51.   Arias-Stella phenomenon ("hypersecretory endometrium") in a patient with ectopic pregnancy. During pregnancy, whether intrauterine or extrauterine, the endometrium undergoes characteristic changes which are evidence of trophoblastic activity. The glands are enlarged and lined by multiple papillary projections consisting of uniform vacuolated epithelial cells, which may show hyperchromatic and pleomorphic nuclei. Secretory material can be identified in the lumenal space.   (hematoxylin-eosin)

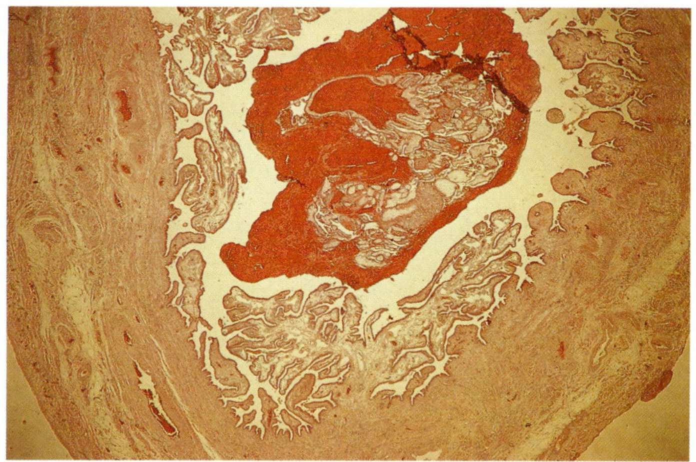

Fig. S52–53.   Tubal gestation. This patient had prior inflammatory disease of the fallopian tubes. After fertilization the egg did not effectively migrate into the uterus and became fixed in the fallopian tube. As the gestational tissue matured, the fallopian tube became enlarged. In the lower photomicrograph the fallopian tube epithelium is to the left. Blood, evidence of hemorrhage, is to the right and there are scattered individual chorionic villi with the usual covering trophoblastic cells. These patients are at risk for fallopian tube perforation and massive hemorrhage into the peritoneal cavity.

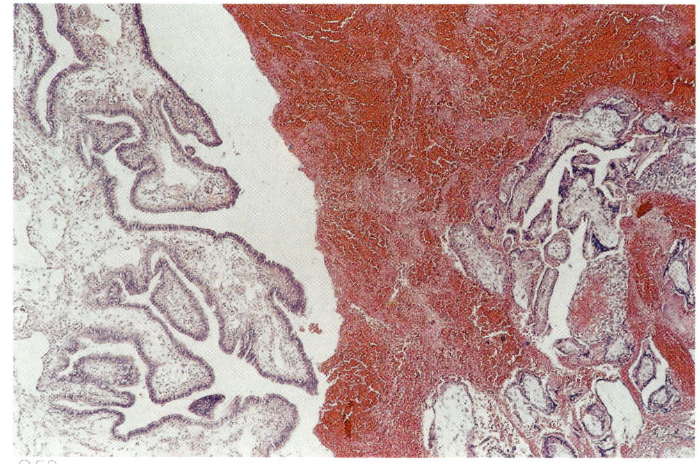

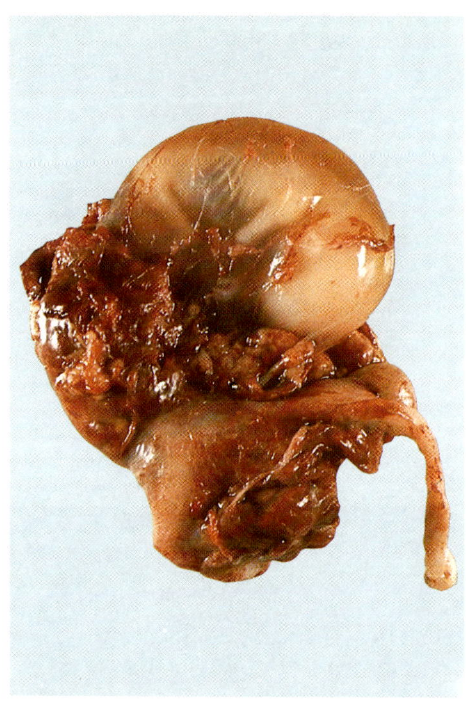

Fig. S54. Tubal gestation with rupture. In most cases of tubal pregnancy there is spontaneous abortion because the fallopian tube does not permit normal growth. In this patient the tubal wall ruptured and placental tissue proliferated on the surface. The fetus, still within the amniotic membrane, can be discerned at the upper portion of the photograph.

T. Diseases of the Breast

J. H. Holzner

The female breast shows changes reflecting hormonal variations. These are obvious during adolescence when the breasts develop, during the reproductive years when there are cyclic variations, during the menstrual cycle, and in the postmenopausal years when the breast tissue involutes. Males may also be subject to breast diseases. Gynecomastia is the condition of mammary gland enlargement in the male which may be idiopathic or may reflect naturally occurring or exogenous excess of estrogens. For example, males treated with estrogens for prostate carcinoma, may develop gynecomastia.

One of the most common conditions affecting the female breast is fibrocystic disease, although there are many who would object to designating this very common change as a disease. Fibrocystic changes occur during the reproductive years, but may persist and manifest post-menopausally. Although there still remains controversy, it would appear that fibrocystic changes in and of themselves do not indicate a propensity for carcinoma.

Many tumors of the breast are benign. One of the most common tumors is the fibroadenoma, in which there is proliferation of epithelial and mesenchymal cells. Breast carcinoma is a particularly important disease, because it is both frequent in industrialized countries and increasing in incidence. It is estimated that one out of every 16 women in North America and Europe will develop carcinoma of the breast. Hormonal and nutritional factors are increasingly incriminated as principal causes. The histopathology continues to be particularly valuable in evaluating these patients and in determining the stage of malignancy. Without excisional biopsy and histologic examination, it is impossible to determine when invasion is present. Lobular carcinoma in-situ remains a somewhat controversial disorder. Paget's disease of the breast is a particularly important clinical entity. Paget's disease of the breast is virtually always associated with an underlying ductal carcinoma and its recognition by the physician is vitally important to assure early treatment.

Mesenchymal tumors of the breast are rare. Cystosarcoma phyllodes is distinctly uncommon and may be biologically benign or malignant. One of the most malignant breast tumors, which is fortunately rare, is the angiosarcoma.

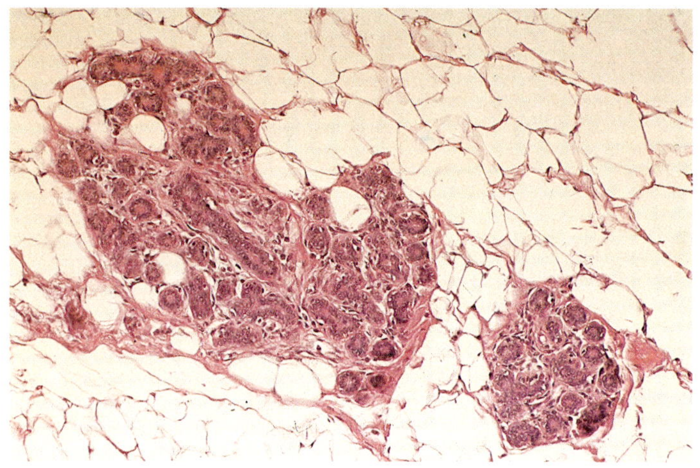

Fig. T1.   Postmenopausal involution of the breast. The usual compact interlobular connective tissue has been replaced by fat. The lobules are absent and the terminal ducts are surrounded by fibrous tissue. These fibrotic areas may be easily palpable in the background of fatty breast tissue and can be clinically mistaken for small carcinomas. Histologically they are easily distinguished from malignancy.   (hematoxylin-eosin)

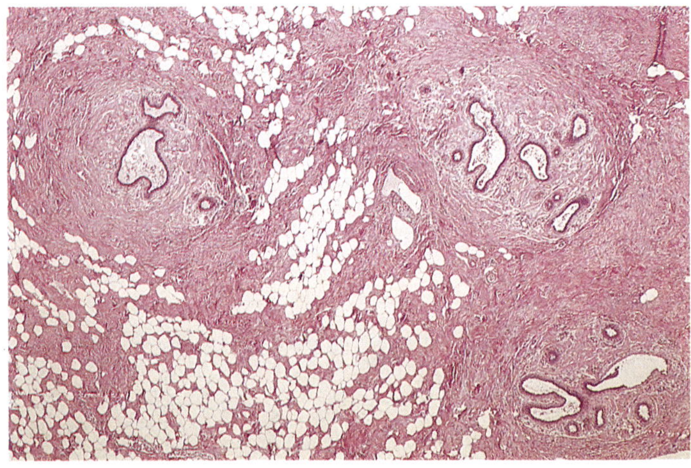

Fig. T2.   Postmenopausal involution of the breast. In this photomicrograph another example of involutional breast tissue is seen. Lobules are completely absent and the terminal ducts show cystic change. The intralobular connective tissue is markedly fibrotic. Unlike the cystic disease that occurs in the reproductive years, this change does not regress.   (hematoxylin-eosin)

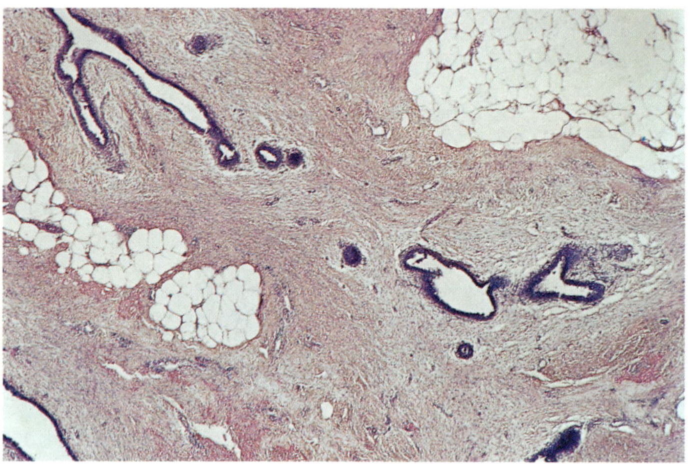

T3

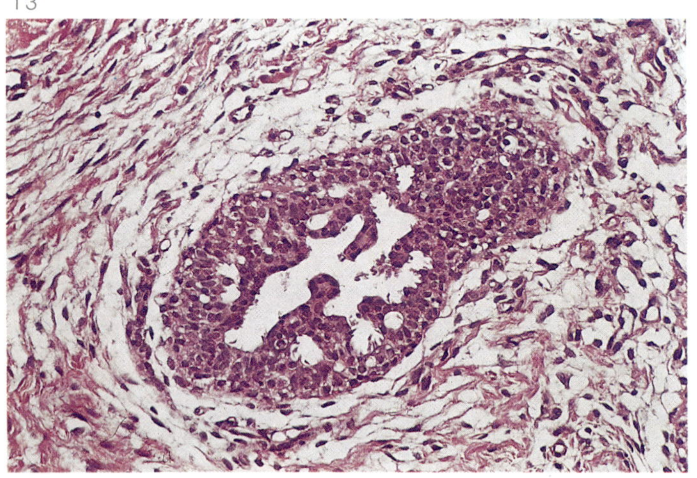

Fig. T3–T4.   Gynecomastia. This breast biopsy was obtained from a male with enlarged breasts. Since the male breast does not usually have lobules, the primary changes involve the ducts and ductules and their surrounding connective tissue. A characteristic finding, apparent even in the low magnification photomicrograph, is the presence of loose, somewhat pale-appearing connective tissue immediately surrounding the ductular structures. This is even more apparent in the lower photomicrograph where the connective tissue appears somewhat edematous. The duct epithelium can proliferate and can form papillary projections, as seen in the high magnification photomicrograph.   (hematoxylin-eosin)

T4

Mastitis and Fibrocystic Disease (T5–T7)

Fig. T5. Granulomatous mastitis. The mammary tissue is extensively destroyed and replaced by a granulomatous infiltrate consisting of accumulations of mononuclear cells and epithelioid cells. This develops in the region of an injured breast duct when there is extravasation of milk or other secretory products. This is a condition of younger women and may, by palpation, mimic carcinoma. (hematoxylin-eosin)

Fig. T6. Fibrocystic disease. Gland architecture is markedly deformed. There is irregular fibrosis of the intralobular stroma and the lobe pattern is altered. The ducts and ductules are irregularly dilated and the epithelium lining these spaces varies considerably. At the upper portion of the photomicrograph the epithelium is low cuboidal, whereas the ducts at the lower portion of the picture are columnar with abundant eosinophilic cytoplasm *(see Fig. T7).* (hematoxylin-eosin)

Fig. T7. Apocrine metaplasia in fibrocystic disease of the breast. This is a not uncommon change in young women. The greatly dilated breast duct is lined by large pale, finely granular eosinophilic cells with small uniform nuclei. Papillary projections are obvious. There is no pleomorphism and no mitoses.   (hematoxylin-eosin)

Tumors (T8–T20)

Fig. T8a–b. Fibroadenoma of the breast. This is the most common benign tumor of the breast, and results from proliferation of epithelial-lined spaces and surrounding mesenchymal tissue. The epithelial-lined spaces are irregularly compressed and form convoluted and branching cleft-like structures. The epithelial cells are uniform, without pleomorphism and mitoses.   (hematoxylin-eosin)

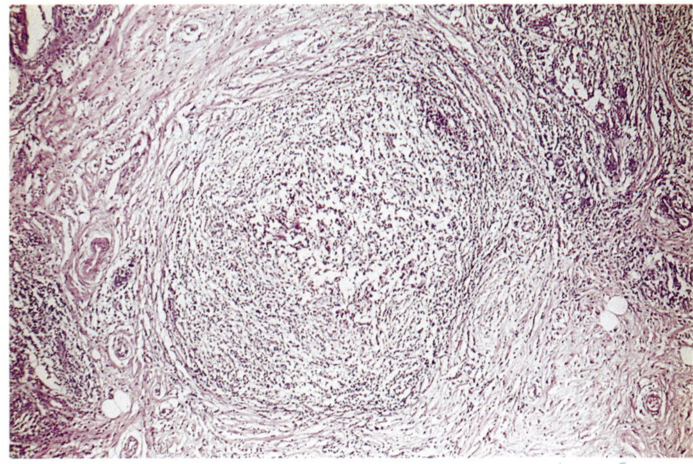

T5

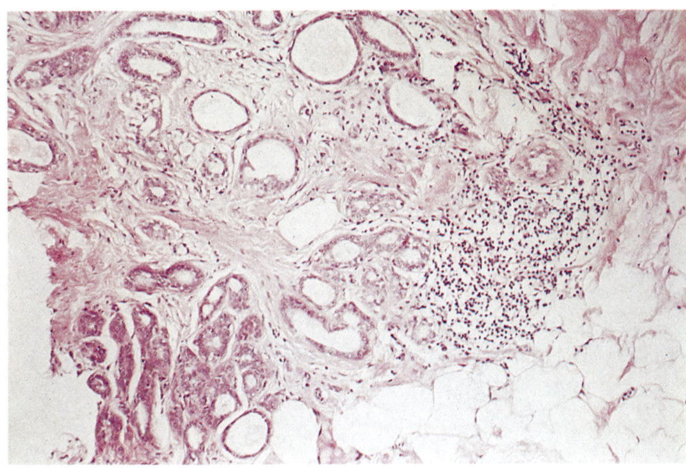

T6

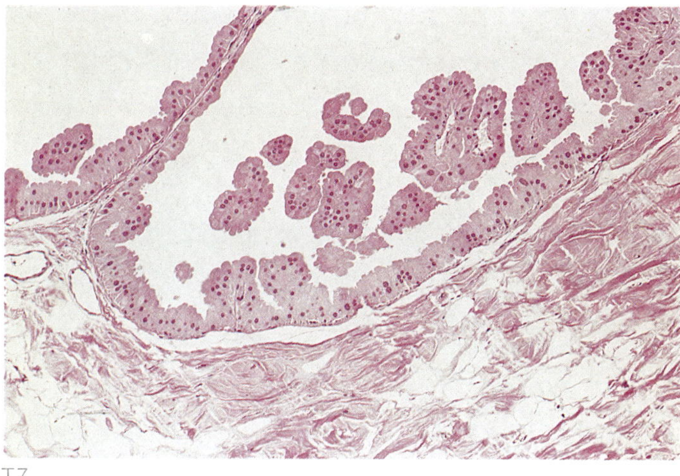

T7

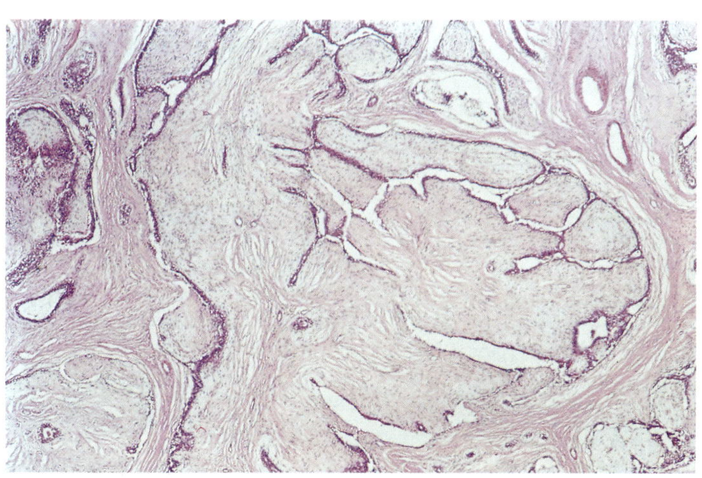

T8a

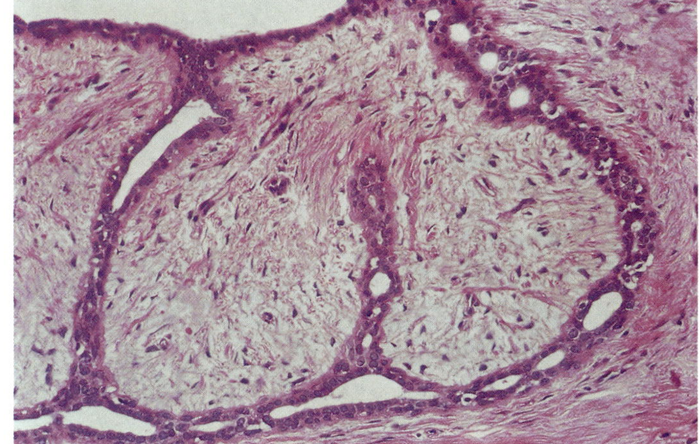

T8b

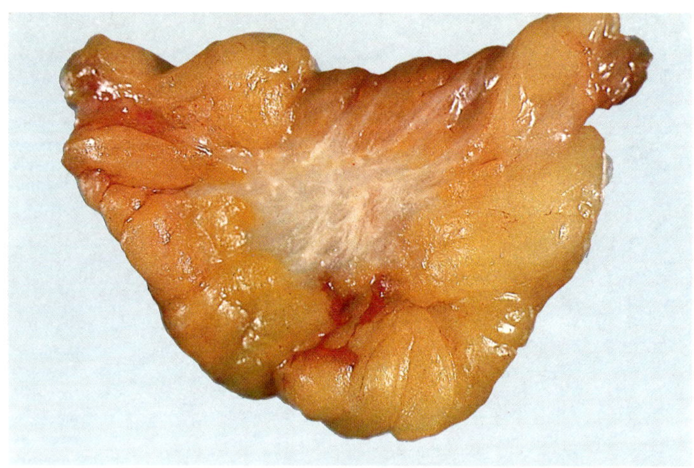

Fig. T9a. Infiltrating duct cell carcinoma of the breast. This is the characteristic gross appearance of duct cell carcinoma of the breast. A poorly defined infiltrating tumor is seen. The interface between tumor and normal fatty breast tissue is difficult to discern. The tumor is quite hard, and there are yellowish streaks, representing proliferation of elastic tissue, throughout.

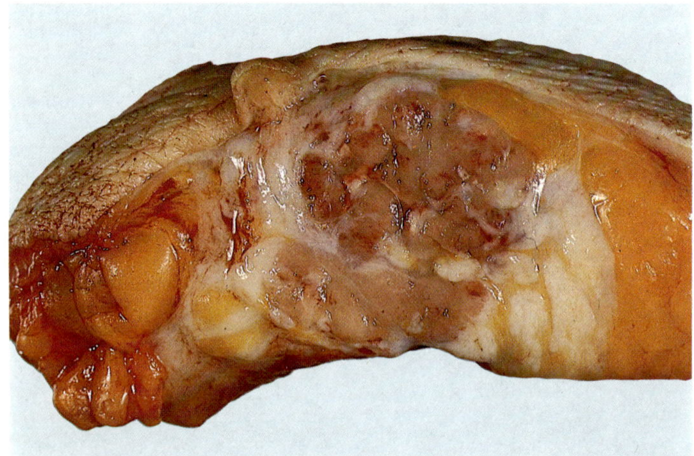

Fig. T9b. Large nodular carcinoma of the breast. This macroscopic appearance may be seen in medullary carcinoma of the breast as well as in mucin-producing ("colloid") carcinoma. The tumor is only moderately firm, poorly defined, multi-nodular, with areas of brownish discoloration, representing prior hemorrhage, and, at the center of the photograph, reddish areas of recent hemorrhage.

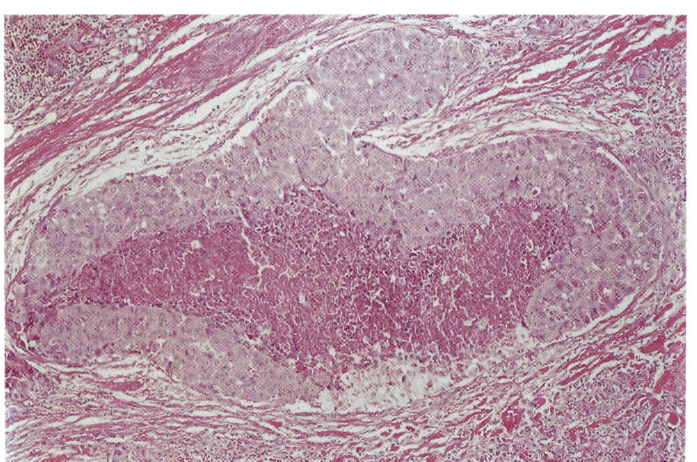

Fig. T10. Intraductal carcinoma of the breast, comedo type. Intraductal carcinoma of the breast tends to be multi-focal, involving all portions of the breast, and may even be bilateral. It tends to develop in relatively large breast ducts. Macroscopically the distended ducts are grossly visible because they are filled with necrotic hemorrhagic material which resembles a brown viscid paste. Histologically the duct is partially filled by fairly uniform tumor cells. The usual myoepithelial cells of breast ducts cannot be identified. There is central necrosis and hemorrhage. Mitoses may be seen but are not uniformly prominent. These tumors are clinically treacherous because of their multi-focal distribution and because, in many cases, sites of infiltration may not be identified, although lymph node metastasis may be present.   (hematoxylin-eosin)

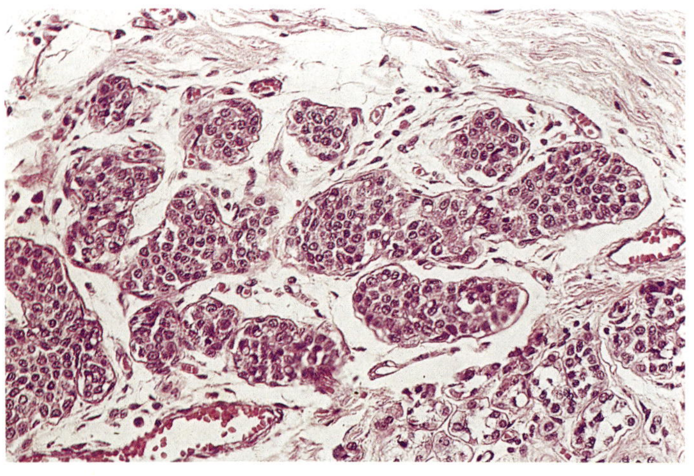

Fig. T11. Lobular carcinoma in-situ ("lobular neoplasia"). The lobules are all enlarged by fairly uniform polyhedral cells. Myoepithelial cells cannot be identified. Mitoses may not necessarily be seen and pleomorphism is not a feature. Patients with lobular carcinoma in-situ are at risk for the development of invasive carcinoma in both the ipsilateral and contralateral breast. This carcinoma may not manifest for as long as 15 years after the identification of the in-situ lesion.   (hematoxylin-eosin)

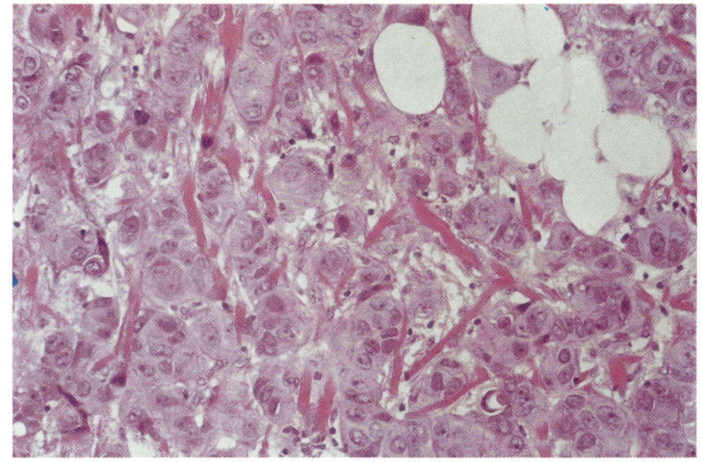

Fig. T12. Duct cell carcinoma of the breast. This is the most common form of breast carcinoma. There is proliferation of highly atypical tumor cells in nests and cords with varying degrees of separating fibrous tissue. In this photomicrograph glandular formation is not seen, and there is relatively poor differentiation. The tumor cells vary in size and shape, nuclei are enlarged, hyperchromatic, and pleomorphic, and there are scattered mitoses. In other cases breast carcinoma may be better differentiated and there may be considerably more prominent desmoplastic reaction. (hematoxylin-eosin)

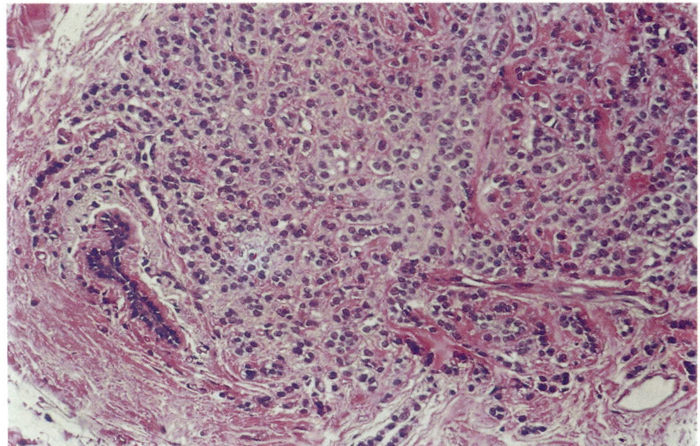

Fig. T13. Infiltrating lobular carcinoma of the breast. Here a terminal duct is surrounded by fairly uniform small tumor cells which are irregularly dispersed or arranged in a linear pattern of one cell behind the other ("indian file"). This is the classical pattern of infiltrating lobular carcinoma.   (hematoxylin-eosin)

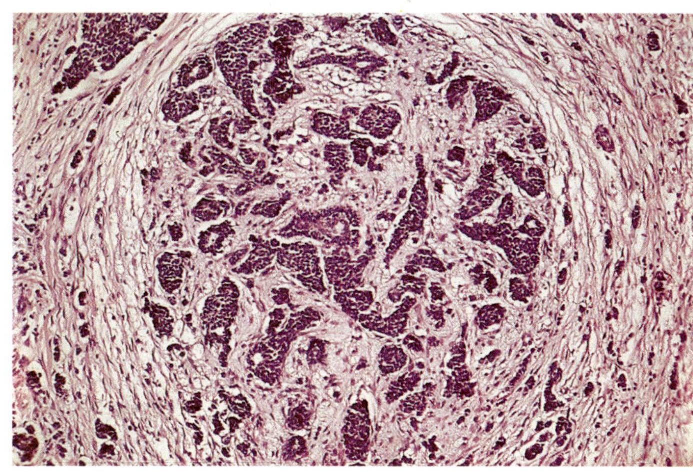

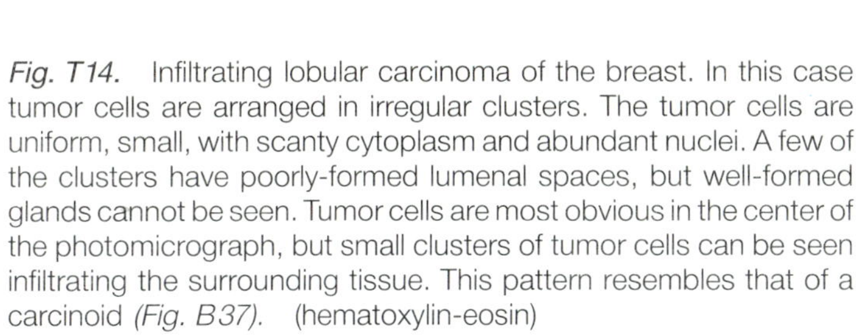

Fig. T14. Infiltrating lobular carcinoma of the breast. In this case tumor cells are arranged in irregular clusters. The tumor cells are uniform, small, with scanty cytoplasm and abundant nuclei. A few of the clusters have poorly-formed lumenal spaces, but well-formed glands cannot be seen. Tumor cells are most obvious in the center of the photomicrograph, but small clusters of tumor cells can be seen infiltrating the surrounding tissue. This pattern resembles that of a carcinoid *(Fig. B37).*   (hematoxylin-eosin)

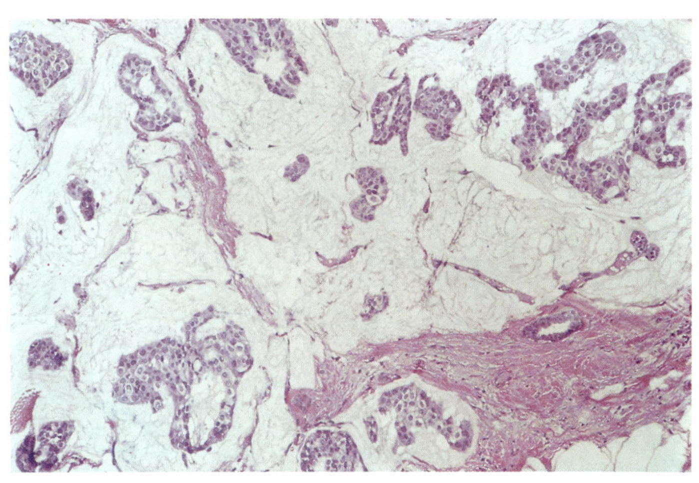

Fig. T15. Mucin-secreting ("colloid") carcinoma of the breast. This mucin-secreting carcinoma of the breast can be recognized macroscopically because of its abundant mucous production. The mucous makes the tumor glistening in appearance and sticky to the touch. Characteristically, tumor cells appear to float in pools of mucous.   (hematoxylin-eosin)

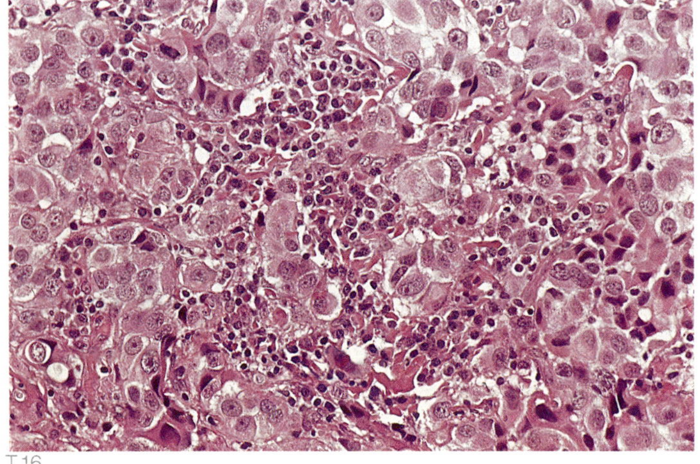

T 16

Fig. T16. Medullary carcinoma of the breast with lymphoid stroma. Tumor cells of medullary carcinoma are characteristically quite large and arranged in poorly-defined sheets. There may be multi-nucleated and syncitial forms. Connective tissue is inconspicuous. The tumor may be infiltrated by variable numbers of lymphocytes and plasma cells. When the lymphocytic component is particularly prominent, prognosis is better.   (hematoxylin-eosin)

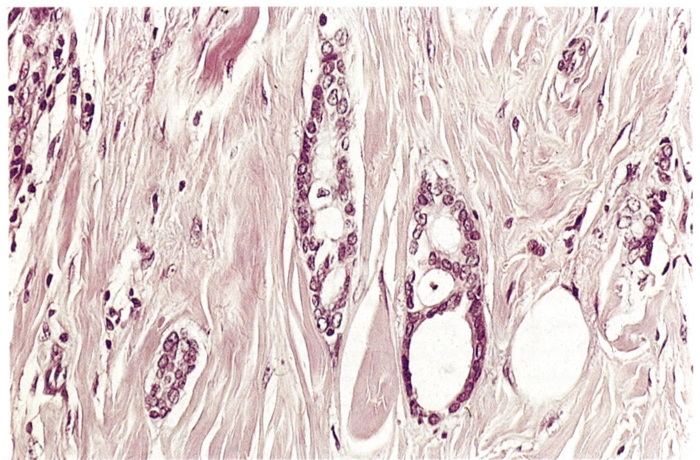

T 17

Fig. T17. Tubular carcinoma of the breast. Tubular carcinoma is a relatively benign form of breast malignancy. Characteristically, there are small single layer tubular structures lined by relatively innocuous appearing uniform epithelial cells. Mitoses are rare. The tumors tend to be small and grow slowly, and lymph node metastases are distinctly uncommon.   (hematoxylin-eosin)

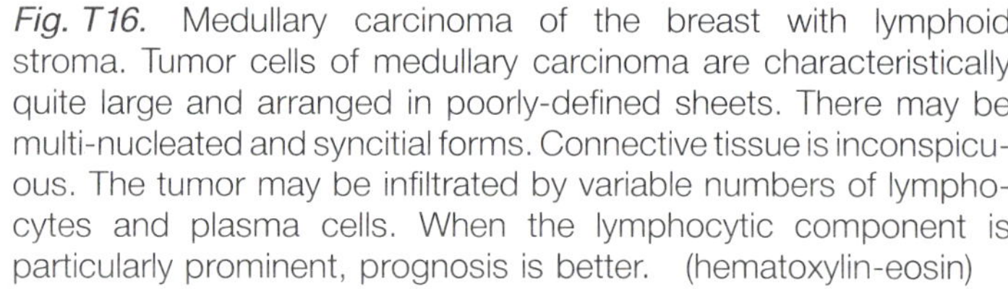

Fig. T18. Paget's disease of the nipple. The skin of the nipple is typically eczematous and may resemble a dermatitis. Large tumor cells with abundant cytoplasm and prominent nuclei, extend up into the epidermis. These tumor cells migrate along breast ducts from an underlying duct cell carcinoma which may be clinically and mammographically difficult to identify. It is important, however, to recognize that this change is associated with carcinoma.

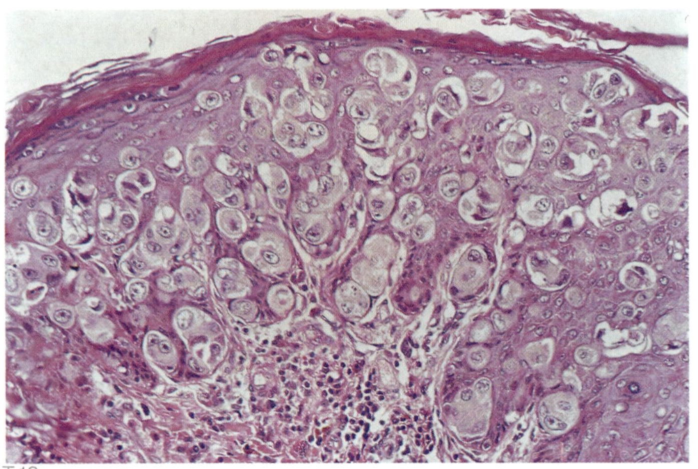

Fig. T19. Cystosarcoma phyllodes of the breast. The general architecture of this tumor is similar to that of a fibroadenoma. In contrast, however, the stromal cells are decidedly atypical with hypochromatic pleomorphic nuclei and many mitoses. A benign variant of cystosarcoma phyllodes exists.   (hematoxylin-eosin)

Fig. T20. Angiosarcoma of the breast. This rare, highly malignant tumor is composed of irregular branching capillary spaces which are lined by fairly uniform endothelial cells which may have intralumenal papillary projections. The tumor cells are generally innocuous in appearance, and the general architecture of the tumor must be recognized to make the diagnosis. Mitoses may be infrequent. Underlying breast tissue, in this photomicrograph, has been completely replaced by tumor.   (hematoxylin-eosin)

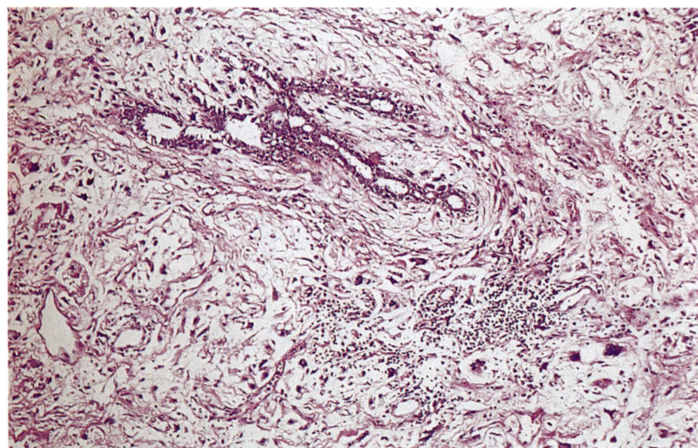

T 18

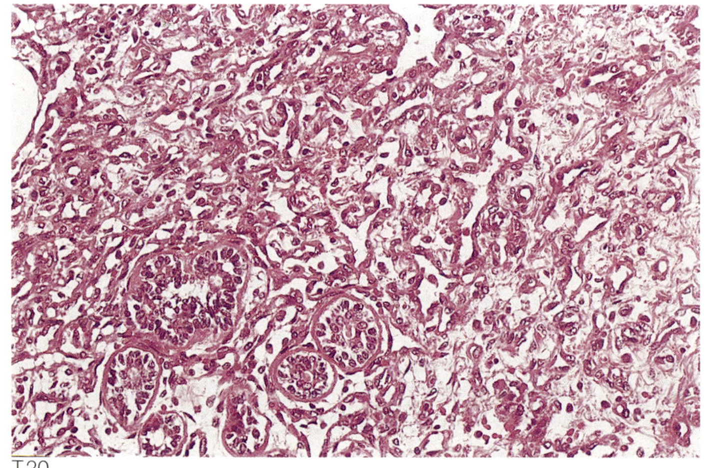

T 19   T 20